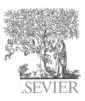

Netter's Neuroscience Fla[sh]

Learn, review, and self-test – anytime, anywhere.

Fun, fast, and in full color, this portable resource is a **perfect study tool** covering everything you need to know for a solid foundation in neuroscience and neuroanatomy. This quick review tool allows you **to test your knowledge on the go**—when and where it's convenient. **More than 220 flash cards with Netter illustrations** on the front and answers to labels and explanatory text on the back emphasize key neuroscience principles and clinical applications for an efficient yet in-depth review.

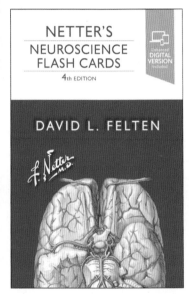

Netter's Neuroscience Flash Cards, 4th Edition
ISBN: 9780323756433

Key Features:

- Cards provide **clinically important correlations** in neuroanatomy, cell biology, neurophysiology, and vascular anatomy; and **clinical discussions and helpful summaries** on the back of each card.

- **New global brain function and dysfunction coverage**, from traumatic brain injury, dementias, and coma to neuropsychiatric disorders such as depression and schizophrenia.

- New access to extensive **cross-sectional anatomy cards online**.

- Coverage of **timely topics** such as cannabinoids, opioids, PTSD, OCD, and aging and the nervous system.

- **Pre-punched holes and convenient binding** ring allow you to carry selected groups of flash cards with you anywhere.

- A perfect study aid and complement to Dr. Felten's related titles: *Netter's Atlas of Neuroscience, 4th Edition* (to which the cards are cross-referenced), and *Netter's Neuroscience Coloring Book.*

NETTER'S ATLAS OF NEUROSCIENCE

4th Edition

David L. Felten, MD, PhD
Associate Dean of Clinical Sciences
University of Medicine and Health Sciences
New York, New York

M. Kerry O'Banion, MD, PhD
Professor and Vice Chair
Department of Neuroscience
Del Monte Neuroscience Institute
Director of the Medical Scientist Training Program
University of Rochester School of Medicine
Rochester, New York

Mary Summo Maida, PhD
Adjunct Professor of Neuroscience
Department of Neuroscience
Del Monte Neuroscience Institute
University of Rochester School of Medicine
Rochester, New York

Illustrations by
Frank H. Netter, MD

Contributing Illustrators
James A. Perkins, MFA, CMI, FAMI
Carlos A.G. Machado, MD
John A. Craig, MD

ELSEVIER

1600 John F. Kennedy Blvd.
Ste. 1600
Philadelphia, PA 19103-2899

NETTER'S ATLAS OF NEUROSCIENCE, FOURTH EDITION　　　　　ISBN: 978-0-323-75654-9

Library of Congress Control Number: 2021932599

Senior Content Strategist: Elyse O'Grady
Senior Content Development Specialist: Marybeth Thiel
Publishing Services Manager: Catherine Jackson
Senior Project Manager/Specialist: Carrie Stetz
Design Direction: Patrick Ferguson

Printed in India

Last digit is the print number:　9　8　7　6　5　4　3

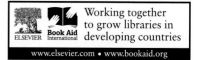

ABOUT THE AUTHORS

DAVID L. FELTEN, MD, PhD, is currently Associate Dean of Clinical Sciences at the University of Medicine and Health Sciences. He counsels and advised MD candidates to assist them in passing the USMLE clinical board exams (Step 2 CK and CS) and the basic sciences board exam (Step 1). He was formerly Vice President for Research and Medical Director of the Research Institute at William Beaumont Health System in Royal Oak, Michigan and the Founding Associate Dean for Research at Oakland University William Beaumont School of Medicine. He previously served as Dean of the School of Graduate Medical Education at Seton Hall University in South Orange, New Jersey; the Founding Executive Director of the Susan Samueli Center for Integrative Medicine and Professor of Anatomy and Neurobiology at the UC Irvine School of Medicine; the Founding Director of the Center for Neuroimmunology at Loma Linda School of Medicine; and the Kilian J. and Caroline F. Schmitt Professor and Chair of the Department of Neurobiology and Anatomy, and Director of the Markey Charitable Trust Institute for Neurobiology and Neurodegenerative Diseases and Aging at the University of Rochester School of Medicine in Rochester, New York. He received a bachelor of science degree from Massachusetts Institute of Technology and MD and PhD degrees (Anatomy, Institute of Neurological Sciences) from the University of Pennsylvania School of Medicine. Dr. Felten carried out pioneering studies of autonomic innervation of lymphoid organs and neural-immune signaling that underlie the mechanistic foundations for psychoneuroimmunology and many aspects of integrative medicine. Dr. Felten is the recipient of numerous honors and awards, including the prestigious John D. and Catherine T. MacArthur Foundation Prize Fellowship, two simultaneous NIH MERIT awards from the National Institutes of Mental Health and the National Institute on Aging, an Alfred P. Sloan Foundation Fellowship, an Andrew W. Mellon Foundation Fellowship, a Robert Wood Johnson Dean's Senior Teaching Scholar Award, the Norman Cousins Award in Mind-Body Medicine, the Building Bridges of Integration Award from the Traditional Chinese Medicine Would Foundation, and numerous teaching awards.

Dr. Felten co-authored the definitive scholarly text in the field of neural-immune interactions, *Psychoneuroimmunology* (Academic Press, 3rd edition, 2001) and was a founding co-editor of the major journal in the field, *Brain, Behavior and Immunity,* with Drs. Robert Ader and Nicholas Cohen of the University of Rochester School of Medicine. He also is the author of three editions of *Netter's Neuroscience Flash Cards* (fourth edition now in process) and, with Dr. Mary Maida, the first edition of *Netter's Neuroscience Coloring Book.* Dr. Felten is the author of more than 210 peer-reviewed journal articles and reviews, many on links between the nervous system and immune system. His work has been featured on Bill Moyer's PBS series and book, "Healing and the Mind," "20/20," and many other media venues. He served for over a decade on the National Board of Medical Examiners, including Chair of the Neurosciences Committee for the US Medical Licensure Examination. He has served on many Study Sections for the National Institutes of Health. Dr. Felten was named one of the "30 Most Influential Neuroscientists Alive Today" by Online Psychology Degree Guide, 2017.

M. KERRY O'BANION, MD, PhD, is Professor and Vice Chair of the Department of Neuroscience, member of the Del Monte Neuroscience Institute, and Director of the Medical Scientist Training Program at the University of Rochester School of Medicine in Rochester, New York. He received a bachelor of science degree and medical and doctoral degrees from the University of Illinois at Champaign-Urbana. As a postdoctoral fellow at the University of Rochester, Dr. O'Banion cloned cyclooxygenase-2 and discovered its critical role in mediating inflammation.

Dr. O'Banion has worked for more than 25 years in the field of neuroinflammation, with particular interests in how cytokines mediate disease pathology. His current work, funded by NIH and NASA, focuses on possible beneficial effects of modulating inflammation in Alzheimer disease, the persistent effects elicited by brain irradiation, and the potential risk of neurodegenerative disease in individuals exposed to cosmic radiation.

Dr. O'Banion has authored over 120 peer-reviewed journal articles and reviews on these and other topics.

Since 1997, Dr. O 'Banion has co-directed the Medical Neural Science course (now called Mind, Brain, and Behavior I) at the University of Rochester School of Medicine, a role he assumed from Dr. Felten. Dr. O'Banion also helped design and direct Mind, Brain, and Behavior II, a basic science course that accompanies medical clerkships in neurology and psychiatry for third-year medical students. He has been program director of the University of Rochester MSTP since 2000 and has served on multiple national committees related to medical and doctoral training.

MARY E.S. MAIDA, PhD, divides her time among research, teaching, mentoring future medical scientists, mentoring future entrepreneurs, and leading a company she founded focused on translational research. She is an adjunct faculty member of the Department of Neuroscience at the University of Rochester School of Medicine, as well as an annually invited MBA Mentor for Entrepreneurship at the University of Rochester Simon School of Business. During her academic training she received bachelor of science degrees in microbiology/immunology, as well as finance and operations management. She returned to academic medicine as a nontraditional student after having raised her children, commencing at the University of Miami School of Medicine and subsequently at the University of Rochester School of Medicine, where she completed a master of science degree in neurobiology and anatomy, and a doctoral degree in molecular neuroscience under the mentorship of Drs. M. Kerry O 'Banion, John Olschowka, Richard Phipps, and Denise Figlewicz.

Because her return to medical and basic sciences training resumed after she raised her children, her interest turned from microbiology/immunology to the broader field of neuroimmunology, which seeks to pinpoint how the CNS and immune systems are intricately involved in a delicate and elaborate dance of connectivity, everyday cross-talk, more elaborate communication when pathogens or damage is involved, give-and-take vs. give- and-go between the two systems (and among other systems), and many more descriptions than words can adequately capture.

Dr. Maida has received several honors and awards across many disciplines, including Outstanding Alumni of Distinction Award from Excelsior College, New York State Hall of Distinction Award, Partners in Lifelong Learning Award, Greater Rochester Excellence in Achievement Technology Award, Winning Mentor for Mark Ain Business Competition, 43North Semifinalist distinction, and winning finalist in several open invitation awards.

A firm proponent of fostering and living the spirit-mind-body relationship that clearly underlies optimal neural-immune health, Dr. Maida is devoted to her family, her Catholic faith, and the privilege of being a Eucharistic Minister. She is honored to be a community volunteer and board member for The EquiCenter, which provides equine therapy and other programs for US military veterans, developmentally and physically disabled children, and their families. She is a member of the board of trustees for Daystar Kids, which provides early education and respite care for medically fragile children and their families. Dr. Maida also serves as a board member for Boots on the Court, which brings weekend tennis fun to military bases across the United States. She has founded a scholarship fund at Excelsior College, named in honor of her parents. Dr. Maida is a fun-loving and enthusiastic competitor in tennis, pickleball, golf, cross-fitness training, and equestrianism and a lover of the arts as a patron, musician, and active performer.

DEDICATION

In memory of Walle J.H. Nauta, MD, PhD, Institute Professor of Neuroscience at the Massachusetts Institute of Technology

>*A distinguished, brilliant, and pioneering neuroscientist*
>*An outstanding and inspirational teacher*
>*A kind, supportive, insightful, and gracious mentor*
>*An incredible role model and human being*

and

To my wife, Mary E.S. Maida, PhD

>*A wonderful wife, partner, and friend*
>*My inspiration and motivation*
>*A superb researcher, teacher, scientific innovator, and business leader*
>*A woman who has it all—brains, beauty, kindness, and accomplishment*

David L. Felten

In memory of Teresa Bellofatto, Joe Summo, Robert Summo, and Nicholas Summo

>*Beloved family and friends who faced overwhelming health challenges with determination and an unwaivering joy for life.*
>*Daily, they demonstrated the strength of the human spirit and unshakable human kindness, even in the face of daunting physiological challenges.*
>*They taught us that it is possible to live life fully, to laugh, and to be the best version of humanity in spite of the absence of a cure.*
>*May their memory forever inspire us to strive for a better understanding of the molecular, physiological, and systemic mechanisms that underlie health and disease.*

David L. Felten
Mary E.S. Maida

In memory of Fred Coyner and Nellie Rogers, sweet souls changed in old age, who turned my attention to brain dysfunction and neuroscience research,

and

To my parents, Terry O'Banion and Mary Rogers, who both served as educators, teaching me the values of service in the name of learning and inspiring me to pursue my love of nature despite the piles of fossils, the stench of chemistry experiments, and some small fires they may still not know about,

and

To my spouse, Dorothy Petrie, also an educator, for her love, her unconditional support through late nights and weekends of writing and looming deadlines, and her consistent reminder that the opportunity to do science is a gift to be shared with all.

M. Kerry O'Banion

In honor of my mother, Mary D. Summo, MS, who endlessly gave her love, time, talent, intellect, and wise advice to the 6 of us, her children, and her 10 grandchildren, and still does to this very day. Thank you, Mom.

and

In memory of my father, Dr. Anthony J. Summo, a true Renaissance man who embraced and promoted the reality of psychobiology, biopsychology, and PTSD well before they became accepted into mainstream medicine. And whose Ciba-Geigy Netter "green books" with the flip-over acetate pages sitting on our living room coffee table fascinated me and formed the basis of my love for science and medicine,

and

To my husband, David L. Felten, MD, PhD, and my sons Michael and Matthew Maida, without whose love, encouragement, and support I would never be the woman I am today. In the spirit and words of our ancestors' family motto: Avanti! Sempre Avanti!

Mary E.S. Maida

ACKNOWLEDGMENTS

For decades, Dr. Frank Netter's beautiful and informative artwork has provided the visual basis for understanding anatomy, physiology, and relationships of great importance in medicine. Generations of physicians and healthcare professionals have "learned from the master" and have carried Dr. Netter's legacy forward through their own knowledge and contributions to patient care. There is no way to compare Dr. Netter's artwork to anything else because it stands in a class of its own. For many decades, the *Netter Collection* volume on the nervous system has been a flagship for the medical profession and for students of neuroscience. It was a great honor to provide the framework, organization, and new information for the updated first, second, and third editions, and now the fourth edition, of *Netter's Alas of Neuroscience*. The opportunity to make a lasting contribution to the next generation of physicians and healthcare professionals is perhaps the greatest honor anyone could receive.

I also gratefully acknowledge Walle J.H. Nauta, MD, PhD, whose inspirational teaching of the nervous system at MIT contributed to the organizational framework for this atlas. Professor Nauta always emphasized the value of an overview; the plates in the beginning of Section II, Regional Neurosciences, on the conceptual organization of sensory, motor, and autonomic systems, especially reflect his approach. I am particularly honored to contribute to these updated editions of *Netter's Atlas of Neuroscience* because I first learned neurosciences as an undergraduate in Professor Nauta's laboratory at MIT through his personal mentorship, masterful insights, and explanations—using the first *Nervous System* "green book" volume by Dr. Frank Netter. It is my hope that continuing generations of students can benefit from the legacy of this wonderful teacher and great scientist.

I thank our outstanding artist and medical illustrator, James Perkins, MS, MFA, for his clear, creative, and beautiful contributions to this revised atlas. Jim is an excellent anatomist, with great insights for bringing otherwise complex systems and mechanisms into understandable illustrations. His accomplishments have received wide acclaim and many awards.

Special thanks go to the outstanding editors at Elsevier Clinical Solutions: Marybeth Thiel, Senior Content Development Specialist, Elyse O'Grady, Senior Content Strategist, and Carrie Stetz, Senior Project Manager. They helped guide the process of the fourth edition and gave us the latitude to introduce new components, such as the new molecular plates (especially in Chapter 1), new additions to forebrain anatomy, a new chapter on Global Neurological Functions, and new clinical correlations.

I also acknowledge and thank my friend, colleague, and co-author of this atlas, Kerry O'Banion. His insights, spanning from the molecular details to the systemic interactions of neural systems, are amazing. For more than 30 years we have had the privilege of working together, both in teaching and research arenas. As one of the premier experts on brain inflammation and a highly knowledgeable molecular neurobiologist, his expertise has been invaluable.

Continuing thanks also go to Ralph Jozefowicz, MD, the consummate neurology educator. It was a delight to work with him in the University of Rochester medical neurosciences course and to learn from him through his amazing insights into clinical neurology, and his ability to make those insights come alive for the benefits of both his students and colleagues.

And finally, to my wife Mary (Mary E.S. Maida), I again thank you for your unwavering love and your support and encouragement to continue this challenging project, and for your patience with the long hours and seemingly endless clutter of papers and folders you tolerated along the way. Your expertise as a molecular neuroscientist and your outstanding ability to take complex plates and explanations and help to clarify and re-express them in understandable terms for the readers has been a valuable addition.

David L. Felten

First, I thank David Felten not only for the opportunity to contribute to this fourth edition but also for his long-standing support, encouragement, and friendship. Second, I thank Ralph Jozefowicz, MD, Professor of Neurology at the University of Rochester, who together with David Felten served as outstanding mentors for how to teach neuroscience. Finally, I am indebted to my professional colleagues and students, past and current, for the opportunity to learn new things as we pursue science together.

M. Kerry O'Banion

To this very day, I remember my fascination with the original Netter "green books" that sat prominently displayed on the coffee table in the living room of my childhood home. I would sit for hours turning each page, which added another colorful layer to the beauty and intricacy of the human body's anatomy and physiology—and day after day trying to recall what I saw, let along make sense of it all. These original tomes that contained the original illustrations of Dr. Frank Netter in part formed the basis of my interest in, and pursuit of, science and medicine.

I thank my parents, Dr. Anthony J. and Mary D. Summo, for having provided us with such an enriched environment at home and for encouraging and allowing us to pursue our dreams.

I thank the University of Rochester School of Medicine and Dentistry Graduate Program in Neuroscience for providing me the opportunity to pursue my dreams as a nontraditional student. I also extend my deepest gratitude to my mentors M. Kerry O'Banion, MD, PhD, John Olschowka, PhD, Richard Phipps, PhD, and Denise Figlewicz, PhD, whom I have the privilege to know as friends as well as research colleagues.

Finally, I express my deepest gratitude to my husband, David Felten, and to my sons Michael and Matthew Maida—my biggest cheerleaders in life—who help me achieve far more than I believe I am capable of achieving and who adeptly help to keep my immune system healthy with the daily dose of humor and laughter we share.

Mary E.S. Maida

PREFACE

As in the three prior editions, *Netter's Atlas of Neuroscience,* 4th edition, combines the richness and beauty of Dr. Frank Netter's illustrations with key information about the many regions and systems of the brain, spinal cord, and periphery. Jim Perkins and John Craig have contributed outstanding illustrations to complement the original Netter illustrations.

The first edition included cross-sectional illustrations through the spinal cord and brainstem, as well as coronal and axial (horizontal) sections. The second edition built on the first edition with several additional illustrations and extensive new imaging using computed tomography (CT), magnetic resonance imaging (MRI), both T1- and T2-weighted, positron emission tomography (PET) scanning, functional MRI (fMRI), and diffusion tensor imaging (DTI), which provides pseudocolor images of central axonal commissural, association, and projection pathways. Full-plate MRIs were included for direct side-by-side comparisons with Dr. John Craig's illustrations of the brainstem cross sections and axial and coronal sections. More than 200 "clinical boxes" were added to offer succinct clinical discussions of the functional importance of key topics. These clinical discussions were intended to assist the reader in bridging the anatomy and physiology depicted in each relevant plate to important related clinical issues.

The third edition added many new components. Chapter 1, in the Overview section, "Neurons and Their Properties," was extensively revised and reorganized. Approximately 15 new plates on molecular and cellular topics such as astrocytes, microglia, oligodendrocytes, axonal transport, growth and trophic factors, nuclear transcription factors, neuronal stem cell biology, and others were added. Almost 50 new plates were added throughout the atlas. Many of these plates reflect Jim Perkins' outstanding ability to represent molecular and cellular concepts in lucid and beautiful form. We added histological cross sections of the spinal cord and brainstem to match the previous illustrations. We also added brainstem sections illustrating the major vascular syndromes of the medulla, pons, and midbrain. Many photomicrographs were introduced to plates throughout the atlas to add clarity to the illustrations. The third edition received three book awards: (1) Highly Commended, British Medical Association (2017); (2) Award of Merit, Association of Medical Illustrators (2016); and (3) Top 10 Neuroscience Textbooks (#2), Wiki Award (2018).

This fourth edition of this Atlas adds significant components that were not present in earlier editions, and are often are minimally covered in other sources. The Systemic Neurosciences Section has a new chapter, Chapter 17, Global Brain Functions. This chapter includes several plates on dementias, neuropsychiatric disorders, traumatic brain injury (TBI) and chronic traumatic encephalopathy (CTE), aphasias, nondominant hemispheric functions and dysfunctions, brain substrates of addictive behaviors, consciousness and coma, and aging and the nervous system.

Chapter 16, on Autonomic-Hypothalamic-Limbic Systems, includes new plates on circumventricular organs and their functions, hypothalamic regulation of sleep, bed nucleus of the stria terminalis, insular cortex, prefrontal cortex, and the functional role of major limbic and cortical regions.

Several other new plates include molecular techniques for studying neurons, genetic models for studying neurons and their diseases, normal pressure hydrocephalus, postnatal and adult neurogenesis, fetal alcohol syndrome, endogenous opioid systems, endogenous cannabinoid systems, somatosensory nuclei neuronal organization (dorsal column and thalamic nuclei), mechanisms of migraine headaches, neural mechanisms of swallowing (central and peripheral), surgical approaches to movement disorders, and others.

The fourth edition retains the organization of the previous three editions: (I) Overview, (II) Regional Neurosciences, and (III) Systemic Neurosciences. Further subdivisions in these sections into component chapters aides in ease of use. We have provided succinct figure legends to point out some of the major functional aspects of each illustration, particularly as they relate to problems that a clinician may encounter in the assessment of a patient with neurological symptoms. We believe that it is important for an atlas of the depth and clarity of *Netter's Atlas of Neuroscience* to let the illustrations provide the focal point for learning, not long and detailed written explanations that constitute a full textbook in itself. However, the figure legends, combined with the excellent illustrations and the clinical discussions, provide content for a thorough understanding of the basic components, organization, and functional aspects of the region or system under consideration.

Netter's Atlas of Neuroscience, 4th edition provides a comprehensive view of the entire nervous system, including the peripheral nerves and their target tissues, central nervous system, ventricular system, meninges, cerebral vascular system, developmental neuroscience, and neuroendocrine regulation. We have provided substantial but not exhaustive details and labels to permit the reader to understand the basics of human neuroscience, including the nervous system information usually presented in medical neurosciences courses, the nervous system components of anatomy courses, and neural components of physiology courses in medical school.

We are confronted with an era of rapid changes in healthcare and exploding knowledge in all fields of medicine, particularly with the continuing revolution in molecular biology. Medical school curricula are under enormous pressure to add more and more non-basic sciences components. It has become dangerously tempting to emphasize high-technology tests, readouts, imaging, and automated EMR drop-down menus as a substitute for the real foundations of medical practice—the history and the physical examination. Many medical schools strive to "decompress" the intensity of teaching and to incorporate more problem-based and small group teaching exercises (which we applaud), with a goal of hastening students into clinical experiences.

In the long run, much of the additional information crammed into the medical curriculum has come at the expense of the basic sciences, particularly anatomy, physiology, histology, and embryology. We believe that there is a fundamental core of knowledge that every physician must know. It is not sufficient for a medical student to learn only 3 of the 12 cranial nerves, their functional importance, and their clinical applications, as "representative examples," in order to further reduce the length of basic sciences courses. Although medical students are always anxious to get into the clinics and see patients, they need a substantial fund of knowledge to be even marginally competent, particularly if they strive to apply evidence-based practice, instead of rote memory, to patient care.

ORGANIZATION OF NETTER'S ATLAS OF NEUROSCIENCE

The Overview section of the atlas is a presentation of the basic components and organization of the nervous system, a "view from 30,000 feet"; this view is an essential foundation for understanding the details of regional and systemic neurosciences. The Overview includes chapters on neurons and their properties, an introduction to the forebrain, brainstem and cerebellum, spinal cord, meninges, ventricular system, cerebral vasculature, and developmental neuroscience.

The Regional Neurosciences section provides the structural components of the peripheral nervous system, the spinal cord, the brainstem and cerebellum, and the forebrain (diencephalon and telencephalon). We begin in the periphery and move from caudal to rostral. The peripheral nervous system section includes details about the somatic and autonomic innervation of peripheral nerves; we do not leave the learner at the boundary of CNS and PNS, and hope that they can find out about peripheral and autonomic nerves from a gross anatomy course. This detailed regional understanding is necessary to diagnose and understand the consequences of a host of lesions whose localization depends on regional knowledge—this includes strokes, local effects of tumors, injuries, specific demyelinating lesions, inflammatory reactions, a host of neuropathies, and many other localized problems. In this section many of the clinical correlations assist the reader in integrating a knowledge of the vascular supply with the consequences of infarcts (e.g., brainstem syndromes), which requires a detailed understanding of brainstem anatomy and relationships.

The Systemic Neurosciences section evaluates the sensory systems, motor systems (including cerebellum and basal ganglia, acknowledging that they also are involved in many other spheres of activity besides motor), autonomic-hypothalamic- limbic systems (including neuroendocrine), and global neural functions and dysfunctions, now named as a fourth section. We have organized each sensory system, when appropriate, with a sequential presentation of reflex channels, cerebellar channels, and lemniscal channels, reflecting Professor Nauta's conceptual organization of sensory systems. For the motor systems, we begin with lower motor neurons and then show the various systems of upper motor neurons followed by cerebellum and basal ganglia, whose major motor influences are ultimately exerted through regulation of upper motor neuronal systems. For the autonomic-hypothalamic-limbic system, we begin with the autonomic preganglionic and postganglionic organization and then show brainstem and hypothalamic regulation of autonomic outflow, and finally limbic and cortical regulation of the hypothalamus and autonomic outflow The newly added Chapter 17 addresses global functions and dysfunctions of the nervous system. The systemic neurosciences constitute the basis for carrying out and interpreting the neurological examination. We believe that it is necessary for a student of neuroscience to understand both regional organization and systemic organization. Without this dual understanding, clinical evaluation of a patient with a neurological problem would be incomplete.

In a discipline as complex as the neurosciences, the acquisition of a solid organization and understanding of the major regions and hierarchies of the nervous system is not just a "nice idea" or a luxury—it is essential. The fact that this approach has been stunningly successful for our students in a course organized and taught for 35 years by both authors of the first edition (David L. Felten, MD, PhD, and Ralph F. Jozefowicz, MD), and by M. Kerry O'Banion, MD, PhD, and Ralph F. Jozefowicz, MD, for more than 15 years is an added benefit but is not why we organized this *Atlas* as we have. A working competence for students in basic and clinical neuroscience, and its value for delivering outstanding patient care, are always the main focus of our efforts. We truly value success in this arena. Knowledgeable and highly competent students are the finest outcome of our teaching that we could ever achieve. We hope that our students will come to appreciate both the beauty and the complexity of the nervous system and be inspired to contribute to the knowledge and functional application to patients of this greatest biological and medical frontier, which constitutes the substrate for human behavior and our loftiest human aspirations and endeavors.

David L. Felten

ABOUT THE ARTISTS

FRANK H. NETTER, MD was born in 1906 in New York City. He studied art at the Art Students League and the National Academy of Design before entering medical school at New York University, where he received his medical degree in 1931. During his student years, Dr. Netter 's notebook sketches attracted the attention of the medical faculty and other physicians, allowing him to augment his income by illustrating articles and textbooks. He continued illustrating as a sideline after establishing a surgical practice in 1933, but he ultimately opted to give up his practice in favor of a full-time commitment to art. After service in the United States Army during World War II, Dr. Netter began his long collaboration with the CIBA Pharmaceutical Company (now Novartis Pharmaceuticals). This 45-year partnership resulted in the production of the extraordinary collection of medical art so familiar to physicians and other medical professionals worldwide.

In 2005, Elsevier, Inc. purchased the Netter Collection and all publications from Icon Learning Systems. There are now more than 50 publications featuring the art of Dr. Netter available through Elsevier, Inc. (in the US: www.us.elsevierhealth.com/Netter; outside the US: www.elsevierhealth.com).

Dr. Netter's works are among the finest examples of the use of illustration in the teaching of medical concepts. The 13-book *Netter Collection of Medical Illustrations,* which includes the greater part of the more than 20,000 paintings created by Dr. Netter, became and remain one of the most famous medical works ever published. Dr. Netter's *Atlas of Human Anatomy,* first published in 1989, presents the anatomical paintings from the *Netter Collection.* Now translated into 16 languages, it is the anatomy atlas of choice among medical and health professions students the world over.

The Netter illustrations are appreciated not only for their aesthetic qualities, but, more important, for their intellectual content. As Dr. Netter wrote in 1949, ". . . clarification of a subject is the aim and goal of illustration. No matter how beautifully painted, how delicately and subtly rendered a subject may be, it is of little value as a medical illustration if it does not serve to make clear some medical point." Dr. Netter's planning, conception, point of view, and approach are what inform his paintings and what makes them so intellectually valuable.

Frank H. Netter, MD, physician and artist, died in 1991.

Learn more about the physician-artist whose work has inspired the Netter Reference collection: http://www.netterimages.com/artist/netter.htm.

CARLOS MACHADO, MD was chosen by Novartis to be Dr. Netter's successor. He continues to be the main artist who contributes to the Netter Collection of medical illustrations.

Self-taught in medical illustration, cardiologist Carlos Machado has contributed meticulous updates to some of Dr. Netter's original plates and has created many paintings of his own in the style of Netter as an extension of the Netter collection. Dr. Machado's photorealistic expertise and his keen insight into the physician/patient relationship inform his vivid and unforgettable visual style. His dedication to researching each topic and subject he paints places him among the premier medical illustrators at work today.

Learn more about his background and see more of his art at: http://www.netterimages.com/artist/machado.htm.

JAMES A. PERKINS, CMI, FAMI is Professor of Medical Illustration at Rochester Institute of Technology (RIT) where he teaches courses in anatomy, digital illustration, and scientific visualization. He is a Board Certified Medical Illustrator and Fellow of the Association of Medical Illustrators.

An expert in visualizing biological processes, Professor Perkins has illustrated more than 40 medical textbooks, particularly in the areas of pathology, physiology, and molecular biology. For more than 20 years, he has been the sole illustrator of the "Robbins" series of pathology texts published by Elsevier, including the flagship of the series, *Robbins and Cotran Pathologic Basis of Disease.* He has been a contributor to the Netter Collection since 2001, creating most of the new art for *Netter's Atlas of Human Physiology, Netter's Illustrated Pharmacology,* and *Netter's Atlas of Neuroscience* and contributing to many other titles.

Professor Perkins received a bachelor degree in biology and geology from Cornell University and studied vertebrate paleontology and anatomy at the University of Texas and University of Rochester. He received a Master of Fine Arts degree in medical illustration from RIT and spent several years working in medical publishing and the medical legal exhibit field before returning to RIT to join the faculty. Learn more about his background and see more of his art at: http://www.netterimages.com/artist/perkins.htm

CONTENTS

VIDEO CONTENTS

Section I OVERVIEW OF THE NERVOUS SYSTEM

1

NEURONS AND THEIR PROPERTIES

Anatomical and Molecular Properties

Electrical Properties

Neurotransmitter and Signaling Properties

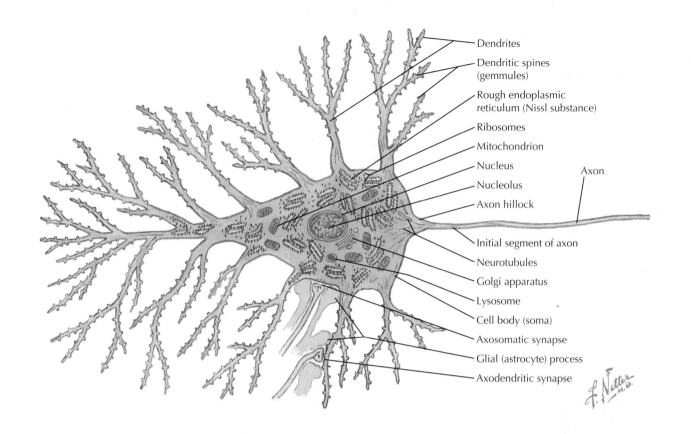

Dendrites

Dendritic spines (gemmules)

Rough endoplasmic reticulum (Nissl substance)

Ribosomes

Mitochondrion

Nucleus

Nucleolus

Axon hillock

Axon

Initial segment of axon

Neurotubules

Golgi apparatus

Lysosome

Cell body (soma)

Axosomatic synapse

Glial (astrocyte) process

Axodendritic synapse

ANATOMICAL AND MOLECULAR PROPERTIES

1.1 NEURONAL STRUCTURE

Neuronal structure reflects the functional characteristics of the individual neuron. Incoming information is projected to a neuron mainly through axonal terminations on the cell body and dendrites. These synapses are isolated and are protected by astrocytic processes. The dendrites usually make up the greatest surface area of the neuron. Some protrusions from dendritic branches (dendritic spines) are sites of specific axodendritic synapses. Each specific neuronal type has a characteristic dendritic branching pattern called the dendritic tree, or dendritic arborizations. The neuronal cell body varies from a few micrometers (μm) in diameter to more than 100 μm. The neuronal cytoplasm contains extensive rough endoplasmic reticulum (rough ER), reflecting the massive amount of protein synthesis necessary to maintain the neuron and its processes. The Golgi apparatus is involved in packaging potential signal molecules for transport and release. Large numbers of mitochondria are necessary to meet the huge energy demands of neurons, particularly those related to the maintenance of ion pumps and membrane potentials. Each neuron has a single (or occasionally no) axon, usually emerging from the cell body or occasionally from a dendrite (e.g., some hippocampal CA neurons). The cell body tapers to the axon at the axon hillock, followed by the initial segment of the axon, which contains the Na^+ channels, the first site where action potentials are initiated. The axon extends for a variable distance from the cell body (up to 1 m or more). An axon larger than 1 to 2 μm in diameter is insulated by a sheath of myelin provided by oligodendroglia in the central nervous system (CNS) or Schwann cells in the peripheral nervous system (PNS). An axon may branch into more than 500,000 axon terminals and may terminate in a highly localized and circumscribed zone (e.g., primary somatosensory axon projections used for fine discriminative touch) or may branch to many disparate regions of the brain (e.g., noradrenergic axonal projections of the locus coeruleus). A neuron whose axon terminates at a distance from its cell body and dendritic tree is called a macroneuron or a Golgi type I neuron; a neuron whose axon terminates locally, close to its cell body and dendritic tree, is called a microneuron, a Golgi type II neuron, a local circuit neuron, or an interneuron. There is no typical neuron because each type of neuron has its own specialization. However, pyramidal cells and lower motor neurons are commonly used to portray a so-called typical neuron.

CLINICAL POINT

Neurons require extraordinary metabolic resources to sustain their functional integrity, particularly that related to the maintenance of membrane potentials for the initiation and propagation of action potentials. Neurons require aerobic metabolism for the generation of adenosine triphosphate (ATP) and have virtually no ATP reserve, so they require continuous delivery of glucose and oxygen, generally in the range of 15% to 20% of the body's resources, which is a disproportionate consumption of resources. During starvation, when glucose availability is limited, the brain can shift gradually to using beta-hydroxybutyrate and acetoacetate as energy sources for neuronal metabolism; however, this is not an instant process and is not available to buffer acute hypoglycemic episodes. An ischemic episode of even 5 minutes, resulting from a heart attack or an ischemic stroke, can lead to permanent damage in some neuronal populations such as pyramidal cells in the CA1 region of the hippocampus. In cases of longer ischemia, widespread neuronal death can occur. Because neurons are postmitotic cells, except for a small subset of interneurons, dead neurons are not replaced. One additional consequence of the postmitotic state of most neurons is that they are not sources of tumor formation. Brain tumors derive mainly from glial cells, ependymal cells, and meningeal cells.

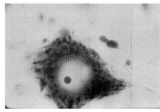

A. Spinal cord lower motor neuron. Nissl substance (rough endoplasmic reticulum) stains purple. The nucleolus is stained in the clear nucleus. Cresyl violet stain.

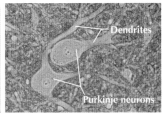

B. Cerebellar Purkinje neurons. Large dendrites branch from the cell body. Intraneuronal neurofibrils and background neural processes (neuropil) stain densely. Silver stain.

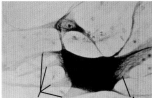

C. Spinal cord neuron. Many large dendrites emerge from the cell body, and the smaller axon extends from the large neuron at the 3 o'clock position. Ink stain.

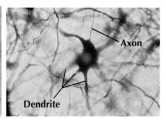

D. Reticular formation neuron. Heavy metal impregnation of selective neurons revealing the cell body and all processes. Golgi stain.

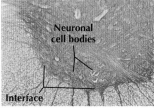

E. Spinal cord ventral horn. Neuronal cell bodies and the tangle of axons and dendrites seen in the neuropil of the ventral horn. The interface between gray matter and white matter is conspicuous. Cajal stain.

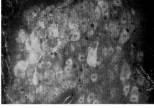

F. Superior mesenteric-celiac ganglion. Glyoxylic acid fluorescence histochemistry demonstrating noradrenergic cell bodies.

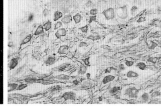

G. Superior mesenteric-celiac ganglion. Immunohistochemical stain demonstrating the presence of interleukin-2 receptors in these neurons.

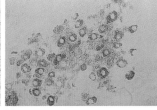

H. Superior mesenteric-celiac ganglion. Acetylcholinesterase (AChE) histochemical stain demonstrating the presence of this enzyme, which cleaves acetylcholine to choline and acetyl coenzyme A.

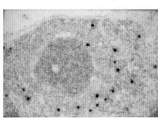

I. Neurons in superior mesenteric-celiac ganglion stained with fluorogold, which has been transported retrogradely from an injection site into immune tissue innervated by NA fibers from these NA ganglion cells in a rat.

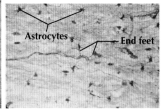

J. Immunocytes in the marginal zone of the spleen. In-situ hybridization demonstrating the presence of corticotropin-releasing factor (CRF) gene in these darkly staining nonneuronal cells. CRF is an important releasing factor secreted by neurons into the hypophyseal portal system in the hypothalamus. CRF also is present in, and secreted by, nonneuronal cells in the immune system.

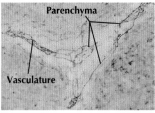

K. CNS astrocytes with processes extending into the gray matter and "end feet" extending to the surface of CNS blood vessels with a blood-brain barrier. Silver stain.

L. Axons from NA sympathetic postganglionic neurons innervating the vasculature and parenchyma (T lymphocyte zone and marginal zone) of the spleen. Immunohistochemical stain for tyrosine hydroxylase (TH), the rate-limiting enzyme for the synthesis of catecholamines from tyrosine.

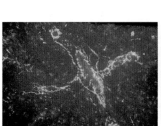

M. Same NA axons as in part L. Stained for norepinephrine with glyoxylic acid fluorescence histochemistry.

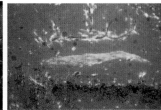

N. Same NA axons as in part M, with added injection of gel ink (dark blue) to demonstrate the vasculature. Gel ink also is picked up by macrophages in the marginal zone.

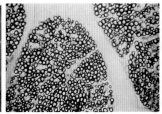

O. Myelinated fascicles in a peripheral nerve cut in cross-section. Osmic acid stain reveals myelinated axons but not unmyelinated axons.

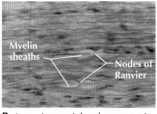

P. Axons in a peripheral nerve cut in longitudinal section. Oil red O stain demonstrating longitudinal axons surrounded by myelin sheaths (light-colored areas), with conspicuous appositions of sheaths at nodes of Ranvier.

1.2 3D NEURONAL STRUCTURE AND NEUROHISTOLOGY

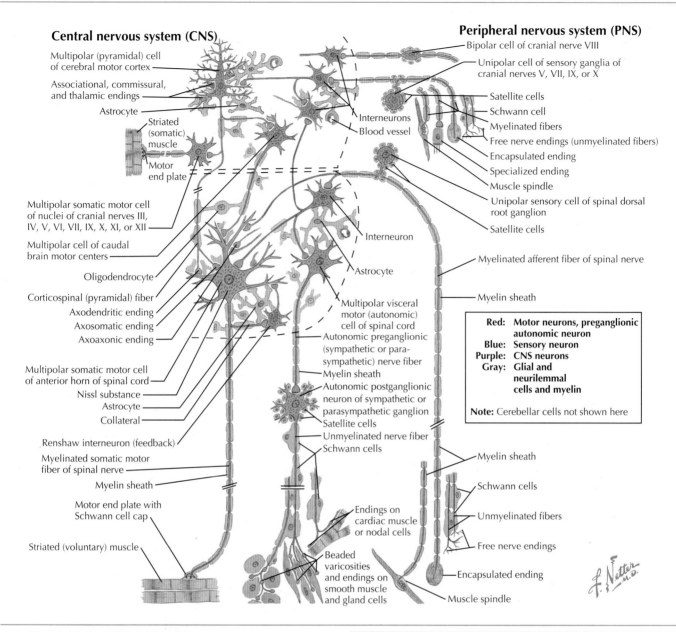

Central nervous system (CNS)

Multipolar (pyramidal) cell of cerebral motor cortex

Associational, commissural, and thalamic endings

Astrocyte

Striated (somatic) muscle

Motor end plate

Multipolar somatic motor cell of nuclei of cranial nerves III, IV, V, VI, VII, IX, X, XI, or XII

Multipolar cell of caudal brain motor centers

Oligodendrocyte

Corticospinal (pyramidal) fiber

Axodendritic ending

Axosomatic ending

Axoaxonic ending

Multipolar somatic motor cell of anterior horn of spinal cord

Nissl substance

Astrocyte

Collateral

Renshaw interneuron (feedback)

Myelinated somatic motor fiber of spinal nerve

Myelin sheath

Motor end plate with Schwann cell cap

Striated (voluntary) muscle

Interneurons

Blood vessel

Interneuron

Astrocyte

Multipolar visceral motor (autonomic) cell of spinal cord

Autonomic preganglionic (sympathetic or parasympathetic) nerve fiber

Myelin sheath

Autonomic postganglionic neuron of sympathetic or parasympathetic ganglion

Satellite cells

Unmyelinated nerve fiber

Schwann cells

Endings on cardiac muscle or nodal cells

Beaded varicosities and endings on smooth muscle and gland cells

Peripheral nervous system (PNS)

Bipolar cell of cranial nerve VIII

Unipolar cell of sensory ganglia of cranial nerves V, VII, IX, or X

Satellite cells

Schwann cell

Myelinated fibers

Free nerve endings (unmyelinated fibers)

Encapsulated ending

Specialized ending

Muscle spindle

Unipolar sensory cell of spinal dorsal root ganglion

Satellite cells

Myelinated afferent fiber of spinal nerve

Myelin sheath

Myelin sheath

Schwann cells

Unmyelinated fibers

Free nerve endings

Encapsulated ending

Muscle spindle

> **Red:** Motor neurons, preganglionic autonomic neuron
> **Blue:** Sensory neuron
> **Purple:** CNS neurons
> **Gray:** Glial and neurilemmal cells and myelin
>
> **Note:** Cerebellar cells not shown here

1.5 NEURONAL CELL TYPES

Local interneurons and projection neurons demonstrate characteristic size, dendritic arborizations, and axonal projections. In the CNS (denoted by dashed lines), glial cells (astrocytes, microglia, oligodendroglia) provide support, protection, and maintenance of neurons. Schwann cells and satellite cells provide these functions in the PNS. The primary sensory neurons (blue) provide sensory transduction of incoming energy or stimuli into electrical signals that are carried into the CNS. The neuronal outflow from the CNS is motor (red) to skeletal muscle fibers via neuromuscular junctions, or is autonomic preganglionic (red) to autonomic ganglia, whose neurons innervate cardiac muscle, smooth muscle, secretory glands, metabolic cells, or cells of the immune system. Neurons other than primary sensory neurons, LMNs, and preganglionic autonomic neurons are located in the CNS in the brain (enclosed by upper dashed lines) or spinal cord (enclosed by lower dashed lines). Neurons and glia are not drawn to scale.

CLINICAL POINT

Neuronal form and configuration provide evidence of the role of that particular type of neuron. Dorsal root ganglion cells have virtually no synapses on the cell body; the sensory receptor is contiguous with the initial segment of the axon to permit direct activation of the initial segment upon reaching a threshold stimulus. This arrangement provides virtually no opportunity for centrifugal control of the initial sensory input; rather, control and analysis of the sensory input occurs in the CNS. Purkinje neurons in the cerebellum have huge planar dendritic trees, with activation occurring via hundreds of parallel fibers and the background excitability influenced by climbing fiber control. This type of array allows network modulation of Purkinje cell output, via neurons of the deep cerebellar nuclei, to UMNs, a control mechanism that permits fine-grained, ongoing adjustments to smooth and coordinated motor activities. Small interneurons in many regions have local and specialized functions that have local circuit connections, whereas large isodendritic neurons of the reticular formation receive widespread, polymodal, nonlocal input, which is important for general arousal of the cerebral cortex and consciousness. Damage to these key neurons may result in coma. LMNs and preganglionic autonomic neurons receive tremendous convergence upon their dendrites and cell bodies to orchestrate the final pattern of activation of these final common pathway neurons through which the peripheral effector tissues are signaled and through which all behavior is achieved.

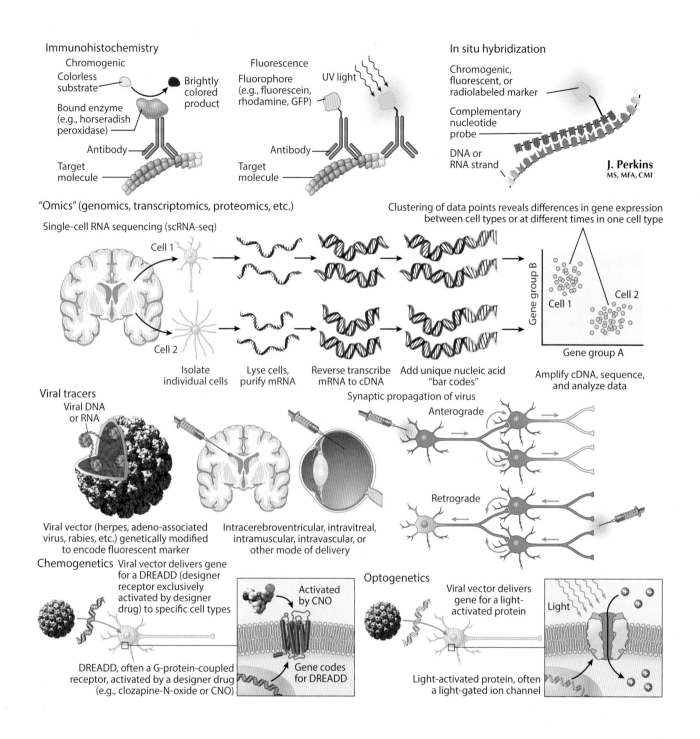

1.6 MOLECULAR TECHNIQUES FOR STUDYING NEURONS

Multiple molecular approaches are used to investigate neurons and their complex interactions. Traditional methods localize specific proteins or mRNA species using immunohistochemistry and in situ hybridization, respectively. New technologies (OMICS) can tag RNA from single cells to investigate patterns of gene expression and their changes in disease states. Some viruses can transduce specific cell types, particularly neurons, and provide precise and efficient means to express molecules in the nervous system.

This technology is used to (1) label neuronal pathways, including transsynaptic connections, and (2) deliver engineered G-protein-coupled receptors or light-sensitive ion channels to modulate neural function directly with exogenous stimuli. Viral vectors are being developed for gene replacement or gene targeting in human disease; some of these therapies are already approved, such as a treatment for **spinal muscular atrophy**.

Transgenic Mouse Models of Human Disease

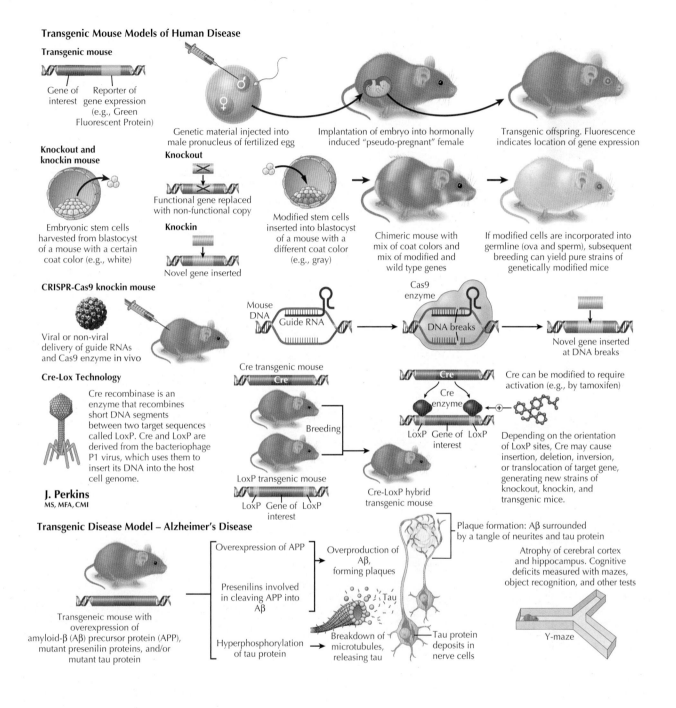

Transgenic mouse

Gene of interest | Reporter of gene expression (e.g., Green Fluorescent Protein)

Genetic material injected into male pronucleus of fertilized egg

Implantation of embryo into hormonally induced "pseudo-pregnant" female

Transgenic offspring. Fluorescence indicates location of gene expression

Knockout and knockin mouse

Embryonic stem cells harvested from blastocyst of a mouse with a certain coat color (e.g., white)

Knockout

Functional gene replaced with non-functional copy

Knockin

Novel gene inserted

Modified stem cells inserted into blastocyst of a mouse with a different coat color (e.g., gray)

Chimeric mouse with mix of coat colors and mix of modified and wild type genes

If modified cells are incorporated into germline (ova and sperm), subsequent breeding can yield pure strains of genetically modified mice

CRISPR-Cas9 knockin mouse

Viral or non-viral delivery of guide RNAs and Cas9 enzyme in vivo

Mouse DNA | Guide RNA

Cas9 enzyme | DNA breaks

Novel gene inserted at DNA breaks

Cre-Lox Technology

Cre recombinase is an enzyme that recombines short DNA segments between two target sequences called LoxP. Cre and LoxP are derived from the bacteriophage P1 virus, which uses them to insert its DNA into the host cell genome.

J. Perkins
MS, MFA, CMI

Cre transgenic mouse

Breeding

LoxP transgenic mouse

LoxP | Gene of interest | LoxP

Cre-LoxP hybrid transgenic mouse

Cre | Cre enzyme

LoxP | Gene of interest | LoxP

Cre can be modified to require activation (e.g., by tamoxifen)

Depending on the orientation of LoxP sites, Cre may cause insertion, deletion, inversion, or translocation of target gene, generating new strains of knockout, knockin, and transgenic mice.

Transgenic Disease Model – Alzheimer's Disease

Transgeneic mouse with overexpression of amyloid-β (Aβ) precursor protein (APP), mutant presenilin proteins, and/or mutant tau protein

Overexpression of APP

Presenilins involved in cleaving APP into Aβ

Hyperphosphorylation of tau protein

Overproduction of Aβ, forming plaques

Breakdown of microtubules, releasing tau

Tau

Tau protein deposits in nerve cells

Plaque formation: Aβ surrounded by a tangle of neurites and tau protein

Atrophy of cerebral cortex and hippocampus. Cognitive deficits measured with mazes, object recognition, and other tests

Y-maze

1.7 GENETIC MODELS FOR STUDYING NEURONS AND THEIR DISORDERS

Genetic manipulation of mammalian DNA, initially in mice, is a powerful experimental tool to explore the effect of the introduction or deletion of specific genes. Transgenic mice, in which a new gene or set of genes is introduced, are widely used in models of human disease. Gene function or disease phenotypes can also be investigated using knockout or knockin technologies, which have been made increasingly efficient by the discovery of systems such as CRISPR-Cas9. This system provides direct, targeted gene insertion or deletion. Other genetic technologies such as Cre-Lox, adapted from bacteriophages, provide methods for cell-specific expression or deletion of genes, depending on which cells express Cre, as well as temporal control of expression or deletion with the use of modified Cre, which can be activated by a drug or hormone. The latter approach is especially useful for avoiding the impact of genetic manipulation during development.

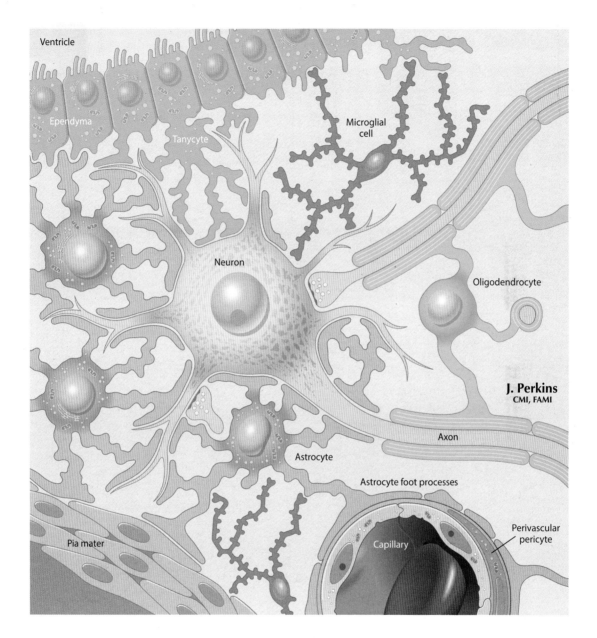

1.8 GLIAL CELL TYPES

Astrocytes provide structural isolation of neurons and their synapses and provide ionic (K⁺) sequestration, trophic support, and support for growth and signaling functions to neurons. Oligodendroglia (oligodendrocytes) provide myelination of axons in the CNS. Microglia are scavenger cells that participate in phagocytosis, inflammatory responses, cytokine and growth factor secretion, and some immune reactivity in the CNS. Perivascular cells participate in similar activities at sites near the blood vessels. Schwann cells provide myelination, ensheathment, trophic support, and actions that contribute to the growth and repair of peripheral neurons. Activated T lymphocytes normally can enter and traverse the CNS for immune surveillance for a period of approximately 24 hours.

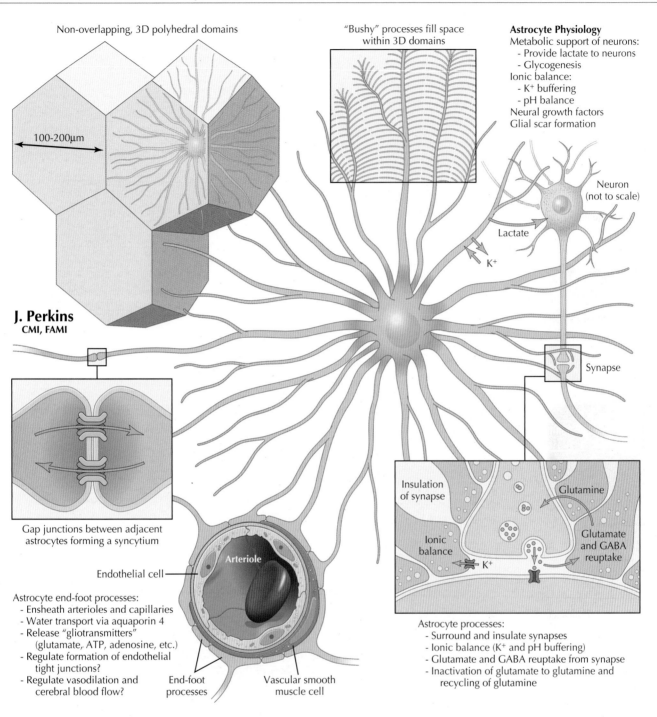

Non-overlapping, 3D polyhedral domains

100-200μm

J. Perkins
CMI, FAMI

"Bushy" processes fill space
within 3D domains

Astrocyte Physiology
Metabolic support of neurons:
- Provide lactate to neurons
- Glycogenesis
Ionic balance:
- K⁺ buffering
- pH balance
Neural growth factors
Glial scar formation

Neuron
(not to scale)

Lactate

K⁺

Synapse

Gap junctions between adjacent
astrocytes forming a syncytium

Endothelial cell

Arteriole

Astrocyte end-foot processes:
- Ensheath arterioles and capillaries
- Water transport via aquaporin 4
- Release "gliotransmitters"
  (glutamate, ATP, adenosine, etc.)
- Regulate formation of endothelial
  tight junctions?
- Regulate vasodilation and
  cerebral blood flow?

End-foot
processes

Vascular smooth
muscle cell

Insulation
of synapse

Glutamine

Ionic
balance

K⁺

Glutamate
and GABA
reuptake

Astrocyte processes:
- Surround and insulate synapses
- Ionic balance (K⁺ and pH buffering)
- Glutamate and GABA reuptake from synapse
- Inactivation of glutamate to glutamine and
  recycling of glutamine

1.9 ASTROCYTE BIOLOGY

Astrocytes are the most abundant glial cells in the CNS. They arise from neuroectoderm and are intimately associated with neural processes, synapses, vasculature, and the pial-glial membrane investing the CNS. Astrocytes in gray matter are called *protoplasmic astrocytes,* and in white matter are called *fibrous astrocytes.* The somas vary in diameter from a few micrometers to 10 or more micrometers. Astrocytes are arrayed in nonoverlapping 3D polyhedral domains of 100–200 μm across (up to 400 μm in hominids). Structurally, astrocytic processes interdigitate, forming a syncytium to protect synapses (as close as 1 μm to these structures). Astrocytic endfeet associate with vascular endothelial cells

and associated smooth muscle cells. Astrocytic processes invest the entire pial membrane from the inside.

Physiologically, astrocytic processes affect ion balance (sequester K⁺), transport water via aquaporin 4 channels, uptake and recycle glutamate and gamma-aminobutyric acid (GABA), provide metabolic support to neurons, and can become reactive after CNS injury and lay down glial scar tissue. Astrocytes also can release growth factors and bioactive molecules (termed *gliotransmitters*) such as glutamate, ATP, and adenosine. In development, specialized astrocytes, called *radial glia,* provide a scaffold for orderly neural migrations in the CNS. Astrocytes are able to transfer mitochondria to neurons damaged by a stroke.

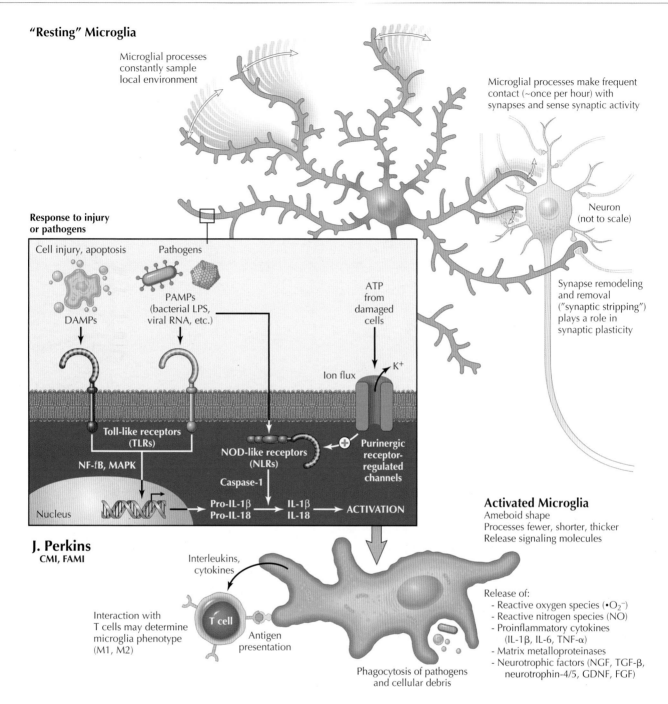

"Resting" Microglia

Microglial processes constantly sample local environment

Microglial processes make frequent contact (~once per hour) with synapses and sense synaptic activity

Neuron (not to scale)

Synapse remodeling and removal ("synaptic stripping") plays a role in synaptic plasticity

Response to injury or pathogens

Cell injury, apoptosis

Pathogens

DAMPs

PAMPs (bacterial LPS, viral RNA, etc.)

ATP from damaged cells

Ion flux

K+

Toll-like receptors (TLRs)

NF-fB, MAPK

NOD-like receptors (NLRs)

Caspase-1

Purinergic receptor-regulated channels

Nucleus

Pro-IL-1β
Pro-IL-18

IL-1β
IL-18

ACTIVATION

J. Perkins
CMI, FAMI

Activated Microglia
Ameboid shape
Processes fewer, shorter, thicker
Release signaling molecules

Interleukins, cytokines

T cell

Interaction with T cells may determine microglia phenotype (M1, M2)

Antigen presentation

Phagocytosis of pathogens and cellular debris

Release of:
- Reactive oxygen species (•O$_2^-$)
- Reactive nitrogen species (NO)
- Proinflammatory cytokines (IL-1β, IL-6, TNF-α)
- Matrix metalloproteinases
- Neurotrophic factors (NGF, TGF-β, neurotrophin-4/5, GDNF, FGF)

1.10 MICROGLIAL BIOLOGY

Microglial cells are mesenchymal cells derived from yolk sac that come to reside in the CNS. They are a unique resident population with the capacity for self-renewal. Microglia provide constant surveillance of the local microenvironment, with processes moving back and forth up to 1.5 μm/min. Microglial processes can grow and shrink up to 2–3 μm/min. They have a territory 15–30 μm wide, with little overlap with each other. Resting microglia have soma of 5–6 μm diameter, and activated microglia are ameboid in appearance, with soma of approximately 10 μm diameter.

Microglia can carry out phagocytosis of debris and apoptotic cells, remodel and remove synapses in developing and adult CNS, and respond to injury or pathogens. Microglia have receptors for multiple types of stimuli, such as ATP (indicator of local damage), toll-like receptors (TLRs) that respond to molecules released from dying cells (DAMPS: damage-associated molecular patterns) or pathogens (PAMPS: pathogen associated molecular patterns) such as LPS on gram-negative bacteria, or double-stranded RNA in viruses. Reactive microglia produce reactive oxygen species (ROS), reactive nitrogen species (RNS, such as NO), proinflammatory cytokines (IL-1β , IL-6, TNF-α), matrix metalloproteinases (MMPs), and neurotrophic factors (such as NGF, TGF-β, neurotrophin 4/5, GDNF, FGF). Such signal molecules from activated microglia can affect neurons and astrocytes, inducing dysfunction. Recent evidence suggests that peripheral macrophages can transfer mitochondria to assist primary sensory neurons in inflamed tissue.

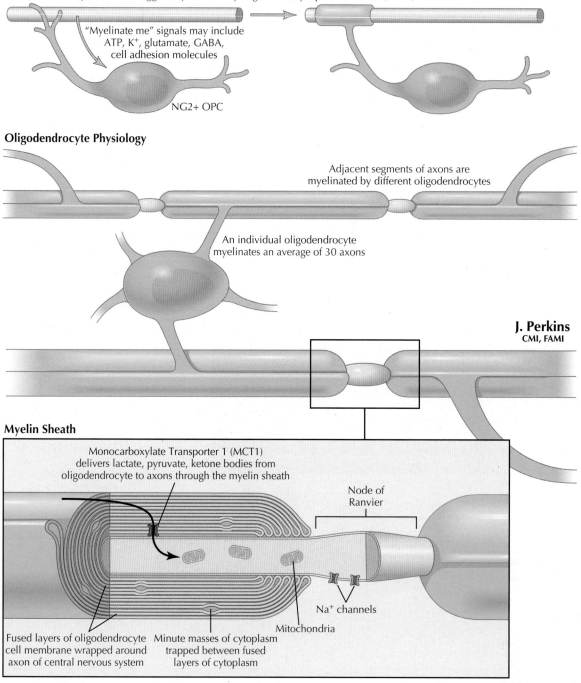

Oligodendrocyte Maturation

Functional activity in neurons triggers myelination by oligodendrocyte precursor cells (OPCs)

"Myelinate me" signals may include ATP, K$^+$, glutamate, GABA, cell adhesion molecules

NG2+ OPC

Oligodendrocyte Physiology

Adjacent segments of axons are myelinated by different oligodendrocytes

An individual oligodendrocyte myelinates an average of 30 axons

J. Perkins
CMI, FAMI

Myelin Sheath

Monocarboxylate Transporter 1 (MCT1) delivers lactate, pyruvate, ketone bodies from oligodendrocyte to axons through the myelin sheath

Node of Ranvier

Na$^+$ channels

Mitochondria

Fused layers of oligodendrocyte cell membrane wrapped around axon of central nervous system

Minute masses of cytoplasm trapped between fused layers of cytoplasm

1.11 OLIGODENDROCYTE BIOLOGY

Oligodendrocytes are neuroectodermally derived glial cells that have the major role of myelinating central axons. The trigger for myelination may include associated axonal size and signal molecules (such as ATP, K$^+$, glutamate, GABA, and some cell adhesion molecules). Each oligodendrocyte can myelinate individual intermodal segments of an average of 30 separate axons (as high as 60 axons); adjacent internodal segments are myelinated by different oligodendrocytes. This pattern of central myelination leaves periodic nodes of Ranvier bare, with sodium channels, at which action potentials (APs) are reinitiated as they travel down the myelinated axon and its branches (called *saltatory conduction*). Oligodendrocytes can be attacked by antibodies directed at specific oligodendrocyte proteins in multiple sclerosis, leading to oligodendrocyte death and axonal dysfunction. Oligodendrocyte precursor cells can replicate following such insults and remyelinate the denuded central axon segments. Oligodendrocyte membranes possess monocarboxylate transporter 1 (MCT 1), which can deliver lactate, pyruvate, and ketone bodies to the axon. Oligodendrocyte precursor cells (OPCs) are present in the adult CNS and have NG2 and PDGFα receptors.

I. Growth (e.g., neuronal differentiation, axonal outgrowth)

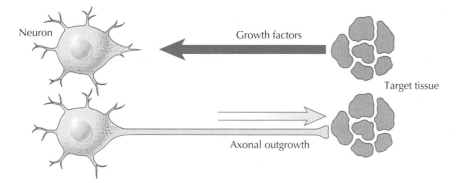

II. Autocrine and paracrine signaling between and among neurons

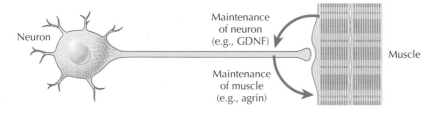

Signaling inhibits apoptosis, promotes neuron survival, maintains synapses

III. Reciprocal signaling (e.g., neuromuscular junction)

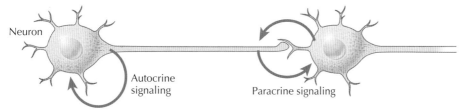

J. Perkins
CMI, FAMI

Growth Factor	Source	Receptor	Critical for:
NGF	Skin, hippocampus?	TrkA, p75	Cutaneous nociceptive neurons (small DRG neurons) Sympathetic neurons Basal forebrain cholinergic neurons (not the only factor required)
BDNF	Many sites	TrkB, p75	Synaptic plasticity In periphery, BDNF KO mice show loss of vestibular ganglion neurons
NT3	Golgi tendon organs and muscle spindles	TrkC, p75	Loss of proprioceptive sensory neurons in DRG No gamma motorneurons; mice die at birth
NT4	Multiple sites	TrkB, p75	No robust phenotype
GDNF	Muscle	Grfα1, Ret	Partial loss of muscles
CNTF	Muscle?	CNTFRα, gp130	KO of CNTFRα partial loss of muscles, but CNTF KO no loss due to LIF working
IGF-1	Muscle	IGFR-1, IGFR-2	Partial loss of muscles
VEGF	Muscle	Flk-1, Flt-1, Flt-4	Embryonic lethal (required for angiogenesis)

NGF, nerve growth factor; BDNF, brain-derived neurotrophic factor; NT3 and NT4, neurotrophic 3 and 4; GDNF, glial cell line–derived neurotrophic factor; CNTF, ciliary neurotrophic factor; IGF-1, insulin-like growth factor 1; VEGF, vascular endothelial growth factor; Trk, tyrosine kinase; KO, knock out; LIF, leukemia inhibitory factor.

1.12 NEURONAL GROWTH FACTORS AND TROPHIC FACTORS

Neuronal growth factors and trophic factors are signal molecules produced by neurons, glia, and target tissues that can influence neuronal differentiation, growth of neurites, establishment of contacts for signaling, maintenance of neural contacts with their central or peripheral targets, and other functions. These factors act through specific receptors and can induce the production of specific molecules, such as agrin for the maintenance of nicotinic cholinergic receptors at the neuromuscular junction. Several identified growth factors, along with their sourced receptors and possible roles, are provided in the table above.

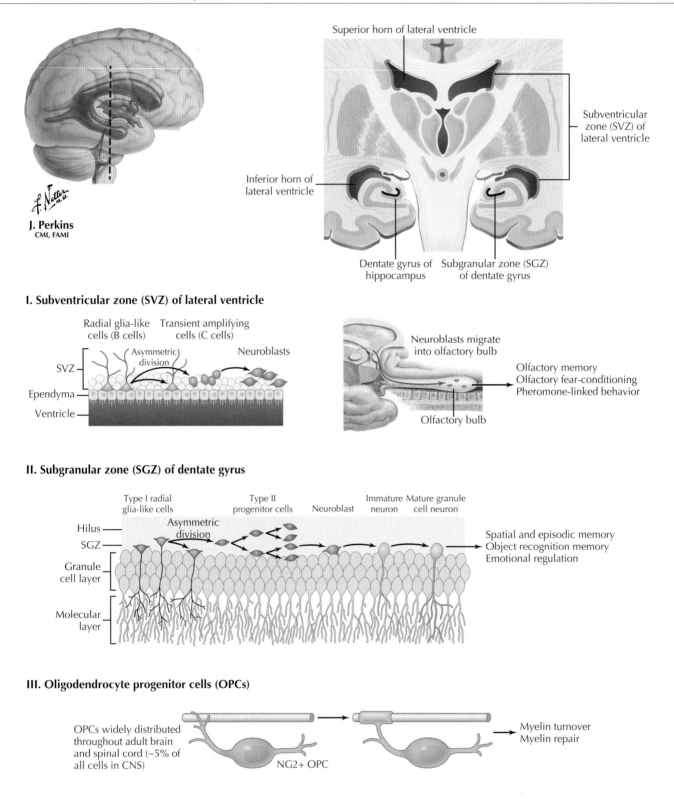

J. Perkins
CMI, FAMI

I. Subventricular zone (SVZ) of lateral ventricle

II. Subgranular zone (SGZ) of dentate gyrus

III. Oligodendrocyte progenitor cells (OPCs)

1.13 STEM CELLS IN THE CNS: INTRINSIC AND EXTRINSIC MECHANISMS

Embryogenesis involves the proliferation of stem cells, followed by differentiation and migration of the resultant cell types. In the CNS, neuronal stem cells, derived from the neural tube, persist in the *subventricular* (or subependymal) *zone* of the lateral ventricles (I). Waves of neuronal proliferation, differentiation, and migration occur during prenatal CNS development. After birth, stem cells in the subventricular zone continue to proliferate and produce granule cells (neurons) for many brain regions; this process is driven by postnatal environmental stimuli. Throughout adulthood radial glial-like cells, in the *subgranular zone* of the dentate gyrus, give rise to neuroblasts that contribute new granule cell neurons (II). In addition, *oligodendroglial progenitor cells* throughout the CNS can proliferate and then differentiate into mature oligodendrocytes (III). This process can occur after a demyelinating lesion and helps to remyelinate CNS axons (e.g., after a multiple sclerosis lesion).

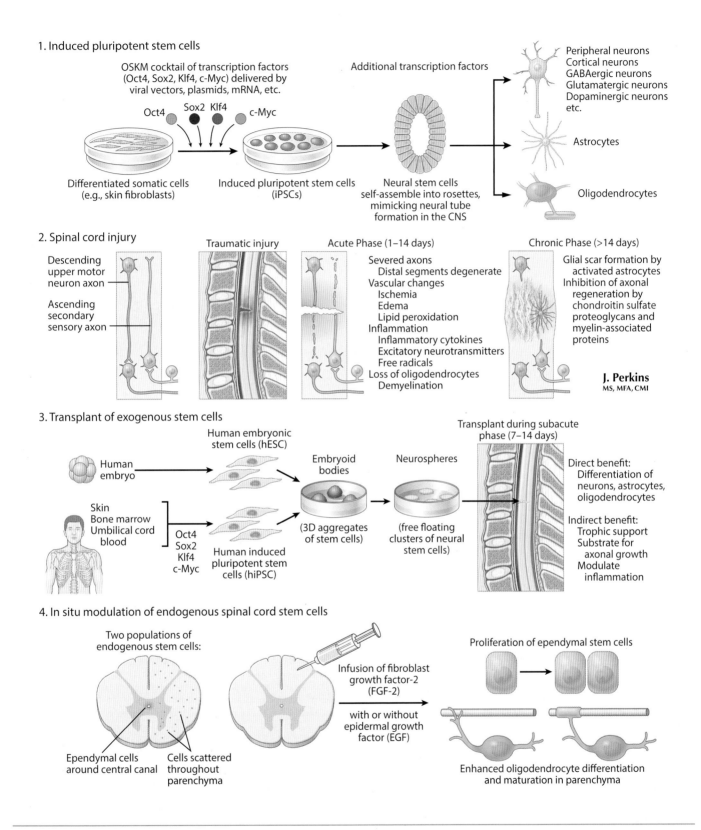

1. Induced pluripotent stem cells

OSKM cocktail of transcription factors
(Oct4, Sox2, Klf4, c-Myc) delivered by
viral vectors, plasmids, mRNA, etc.

Oct4 Sox2 Klf4 c-Myc

Additional transcription factors

Differentiated somatic cells
(e.g., skin fibroblasts)

Induced pluripotent stem cells
(iPSCs)

Neural stem cells
self-assemble into rosettes,
mimicking neural tube
formation in the CNS

Peripheral neurons
Cortical neurons
GABAergic neurons
Glutamatergic neurons
Dopaminergic neurons
etc.

Astrocytes

Oligodendrocytes

2. Spinal cord injury

Descending
upper motor
neuron axon

Ascending
secondary
sensory axon

Traumatic injury

Acute Phase (1–14 days)

Severed axons
Distal segments degenerate
Vascular changes
Ischemia
Edema
Lipid peroxidation
Inflammation
Inflammatory cytokines
Excitatory neurotransmitters
Free radicals
Loss of oligodendrocytes
Demyelination

Chronic Phase (>14 days)

Glial scar formation by
activated astrocytes
Inhibition of axonal
regeneration by
chondroitin sulfate
proteoglycans and
myelin-associated
proteins

J. Perkins
MS, MFA, CMI

3. Transplant of exogenous stem cells

Human embryonic
stem cells (hESC)

Human
embryo

Embryoid
bodies

Neurospheres

Transplant during subacute
phase (7–14 days)

Skin
Bone marrow
Umbilical cord
blood

Oct4
Sox2
Klf4
c-Myc

Human induced
pluripotent stem
cells (hiPSC)

(3D aggregates
of stem cells)

(free floating
clusters of neural
stem cells)

Direct benefit:
Differentiation of
neurons, astrocytes,
oligodendrocytes

Indirect benefit:
Trophic support
Substrate for
axonal growth
Modulate
inflammation

4. In situ modulation of endogenous spinal cord stem cells

Two populations of
endogenous stem cells:

Proliferation of ependymal stem cells

Infusion of fibroblast
growth factor-2
(FGF-2)

with or without
epidermal growth
factor (EGF)

Ependymal cells
around central canal

Cells scattered
throughout
parenchyma

Enhanced oligodendrocyte differentiation
and maturation in parenchyma

1.14 STEM CELL THERAPY

Recent approaches to stem cell therapy after a spinal cord injury are depicted here. 1. *Induced pluripotent stem cells* can be generated from somatic cells (e.g., skin biopsy) and differentiated into neural lineage cells for therapy. 2. *The pathologic process of spinal cord injury* shows acute and chronic responses. 3. *Use of exogenous stem cells* transplanted during the subacute phase leads to differentiation of neurons and glia, and trophic support and modulation of inflammation. 4. *In situ modulation of endogenous stem cells* uses infusion of growth factors. These approaches remain experimental but offer possible applications of knowledge derived from stem cell biology to treat devastating conditions such as spinal cord injury.

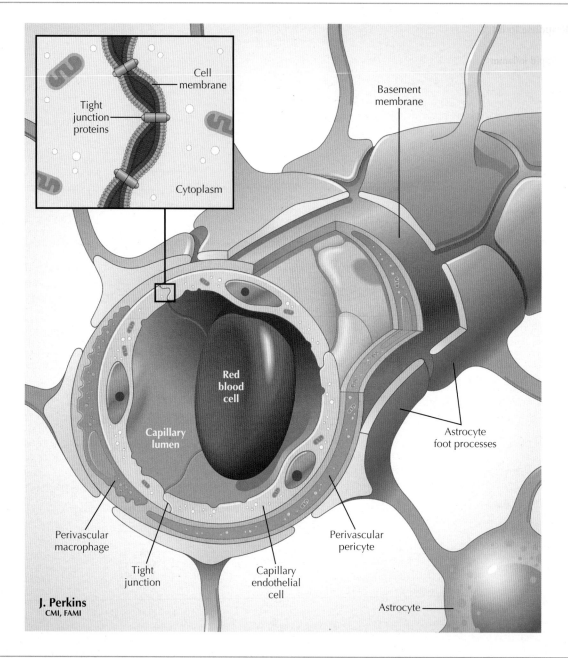

Cell membrane

Tight junction proteins

Cytoplasm

Basement membrane

Red blood cell

Astrocyte foot processes

Capillary lumen

Perivascular pericyte

Perivascular macrophage

Tight junction

Capillary endothelial cell

Astrocyte

J. Perkins
CMI, FAMI

1.15 **BLOOD-BRAIN BARRIER**

The blood-brain barrier (BBB) is the cellular interface between the blood and the CNS. It serves to protect the brain from unwanted intrusion by many large molecules and potentially toxic substances and to maintain the interstitial fluid environment to ensure optimal functioning of the neurons and their associated glial cells. The major cellular basis for the BBB consists of the capillary endothelial cells, which have an elaborate network of tight junctions; these tight junctions restrict access by many large molecules, including many drugs, to the CNS. Endothelial cells in the CNS also exhibit a low level of pinocytotic activity across the cell, providing selected specific carrier systems for the transport of essential substrates of energy production and amino acid metabolism into the CNS. Astrocytic endfoot processes abut the endothelial cells and their basement membranes; these processes help to transfer important metabolites from the blood to neurons and can influence the expression of some specific gene products in the endothelial cells. These astrocytic processes also can remove excess K^+ and some neurotransmitters from the interstitial fluid.

CLINICAL POINT

The BBB, anatomically consisting mainly of the capillary tight junctions of the vascular endothelial cells, serves to protect the CNS from the intrusion of large molecules and potentially damaging agents from the peripheral circulation. The neurons need protection of their ionic and metabolic environment, which is aided by glial cells and the BBB. There are selected areas (windows on the brain) where the BBB is not present, such as the median eminence, the area postrema, the organum vasculosum of the lamina terminalis, and others, and where specialized cells can sample the peripheral circulation and can initiate corrective brain mechanisms to protect the neuronal environment. The presence of the BBB presents a challenge for pharmacotherapy aimed at the CNS; many antibiotics and other agents will not penetrate the BBB and must be coupled to a carrier molecule that does cross or must be injected intrathecally. In some pathological circumstances, such as the presence of a brain tumor, neuronal degeneration resulting from a neurodegenerative disease, the presence of a high concentration of a solute, or a stroke, the BBB is disrupted extensively, exposing the internal CNS milieu to molecules in the peripheral circulation. Therapeutic strategies now are being tested that will achieve transport of desired pharmacotherapeutic agents across the BBB and will protect the brain from unwanted disruption of the BBB in pathological circumstances.

I. Response to intrinsic damage (acute stroke, trauma, bacterial infection, etc.)

A. Rapid inflammatory response

B. Delayed inflammatory response

C. Healing

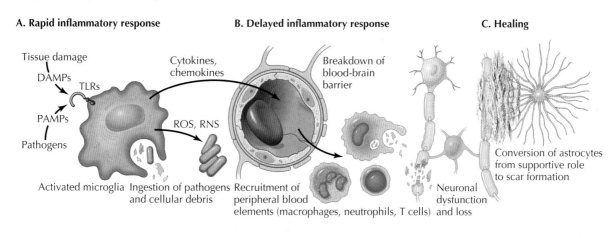

Tissue damage

DAMPs

TLRs

PAMPs

Pathogens

Cytokines, chemokines

ROS, RNS

Activated microglia | Ingestion of pathogens and cellular debris

Breakdown of blood-brain barrier

Recruitment of peripheral blood elements (macrophages, neutrophils, T cells)

Neuronal dysfunction and loss

Conversion of astrocytes from supportive role to scar formation

II. Response to extrinsic stimuli

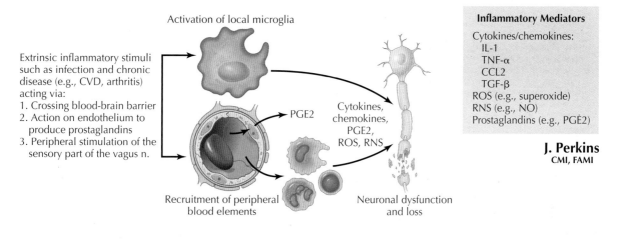

Activation of local microglia

Extrinsic inflammatory stimuli such as infection and chronic disease (e.g., CVD, arthritis) acting via:
1. Crossing blood-brain barrier
2. Action on endothelium to produce prostaglandins
3. Peripheral stimulation of the sensory part of the vagus n.

PGE2

Cytokines, chemokines, PGE2, ROS, RNS

Recruitment of peripheral blood elements

Neuronal dysfunction and loss

Inflammatory Mediators

Cytokines/chemokines:
 IL-1
 TNF-α
 CCL2
 TGF-β
ROS (e.g., superoxide)
RNS (e.g., NO)
Prostaglandins (e.g., PGE2)

J. Perkins
CMI, FAMI

III. Response to intrinsic proteinopathy or neurodegenerative process (e.g., Alzheimer's disease)

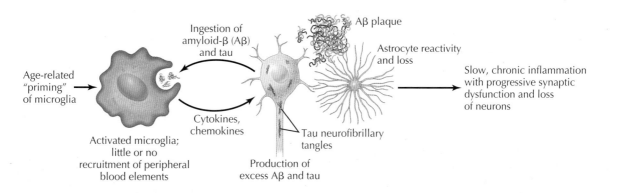

Ingestion of amyloid-β (Aβ) and tau

Aβ plaque

Astrocyte reactivity and loss

Age-related "priming" of microglia

Slow, chronic inflammation with progressive synaptic dysfunction and loss of neurons

Cytokines, chemokines

Tau neurofibrillary tangles

Activated microglia; little or no recruitment of peripheral blood elements

Production of excess Aβ and tau

1.16 INFLAMMATION IN THE CNS

Inflammatory responses in the CNS occur under several different conditions. *I. Inflammatory response to intrinsic damage* such as stroke, trauma, or infection involves an acute inflammatory response, a delayed inflammatory response, and a healing phase. *II. Response to extrinsic inflammatory stimuli* such as infection and chronic disease usually involves a host of inflammatory mediators crossing the blood-brain barrier, triggering release of prostaglandins and central neuronal dysfunction and loss. *III. Response to intrinsic proteinopathy or neurodegenerative processes* such as aberrant amyloid-β plaque or tau neurofibrillary tangles in Alzheimer's disease is a slow, chronic inflammatory response that leads to synaptic dysfunction and neuronal loss.

I. Fast Anterograde Axonal Transport

100–400 mm/day in a saltatory
fashion (start-stop-start)

Cargo includes:
- Synaptic vesicles and
  synaptic vesicle precursors
- Mitochondria and other
  membrane organelles
- Integral membrane proteins
- Secretory polypeptides
- Neurotransmitters
- Elements of smooth
  endoplasmic reticulum

II. Fast Retrograde Axonal Transport

200–270 mm/day

Cargo includes:
- Endosomes
- Damaged mitochondria and
  other organelles
- Elements of smooth
  endoplasmic reticulum
- Regulatory signals (growth
  factors and neurotrophins)
- Viruses and toxins (e.g., tetanus,
  herpes simplex, rabies, polio)

III. Slow Axonal Transport (Anterograde Only)

Different substances move at
two different speeds:

Slow component a (SCa)
0.2–2.5 mm/day (rate of neurite
  elongation)
- Microtubules
- Neurofilaments
- Cytoskeletal proteins
  (e.g., α- and β-tubulin)

Slow component b (SCb)
5.0–6.0 mm/day
- Cytosolic proteins
- Clathrin
- Calmodulin
- Soluble enzymes and other proteins

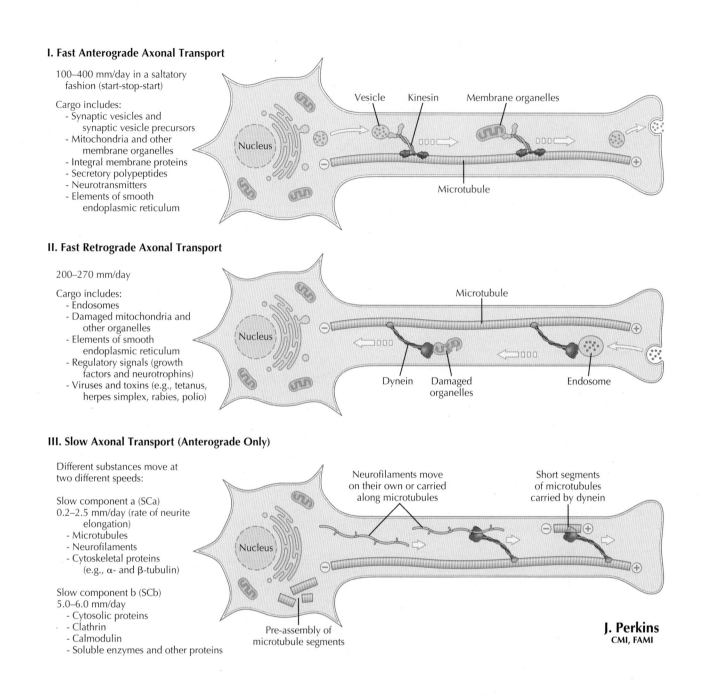

J. Perkins
CMI, FAMI

1.17 AXONAL TRANSPORT IN THE CNS AND PNS

Intracellular organelles and molecules are transported both away from the cell body down the axon (anterograde transport) and toward the cell body from the axon (retrograde transport). *I. Fast anterograde transport* moves vesicles, organelles, membrane proteins, neurotransmitter elements, and smooth endoplasmic reticulum components at a rate of 100–400 mm/day in a stop-start fashion, using kinesin as a transport mechanism. *II. Fast retrograde transport* returns endosomes, damaged organelles, growth factors and trophic factors, and some viruses and toxins at a rate of 200–270 mm/day, using dynein as a transport mechanism. Fast anterograde and retrograde transport mechanisms have been exploited in experimental neuroanatomical studies using labeled compounds (e.g., horseradish peroxidase, fluorogold) for retrograde tract tracing and radiolabeled proteins for anterograde tract tracing. *III. Slow anterograde transport* carries microtubules, neurofilaments, and some cytoskeletal proteins at 0.2–2.5 mm/day (slow component a) and other enzymes and proteins at 5.0–6.0 mm/day (slow component b). This slow transport process is the rate-limiting factor governing axonal recovery after injury or insult; recovery usually proceeds (if it occurs at all) at approximately 1 mm/day.

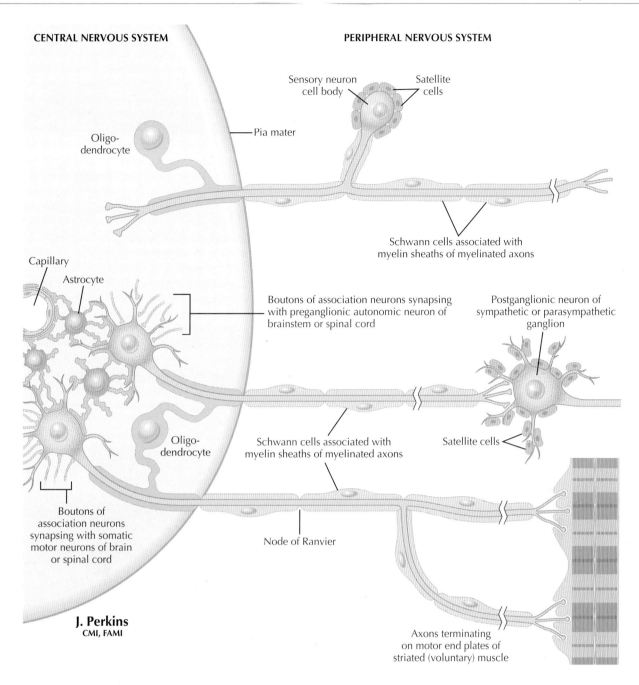

CENTRAL NERVOUS SYSTEM

PERIPHERAL NERVOUS SYSTEM

Sensory neuron cell body

Satellite cells

Oligo-dendrocyte

Pia mater

Schwann cells associated with myelin sheaths of myelinated axons

Capillary

Astrocyte

Boutons of association neurons synapsing with preganglionic autonomic neuron of brainstem or spinal cord

Postganglionic neuron of sympathetic or parasympathetic ganglion

Oligo-dendrocyte

Schwann cells associated with myelin sheaths of myelinated axons

Satellite cells

Boutons of association neurons synapsing with somatic motor neurons of brain or spinal cord

Node of Ranvier

J. Perkins
CMI, FAMI

Axons terminating on motor end plates of striated (voluntary) muscle

1.18 MYELINATION OF CNS AND PNS AXONS

Central myelination of axons is provided by oligodendroglia. Each oligodendroglial cell can myelinate a single segment of several separate central axons. In the PNS, sensory, motor, and preganglionic autonomic axons are myelinated by Schwann cells. A Schwann cell myelinates only a single segment of one axon. Unmyelinated sensory and autonomic postganglionic autonomic axons are ensheathed by a Schwann cell, which provides a single enwrapping arm of cytoplasm around each of several such axons. The space between adjacent myelin segments of an axon is called a node of Ranvier; this site of axon membrane contains sodium channels and allows the reinitiation of action potentials in the course of propagation down the axon, a process called saltatory conduction.

CLINICAL POINT

The integrity of the **myelin sheath** is essential for proper neuronal function in both the CNS and the PNS. Disruption of the myelin sheath around axons in either system results in the inability of the formerly myelinated axons to carry out their functional activities. In the CNS, the myelin sheath of central axons can be attacked in an autoimmune disease such as multiple sclerosis, resulting in a variety of symptoms, such as blindness, diplopia caused by discoordinated eye movements, loss of sensation, loss of coordination, paresis, and others. This condition may occur episodically, with intermittent remyelination occurring as the result of oligodendroglia proliferation and remyelination. In the PNS, a wide variety of insults, including exposure to toxins and the presence of diabetes or autoimmune Guillain-Barré syndrome, result in peripheral axonal demyelination, which is manifested mainly as sensory loss and paralysis or weakness. Remyelination also can occur around peripheral axons, initiated by the Schwann cells. Clinically, the status of axonal conduction is assessed by examining sensory evoked potentials in the CNS and by conduction velocity studies in the PNS.

SHEATH AND SATELLITE CELL FORMATION

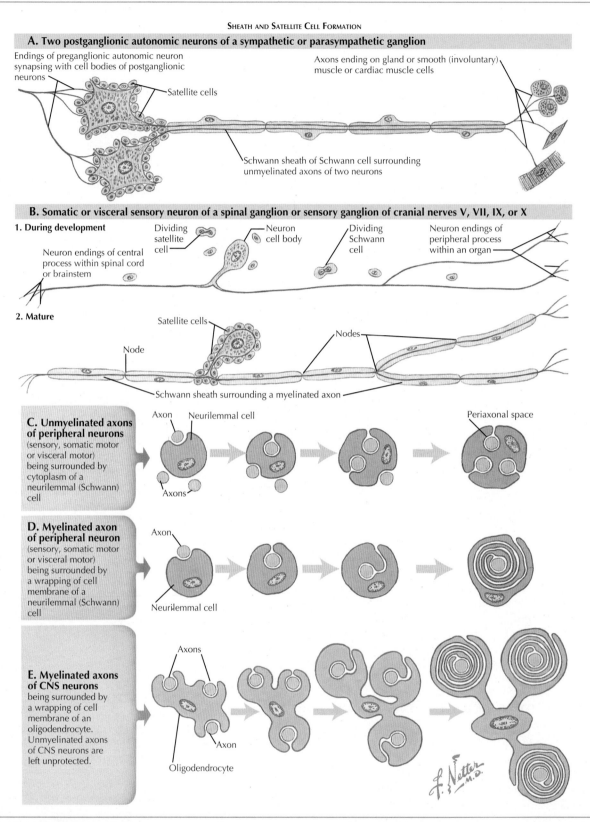

A. Two postganglionic autonomic neurons of a sympathetic or parasympathetic ganglion

Endings of preganglionic autonomic neuron synapsing with cell bodies of postganglionic neurons

Satellite cells

Axons ending on gland or smooth (involuntary) muscle or cardiac muscle cells

Schwann sheath of Schwann cell surrounding unmyelinated axons of two neurons

B. Somatic or visceral sensory neuron of a spinal ganglion or sensory ganglion of cranial nerves V, VII, IX, or X

1. During development

Dividing satellite cell

Neuron cell body

Dividing Schwann cell

Neuron endings of peripheral process within an organ

Neuron endings of central process within spinal cord or brainstem

2. Mature

Satellite cells

Nodes

Node

Schwann sheath surrounding a myelinated axon

C. Unmyelinated axons of peripheral neurons (sensory, somatic motor or visceral motor) being surrounded by cytoplasm of a neurilemmal (Schwann) cell

Axon

Neurilemmal cell

Periaxonal space

Axons

D. Myelinated axon of peripheral neuron (sensory, somatic motor or visceral motor) being surrounded by a wrapping of cell membrane of a neurilemmal (Schwann) cell

Axon

Neurilemmal cell

E. Myelinated axons of CNS neurons being surrounded by a wrapping of cell membrane of an oligodendrocyte. Unmyelinated axons of CNS neurons are left unprotected.

Axons

Axon

Oligodendrocyte

1.19 DEVELOPMENT OF MYELINATION AND AXON ENSHEATHMENT

Myelination requires a cooperative interaction between the neuron and its myelinating support cell. Unmyelinated peripheral axons are invested with a single layer of Schwann cell cytoplasm. When a peripheral axon at least 1 to 2 μm in diameter triggers myelination, a Schwann cell wraps many layers of tightly packed cell membrane around a single segment of that axon. In the CNS, an oligodendroglia cell extends several arms of cytoplasm, which then wrap multiple layers of tightly packed membrane around a single segment of each of several axons (or occasionally two autonomic preganglionic axons). Although myelination is a process that occurs most intensely during development, Schwann cells may remyelinate peripheral axons following injury, and oligodendroglial cells may proliferate and remyelinate injured or demyelinated central axons in diseases such as multiple sclerosis.

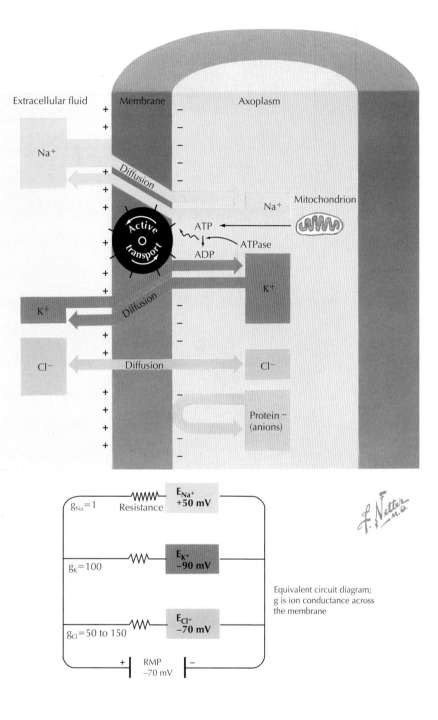

Equivalent circuit diagram; g is ion conductance across the membrane

ELECTRICAL PROPERTIES

1.20 NEURONAL RESTING POTENTIAL

Cations (+) and anions (−) are distributed unevenly across the neuronal cell membrane because the membrane is differentially permeable to these ions. The uneven distribution depends on the forces of charge separation and diffusion. The permeability of the membrane to ions changes with depolarization (toward 0) or hyperpolarization (away from 0). The typical neuronal resting potential is approximately −90 mV with respect to the extracellular fluid. The extracellular concentrations of Na^+ and Cl^- of 145 and 105 mEq/L, respectively, are high compared to the intracellular concentrations of 15 and 8 mEq/L. The extracellular concentration of K^+ of 3.5 mEq/L is low compared to the intracellular concentration of 130 mEq/L. The resting potential of neurons is close to the equilibrium potential for K^+ (as if the membrane were permeable only to K^+). Na^+ is actively pumped out of the cell in exchange for inward pumping of K^+ by the Na^+-K^+-ATPase membrane pump. Equivalent circuit diagrams for Na^+, K^+, and Cl^-, calculated using the Nernst equation, are illustrated in the lower diagram.

A. The movement of ions across the cell membrane is dependent upon both concentration and electrostatic forces. Ions flow from high concentrations to lower concentrations as depicted by the flow of K^+ ions from inside the cell, where the concentration is high, to outside the cell, where the concentrations is lower.

B. Ions are attracted to charges of the opposite polarity. In this example, K^+ ions flow from the extracellular environment, which is positive in relationship to the intracellular space, which is negative. Both concentration and electrostatic forces determine flow of ions. The equilibrium potential for the ion is the membrane potential at which a particular ion does not diffuse through the membrane in either direction.

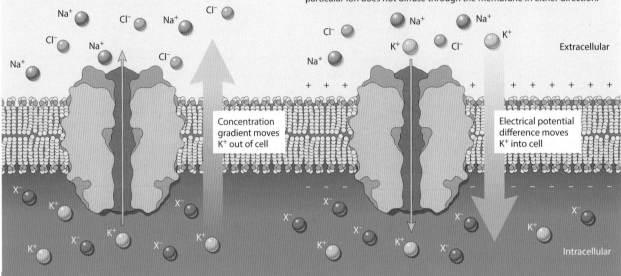

Three states of the sodium channel. **C.** In the resting state, no ion flow occurs due to closure of the activation gate. **D.** When the membrane begins to depolarize, the activation channel opens and ion flow occurs. **E.** As the cell becomes depolarized, the inactivation gate closes and no further ion flow occurs. Only when the cell repolarizes does the sodium channel return to the resting state.

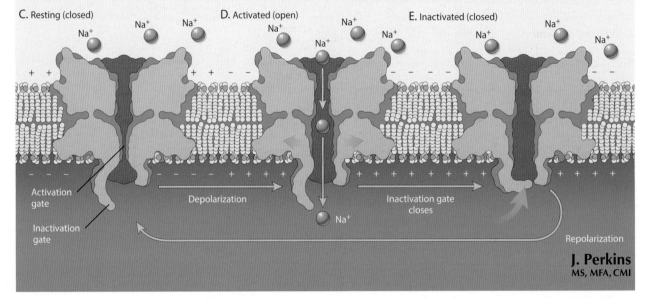

J. Perkins
MS, MFA, CMI

1.21 NEURONAL MEMBRANE POTENTIAL AND SODIUM CHANNELS

Illustrations of ion flow contributing to the neuronal resting potential and three states of the sodium channel in neuronal excitability.

Chemical Synaptic Transmission

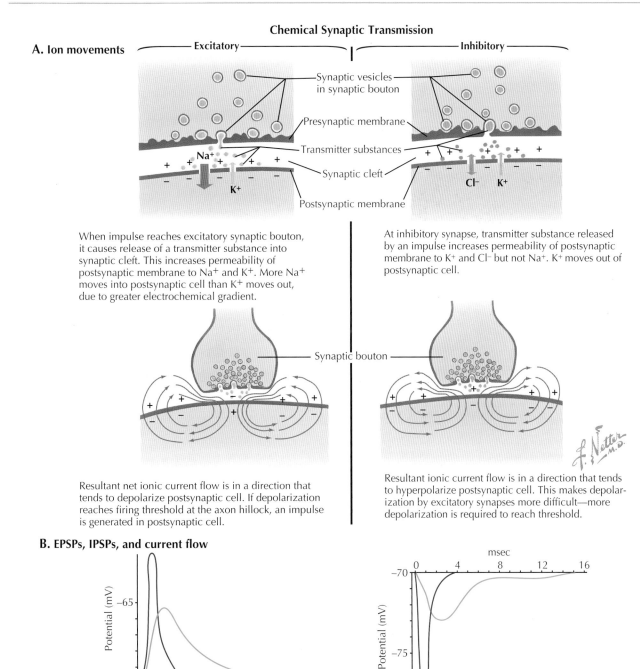

A. Ion movements

Excitatory — | — Inhibitory

Synaptic vesicles in synaptic bouton

Presynaptic membrane

Transmitter substances

Synaptic cleft

Postsynaptic membrane

Na⁺   K⁺   Cl⁻   K⁺

When impulse reaches excitatory synaptic bouton, it causes release of a transmitter substance into synaptic cleft. This increases permeability of postsynaptic membrane to Na⁺ and K⁺. More Na⁺ moves into postsynaptic cell than K⁺ moves out, due to greater electrochemical gradient.

At inhibitory synapse, transmitter substance released by an impulse increases permeability of postsynaptic membrane to K⁺ and Cl⁻ but not Na⁺. K⁺ moves out of postsynaptic cell.

Synaptic bouton

Resultant net ionic current flow is in a direction that tends to depolarize postsynaptic cell. If depolarization reaches firing threshold at the axon hillock, an impulse is generated in postsynaptic cell.

Resultant ionic current flow is in a direction that tends to hyperpolarize postsynaptic cell. This makes depolarization by excitatory synapses more difficult—more depolarization is required to reach threshold.

B. EPSPs, IPSPs, and current flow

Current flow and potential change

Current flow and potential change

Current flow
Potential change

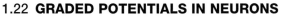

1.22 GRADED POTENTIALS IN NEURONS

A, Ion movements. Excitatory and inhibitory neurotransmissions are processes by which released neurotransmitter, acting on postsynaptic membrane receptors, elicits a local or regional perturbation in the membrane potential: (1) toward 0 (depolarization, excitatory postsynaptic potential; EPSP) via an inward flow of Na⁺ caused by increased permeability of the membrane to positively charged ions; or (2) away from 0 (hyperpolarization, inhibitory postsynaptic potential; IPSP) via an inward flow of Cl⁻ and a compensatory outward flow of K⁺ caused by increased membrane permeability to Cl⁻. Following the action of neurotransmitters on the postsynaptic membrane, the resultant EPSPs and IPSPs exert local influences that dissipate over time and distance but contribute to the overall excitability and ion distribution in the neuron. It is unusual for a single excitatory input to generate sufficient EPSPs to bring about depolarization of the initial segment of the axon above threshold so that an action potential is fired. However, the influence of multiple EPSPs, integrated over space and time, may sum to collectively reach threshold. IPSPs reduce the ability of EPSPs to bring the postsynaptic membrane to threshold. **B,** EPSPs, IPSPs, and current flow. EPSP- and IPSP-induced changes in postsynaptic current (red) and potential (blue).

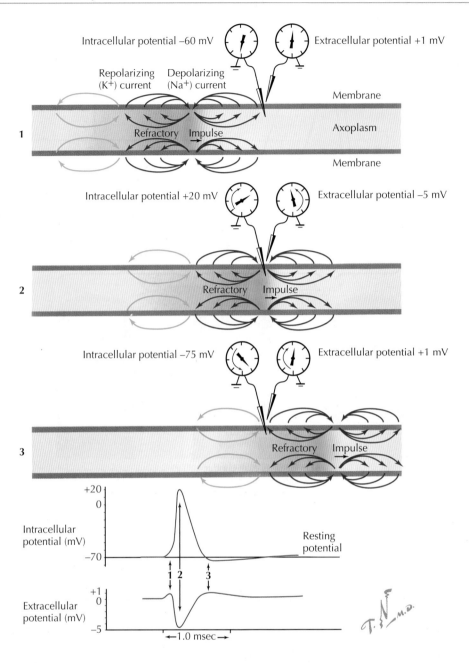

1.25 PROPAGATION OF THE ACTION POTENTIAL

When an AP is initiated at a specific site of the axonal membrane (usually the initial segment), the inward flow of Na^+ alters the extracellular ion environment, causing a local flow of charge from adjacent regions of the axon. This induces a depolarized state in the adjacent node of Ranvier (myelinated axon) or patch of axonal membrane (unmyelinated axon), bringing that region to threshold and resulting in the reinitiation of the action potential. The presence of myelination along axonal segments results in the reinitiation of the action potential at the next node, thus hastening the velocity of conduction of the AP. The resultant appearance of the AP skipping from node to node down the axon is called *saltatory conduction*.

CLINICAL POINT

An **action potential** is an explosive reversal of the neuronal membrane potential that takes place because of an increase in Na^+ conductance induced by depolarization, usually due to the cumulative effects of graded potentials from incoming neurotransmitters; this explosive reversal is followed later by an increase in K^+ conductance, restoring the membrane back toward the resting potential. This process normally takes place at the initial segment of an axon. The conduction of an AP down a myelinated axon, saltatory conduction, requires the reinitiation of the AP at each bare patch of axonal membrane, a node of Ranvier. The reinitiation of the AP occurs because of a voltage change at the next node brought about by passive current flow from the AP at its present site. If several nodes distal to the site of AP propagation are blocked with a local anesthetic, preventing Na^+ conductance, then the AP will die, or cease, because the closest fully functional, nonblocked node is too far from the point of AP propagation to reach threshold by means of passive current flow. This mechanism of blocking reinitiation of the action potential at nodes of Ranvier underlies the use of the -*caine* derivatives, as in novocaine and xylocaine, for local anesthesia during surgical and dental procedures.

A. Anatomic organization of myelinated nerve fibers and its subdivisions

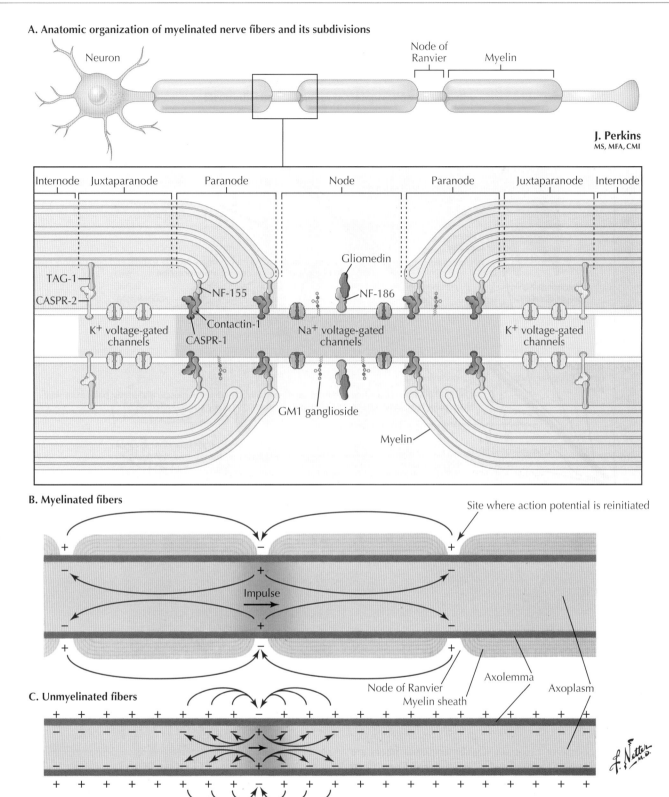

J. Perkins
MS, MFA, CMI

B. Myelinated fibers

Site where action potential is reinitiated

Impulse

Node of Ranvier
Myelin sheath
Axolemma
Axoplasm

C. Unmyelinated fibers

1.26 NODE OF RANVIER AND CONDUCTION VELOCITY

A, Intra-axonal and membrane components of an axon associated with Na+ and K+ ion channels. **B,** The speed of propagation increases with larger axonal diameter and in the presence of a myelin sheath. In myelinated axons the AP is propagated from node to node by saltatory conduction. **C,** The AP travels down the unmyelinated axon by depolarizing adjacent patches of membrane, leading to reinitiation of the action potential.

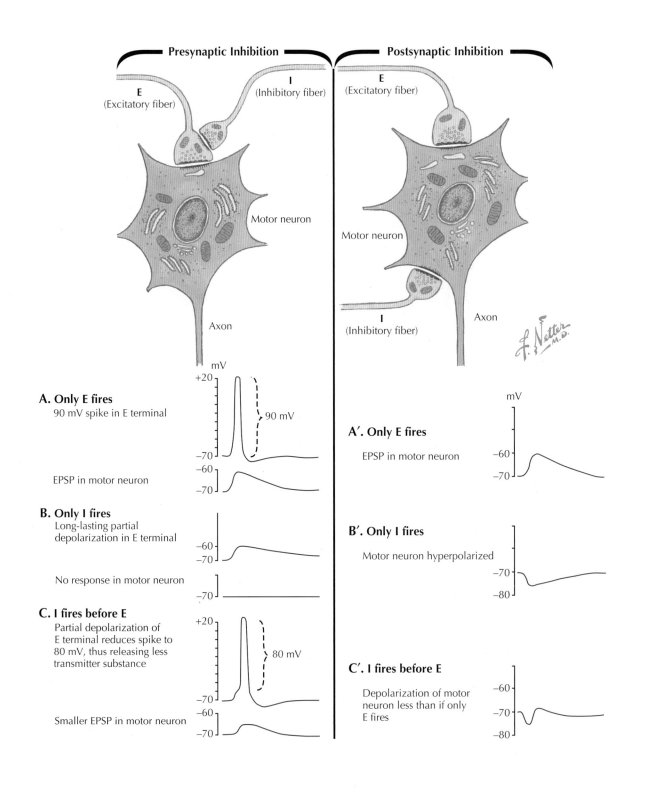

Presynaptic Inhibition

E (Excitatory fiber)

I (Inhibitory fiber)

Postsynaptic Inhibition

E (Excitatory fiber)

Motor neuron

Motor neuron

Axon

I (Inhibitory fiber)

Axon

mV

A. Only E fires
90 mV spike in E terminal

90 mV

EPSP in motor neuron

mV

A′. Only E fires

EPSP in motor neuron

B. Only I fires
Long-lasting partial depolarization in E terminal

No response in motor neuron

B′. Only I fires

Motor neuron hyperpolarized

C. I fires before E
Partial depolarization of E terminal reduces spike to 80 mV, thus releasing less transmitter substance

80 mV

Smaller EPSP in motor neuron

C′. I fires before E

Depolarization of motor neuron less than if only E fires

1.29 PRESYNAPTIC AND POSTSYNAPTIC INHIBITION

Inhibitory synapses modulate neuronal excitability. Presynaptic inhibition (left) and postsynaptic inhibition (right) are shown in relation to a motor neuron. Postsynaptic inhibition causes local hyperpolarization at the postsynaptic site. Presynaptic inhibition involves the depolarization of an excitatory axon terminal, which decreases the amount of Ca^{2+} influx that occurs with depolarization of that excitatory terminal, thus reducing the resultant EPSP at the postsynaptic site.

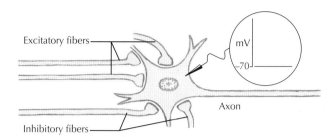

A. Resting state: motor nerve cell shown with synaptic boutons of excitatory and inhibitory nerve fibers ending close to it

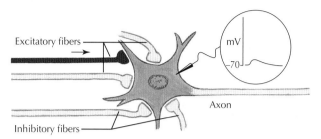

B. Partial depolarization: impulse from one excitatory fiber has caused partial (below firing threshold) depolarization of motor neuron

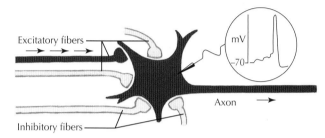

C. Temporal excitatory summation: a series of impulses in one excitatory fiber together produce a suprathreshold depolarization that triggers an action potential

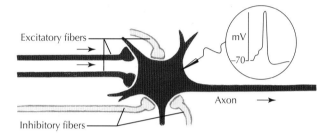

D. Spatial excitatory summation: impulses in two excitatory fibers cause two synaptic depolarizations that together reach firing threshold, triggering an action potential

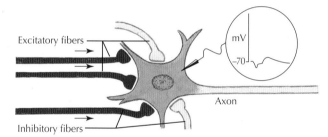

E. Spatial excitatory summation with inhibition: impulses from two excitatory fibers reach motor neuron but impulses from inhibitory fiber prevent depolarization from reaching threshold

■ Axon(s) activated in each scenario

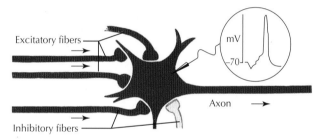

E. (continued): motor neuron now receives additional excitatory impulses and reaches firing threshold despite a simultaneous inhibitory impulse; additional inhibitory impulses might still prevent firing

1.30 SPATIAL AND TEMPORAL SUMMATION

A, In the resting state, the resting potential of the membrane reflects the balance of negative and positive charges and the diffusion of ion species. **B,** Neurons receive multiple excitatory and inhibitory inputs. Stimulation of a neuron by an excitatory neurotransmitter from an incoming nerve fiber results in partial depolarization of that neuron. **C,** Temporal summation occurs when a series of subthreshold EPSPs in one excitatory fiber produce an AP in the postsynaptic cell. This occurs because the EPSPs are superimposed on each other temporally before the local region of membrane has completely returned to its resting state. **D,** Spatial summation occurs when subthreshold impulses from two or more synapses trigger an AP because of synergistic interactions. **E,** Both temporal and spatial summation can be modulated by simultaneous inhibitory input. Inhibitory and excitatory neurons use a wide variety of neurotransmitters, whose actions depend on the ion channels opened by the ligand-receptor interactions.

Origin and Spread of Seizures

A. Normal firing pattern of cortical neurons

Thalamus

Recurrent inhibitory circuit

Cerebral cortex

Single stimulus

Recurrent excitatory circuit

Action potentials (nonsynchronous)

Substantia nigra

Corpus striatum

Normal activation of cortical neurons (P) modulated by excitatory (E) and inhibitory (I) feedback circuits.

Excitatory pathways between cerebral cortex and thalamus modulated by tonic midbrain inhibitory stimuli.

B. Epileptic firing pattern of cortical neurons

Depolarization ↑ field potential

Depressed inhibition

Cortex

High frequency

Repetitive stimuli

Increased excitation

Depolarization ↑ extracellular K⁺

Burst firing action potentials (hypersynchronous)

Thalamus

Substantia nigra

Corpus striatum

Repetitive cortical activation potentiates excitatory transmission and depresses inhibitory transmission, creating self-perpetuating excitatory circuit (burst) and facilitating excitation (recruitment) of neighboring neurons.

Cortical bursts to corpus striatum and thalamus block inhibitory projections and create self-perpetuating feedback circuit.

JOHN A. CRAIG—AD

1.31 NORMAL ELECTRICAL FIRING PATTERNS OF CORTICAL NEURONS AND THE ORIGIN AND SPREAD OF SEIZURES

The collective electrical activity of the cerebral cortex can be monitored by electroencephalography (EEG). Normal cortical electrical activity reflects the summation of excitatory and inhibitory actions, which is modulated through feedback circuits.

Thalamic inputs to the cortex can drive electrical excitability; the midbrain can provide inhibitory control over this process. Repetitive cortical activation can dampen inhibition, enhance excitatory feedback circuits, and recruit repetitive excitatory circuitry in adjacent cortical neurons. These self-perpetuating excitatory feedback circuits can initiate and spread seizure activity.

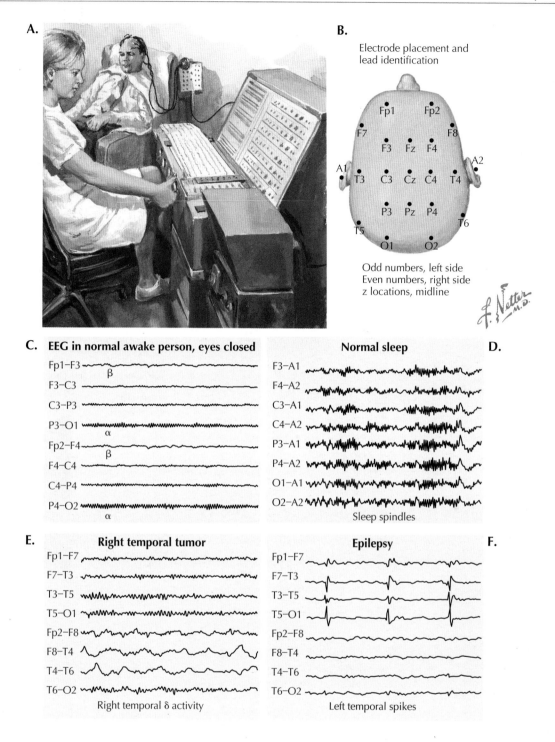

A.

B.

Electrode placement and lead identification

Fp1 Fp2
F7 F8
F3 Fz F4
A1 A2
T3 C3 Cz C4 T4
P3 Pz P4
T5 T6
O1 O2

Odd numbers, left side
Even numbers, right side
z locations, midline

C.   EEG in normal awake person, eyes closed

Fp1–F3
β
F3–C3
C3–P3
P3–O1
α
Fp2–F4
β
F4–C4
C4–P4
P4–O2
α

Normal sleep   **D.**

F3–A1
F4–A2
C3–A1
C4–A2
P3–A1
P4–A2
O1–A1
O2–A2

Sleep spindles

E.   Right temporal tumor

Fp1–F7
F7–T3
T3–T5
T5–O1
Fp2–F8
F8–T4
T4–T6
T6–O2

Right temporal δ activity

Epilepsy   **F.**

Fp1–F7
F7–T3
T3–T5
T5–O1
Fp2–F8
F8–T4
T4–T6
T6–O2

Left temporal spikes

1.32 ELECTROENCEPHALOGRAPHY

EEG permits the recording of the collective electrical activity of the cerebral cortex as a summation of activity measured as a difference between two recording electrodes. Recording electrodes (leads) are placed on the scalp on at least 16 standard sites, and recordings of potential differences between key electrodes are obtained. The principal waveforms recorded in the EEG are alpha (9 to 10 Hz, occipital location, predominant activity in adults, awake in resting state with eyes closed), beta (20 to 25 Hz, frontal and precentral locations, prominent in wakefulness, seen in light sleep), delta (2 to 2.5 Hz, frontal and central location, not prominent in wakefulness, generalized in deep sleep and coma or toxic states), and theta (5 to 6 Hz, central location, constant and not prominent when awake and active, sometimes generalized when drowsy). Electrode placement is shown in part **B**. Examples are provided of a normal EEG taken when the patient is awake with eyes closed (**C**) and when sleeping normally (**D**). Abnormal patterns of activity can be seen in the presence of tumors (**E**) and in seizures (**F**); for example, the spike-and-wave appearance in a generalized tonic-clonic seizure (generalized fast repetitive spikes and generalized spikes and slow waves, respectively) and a 3 Hz spike-and-wave EEG in the case of an absence seizure.

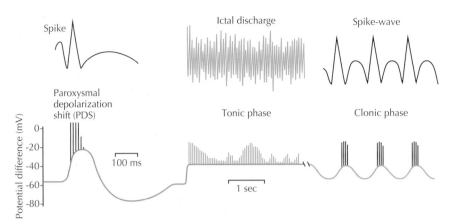

A. Paroxysmal depolarization shift (PDS) is a cellular marker of epilepsy and consists of a large depolarization of a group of neurons with action potentials, as indicated by the vertical lines on the large depolarization. The PDS is followed by repolarization. The PDS and repolarization correspond to a spike and wave on the EEG. A seizure occurs when there is a massive depolarization of cells without intervening periods of repolarization. This would correspond to the tonic phase of the seizure. As inhibition increases during the seizure, there is a cycle of PDS followed by repolarization. This corresponds to the clonic phase of the seizure.

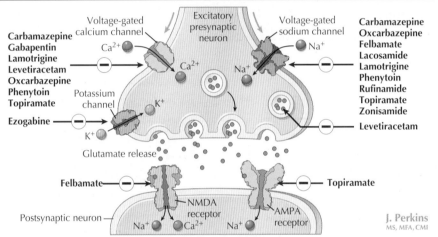

B. Examples of molecular targets of antiepileptic drugs that reduce excitability. This may occur through blockage of calcium, sodium, and potassium channels or through reducing ion flow through NMDA and AMPA receptors. Levetiracetam binds to synaptic vesicles, which may lead to reduced neurotrasnmiter release.

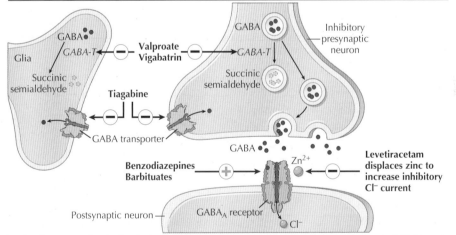

C. Examples of molecular targets of antiepileptic drugs that enhance inhibition. Drugs may increase amount of GABA postsynaptically by blocking GABA uptake or increase intracellular GABA by reducing degradation of GABA. Enhancing chloride flow through the GABA receptor is a common mechanism of inhibitory drugs, such as barbiturates and benzodiazepines. Levetiracetam displaces zinc from the GABA receptor, which results in increased chloride currents.

1.33 TYPES OF ELECTRICAL DISCHARGES IN GENERALIZED SEIZURES AND SITES OF ACTION OF ANTISEIZURE MEDICATIONS

Illustrations of types of electrical discharges in generalized seizures and the sites of action for antiseizure medications that reduce excitability or that enhance inhibition.

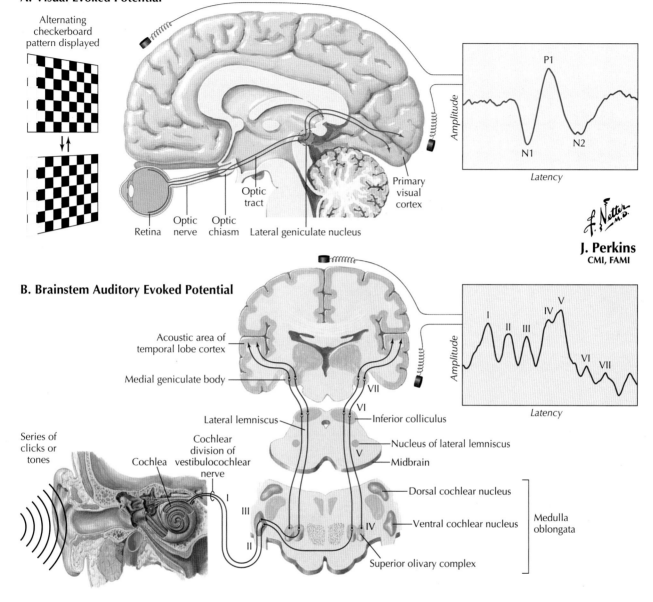

A. Visual Evoked Potential

Alternating checkerboard pattern displayed

Retina
Optic nerve
Optic chiasm
Optic tract
Lateral geniculate nucleus
Primary visual cortex

Amplitude

P1

N1   N2

Latency

f. Netter
M.D.

J. Perkins
CMI, FAMI

B. Brainstem Auditory Evoked Potential

Acoustic area of temporal lobe cortex

Medial geniculate body

Lateral lemniscus

Series of clicks or tones

Cochlea

Cochlear division of vestibulocochlear nerve

VII
VI
Inferior colliculus
Nucleus of lateral lemniscus
V
Midbrain
Dorsal cochlear nucleus
Ventral cochlear nucleus
Superior olivary complex

Medulla oblongata

Amplitude

I   II   III   IV   V   VI   VII

Latency

1.34 VISUAL AND AUDITORY EVOKED POTENTIALS

Electrophysiological recordings can be used to evaluate the intactness of specific sensory systems, including the visual system and the auditory system. **A,** Visual evoked potentials. The visual stimulus is often an alternating flashing checkerboard (2 Hz), with recording done over the primary visual cortex in the midline. The normal latencies for recordings are 70 msec for N1 (negative 1), 100 msec for P1 (positive 1), and 140 msec for N2 (negative 2). Damage to the retino-geniculo-calcarine pathway may result in altered latencies and amplitudes. **B,** Brainstem auditory evoked responses or potentials (BAERs). The auditory stimulus is a series of clicks or tones, with recording done over the temporal lobe auditory cortex. Seven distinctive peak latencies occur: I. distal auditory nerve; II. proximal auditory nerve; III. cochlear nuclei; IV. superior olivary complex; V. nucleus of the lateral lemniscus; VI. inferior colliculus; and VII. medial geniculate nucleus. Altered latencies and amplitudes may indicate damage or disruption to the auditory pathway at specific sites.

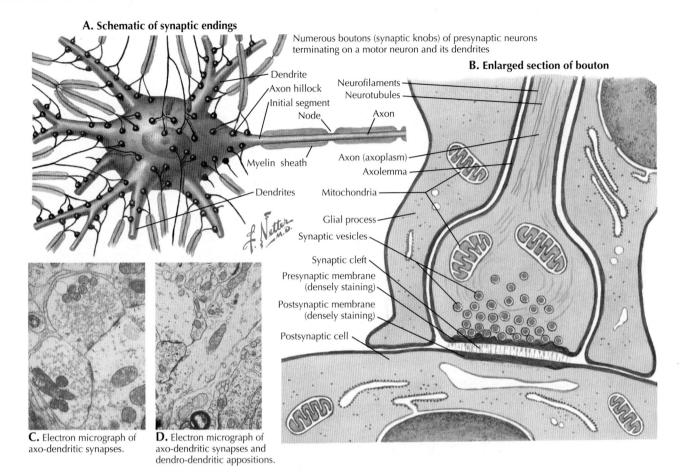

A. Schematic of synaptic endings

Numerous boutons (synaptic knobs) of presynaptic neurons terminating on a motor neuron and its dendrites

Dendrite
Axon hillock
Initial segment
Node
Myelin sheath
Dendrites

B. Enlarged section of bouton

Neurofilaments
Neurotubules
Axon
Axon (axoplasm)
Axolemma
Mitochondria
Glial process
Synaptic vesicles
Synaptic cleft
Presynaptic membrane (densely staining)
Postsynaptic membrane (densely staining)
Postsynaptic cell

C. Electron micrograph of axo-dendritic synapses.

D. Electron micrograph of axo-dendritic synapses and dendro-dendritic appositions.

NEUROTRANSMITTER AND SIGNALING PROPERTIES

1.35 SYNAPTIC MORPHOLOGY

Synapses are specialized sites where neurons communicate with each other and with effector or target cells. **A,** A typical neuron that receives numerous synaptic contacts on its cell body and associated dendrites. The contacts are derived from both myelinated and unmyelinated axons. Incoming myelinated axons lose their myelin sheaths, exhibit extensive branching, and terminate as synaptic boutons (terminals) on the target (in this example, motor) neuron. **B,** An enlargement of an axosomatic terminal. Chemical neurotransmitters are packaged in synaptic vesicles. When an action potential invades the terminal region, depolarization triggers Ca^{2+} influx into the terminal, causing numerous synaptic vesicles to fuse with the presynaptic membrane, releasing their packets of neurotransmitter into the synaptic cleft. The neurotransmitter can bind to receptors on the postsynaptic membrane, resulting in graded excitatory or inhibitory postsynaptic potentials or in neuromodulatory effects on intracellular signaling systems in the target cell. There is sometimes a mismatch between the site of release of a neurotransmitter and the location of target neurons possessing receptors for the neurotransmitter (can be immediately adjacent or at a distance). Many nerve terminals can release multiple neurotransmitters; the process is regulated by gene activation and by the frequency and duration of axonal activity. Some nerve terminals possess presynaptic receptors for their released neurotransmitters. Activation of these presynaptic receptors regulates neurotransmitter release. Some nerve terminals also possess high-affinity uptake carriers for transport of the neurotransmitters (e.g., dopamine, norepinephrine, serotonin) back into the nerve terminal for repackaging and reuse.

CLINICAL POINT

Synaptic endings, particularly axodendritic and axosomatic endings, terminate abundantly on some neuronal cell types such as LMNs. The distribution of synapses, based on a hierarchy of descending pathways and interneurons, orchestrates the excitability of the target neuron. If one of the major sources of input is disrupted (such as the corticospinal tract in an internal capsule lesion, which may occur in an ischemic stroke) or if damage has occurred to the collective descending UMN pathways (as in a spinal cord injury), the remaining potential sources of input can sprout and occupy regional sites left bare because of the degeneration of the normal complement of synapses. As a result, primary sensory inputs from Ia afferents and other sensory influences, via interneurons, can take on a predominant influence over the excitability of the target motor neurons, leading to a hyperexcitable state. This may account in part for the hypertonic state and hyperreflexic responses to stimulation of primary muscle spindle afferents (muscle stretch reflex) and of flexor reflex afferents (nociceptive stimulation). Recent studies indicate that synaptic growth, plasticity, and remodeling can continue into adulthood and even into old age.

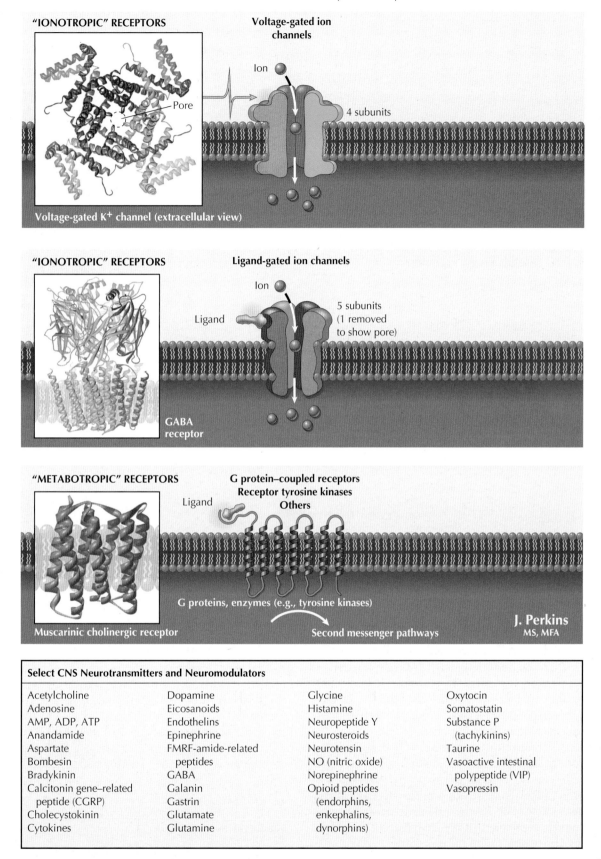

"IONOTROPIC" RECEPTORS

Voltage-gated ion channels

Ion

4 subunits

Pore

Voltage-gated K+ channel (extracellular view)

"IONOTROPIC" RECEPTORS

Ligand-gated ion channels

Ion

Ligand

5 subunits
(1 removed
to show pore)

GABA
receptor

"METABOTROPIC" RECEPTORS

G protein–coupled receptors
Receptor tyrosine kinases
Others

Ligand

G proteins, enzymes (e.g., tyrosine kinases)

Muscarinic cholinergic receptor

Second messenger pathways

J. Perkins
MS, MFA

Select CNS Neurotransmitters and Neuromodulators

Acetylcholine	Dopamine	Glycine	Oxytocin
Adenosine	Eicosanoids	Histamine	Somatostatin
AMP, ADP, ATP	Endothelins	Neuropeptide Y	Substance P
Anandamide	Epinephrine	Neurosteroids	(tachykinins)
Aspartate	FMRF-amide-related	Neurotensin	Taurine
Bombesin	peptides	NO (nitric oxide)	Vasoactive intestinal
Bradykinin	GABA	Norepinephrine	polypeptide (VIP)
Calcitonin gene–related	Galanin	Opioid peptides	Vasopressin
peptide (CGRP)	Gastrin	(endorphins,	
Cholecystokinin	Glutamate	enkephalins,	
Cytokines	Glutamine	dynorphins)	

1.36 MECHANISMS OF MOLECULAR SIGNALING IN NEURONS

Types of molecular signaling in neurons are shown, including ionotropic receptors (both voltage-gated ion channels and ligand-gated channels) and metabotropic receptors.

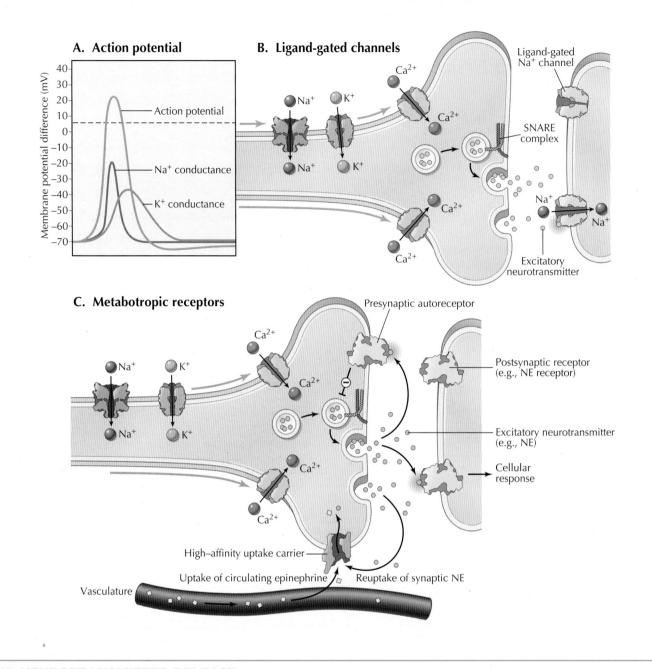

A. Action potential

Membrane potential difference (mV)

Action potential

Na⁺ conductance

K⁺ conductance

B. Ligand-gated channels

Ca²⁺

Na⁺ K⁺

Na⁺ K⁺

Ca²⁺

Ca²⁺

Ca²⁺

Ligand-gated Na⁺ channel

SNARE complex

Na⁺

Na⁺

Excitatory neurotransmitter

C. Metabotropic receptors

Presynaptic autoreceptor

Ca²⁺

Na⁺ K⁺

Ca²⁺

Na⁺ K⁺

Ca²⁺

Ca²⁺

Postsynaptic receptor (e.g., NE receptor)

Excitatory neurotransmitter (e.g., NE)

Cellular response

High–affinity uptake carrier

Uptake of circulating epinephrine

Reuptake of synaptic NE

Vasculature

1.37 NEUROTRANSMITTER RELEASE

A, Major ion conductances are triggered by an action potential (AP). **B,** Their effects on neurotransmitter (NT) release as related to ligand-gated channels influencing postsynaptic excitability. NT is packaged in synaptic vesicles; these vesicles, in response to nerve terminal depolarization and Ca²⁺ influx, merge with the nerve terminal membrane through a mechanism involving the SNARE complex. Through this mechanism of docking proteins, membrane fusion, and NT exocytosis, multiple vesicles simultaneously release their NT content, called *quantal release,* allowing postsynaptic stimulation. SNARE proteins represent a large superfamily of soluble NSF (N-ethylmaleimide-sensitive factor) attachment protein receptors that are composed of four alpha helices that mediate vesicle fusion and exocytosis.

C, Metabotropic receptors responding to nerve terminal depolarization with SNARE complex–mediated vesicle membrane fusion and exocytosis. Both postsynaptic and presynaptic receptors bind with NT (in this case norepinephrine, NE) and transduce the receptor-ligand binding into intracellular signaling. The presynaptic receptor can modulate nerve terminal excitability and subsequent NT release. The postsynaptic receptor can modulate postsynaptic excitability and the postsynaptic membrane responsiveness to other NTs. High-affinity uptake carriers remove NE from the synaptic cleft back into the nerve terminal for repackaging into synaptic vesicles. This NE uptake carrier also can take up epinephrine (E) from the circulation. Uptaken E also is repackaged into the NE synaptic vesicles and is preferentially released on subsequent nerve terminal depolarization. This E substitute-NT mechanism provides augmented receptor activation (especially beta receptor activation by E) during sympathetic responses.

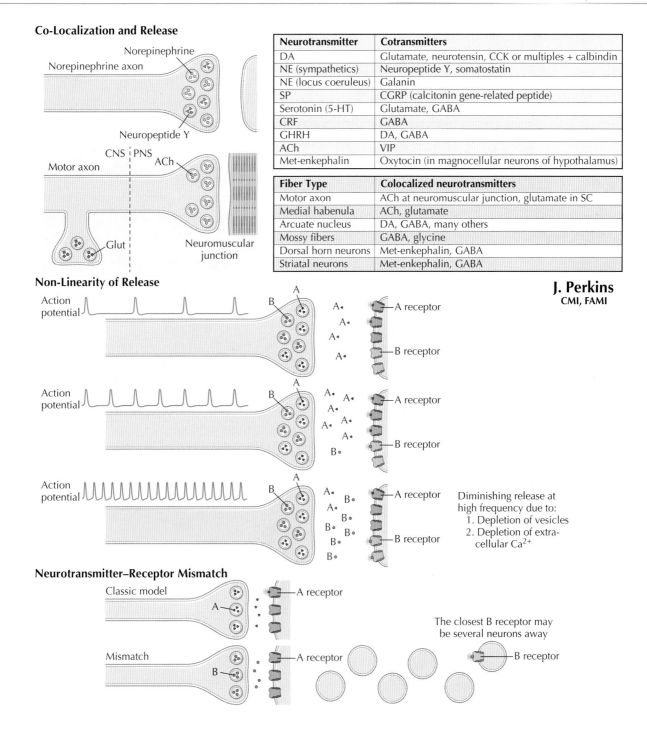

Co-Localization and Release

Neurotransmitter	Cotransmitters
DA	Glutamate, neurotensin, CCK or multiples + calbindin
NE (sympathetics)	Neuropeptide Y, somatostatin
NE (locus coeruleus)	Galanin
SP	CGRP (calcitonin gene-related peptide)
Serotonin (5-HT)	Glutamate, GABA
CRF	GABA
GHRH	DA, GABA
ACh	VIP
Met-enkephalin	Oxytocin (in magnocellular neurons of hypothalamus)

Fiber Type	Colocalized neurotransmitters
Motor axon	ACh at neuromuscular junction, glutamate in SC
Medial habenula	ACh, glutamate
Arcuate nucleus	DA, GABA, many others
Mossy fibers	GABA, glycine
Dorsal horn neurons	Met-enkephalin, GABA
Striatal neurons	Met-enkephalin, GABA

J. Perkins
CMI, FAMI

Non-Linearity of Release

Diminishing release at high frequency due to:
1. Depletion of vesicles
2. Depletion of extra-cellular Ca^{2+}

Neurotransmitter–Receptor Mismatch

The closest B receptor may be several neurons away

1.38 MULTIPLE NEUROTRANSMITTER SYNTHESIS, RELEASE, AND SIGNALING FROM INDIVIDUAL NEURONS

Many, perhaps most, nerve terminals co-localize and release multiple neurotransmitters (NTs), each presumably packaged in its own synaptic vesicles. Major co-localized NTs, sorted by transmitter and by fiber type, are presented in the table. Some authors have noted as many as seven or more NTs present in a single type of nerve terminal. It should be noted that some NTs are present in the presynaptic cytoplasm and are not released by quantal (vesicle-based) release. Some NTs are packaged in vesicles in the cell body and transported by axonal transport (e.g., neuropeptides), while other NTs are synthesized and/or packaged locally in the nerve terminals (e.g., amino acids, monoamines).

NT release is usually nonlinear, with some NTs diminishing their quantal release at higher action potential (AP) frequencies, while other co-localized NTs (especially some neuropeptides) are released only at much higher AP frequencies. A further phenomenon affecting the functional consequence of NT release is the frequent NT-receptor mismatch. Some NTs are released into a synaptic cleft and immediately activate receptors on the postsynaptic site (e.g., ACh at the neuromuscular junction). However, some NTs, when released, have no local receptors with which to interact, except at distant sites. Hence, NT-receptor activation in these circumstances may occur only during particularly robust or prolonged NT transmitter release.

Hypothalamic-Pituitary Axis (HPA)

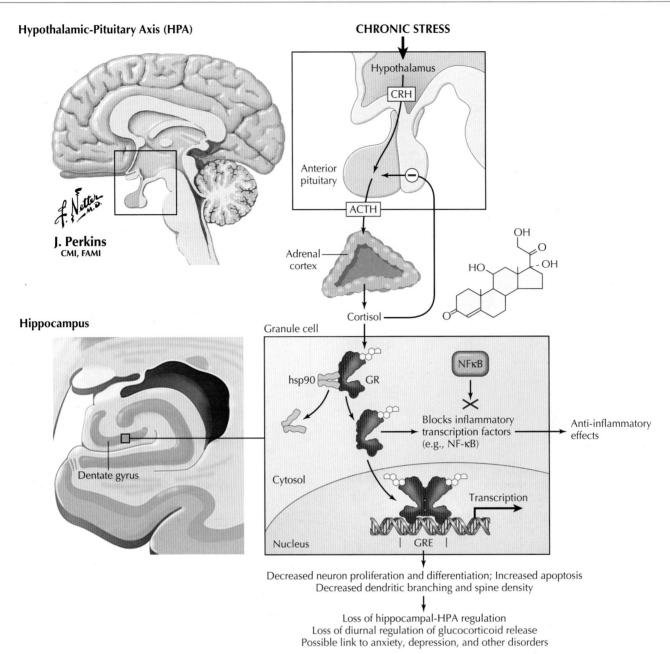

J. Perkins
CMI, FAMI

CHRONIC STRESS

Hypothalamus

CRH

Anterior pituitary

ACTH

Adrenal cortex

Cortisol

Hippocampus

Dentate gyrus

Granule cell

hsp90   GR

NFκB

Blocks inflammatory transcription factors (e.g., NF-κB)

Anti-inflammatory effects

Cytosol

Transcription

Nucleus | GRE |

Decreased neuron proliferation and differentiation; Increased apoptosis
Decreased dendritic branching and spine density

Loss of hippocampal-HPA regulation
Loss of diurnal regulation of glucocorticoid release
Possible link to anxiety, depression, and other disorders

1.41 GLUCOCORTICOID REGULATION OF NEURONS AND APOPTOSIS

Glucocorticoid production is controlled by the hypothalamic-pituitary-adrenal (HPA) axis in which hypothalamic corticotropin-releasing hormone (CRH) stimulates cells in the anterior pituitary via the hypophyseal-portal circulation to produce adrenocorticotropic hormone (ACTH). ACTH, in turn, stimulates the adrenal cortices to produce the glucocorticoid hormone cortisol. Cortisol interacts with glucocorticoid receptors (GR) in the cytoplasm of some neurons to effect dissociation from chaperone proteins such as heat shock protein (hsp) 90 and translocation to the nucleus, where the activated GR interacts with glucocorticoid response elements (GREs) to effect gene transcription. Cortisol acts on many body tissues to promote metabolic and antiinflammatory effects, in the latter case by blocking inflammatory transcription factors such as nuclear factor κB (NF-κB). Under normal conditions, the HPA axis is regulated by feedback at several levels, including regulation of CRH release via the hippocampus, resulting in normal diurnal regulation of systemic cortisol levels. In the hippocampus, low to moderate levels of cortisol provide optimal memory acquisition and consolidation by supporting synaptic plasticity. However, under conditions of chronic stress, sustained high levels of cortisol can negatively affect hippocampal neurons, particularly the granule cells of the dentate gyrus, resulting in decreased neurogenesis, decreased dendritic complexity, and cell death via apoptosis. Hippocampal cell loss and dysfunction can lead to loss of hippocampal control over cortisol release, resulting in loss of normal diurnal release patterns, which is seen in old age and in diseases such as Alzheimer's. Such changes have also been linked to psychiatric disorders. Loss of diurnal cortisol rhythms also contributes to metabolic dysfunction and truncal obesity in the periphery.

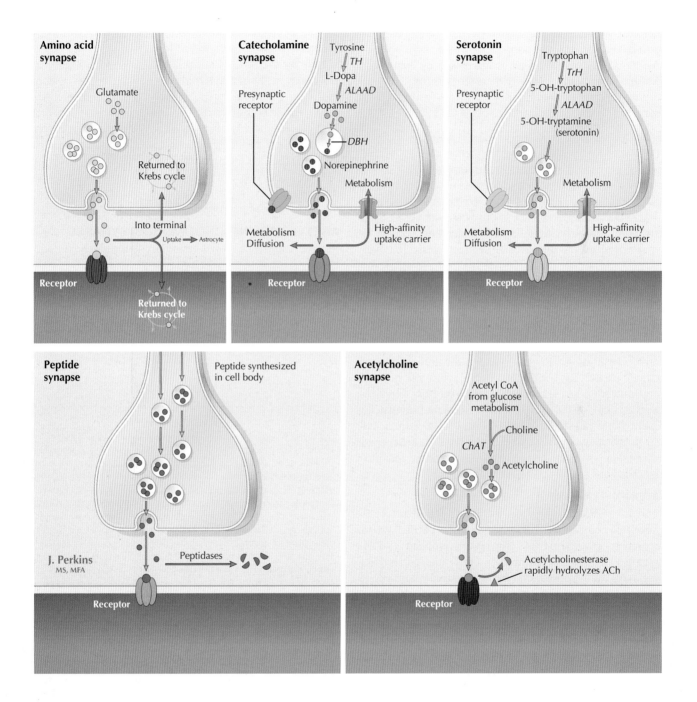

Amino acid synapse
Glutamate
Returned to Krebs cycle
Into terminal
Uptake → Astrocyte
Receptor
Returned to Krebs cycle

Catecholamine synapse
Tyrosine
TH
L-Dopa
ALAAD
Dopamine
Presynaptic receptor
DBH
Norepinephrine
Metabolism
Metabolism
Diffusion
High-affinity uptake carrier
Receptor

Serotonin synapse
Tryptophan
TrH
5-OH-tryptophan
ALAAD
5-OH-tryptamine (serotonin)
Presynaptic receptor
Metabolism
Metabolism
Diffusion
High-affinity uptake carrier
Receptor

Peptide synapse
Peptide synthesized in cell body
J. Perkins
MS, MFA
Peptidases
Receptor

Acetylcholine synapse
Acetyl CoA from glucose metabolism
Choline
ChAT
Acetylcholine
Acetylcholinesterase rapidly hydrolyzes ACh
Receptor

1.42 CHEMICAL NEUROTRANSMISSION

See next page.

1.42 CHEMICAL NEUROTRANSMISSION (CONTINUED)

AMINO ACID SYNAPSE

Amino acids used by a neuron as neurotransmitters are compartmentalized for release as neurotransmitters in synaptic vesicles. The amino acid glutamate (depicted in this diagram) is the most abundant excitatory neurotransmitter in the CNS. Following release from synaptic vesicles, some glutamate binds to postsynaptic receptors. Released glutamate is inactivated by uptake into both pre- and postsynaptic neurons, where the amino acid is incorporated into the Krebs cycle or reused for a variety of functions. Glutamate also is taken up and recycled in the CNS by astrocytes.

CATECHOLAMINE SYNAPSE

Catecholamines are synthesized from the dietary amino acid tyrosine, which is taken up competitively into the brain by a carrier system. Tyrosine is synthesized into L-dopa by tyrosine hydroxylase (TH), the rate-limiting synthetic enzyme. Additional conversion into dopamine takes place in the cytoplasm via aromatic L-amino acid decarboxylase (ALAAD). Dopamine is taken up into synaptic vesicles and stored for subsequent release. In noradrenergic nerve terminals, dopamine beta-hydroxylase (DBH) further hydroxylates dopamine into norepinephrine in the synaptic vesicles. In adrenergic nerve terminals, norepinephrine is methylated to epinephrine by phenolethanolamine N-methyl transferase (PNMT). Following release, the catecholamine neurotransmitter binds to appropriate receptors (dopamine and alpha- and beta-adrenergic receptors) on the postsynaptic membrane, altering postsynaptic excitability, second messenger activation, or both. Catecholamines also can act on presynaptic receptors, modulating the excitability of the presynaptic terminal and influencing subsequent neurotransmitter release. Catecholamines are inactivated by presynaptic reuptake (high-affinity uptake carrier) and, to a lesser extent, by metabolism (monoamine oxidase deamination and catechol-O-methyltransferase) and diffusion.

SEROTONIN SYNAPSE

Serotonin is synthesized from the dietary amino acid tryptophan, taken up competitively into the brain by a carrier system. Tryptophan is synthesized to 5-hydroxytryptophan (5-OH-tryptophan) by tryptophan hydroxylase (TrH), the rate-limiting synthetic enzyme. Conversion of 5-hydroxytryptophan to 5-hydroxytryptamine (5-HT, serotonin) takes place in the cytoplasm by means of ALAAD. Serotonin is stored in synaptic vesicles. Following release, serotonin can bind to receptors on the postsynaptic membrane, altering postsynaptic excitability, second messenger activation, or both. Serotonin also can act on presynaptic receptors (5-HT receptors), modulating the excitability of the presynaptic terminal and influencing subsequent

neurotransmitter release. Serotonin is inactivated by presynaptic reuptake (high-affinity uptake carrier) and to a lesser extent by metabolism and diffusion.

PEPTIDE SYNAPSES

Neuropeptides are synthesized from prohormones, large peptides synthesized in the cell body from mRNA. The larger precursor peptide is cleaved posttranslationally to active neuropeptides, which are packaged in synaptic vesicles and transported anterogradely by the process of axoplasmic transport. These vesicles are stored in the nerve terminals until released by appropriate excitation-secretion coupling induced by an action potential. The neuropeptide binds to receptors on the postsynaptic membrane. In the CNS, there is often an anatomic mismatch between the localization of peptidergic nerve terminals and the localization of cells possessing membrane receptors responsive to that neuropeptide, suggesting that the amount of release and the extent of diffusion may be important factors in neuropeptide neurotransmission. Released neuropeptides are inactivated by peptidases.

ACETYLCHOLINE (CHOLINERGIC) SYNAPSE

Acetylcholine (ACh) is synthesized from dietary choline and acetyl coenzyme A (CoA), derived from the metabolism of glucose by the enzyme choline acetyltransferase (ChAT). ACh is stored in synaptic vesicles; following release, it binds to cholinergic receptors (nicotinic or muscarinic) on the postsynaptic membrane, influencing the excitability of the postsynaptic cell. Enzymatic hydrolysis (cleavage) by acetylcholine esterase rapidly inactivates ACh.

CLINICAL POINT

Synthesis of catecholamines in the brain is rate limited by the availability of the precursor amino acid tyrosine; synthesis of serotonin, an indoleamine, is rate limited by the availability of the precursor amino acid tryptophan. Tyrosine and tryptophan compete with other amino acids—phenylalanine, leucine, isoleucine, and valine—for uptake into the brain through a common carrier mechanism. When a good protein source is available in the diet, tyrosine is present in abundance, and robust catecholamine synthesis occurs; when a diet lacks sufficient protein, tryptophan is competitively abundant compared with tyrosine, and serotonin synthesis is favored. This is one mechanism by which the composition of the diet can influence the synthesis of serotonin as opposed to catecholamine and influence mood and affective behavior. During critical periods of development, if low availability of tyrosine occurs because of protein malnourishment, central noradrenergic axons cannot exert their trophic influence on cortical neuronal development such as the visual cortex; stunted dendritic development occurs, and the binocular responsiveness of key cortical neurons is prevented. Thus, nutritional content and balance are important to both proper brain development and ongoing affective behavior.

2

SKULL AND MENINGES

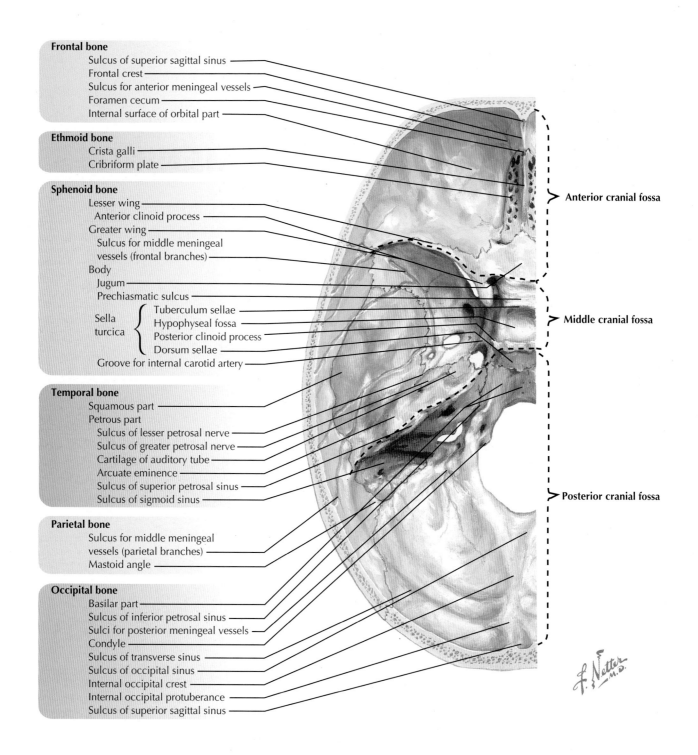

Frontal bone
Sulcus of superior sagittal sinus
Frontal crest
Sulcus for anterior meningeal vessels
Foramen cecum
Internal surface of orbital part

Ethmoid bone
Crista galli
Cribriform plate

Sphenoid bone
Lesser wing
Anterior clinoid process
Greater wing
Sulcus for middle meningeal
vessels (frontal branches)
Body
Jugum
Prechiasmatic sulcus
Sella turcica {
Tuberculum sellae
Hypophyseal fossa
Posterior clinoid process
Dorsum sellae
}
Groove for internal carotid artery

Temporal bone
Squamous part
Petrous part
Sulcus of lesser petrosal nerve
Sulcus of greater petrosal nerve
Cartilage of auditory tube
Arcuate eminence
Sulcus of superior petrosal sinus
Sulcus of sigmoid sinus

Parietal bone
Sulcus for middle meningeal
vessels (parietal branches)
Mastoid angle

Occipital bone
Basilar part
Sulcus of inferior petrosal sinus
Sulci for posterior meningeal vessels
Condyle
Sulcus of transverse sinus
Sulcus of occipital sinus
Internal occipital crest
Internal occipital protuberance
Sulcus of superior sagittal sinus

Anterior cranial fossa

Middle cranial fossa

Posterior cranial fossa

2.1 INTERIOR VIEW OF THE BASE OF THE ADULT SKULL

The anterior, middle, and posterior cranial fossae house the anterior frontal lobe, temporal lobe, and cerebellum and brainstem, respectively. The fossae are separated from each other by bony structures and dural membranes. A swelling of the brain or the presence of mass lesions can selectively exert pressure within an individual fossa. The perforated cribriform plate allows the olfactory nerves to penetrate into the olfactory bulb, a site where head trauma can result in the tearing of the penetrating olfactory nerve fibers.

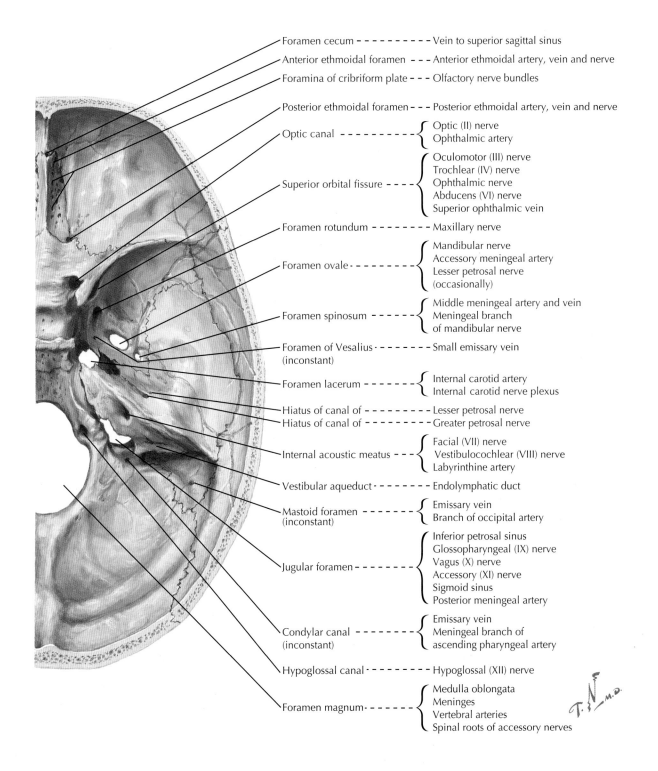

Foramen cecum – – – – – – – – – Vein to superior sagittal sinus

Anterior ethmoidal foramen – – – Anterior ethmoidal artery, vein and nerve

Foramina of cribriform plate – – – Olfactory nerve bundles

Posterior ethmoidal foramen – – – Posterior ethmoidal artery, vein and nerve

Optic canal – – – – – – – – {
Optic (II) nerve
Ophthalmic artery

Superior orbital fissure – – – – {
Oculomotor (III) nerve
Trochlear (IV) nerve
Ophthalmic nerve
Abducens (VI) nerve
Superior ophthalmic vein

Foramen rotundum – – – – – – – Maxillary nerve

Foramen ovale – – – – – – – {
Mandibular nerve
Accessory meningeal artery
Lesser petrosal nerve
(occasionally)

Foramen spinosum – – – – – – {
Middle meningeal artery and vein
Meningeal branch
of mandibular nerve

Foramen of Vesalius – – – – – – – Small emissary vein
(inconstant)

Foramen lacerum – – – – – – – {
Internal carotid artery
Internal carotid nerve plexus

Hiatus of canal of – – – – – – – – Lesser petrosal nerve
Hiatus of canal of – – – – – – – – Greater petrosal nerve

Internal acoustic meatus – – – {
Facial (VII) nerve
Vestibulocochlear (VIII) nerve
Labyrinthine artery

Vestibular aqueduct – – – – – – – Endolymphatic duct

Mastoid foramen – – – – – – – {
Emissary vein
(inconstant)   Branch of occipital artery

Jugular foramen – – – – – – – {
Inferior petrosal sinus
Glossopharyngeal (IX) nerve
Vagus (X) nerve
Accessory (XI) nerve
Sigmoid sinus
Posterior meningeal artery

Condylar canal – – – – – – – {
Emissary vein
Meningeal branch of
(inconstant)   ascending pharyngeal artery

Hypoglossal canal – – – – – – – Hypoglossal (XII) nerve

Foramen magnum – – – – – – {
Medulla oblongata
Meninges
Vertebral arteries
Spinal roots of accessory nerves

2.2 FORAMINA IN THE BASE OF THE ADULT SKULL

The foramina in the base of the skull allow major nerves and blood vessels to course through the skull. Pressure, traction, and masses can damage structures traversing these small spaces that snugly confine the structures.

CLINICAL POINT

The foramina of the skull are narrow openings that allow the passage of nerves and blood vessels. Under normal circumstances, there is enough room for comfortable passage of these structures without traction or pressure. However, with the presence of a tumor at a foramen, the passing structures can be compressed or damaged. For example, a tumor at the internal acoustic meatus can result in ipsilateral facial and vestibuloacoustic nerve damage, and a tumor at the jugular foramen can result in damage to the glossopharyngeal, vagus, and spinal accessory nerves.

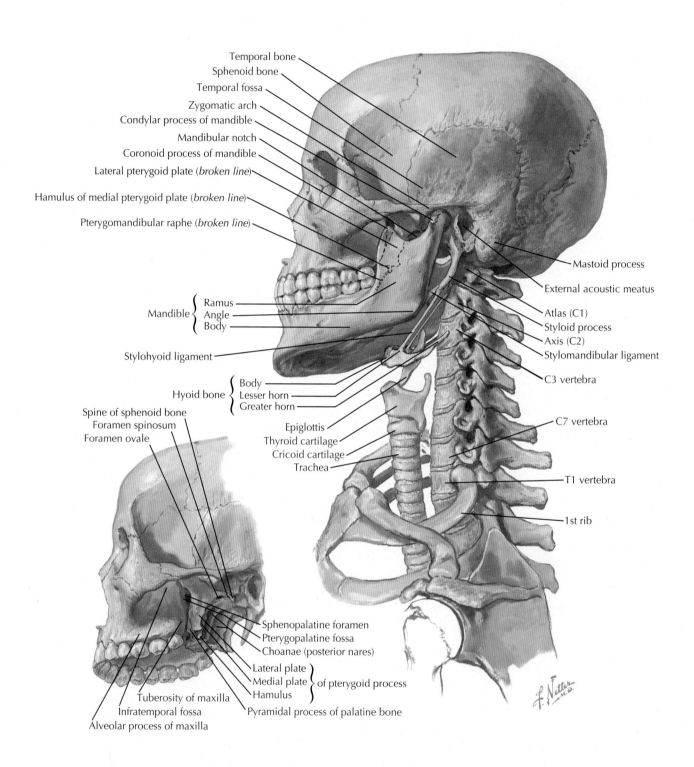

Temporal bone
Sphenoid bone
Temporal fossa
Zygomatic arch
Condylar process of mandible
Mandibular notch
Coronoid process of mandible
Lateral pterygoid plate (*broken line*)
Hamulus of medial pterygoid plate (*broken line*)
Pterygomandibular raphe (*broken line*)

Mastoid process
External acoustic meatus
Atlas (C1)
Styloid process
Axis (C2)
Stylomandibular ligament
C3 vertebra

Mandible { Ramus
Angle
Body
Stylohyoid ligament

C7 vertebra

Body
Hyoid bone { Lesser horn
Greater horn

Spine of sphenoid bone
Foramen spinosum
Foramen ovale

Epiglottis
Thyroid cartilage
Cricoid cartilage
Trachea

T1 vertebra

1st rib

Sphenopalatine foramen
Pterygopalatine fossa
Choanae (posterior nares)
Lateral plate }
Medial plate } of pterygoid process
Hamulus }
Tuberosity of maxilla
Infratemporal fossa
Alveolar process of maxilla
Pyramidal process of palatine bone

2.3 BONY FRAMEWORK OF THE HEAD AND NECK

The skull provides bony protection for the brain. The spine, consisting of vertebrae and their intervertebral disks, provides bony protection for the spinal cord. The spine and skull articulate at the foramen magnum, where the C1 vertebral body (the atlas) abuts the occipital bone.

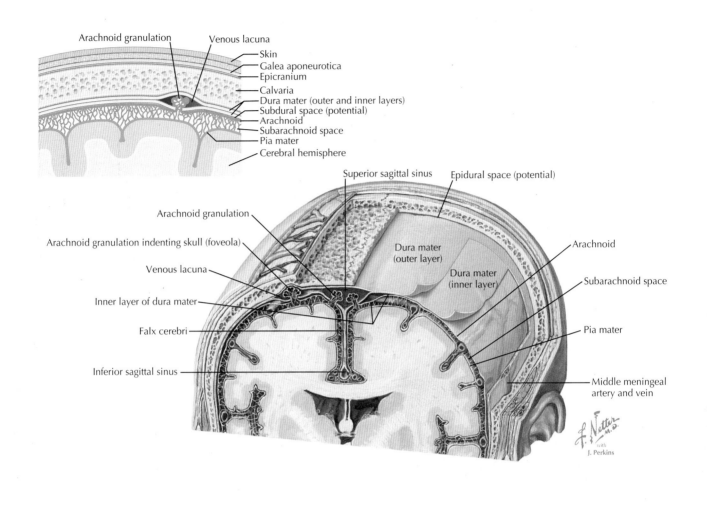

2.4 SCHEMATIC OF THE MENINGES AND THEIR RELATIONSHIPS TO THE BRAIN AND SKULL

The meninges provide protection and support for neural tissue in the central nervous system. The innermost membrane, the pia mater, adheres to every contour of neural tissue, including sulci, folia, and other infoldings. It adheres tightly to glial endfoot processes of astrocytes; this association is called the pial-glial membrane. The arachnoid mater, a fine, lacy membrane external to the pia, extends across the neural sulci and foldings. The space between these two membranes is the subarachnoid space, a space into which the cerebrospinal fluid flows, providing buoyancy and protection for the brain. Arteries and veins run through the subarachnoid space to and from the central nervous system. The rupture of an arterial aneurysm in a cerebral artery results in a subarachnoid hemorrhage. The dura mater, usually adherent to the inner arachnoid, is a tough protective outer membrane. It splits into two layers in some locations to provide channels, the venous sinuses, for return flow of the venous blood. The arachnoid granulations, one-way valves, extend from the subarachnoid space into the venous sinuses, especially the superior sagittal sinus, allowing cerebrospinal fluid to

drain into the venous blood and return to the heart. Blockage of these arachnoid granulations (e.g., in acute purulent meningitis) can result in increased intracranial pressure. Cerebral arteries and veins traverse the subarachnoid space. The veins, called bridging veins, drain into the dural sinuses. As they enter the sinus, these bridging veins are subject to tearing in cases of head trauma. If there is atrophy in the brain, as occurs with age, these veins may tear with relatively minor head trauma; in younger adults, more severe head trauma is needed to tear these bridging veins. Such tearing permits venous blood to accumulate in the subdural space as it dissects the inner dura from the arachnoid. This process may be gradual (chronic subdural hematoma) in older individuals or may be abrupt (acute subdural hematoma) with severe head trauma. A sub- dural hematoma, especially when it occurs acutely, may be life-threatening as the result of increased intracranial pressure caused by accompanying edema and by the accumulation of the blood in the hematoma itself. The dura is closely adherent to the inner table of the skull. A skull fracture may tear a branch of the middle meningeal artery, permitting arterial blood to dissect the dura from the skull, resulting in an epidural hematoma.

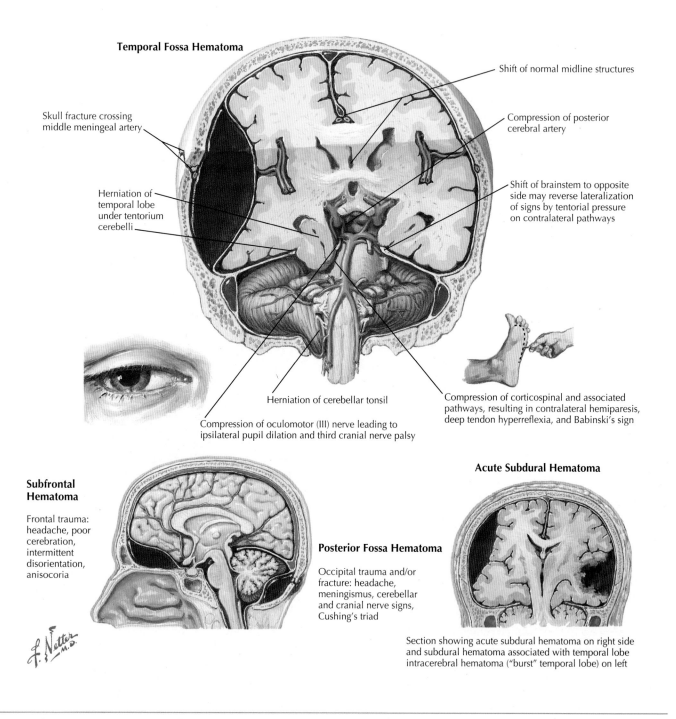

Temporal Fossa Hematoma

Shift of normal midline structures

Skull fracture crossing middle meningeal artery

Compression of posterior cerebral artery

Herniation of temporal lobe under tentorium cerebelli

Shift of brainstem to opposite side may reverse lateralization of signs by tentorial pressure on contralateral pathways

Compression of oculomotor (III) nerve leading to ipsilateral pupil dilation and third cranial nerve palsy

Herniation of cerebellar tonsil

Compression of corticospinal and associated pathways, resulting in contralateral hemiparesis, deep tendon hyperreflexia, and Babinski's sign

Subfrontal Hematoma

Frontal trauma: headache, poor cerebration, intermittent disorientation, anisocoria

Posterior Fossa Hematoma

Occipital trauma and/or fracture: headache, meningismus, cerebellar and cranial nerve signs, Cushing's triad

Acute Subdural Hematoma

Section showing acute subdural hematoma on right side and subdural hematoma associated with temporal lobe intracerebral hematoma ("burst" temporal lobe) on left

2.5 HEMATOMAS

Epidural hematomas occur with trauma or skull fractures that tear meningeal arteries (especially middle meningeal artery branches). Blood from the tear dissects the outer layer of the dura from the skull, forming a space-occupying mass in what was normally only a potential space. The hematoma may compress adjacent brain tissue, producing localized signs, and may also cause herniation of distant brain regions across the free edge of the tentorium cerebelli (a transtentorial herniation) or across the falx cerebri (a subfalcial herniation). Such herniation may produce changes in consciousness, breathing, and blood pressure, and altered motor, pupillary, and other neurological signs. It may be fatal. Severe head trauma in an adult may tear bridging veins that lead from the brain through the subarachnoid space and into the dural sinuses, especially the superior sagittal sinus. The subsequent venous bleeding dissects the arachnoid membrane from the inner layer of the dura, and the blood accumulates as a subdural hematoma. The subdural space is normally only a potential space. Some of the proteins and other solutes in the hematoma attract edema, adding fluid accumulation to the hematoma and further exacerbating the space-occupying nature of the bleed. A subdural hematoma also may be associated with bleeding directly into the brain, an intracerebral hematoma.

3

BRAIN

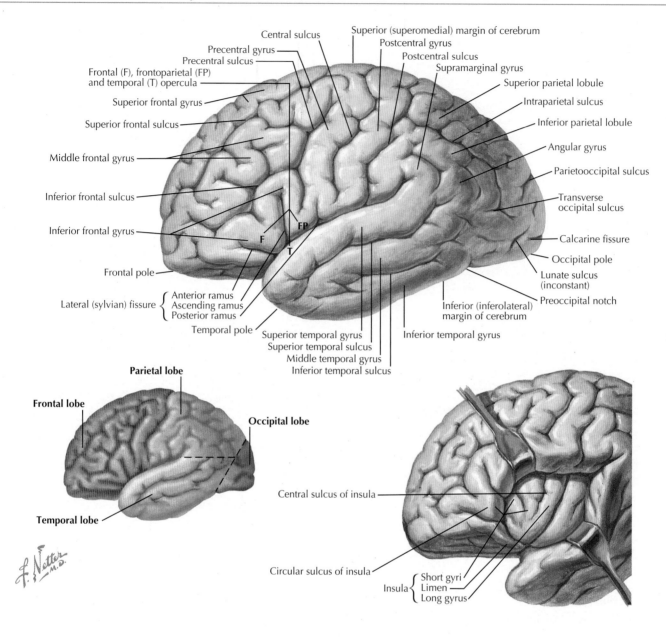

Central sulcus
Precentral gyrus
Precentral sulcus
Frontal (F), frontoparietal (FP) and temporal (T) opercula
Superior frontal gyrus
Superior frontal sulcus
Middle frontal gyrus
Inferior frontal sulcus
Inferior frontal gyrus
Frontal pole
Lateral (sylvian) fissure { Anterior ramus / Ascending ramus / Posterior ramus
Temporal pole
Superior temporal gyrus
Superior temporal sulcus
Middle temporal gyrus
Inferior temporal sulcus

Superior (superomedial) margin of cerebrum
Postcentral gyrus
Postcentral sulcus
Supramarginal gyrus
Superior parietal lobule
Intraparietal sulcus
Inferior parietal lobule
Angular gyrus
Parietooccipital sulcus
Transverse occipital sulcus
Calcarine fissure
Occipital pole
Lunate sulcus (inconstant)
Preoccipital notch
Inferior (inferolateral) margin of cerebrum
Inferior temporal gyrus

FP
F
T

Parietal lobe
Frontal lobe
Occipital lobe
Temporal lobe

Central sulcus of insula
Circular sulcus of insula
Insula { Short gyri / Limen / Long gyrus

3.1 SURFACE ANATOMY OF THE FOREBRAIN: LATERAL VIEW

The convolutions of the cerebral cortex permit a large expanse of cortex to be compactly folded into a small volume, an adaptation particularly prominent in primates. Major dependable landmarks separate the forebrain into lobes; the lateral (sylvian) fissure separates the temporal lobe below from the parietal and frontal lobes above, and the central sulcus separates the parietal and frontal lobes from each other. Several of the named gyri are associated with specific functional activities, such as the precentral gyrus (motor cortex) and the postcentral gyrus (primary sensory cortex). Some gyri, such as the superior, middle, and inferior frontal and temporal gyri, serve as anatomical landmarks of the cerebral cortex. The insula, the fifth lobe of the cerebral cortex, is deep to the outer cortex and can be seen by opening the lateral fissure.

CLINICAL POINT
Some **functional characteristics of the cerebral cortex**, such as long-term memory and some cognitive capabilities, cannot be localized easily to a particular gyrus or region of cortex. However, other functional capabilities are regionally localized. For example, the inferior frontal gyrus on the left contains the neuronal machinery for expressive language capabilities; the occipital pole, particularly along the upper and lower banks of the calcarine fissure, is specialized for visual processing from the retino-geniculo-calcarine system. Some very discrete lesions in further processing sites such as vision-related regions of the temporal lobe can result in specific deficits, such as agnosia for the recognition of faces or the inability to distinguish animate objects. This knowledge provides some clues about how feature extraction in sensory systems might be achieved in neuronal networks.

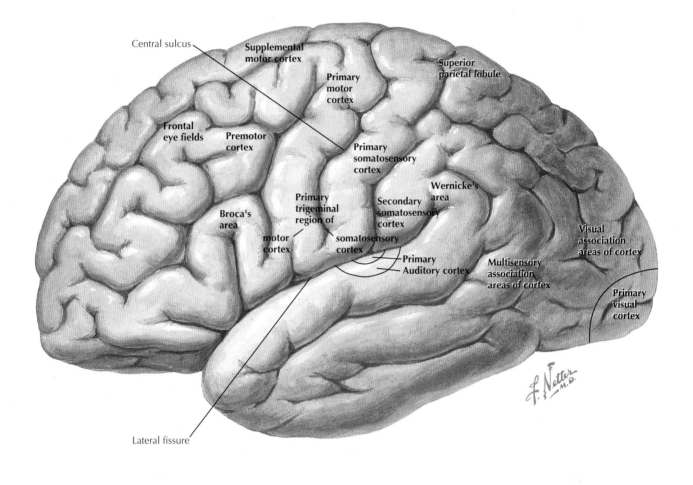

3.2 **LATERAL VIEW OF THE FOREBRAIN: FUNCTIONAL REGIONS**

Some circumscribed regions of the cerebral hemisphere are associated with specific functional activities, including the motor cortex, the supplemental and premotor cortices, the frontal eye fields, the primary sensory cortex, and other association regions of the sensory cortex. Part of the auditory cortex is visible at the inferior edge of the lateral fissure (the transverse temporal gyrus of Heschl). Part of the visual cortex is visible at the occipital pole. Language areas of the left hemisphere include Broca's area (expressive language) and Wernicke's area (receptive language). Damage to these cortical regions results in loss of specific functional capabilities. There is some overlap between functional areas and named gyri (e.g., the motor cortex and the precentral gyrus), but there is no absolute concordance.

CLINICAL POINT

Some **specific regions (gyri) of the cerebral cortex**, such as the precentral gyrus (primary motor cortex) and the postcentral gyrus (primary somatosensory cortex), demonstrate topographic organization. Thus, information from the contralateral hand and arm is localized laterally, the body is represented more medially, and the lower extremity is represented along the midline and over the edge into the paracentral lobule. The face and head are represented in far lateral regions of these gyri, just above the lateral fissure. This has important functional implications; damage to selected regions such as the midline territory, which is supplied with blood from the anterior cerebral artery, results in somatosensory loss and paresis in the contralateral lower extremity, while sparing the upper extremity.

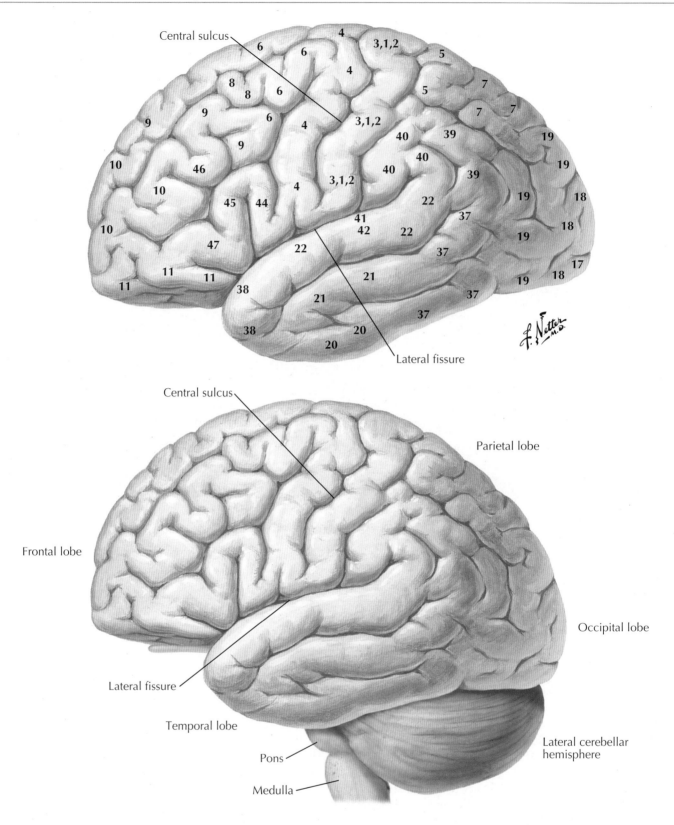

3.3 LATERAL VIEW OF THE FOREBRAIN: BRODMANN'S AREAS

Brodmann's areas of the cerebral cortex have unique architectural characteristics in terms of the thickness and layering of the cerebral cortex; this knowledge is based on histological observations originally made by Korbinian Brodmann in 1909. His numbering of cortical areas is still used as a shorthand for describing the functional regions of the cortex, particularly those related to sensory functions. Some overlap exists among functional areas. For example, the motor cortex is area 4; the primary sensory cortex includes areas 3, 1, and 2; and the primary visual cortex is area 17. In this lateral view, the lateral surface of the spinal cord, medulla, and caudal pons can be seen, as well as the lateral surface of the cerebellum. The temporal lobe overlies the more rostral portions of the brainstem.

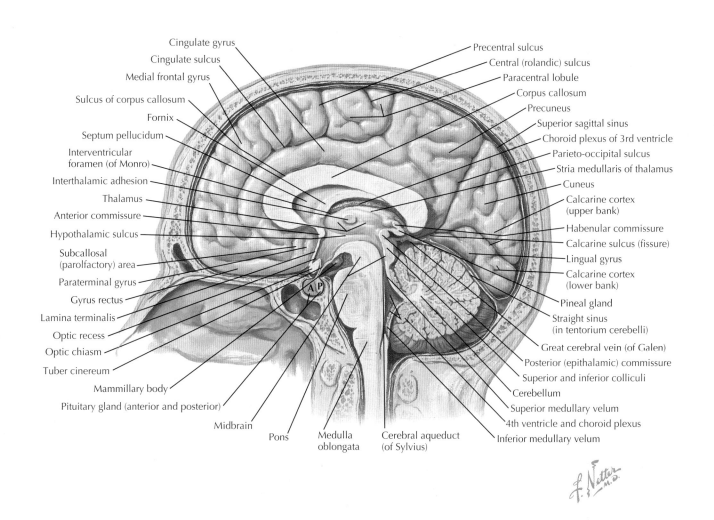

Cingulate gyrus
Cingulate sulcus
Medial frontal gyrus
Sulcus of corpus callosum
Fornix
Septum pellucidum
Interventricular foramen (of Monro)
Interthalamic adhesion
Thalamus
Anterior commissure
Hypothalamic sulcus
Subcallosal (parolfactory) area
Paraterminal gyrus
Gyrus rectus
Lamina terminalis
Optic recess
Optic chiasm
Tuber cinereum
Mammillary body
Pituitary gland (anterior and posterior)
Midbrain
Pons
Medulla oblongata
Cerebral aqueduct (of Sylvius)

Precentral sulcus
Central (rolandic) sulcus
Paracentral lobule
Corpus callosum
Precuneus
Superior sagittal sinus
Choroid plexus of 3rd ventricle
Parieto-occipital sulcus
Stria medullaris of thalamus
Cuneus
Calcarine cortex (upper bank)
Habenular commissure
Calcarine sulcus (fissure)
Lingual gyrus
Calcarine cortex (lower bank)
Pineal gland
Straight sinus (in tentorium cerebelli)
Great cerebral vein (of Galen)
Posterior (epithalamic) commissure
Superior and inferior colliculi
Cerebellum
Superior medullary velum
4th ventricle and choroid plexus
Inferior medullary velum

3.4 ANATOMY OF THE MEDIAL (MIDSAGITTAL) SURFACE OF THE BRAIN IN SITU

The entire extent of the neuraxis, from the spinomedullary junction through the brainstem, diencephalon, and telencephalon, is visible in a midsagittal section. The corpus callosum, a major commissural fiber bundle interconnecting the two hemispheres, is a landmark separating the cerebral cortex above from the thalamus, fornix, and subcortical forebrain below. The ventricular system, including the interventricular foramen (of Munro); the third ventricle (diencephalon); the cerebral aqueduct (midbrain); and the fourth ventricle (pons and medulla), is visible in a midsagittal view. This subarachnoid fluid system provides internal (the ventricular system) and external (cerebrospinal fluid in the subarachnoid space) protection to the brain and also may serve as a fluid transport system for important regulatory molecules. The thalamus serves as a gateway to the cortex. The hypothalamic proximity to the median eminence (tuber cinereum) and the pituitary gland reflects the

important role of the hypothalamus in regulating neuroendocrine function. A midsagittal view also reveals the midbrain colliculi, sometimes called the visual (superior) and auditory (inferior) tecta. See Video 3.1.

CLINICAL POINT

The right and left hemispheres are interconnected by **commissural fiber bundles**. The largest is the corpus callosum, which interconnects all lobes with their counterparts. The anterior commissure interconnects regions of the temporal lobes. When these commissural fiber bundles are disconnected (split brain), the hemispheres do not know what their counterparts are doing, and inputs to one hemisphere cannot produce an appropriate response from the opposite hemisphere. With a split brain, only a more generalized recognition of mood states occurs between the two hemispheres, presumably communicated through interconnections between lower structures, such as the diencephalon and brainstem.

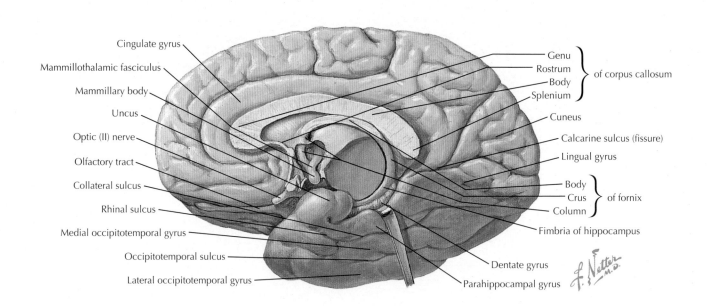

Cingulate gyrus

Mammillothalamic fasciculus

Mammillary body

Uncus

Optic (II) nerve

Olfactory tract

Collateral sulcus

Rhinal sulcus

Medial occipitotemporal gyrus

Occipitotemporal sulcus

Lateral occipitotemporal gyrus

Genu

Rostrum

Body

Splenium

of corpus callosum

Cuneus

Calcarine sulcus (fissure)

Lingual gyrus

Body

Crus

Column

of fornix

Fimbria of hippocampus

Dentate gyrus

Parahippocampal gyrus

3.5 ANATOMY OF THE MEDIAL (MIDSAGITTAL) SURFACE OF THE BRAIN, WITH BRAINSTEM REMOVED

When the brainstem is removed, a midsagittal view reveals the C-shaped course of the fornix, extending from the hippocampal formation in the temporal lobe to the septum and hypothalamus. Temporal lobe structures, such as the parahippocampal cortex, the dentate gyrus and fimbria of the hippocampus, and the uncus (olfactory cortex) also are visible. In the hypothalamus, the caudal mammillary bodies and the interconnecting pathway to the thalamus, the mammillothalamic tract, are revealed.

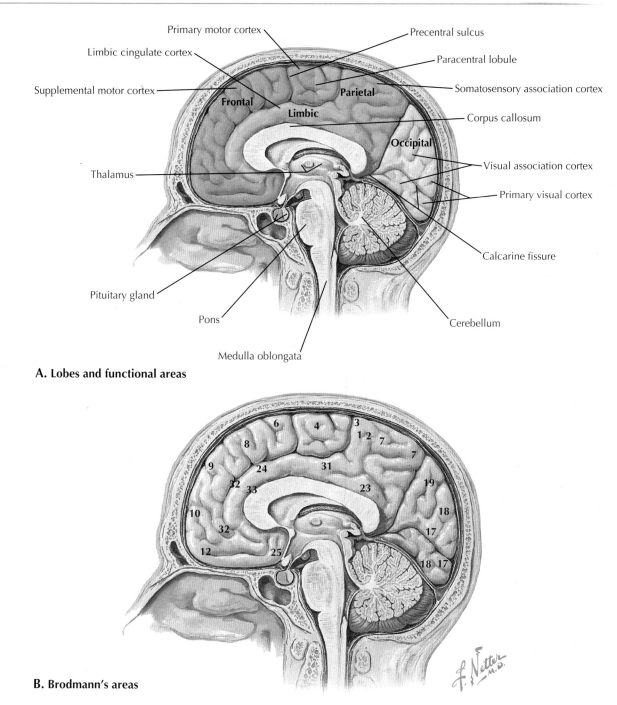

A. Lobes and functional areas

Primary motor cortex
Limbic cingulate cortex
Supplemental motor cortex
Frontal
Limbic
Parietal
Precentral sulcus
Paracentral lobule
Somatosensory association cortex
Corpus callosum
Occipital
Thalamus
Visual association cortex
Primary visual cortex
Calcarine fissure
Pituitary gland
Pons
Cerebellum
Medulla oblongata

B. Brodmann's areas

3.6 MEDIAL SURFACE OF THE BRAIN

A, Lobes and functional areas. The cingulate cortex is labeled the limbic lobe, reflecting its association with other limbic forebrain structures and with hypothalamic control of the autonomic nervous system. Functional areas of the cortex, particularly those involved with vision, are best seen on a midsagittal view. The sensory and motor cortices associated with the lower extremities are located medially and are supplied with blood by the anterior cerebral artery. This region is selectively vulnerable to specific vascular (anterior cerebral artery infarct) and mass (parasagittal meningioma) lesions that result in contralateral motor and sensory deficits of the lower extremity. **B,** Brodmann's areas of the cerebral cortex are labeled on this midsagittal view of the brain. The major regions are the primary (17) and associative (18, 19) visual cortices and the continuation of areas 4 (motor) and areas 3, 1, and 2 (primary sensory) onto the paracentral lobule in the midline.

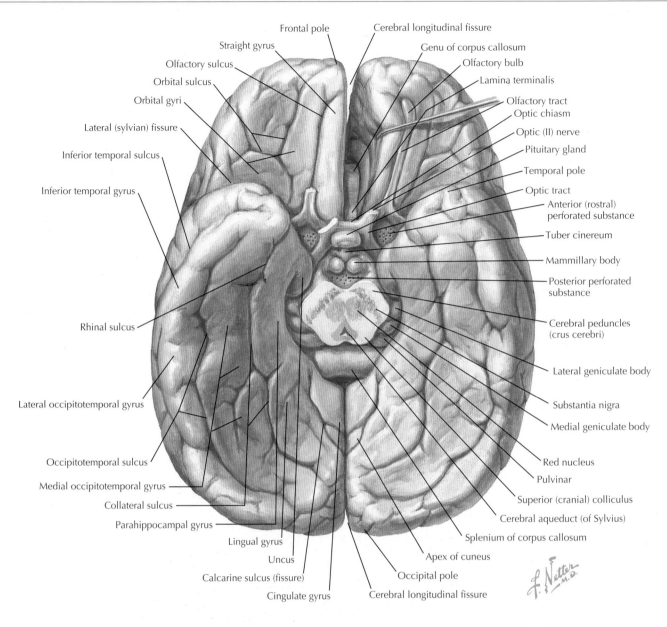

Frontal pole
Cerebral longitudinal fissure
Straight gyrus
Genu of corpus callosum
Olfactory sulcus
Olfactory bulb
Orbital sulcus
Lamina terminalis
Orbital gyri
Olfactory tract
Lateral (sylvian) fissure
Optic chiasm
Inferior temporal sulcus
Optic (II) nerve
Pituitary gland
Inferior temporal gyrus
Temporal pole
Optic tract
Anterior (rostral) perforated substance
Tuber cinereum
Mammillary body
Posterior perforated substance
Rhinal sulcus
Cerebral peduncles (crus cerebri)
Lateral geniculate body
Lateral occipitotemporal gyrus
Substantia nigra
Medial geniculate body
Occipitotemporal sulcus
Red nucleus
Medial occipitotemporal gyrus
Pulvinar
Collateral sulcus
Superior (cranial) colliculus
Parahippocampal gyrus
Cerebral aqueduct (of Sylvius)
Lingual gyrus
Splenium of corpus callosum
Uncus
Apex of cuneus
Calcarine sulcus (fissure)
Occipital pole
Cingulate gyrus
Cerebral longitudinal fissure

3.7 ANATOMY OF THE BASAL SURFACE OF THE BRAIN, WITH THE BRAINSTEM AND CEREBELLUM REMOVED

Removal of the brainstem and cerebellum by a cut through the midbrain exposes the underlying cerebral cortex, the base of the diencephalon, and the basal forebrain. Basal hypothalamic landmarks, from caudal to rostral, include the mammillary bodies, tuber cinereum, pituitary gland, and optic chiasm. The proximity of the pituitary to the optic chiasm is important because bitemporal hemianopsia can result from optic chiasm fiber damage, often an early sign of a pituitary tumor. The genu and splenium of the corpus callosum are revealed in this view. In the cross-section of the midbrain, the superior colliculus, cerebral aqueduct, periaqueductal gray, red nucleus, substantia nigra, and cerebral peduncles are shown.

CLINICAL POINT

The **olfactory bulb and tract** send connections directly into limbic forebrain structures, such as the uncus (the primary olfactory cortex), amygdala, and other limbic regions. This is the only sensory system with direct access to forebrain structures without prior screening through the diencephalon. This reflects the evolutionary importance of olfaction to functions vital for survival, such as detection of food, defense, and reproduction. Olfactory damage can alter emotional behavior. In addition, complex partial seizures involving the temporal lobe frequently are accompanied by an olfactory aura. Changes in olfactory function and gene expression may be among the earliest signs of Alzheimer's disease.

The **optic nerve, chiasm, and tract** can be seen extending toward the lateral geniculate body (nucleus), the pulvinar, and the superior colliculus. Optic nerve damage can result in ipsilateral blindness; optic chiasm damage can result in bitemporal visual field deficits; and optic tract damage can result in contralateral hemianopsia. Additional visual input from the optic tract enters the hypothalamus and ends in the suprachiasmatic nucleus. This visual input conveys information of total light flux and exposure, permitting visual influence over diurnal rhythms such as the cortisol rhythm. Disruption of this diurnal input can produce altered production of hormones such as melatonin, and metabolic consequences such as the propensity for abdominal obesity resulting from disruption of the diurnal cortisol rhythm.

Brodmann's areas

Structures

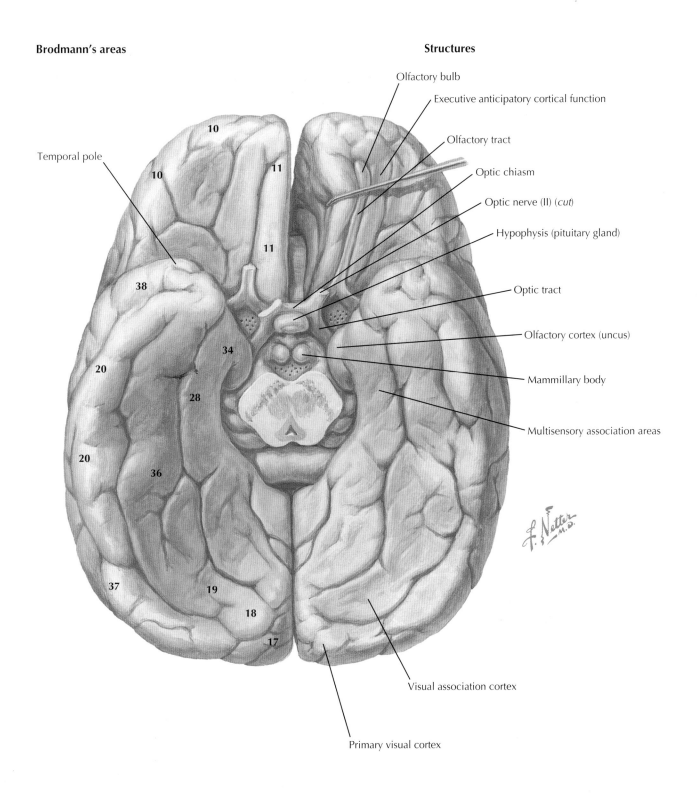

Olfactory bulb

Executive anticipatory cortical function

Olfactory tract

Optic chiasm

Optic nerve (II) (*cut*)

Hypophysis (pituitary gland)

Optic tract

Olfactory cortex (uncus)

Mammillary body

Multisensory association areas

Temporal pole

10

10

11

11

38

34

20

28

20

36

37

19

18

17

Visual association cortex

Primary visual cortex

3.8 BASAL SURFACE OF THE BRAIN: FUNCTIONAL AREAS AND BRODMANN'S AREAS

This view provides information about the medial temporal lobe on the left side of the brain, especially cortical regions associated with the hippocampal formation, the amygdaloid nuclei, and the olfactory system. On the right side of the brain, Brodmann's areas are noted.

A. Axial view

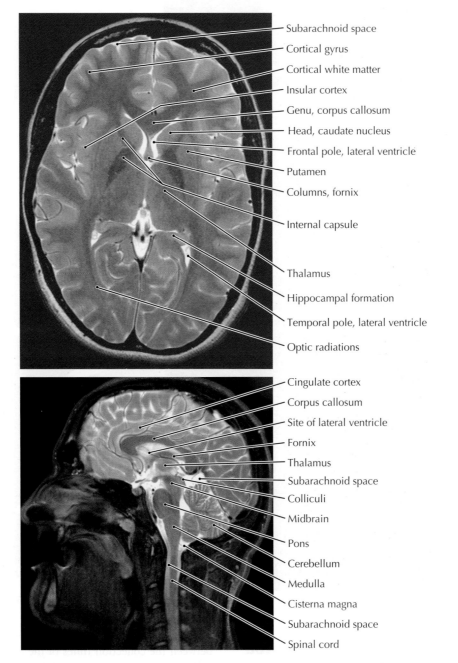

- Subarachnoid space
- Cortical gyrus
- Cortical white matter
- Insular cortex
- Genu, corpus callosum
- Head, caudate nucleus
- Frontal pole, lateral ventricle
- Putamen
- Columns, fornix
- Internal capsule
- Thalamus
- Hippocampal formation
- Temporal pole, lateral ventricle
- Optic radiations

- Cingulate cortex
- Corpus callosum
- Site of lateral ventricle
- Fornix
- Thalamus
- Subarachnoid space
- Colliculi
- Midbrain
- Pons
- Cerebellum
- Medulla
- Cisterna magna
- Subarachnoid space
- Spinal cord

B. Sagittal view

3.11 BRAIN IMAGING: MAGNETIC RESONANCE IMAGING, AXIAL AND SAGITTAL T2-WEIGHTED IMAGES

A, Axial view. **B,** Sagittal view. T2-weighted images are particularly useful for imaging the ventricular system and the cisterns of cerebrospinal fluid. The ventricular system and subarachnoid space in T2-weighted images appear white.

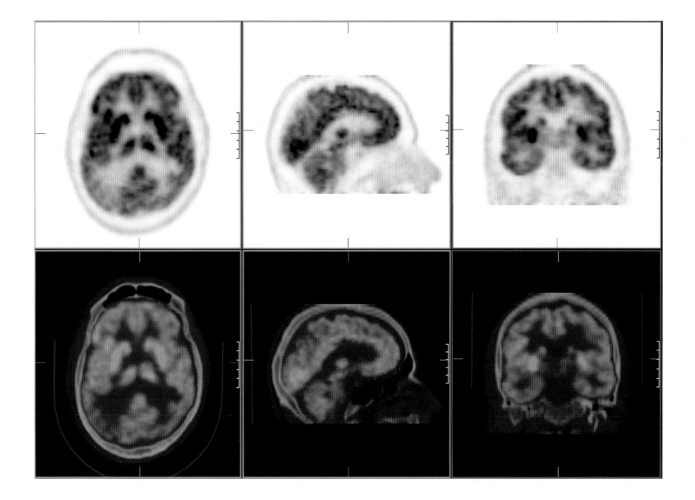

3.12 **POSITRON EMISSION TOMOGRAPHY SCANNING**

Positron emission tomography (PET) scanning is designed to assess the distribution of tracers labeled with positron-emitting nuclides, such as carbon-11 (^{11}C), nitrogen-13 (^{13}N), oxygen-15 (^{15}O), and fluorine-18 (^{18}F). Fluorodeoxyglucose (FDG), a glucose analogue labeled with ^{18}F, can cross the blood-brain barrier. The metabolic products of FDG become immobile and trapped where the molecule is first used, thereby permitting FDG to be used to map glucose uptake in the brain.

This is a valuable tool for investigating subtle physiological processes related to neurological diseases. The distribution of FDG can be localized and reconstructed using standard tomographic techniques that show the tracer distribution throughout the body or brain. In this example of axial, sagittal, and coronal views, the transmission measurement and correction was performed immediately following PET acquisition using a 16-slice CT unit. The PET and CT images were automatically fused by anatomical coregistration software (shown as colored images).

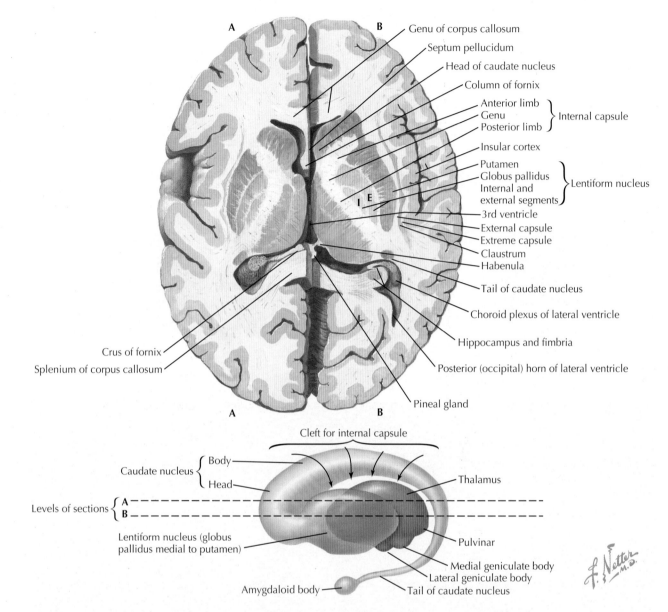

Schematic illustration showing interrelationship of thalamus, lentiform nucleus, caudate nucleus, and amygdaloid body (viewed from side).

3.13 HORIZONTAL BRAIN SECTIONS SHOWING THE BASAL GANGLIA

Two levels of horizontal sections through the forebrain reveal the major anatomical features and the relationships among the basal ganglia, the internal capsule, and the thalamus (schematically shown in the lower illustration). The caudate nucleus is a C-shaped structure that sweeps from the frontal lobe into the temporal lobe; a horizontal section passes through this nucleus in two distinct places (head and tail). The anterior limb, genu, and posterior limb of the internal capsule contain major connections into and out of the cerebral cortex. The head and body of the caudate are medial to the anterior limb, whereas the thalamus is medial to the posterior limb. These relationships are important for understanding imaging studies and for understanding the involvement of specific functional systems in vascular lesions or strokes. The internal and external segments of the globus pallidus are located medial to the putamen. The external capsule, claustrum, extreme capsule,

and insular cortex, from medial to lateral, are located lateral to the putamen. The fornix, also a C-shaped bundle, is sectioned in two sites, the crus and the column.

CLINICAL POINT

The **basal ganglia** (caudate nucleus, putamen, and globus pallidus) form characteristic anatomical relationships with the internal capsule. The head and body of the caudate nucleus are found medial to the anterior limb; the thalamus is found medial to the posterior limb; and the globus pallidus and putamen are found lateral to the anterior and posterior limbs. Basal ganglia disorders are characterized by movement disorders, although emotional and cognitive symptoms also are seen. Some movement disorders involve actual degeneration of basal ganglia and related structures; these disorders include Huntington's chorea and degeneration of the head of the caudate nucleus as well as Parkinson's disease and degeneration of the dopaminergic pars compacta of substantia nigra. Other movement disorders involve altered inhibitory and excitatory activity of specific portions of basal ganglia circuitry; reordering this circuitry may require pharmacologic treatment, therapeutic ablation procedures, or deep brain stimulation.

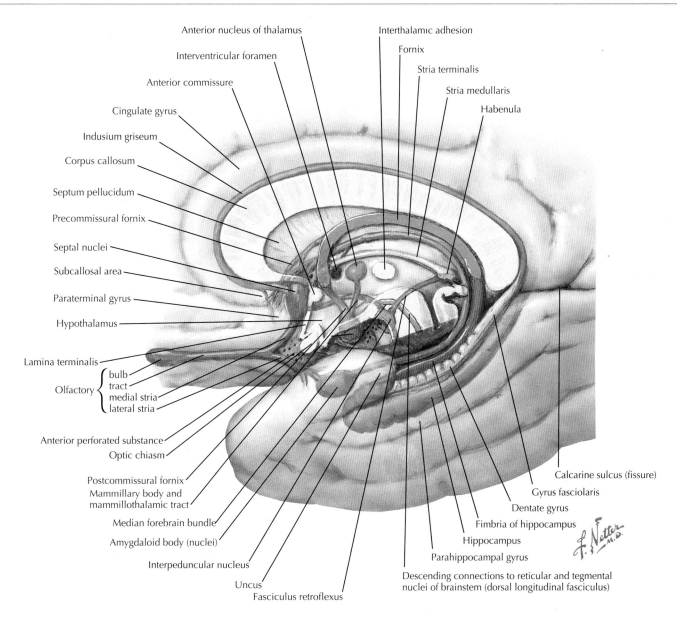

Anterior nucleus of thalamus
Interventricular foramen
Anterior commissure
Cingulate gyrus
Indusium griseum
Corpus callosum
Septum pellucidum
Precommissural fornix
Septal nuclei
Subcallosal area
Paraterminal gyrus
Hypothalamus
Lamina terminalis
Olfactory { bulb / tract / medial stria / lateral stria
Anterior perforated substance
Optic chiasm
Postcommissural fornix
Mammillary body and mammillothalamic tract
Median forebrain bundle
Amygdaloid body (nuclei)
Interpeduncular nucleus
Uncus
Fasciculus retroflexus

Interthalamic adhesion
Fornix
Stria terminalis
Stria medullaris
Habenula

Calcarine sulcus (fissure)
Gyrus fasciolaris
Dentate gyrus
Fimbria of hippocampus
Hippocampus
Parahippocampal gyrus
Descending connections to reticular and tegmental nuclei of brainstem (dorsal longitudinal fasciculus)

3.14 MAJOR LIMBIC FOREBRAIN STRUCTURES

The term *limbic* is derived from *limbus,* meaning ring. Many of these structures and their pathways in the limbic system form a ring around the diencephalon. They are involved in emotional behavior and individualized interpretations of external and internal stimuli. The hippocampal formation and its major pathway, the fornix, curve into the anterior pole of the diencephalon, forming precommissural (to the septum) and postcommissural (to the hypothalamus) connections in relation to the anterior commissure. The amygdaloid nuclei give rise to several pathways; one, the stria terminalis, extends in a C-shaped course around the diencephalon into the hypothalamus and basal forebrain. The olfactory tract communicates directly with several limbic forebrain areas; it is the only sensory system to entirely bypass the thalamus and terminate directly in cortical and subcortical zones of the telencephalon. Connections from the septal nuclei to the habenula (stria medullaris thalami) connect the limbic forebrain to the brainstem. The amygdaloid nuclei and hippocampus (shaded) are deep to the cortex.

CLINICAL POINT

Many of the **limbic forebrain structures** are connected with the hypothalamus by C-shaped structures, such as the hippocampus and the fornix, and with the amygdala and the stria terminalis. The amygdala has additional direct connections into the hypothalamus via the ventral amygdalofugal pathway. The amygdaloid nuclei receive multimodal sensory information from cortical regions and provide context for this input, particularly emotions related to fear responses. Bilateral amygdaloid damage results in the loss of the fear response and also in failure to recognize facial responses of fear in others.

The hippocampal formation processes abundant information from the temporal lobe, subiculum, and entorhinal cortex and sends connections through the fornix to the hypothalamus and septal nuclei, with subsequent connections through the thalamus to the cingulate cortex. These structures are part of the so-called Papez circuit. The hippocampal formation is particularly vulnerable to ischemia; damage bilaterally results in the inability to consolidate new information into long-term memory. A common pattern may be observed in older persons who forget who has talked with them minutes before or forget what they had for breakfast (or even whether they had breakfast) but can recall details from the past that have some degree of accuracy.

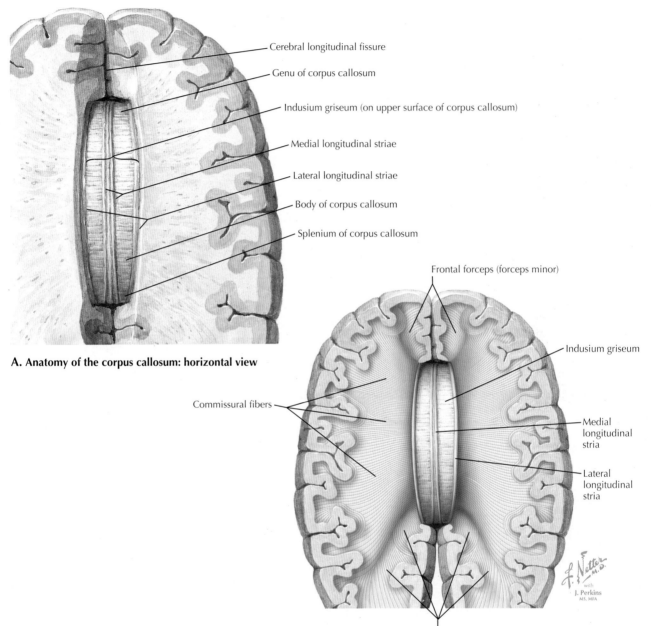

A. Anatomy of the corpus callosum: horizontal view

Cerebral longitudinal fissure

Genu of corpus callosum

Indusium griseum (on upper surface of corpus callosum)

Medial longitudinal striae

Lateral longitudinal striae

Body of corpus callosum

Splenium of corpus callosum

Frontal forceps (forceps minor)

Indusium griseum

Medial longitudinal stria

Lateral longitudinal stria

Commissural fibers

B. Schematic view of the lateral extent of major components

Occipital forceps (forceps major)

3.15 CORPUS CALLOSUM

A, Anatomy of the corpus callosum, horizontal view. The corpus callosum, the major fiber commissure between the hemispheres, is a conspicuous landmark in imaging studies. It is viewed from above after dissection of tissue just dorsal to its upper surface. Horizontal cuts taken deeper (more ventrally) section the genu anteriorly and the splenium posteriorly (see Fig. 3.13). **B,** Schematic view of the lateral extent of major components. Many of the commissural fibers of the corpus callosum, particularly the forceps of commissural fibers that interconnect frontal areas with each other and occipital areas with each other, extend rostrally and caudally, respectively, after crossing the midline. These interconnections allow communication between the hemispheres for coordinated activity of these two "separate" hemispheres.

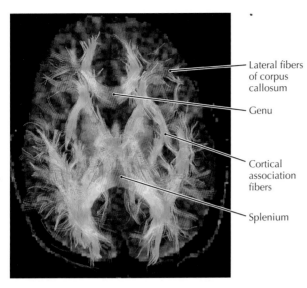

A. Axial view

- Lateral fibers of corpus callosum
- Genu
- Cortical association fibers
- Splenium

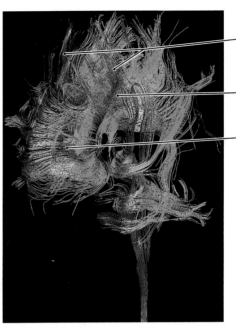

B. Oblique sagittal view

- Lateral corpus callosum fibers radiating to cortical gyri
- Midline fibers, body of corpus callosum
- Midline fibers, genu of corpus callosum

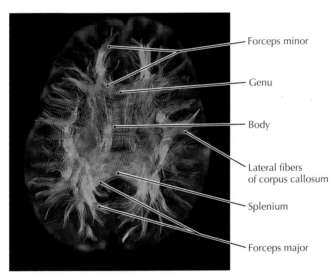

C. Axial view

- Forceps minor
- Genu
- Body
- Lateral fibers of corpus callosum
- Splenium
- Forceps major

3.16 COLOR IMAGING OF THE CORPUS CALLOSUM BY DIFFUSION TENSOR IMAGING

A–C, Diffusion-weighted imaging (DWI), also called diffusion tensor imaging (DTI), provides unique information about tissue viability, architecture, and cellular function. In many tissues, restricted water diffusion is isotropic or independent of direction. In structured tissues, such as cerebral white matter and peripheral nerves, diffusion is anisotropic because of cellular arrangements. By using diffusion sensitivity that projects in multiple directions, such diffusion can be evaluated in the form of a tensor. Tensor field calculations for six or more diffusion-weighted measurements are based on an analytical solution of the Stejskal and Tanner diffusion equation system. Diffusion tensor imaging permits reconstruction of axonal tracts in brain and spinal cord; the three-dimensional architecture of the white matter tracts can be traced based on eigenvectors of the diffusion tensor. To discriminate fiber bundles that radiate in different directions, a color scheme is adopted in which green represents eigenvectors pointing in anteroposterior directions; red represents eigenvectors radiating in left-right directions; and blue represents eigenvectors pointing in the superoinferior direction. In these images of the corpus callosum, components of this major commissural bundle are represented in red. See Video 3.2.

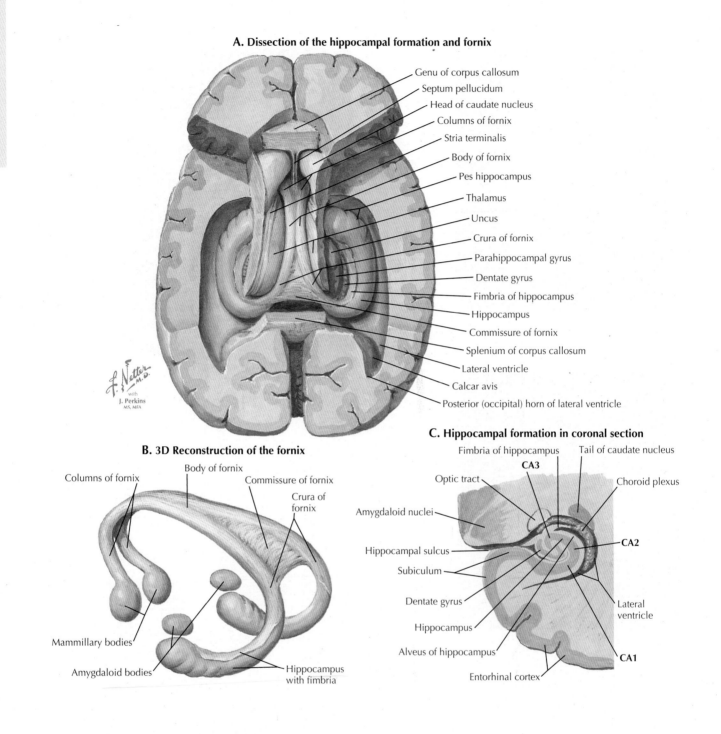

A. Dissection of the hippocampal formation and fornix

- Genu of corpus callosum
- Septum pellucidum
- Head of caudate nucleus
- Columns of fornix
- Stria terminalis
- Body of fornix
- Pes hippocampus
- Thalamus
- Uncus
- Crura of fornix
- Parahippocampal gyrus
- Dentate gyrus
- Fimbria of hippocampus
- Hippocampus
- Commissure of fornix
- Splenium of corpus callosum
- Lateral ventricle
- Calcar avis
- Posterior (occipital) horn of lateral ventricle

B. 3D Reconstruction of the fornix

- Columns of fornix
- Body of fornix
- Commissure of fornix
- Crura of fornix
- Mammillary bodies
- Amygdaloid bodies
- Hippocampus with fimbria

C. Hippocampal formation in coronal section

- Fimbria of hippocampus
- CA3
- Tail of caudate nucleus
- Optic tract
- Choroid plexus
- Amygdaloid nuclei
- CA2
- Hippocampal sulcus
- Subiculum
- Dentate gyrus
- Lateral ventricle
- Hippocampus
- Alveus of hippocampus
- CA1
- Entorhinal cortex

3.17 HIPPOCAMPAL FORMATION AND FORNIX

In this dissection, the cortex, white matter, and corpus callosum have been removed. The lateral ventricles have been opened, and the head of the caudate nucleus and the thalamus have been dissected away quite close to the midline, allowing a downward view of the full extent of the hippocampal formation, including the dentate gyrus and the associated fornix. This view reveals the relationship between the hippocampus proper and the dentate gyrus. The two limbs of the fornix sweep upward medially, eventually running side by side at their most dorsal position, just beneath the corpus callosum. The full extent of this arching, C-shaped bundle is shown in the left lower image. The hippocampal formation occupies a large portion of the temporal pole of the lateral ventricle. The dentate gyrus is adjacent to subcomponents of the cornu ammonis (CA) regions of the hippocampus proper (the CA1 and CA3 regions), the subiculum, and the entorhinal cortex). Pyramidal neurons in the CA1 region are particularly sensitive to ischemic damage, and their counterparts in the CA3 region are sensitive to damage from high levels of corticosteroids (cortisol). Damage to pyramidal cells in both regions that has been caused by ischemia and/or high levels of corticosteroids is synergistic.

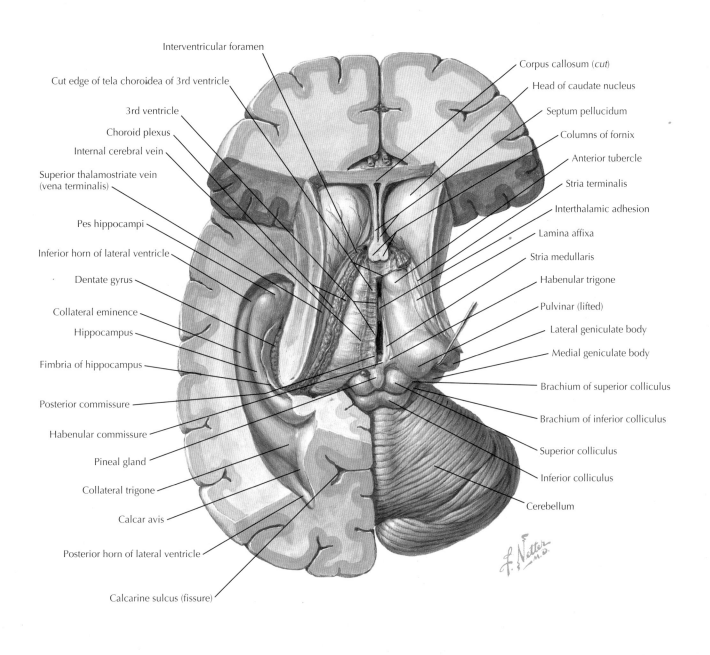

Interventricular foramen

Cut edge of tela choroidea of 3rd ventricle

3rd ventricle

Choroid plexus

Internal cerebral vein

Superior thalamostriate vein
(vena terminalis)

Pes hippocampi

Inferior horn of lateral ventricle

Dentate gyrus

Collateral eminence

Hippocampus

Fimbria of hippocampus

Posterior commissure

Habenular commissure

Pineal gland

Collateral trigone

Calcar avis

Posterior horn of lateral ventricle

Calcarine sulcus (fissure)

Corpus callosum (cut)

Head of caudate nucleus

Septum pellucidum

Columns of fornix

Anterior tubercle

Stria terminalis

Interthalamic adhesion

Lamina affixa

Stria medullaris

Habenular trigone

Pulvinar (lifted)

Lateral geniculate body

Medial geniculate body

Brachium of superior colliculus

Brachium of inferior colliculus

Superior colliculus

Inferior colliculus

Cerebellum

3.18 THALAMIC ANATOMY

The thalamus is viewed from above. The entire right side of the brain, just lateral to the thalamus, has been removed, the head of the caudate nucleus has been sectioned, the corpus callosum and all tissue dorsal to the thalamus have been removed, and the third ventricle has been opened from its dorsal surface. The pineal gland is present in the midline, just caudal to the third ventricle; it produces melatonin, a hormone that helps regulate circadian rhythms, sleep, and immune responses. The superior and inferior colliculi are shown, depicting the dorsal surface of the midbrain. On the left, the temporal horn of the lateral ventricle, with the hippocampal formation, has been exposed to show the relationship of these structures to the thalamus. The terminal vein and choroid plexus accompany the stria terminalis along the lateral margin of the thalamus. The stria medullaris runs along the medial surface of the dorsal thalamus.

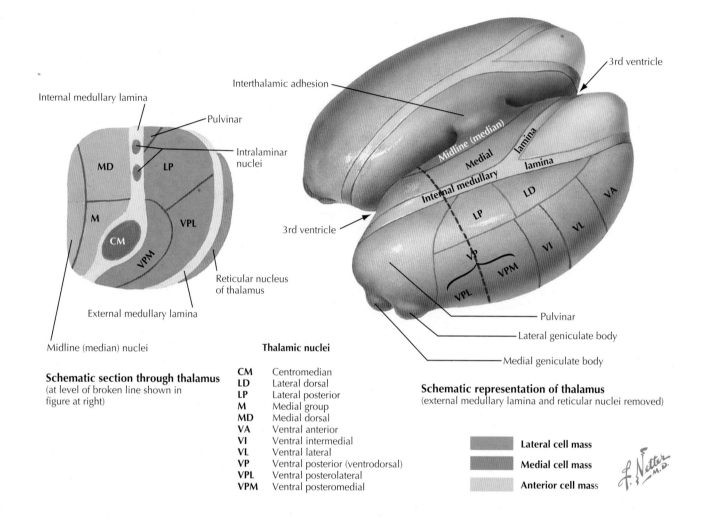

Internal medullary lamina

Pulvinar

Intralaminar nuclei

MD

LP

M

VPL

CM

VPM

Reticular nucleus of thalamus

External medullary lamina

Midline (median) nuclei

Schematic section through thalamus
(at level of broken line shown in figure at right)

Interthalamic adhesion

3rd ventricle

Midline (median)

Medial

lamina

Internal medullary

lamina

LD

VA

LP

VL

VI

VP

VPM

VPL

Pulvinar

Lateral geniculate body

Medial geniculate body

3rd ventricle

Thalamic nuclei

CM	Centromedian
LD	Lateral dorsal
LP	Lateral posterior
M	Medial group
MD	Medial dorsal
VA	Ventral anterior
VI	Ventral intermedial
VL	Ventral lateral
VP	Ventral posterior (ventrodorsal)
VPL	Ventral posterolateral
VPM	Ventral posteromedial

Schematic representation of thalamus
(external medullary lamina and reticular nuclei removed)

Lateral cell mass

Medial cell mass

Anterior cell mass

3.19 **THALAMIC NUCLEI**

The thalamus is subdivided into nuclear groups (medial, lateral, and anterior) that are separated by medullary (white matter) lamina. Many of these thalamic nuclei are "specific" thalamic nuclei that are reciprocally connected with discrete regions of the cerebral cortex. Some nuclei, such as those embedded within the internal medullary lamina (intralaminar nuclei such as the centromedian and parafascicular nuclei) and the outer, lateral shell nucleus (reticular nucleus of the thalamus), have very diffuse, nonspecific associations with the cerebral cortex.

CLINICAL POINT

Thalamic syndrome (posterolateral thalamic syndrome, or Dejerine-Roussy syndrome) results from obstruction of the thalamogeniculate arterial supply to the region of the thalamus where the ventral posterolateral nucleus is located. Initially, all sensation is lost in the contralateral body, epicritic more completely than protopathic. Commonly, severe spontaneous pain occurs contralaterally, described as stabbing, burning, or tearing pain; it is diffuse and persistent. Even light stimulation can evoke such pain (hyperpathia), and other sensory stimuli or emotionally charged situations can result in these painful sensations. Even when the threshold for pain and temperature sensation (protopathic sensations) is elevated, the thalamic pain may be present; it is called analgesic dolorosa. If the vascular lesion includes the subthalamic nucleus or associated basal ganglia circuitry, the patient may also experience hemiballismus (or choreiform or athetoid) movements in addition to the sensory deficits.

4

BRAINSTEM AND CEREBELLUM

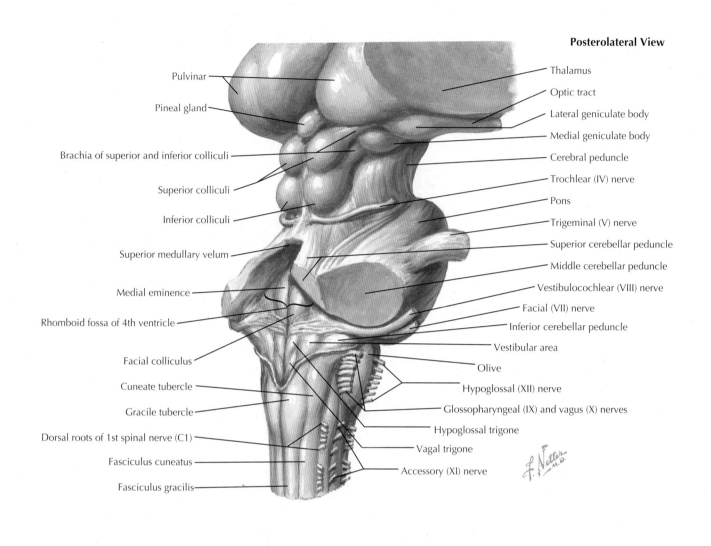

Posterolateral View

Pulvinar

Pineal gland

Brachia of superior and inferior colliculi

Superior colliculi

Inferior colliculi

Superior medullary velum

Medial eminence

Rhomboid fossa of 4th ventricle

Facial colliculus

Cuneate tubercle

Gracile tubercle

Dorsal roots of 1st spinal nerve (C1)

Fasciculus cuneatus

Fasciculus gracilis

Thalamus

Optic tract

Lateral geniculate body

Medial geniculate body

Cerebral peduncle

Trochlear (IV) nerve

Pons

Trigeminal (V) nerve

Superior cerebellar peduncle

Middle cerebellar peduncle

Vestibulocochlear (VIII) nerve

Facial (VII) nerve

Inferior cerebellar peduncle

Vestibular area

Olive

Hypoglossal (XII) nerve

Glossopharyngeal (IX) and vagus (X) nerves

Hypoglossal trigone

Vagal trigone

Accessory (XI) nerve

4.1 BRAINSTEM SURFACE ANATOMY: POSTEROLATERAL VIEW

The entire telencephalon, most of the diencephalon, and the cerebellum are removed to reveal the dorsal surface of the brainstem. The three cerebellar peduncles (superior, middle, and inferior) are sectioned and the cerebellum removed. The dorsal roots provide input into the spinal cord, and the cranial nerves provide input into and receive output from the brainstem. The fourth nerve (trochlear) is the only cranial nerve to exit dorsally from the brainstem. The tubercles and trigones on the floor of the fourth ventricle are named for nuclei just beneath them. The superior and inferior colliculi form the dorsal surface of the midbrain, and the medial and lateral geniculate bodies (nuclei), associated with auditory and visual processing, respectively, are shown at the caudalmost region of the diencephalon.

CLINICAL POINT

The **facial colliculus** is an elevation on the floor of the fourth ventricle in the pons under which is located the abducens nucleus (cranial nerve VI) and the axons of the facial nerve nucleus (VII), which arc around the abducens nucleus. A tumor or other lesion on one side of the floor of the fourth ventricle may induce symptoms related to cranial nerves VI and VII, including (1) ipsilateral paralysis of lateral gaze (lateral rectus) and medial gaze (resulting from damage to interneurons of the abducens nucleus, whose axons ascend to the nucleus of CN III via the medial longitudinal fasciculus), and (2) ipsilateral facial palsy resulting from damage to the axons in the genu of the facial nerve.

The **cerebellar peduncles** convey the cerebellar afferent and efferent fibers. The superior peduncle conveys the major efferents to the red nucleus and thalamus (especially the ventrolateral nucleus), whereas the inferior peduncle conveys the major efferents to the vestibular and reticular nuclei. The middle peduncle conveys the corticopontocerebellar fibers. Afferents enter the cerebellum especially through the inferior peduncle but also through the superior peduncle. Damage to the lateral hemisphere of the cerebellum or its associated peduncles results in ipsilateral symptoms, including limb ataxia, mild hypotonia, dysmetria (misjudgment of distance), decomposition of movement (especially movement involving several joints), intention tremor (with movement), dysdiadochokinesia (inability to perform rapid alternating movements), and inability to dampen movements appropriately (rebound phenomena).

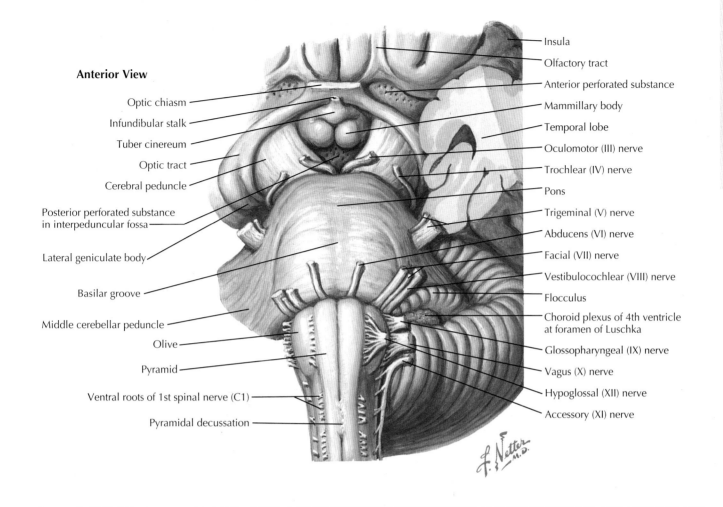

Anterior View

Optic chiasm

Infundibular stalk

Tuber cinereum

Optic tract

Cerebral peduncle

Posterior perforated substance
in interpeduncular fossa

Lateral geniculate body

Basilar groove

Middle cerebellar peduncle

Olive

Pyramid

Ventral roots of 1st spinal nerve (C1)

Pyramidal decussation

Insula

Olfactory tract

Anterior perforated substance

Mammillary body

Temporal lobe

Oculomotor (III) nerve

Trochlear (IV) nerve

Pons

Trigeminal (V) nerve

Abducens (VI) nerve

Facial (VII) nerve

Vestibulocochlear (VIII) nerve

Flocculus

Choroid plexus of 4th ventricle
at foramen of Luschka

Glossopharyngeal (IX) nerve

Vagus (X) nerve

Hypoglossal (XII) nerve

Accessory (XI) nerve

4.2 BRAINSTEM SURFACE ANATOMY: ANTERIOR VIEW

The left temporal lobe is dissected to show the anterior (ventral) surface of the brainstem. The cerebral peduncles, direct caudal extensions of the posterior limbs of the internal capsules, carry corticospinal and corticobulbar fibers from the internal capsule to the spinal cord and brainstem, respectively. The decussation of the pyramids marks the boundary between the caudal medulla and the cervical spinal cord. Cranial nerve XI (accessory) is associated with the lateral margin of the upper cervical spinal cord. Cranial nerves XII (hypoglossal), X (vagus), and IX (glossopharyngeal) emerge from the ventrolateral margin of the medulla. Cranial nerves VI (abducens), VII (facial), and VIII (vestibulocochlear) emerge from the boundary between the medulla and the pons. Cranial nerve V (trigeminal) emerges from the lateral margin of the upper pons. Cranial nerve III (oculomotor) emerges from the interpeduncular fossa in the medial portion of the caudal midbrain. The optic nerve, chiasm, and tract (cranial nerve II) and the olfactory tract (cranial nerve I) are not peripheral nerves; they are central nervous system tracts that were identified as cranial nerves by anatomists in centuries past.

CLINICAL POINT
The **oculomotor nerve (III)** emerges from the ventral surface of the brainstem in the interpeduncular fossa, at the medial edge of the cerebral peduncle. In conditions of increased intracranial pressure in the anterior and middle cranial fossa, such as that caused by a tumor, edema from injury, or other space-occupying lesions, the brainstem can herniate through the tentorium cerebelli, a rigid wing of dura. The resultant transtentorial herniation can compress the third nerve on one side (ipsilateral fixed and dilated pupil resulting from parasympathetic disruption and paralysis of medial gaze resulting from motor fiber disruption) and compress the cerebral peduncle on that same side, resulting in contralateral hemiparesis.

The **medullary pyramids** contain the descending corticospinal tract fibers from the ipsilateral cerebral cortex, particularly from the motor and premotor cortex. The major crossing of the corticospinal tract takes place in the decussation of the pyramids (80%), producing the crossed, descending, lateral corticospinal tract in the spinal cord. An infarct in the upper reaches of the anterior spinal artery or the paramedian branches of the vertebral artery can result in damage to the ipsilateral pyramid (contralateral hemiparesis); to the ipsilateral medial lemniscus (contralateral loss of epicritic somatosensory sensations such as fine, discriminative touch, vibratory sensation, and joint position sense); and the ipsilateral hypoglossal nerve (cranial nerve XII; paralysis of the ipsilateral tongue, which deviates toward the weak side when protruded). This condition is called Dejerine's syndrome. The hemiparesis is not spastic and is characterized by mild loss of tone, loss of fine hand movements, and a plantar extensor response (Babinski's sign). It appears that isolated damage to the pyramids does not result in spasticity. Damage to other descending systems, from either the motor-related cortices or other upper motor neurons in the brainstem, must accompany pyramidal tract damage to produce spasticity. Thus, the term *pyramidal tract syndrome,* when used to describe spastic hemiplegia, is a misnomer and is anatomically incorrect.

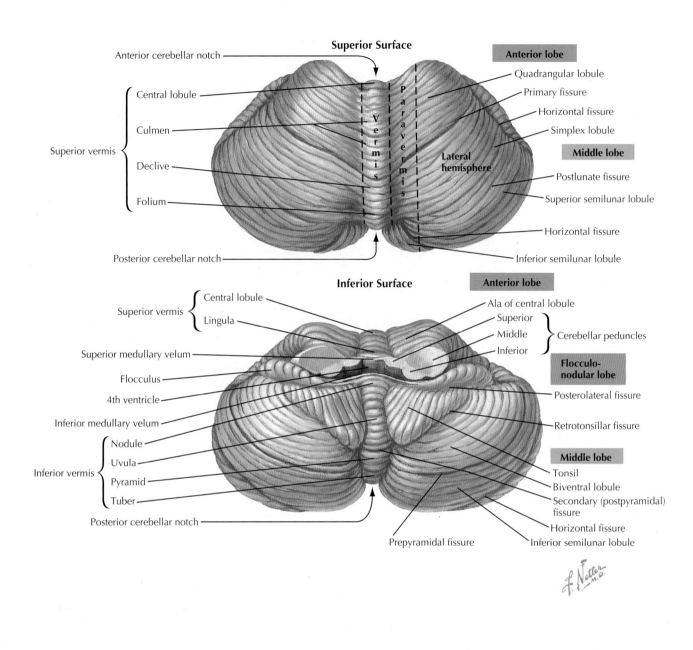

Superior Surface

Anterior cerebellar notch

Central lobule — Superior vermis

Culmen

Declive

Folium

Posterior cerebellar notch

Vermis

Paravermis

Lateral hemisphere

Anterior lobe

Quadrangular lobule

Primary fissure

Horizontal fissure

Simplex lobule

Middle lobe

Postlunate fissure

Superior semilunar lobule

Horizontal fissure

Inferior semilunar lobule

Inferior Surface

Central lobule — Superior vermis

Lingula

Superior medullary velum

Flocculus

4th ventricle

Inferior medullary velum

Nodule

Uvula — Inferior vermis

Pyramid

Tuber

Posterior cerebellar notch

Prepyramidal fissure

Anterior lobe

Ala of central lobule

Superior

Middle — Cerebellar peduncles

Inferior

Flocculo-nodular lobe

Posterolateral fissure

Retrotonsillar fissure

Middle lobe

Tonsil

Biventral lobule

Secondary (postpyramidal) fissure

Horizontal fissure

Inferior semilunar lobule

F. Netter M.D.

4.3 CEREBELLAR ANATOMY: EXTERNAL FEATURES

These color-coded illustrations show the superior (dorsal) surface and the inferior (ventral) surface of the cerebellum. The cerebellar peduncles are cut to provide this view. The ventral surface of the cerebellum is the roof of the fourth ventricle. The anterior, middle, and flocculo-nodular lobes of the cerebellum are traditional anatomic subdivisions with well-described syndromes derived from lesions. The vermis, paravermis, and lateral hemispheres are cerebellar cortical zones that have specific projection relationships with deep cerebellar nuclei (vermis with fastigial nucleus and lateral vestibular nucleus; paravermis with globose and emboliform nuclei; lateral hemispheres with dentate nucleus), which, in turn, provide neuronal feedback to specific upper motor neuronal systems that regulate specific types of motor responses. These relationships are key to understanding how the major upper motor neuronal systems are coordinated for specific functional tasks.

CLINICAL POINT

The **anterior lobe of the cerebellum (paleocerebellum)** receives extensive input from the proprioceptors of the body, particularly the limbs, via the spinocerebellar tracts. This region is particularly important for coordination of the lower limbs. The anterior cerebellum also helps to regulate tone in the limbs via connections to the lateral vestibular nucleus. In some alcoholic patients, the anterior lobe of the cerebellum shows selective cortical degeneration. The patient shows a wide-based stance and gait with some ataxia but little involvement of dysarthria or oculomotor dysfunction. The gait tends to be stiff-legged, probably reflecting disinhibition of the extensor-dominant lateral vestibular nucleus. Typically, heel to shin testing is not severely impaired when the patient is tested while lying down. Few treatment options are available.

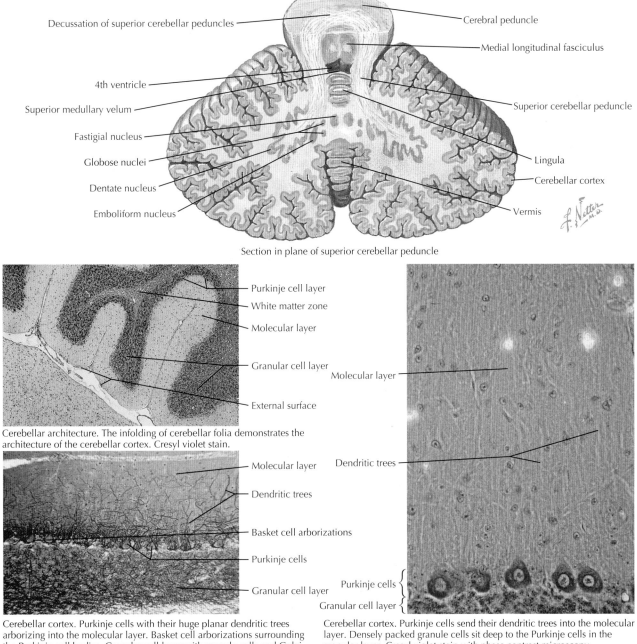

Decussation of superior cerebellar peduncles

Cerebral peduncle

Medial longitudinal fasciculus

4th ventricle

Superior medullary velum

Fastigial nucleus

Superior cerebellar peduncle

Globose nuclei

Dentate nucleus

Lingula

Emboliform nucleus

Cerebellar cortex

Vermis

Section in plane of superior cerebellar peduncle

Purkinje cell layer

White matter zone

Molecular layer

Granular cell layer

External surface

Cerebellar architecture. The infolding of cerebellar folia demonstrates the architecture of the cerebellar cortex. Cresyl violet stain.

Molecular layer

Dendritic trees

Basket cell arborizations

Purkinje cells

Granular cell layer

Cerebellar cortex. Purkinje cells with their huge planar dendritic trees arborizing into the molecular layer. Basket cell arborizations surrounding the Purkinje cell bodies. Granular cell layer with granule cells and Golgi cells. The molecular layer contains outer stellate cells and basket cells. Cajal stain–fiber stain.

Molecular layer

Dendritic trees

Purkinje cells

Granular cell layer

Cerebellar cortex. Purkinje cells send their dendritic trees into the molecular layer. Densely packed granule cells sit deep to the Purkinje cells in the granular layer. Cresyl violet stain with phase contrast microscopy.

4.4 CEREBELLAR ANATOMY: INTERNAL FEATURES

The major internal subdivisions of the cerebellum are shown in this transverse section. The outer zone, the cerebellar cortex (three-layered), is infolded to form numerous folia. Deep to the folia is the white matter, carrying afferent and efferent fibers associated with the cerebellar cortex. Deep to the white matter are the deep cerebellar nuclei, cell groups that receive most of the output from the cerebellar cortex via Purkinje cell axon projections. The deep cerebellar nuclei also receive collaterals from mossy fiber and climbing fiber inputs to the cerebellum. These direct afferent inputs to the deep nuclei provide a coarse adjustment for their output to upper motor neurons, whereas the loop of afferent input through the cerebellar cortex back to the deep nuclei provides fine adjustments for their output to upper motor neurons. The cerebellar peduncles are interior to the deep nuclei; these massive fiber bundles interconnect the cerebellum with the brainstem and the thalamus.

5

SPINAL CORD

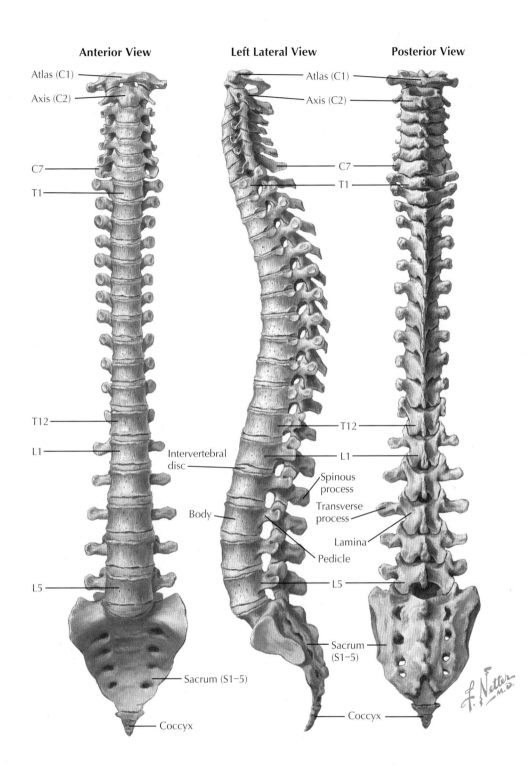

Anterior View

Atlas (C1)
Axis (C2)
C7
T1
T12
L1
L5
Sacrum (S1–5)
Coccyx

Left Lateral View

Atlas (C1)
Axis (C2)
C7
T1
Intervertebral disc
Body
T12
L1
Spinous process
Transverse process
Lamina
Pedicle
L5
Sacrum (S1–5)
Coccyx

Posterior View

Atlas (C1)
Axis (C2)
C7
T1
T12
L1
L5
Sacrum (S1–5)
Coccyx

5.1 SPINAL COLUMN: BONY ANATOMY

Anterior, lateral, and posterior views of the bony spinal column show the relationships of the intervertebral discs with the vertebral bodies. The discs' proximity to the intervertebral foramina provides an anatomical substrate for understanding the possible impingement of a herniated nucleus pulposus on spinal roots. Such impingement can cause excruciating, radiating pain if dorsal roots are involved and can cause loss of motor control of affected muscles if ventral roots are involved. In the adult, the spinal cord extends caudally only as far as the L1 vertebral body, leaving the lumbar cistern (the subarachnoid space) accessible for withdrawal of cerebrospinal fluid.

Anteroposterior Radiograph

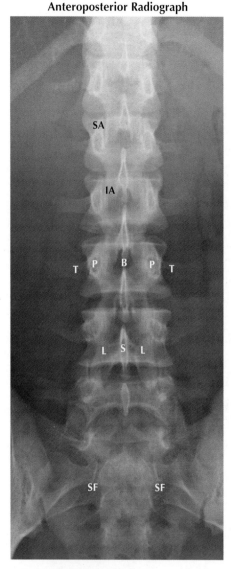

Lateral Radiograph

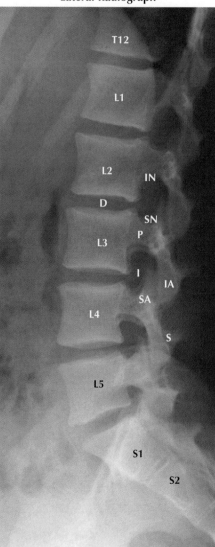

B	Body of L3 vertebra
IA	Inferior articular process of L1 vertebra
L	Lamina of L4 vertebra
P	Pedicle of L3 vertebra
S	Spinous process of L4 vertebra
SA	Superior articular process of L1 vertebra
SF	Sacral foramen
T	Transverse process of L3 vertebra

D	Intervertebral disc space
I	Intervertebral foramen
IA	Inferior articular process of L3 vertebra
IN	Inferior vertebral notch of L2 vertebra
P	Pedicle of L3 vertebra
S	Spinous process of L4 vertebra
SA	Superior articular process of L4 vertebra
SN	Superior vertebral notch of L3 vertebra
Note:	The vertebral bodies are numbered

5.2 LUMBAR VERTEBRAE: RADIOGRAPHY

These lumbar radiographs show the lumbar spine in an antero-posterior view and a lateral view. The vertebral bodies, with their spinous and transverse processes, are visible, and the spaces occupied by the intervertebral discs are uniform and symmetrical in a normal radiograph. A herniated disc may show a disruption of that symmetry. However, the presence of lumbar radiculopathy and a herniated disc is not always accompanied by radiographic abnormalities.

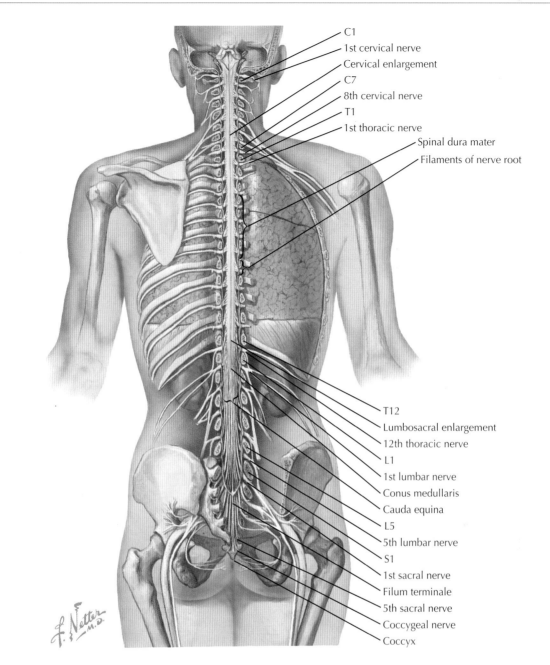

C1
1st cervical nerve
Cervical enlargement
C7
8th cervical nerve
T1
1st thoracic nerve
Spinal dura mater
Filaments of nerve root

T12
Lumbosacral enlargement
12th thoracic nerve
L1
1st lumbar nerve
Conus medullaris
Cauda equina
L5
5th lumbar nerve
S1
1st sacral nerve
Filum terminale
5th sacral nerve
Coccygeal nerve
Coccyx

5.3 SPINAL CORD: GROSS ANATOMY IN SITU

The posterior portions of the vertebrae have been removed to show the posterior (dorsal) surface of the spinal cord. Cervical and lumbosacral enlargements of the spinal cord reflect innervation of the limbs. The spinal cord extends rostrally through the foramen magnum, continuous with the medulla. The conus medullaris is located under the L1 vertebral body. The longitudinal growth of the spinal column exceeds that of the spinal cord, causing the spinal cord to end considerably more rostrally in the adult than in the newborn. The associated nerve roots traverse a considerable distance through the subarachnoid space, particularly more caudally in the lumbar cistern, to reach the appropriate intervertebral foramina of exit. In the lumbar cistern, this collection of nerve roots is called the cauda equina (horse's tail). The lumbar cistern is a large reservoir of subarachnoid space from which cerebrospinal fluid can be withdrawn. The filum terminale helps to anchor the spinal cord caudally to the coccyx.

CLINICAL POINT

In the adult, the spinal cord ends at the level of the L1 vertebral body, and the roots extend caudally in the cauda equina to exit in the appropriate intervertebral foramina. As a consequence, a large **lumbar cistern** is filled with cerebrospinal fluid (CSF); from this cistern, samples can be drawn in a spinal tap with little risk for neurological damage by the needle. Analysis of CSF is a vitally important part of neurological assessment in many conditions, such as infections, bleeds, inflammatory conditions, some degenerative conditions, and other disorders. The CSF is commonly analyzed for color and appearance, viscosity, cytology, and the presence of red and white blood cells, protein, and glucose. It should be noted that in some conditions in which intracranial pressure is elevated, withdrawal of CSF from the lumbar cistern may encourage brainstem herniation through the foramen magnum.

A. Sections through spinal cord at various levels

C5   T2   T8   L1   L3   S1   S3

B. Principal fiber tracts of spinal cord (composite)

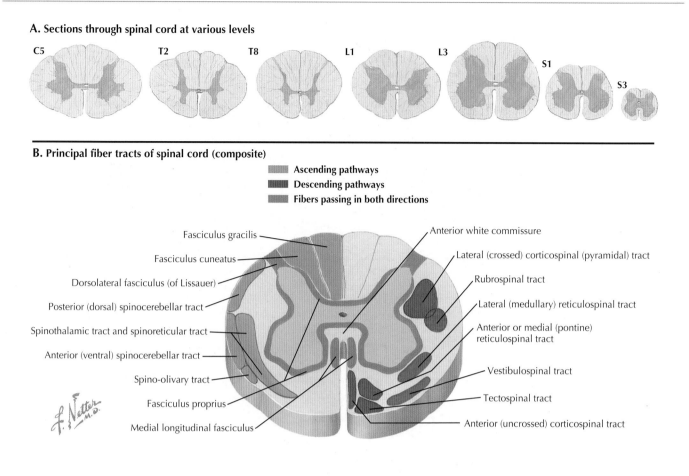

Ascending pathways
Descending pathways
Fibers passing in both directions

Fasciculus gracilis

Fasciculus cuneatus

Dorsolateral fasciculus (of Lissauer)

Posterior (dorsal) spinocerebellar tract

Spinothalamic tract and spinoreticular tract

Anterior (ventral) spinocerebellar tract

Spino-olivary tract

Fasciculus proprius

Medial longitudinal fasciculus

Anterior white commissure

Lateral (crossed) corticospinal (pyramidal) tract

Rubrospinal tract

Lateral (medullary) reticulospinal tract

Anterior or medial (pontine) reticulospinal tract

Vestibulospinal tract

Tectospinal tract

Anterior (uncrossed) corticospinal tract

5.6 SPINAL CORD: WHITE AND GRAY MATTER

A, Seven representative spinal cord levels. The images depict their relative sizes and the variability in the amount of gray matter at each level. Levels associated with the limbs have greater amounts of gray matter. White matter increases in absolute amount from caudal to rostral, reflecting the level-by-level addition of ascending tracts and the termination of descending tracts. **B,** The gray matter consists of dorsal and ventral horns, and in the T1–L2 segments, there is an intermediolateral cell column (lateral horn) where preganglionic sympathetic neurons reside. The white matter is subdivided into dorsal, lateral, and ventral funiculi, each containing multiple tracts (fasciculi, bundles). The tracts conveying pain and temperature information rostrally travel in the anterolateral funiculus, the spinothalamic/spinoreticular system. Fine discriminative sensation is conveyed through the dorsal funiculus. The major descending upper motor neuronal tract, the corticospinal tract, travels mainly in the lateral funiculus, with a component present in the medial part of the anterior funiculus. Dorsal root entry zones and ventral root exit zones are present at each cross-sectional level.

CLINICAL POINT

The spinal cord levels show considerable variation in the size of the dorsal and ventral horns. The cervical and lumbosacral enlargements reflect the large number of sensory, intermediate, and motor neurons necessary for the afferent and efferent innervation of the limbs. The lower motor neurons (LMNs) in these enlargements are particularly vulnerable to poliovirus. **Acute poliomyelitis** results in the death of some LMNs, with resultant denervation of corresponding muscles, atrophy, flaccid paralysis, and loss of tone and reflexes. Remaining LMNs that survive the viral infection may sprout axons to reoccupy the sites on skeletal muscles left denuded by death of their original LMNs. These remaining LMNs then possess larger motor units (innervate more muscle fibers per cell body); this extra burden may account for some of the later degeneration and weakness seen in postpolio syndrome many decades after the acute disease. Polio is unusual in the United States and Western countries because of widespread vaccination programs, but still occurs in some developing nations.

The ascending and descending tracts are clustered in specific zones of the dorsal (posterior), lateral, and ventral (anterior) funiculi. Some regions of these funiculi are selectively vulnerable to vitamin B_{12} (cobalamin) deficiency; impairment of methylmalonyl-CoA mutase results in damage to myelinated fibers. Pernicious anemia may precede neurological symptoms by months or years. Damage involves the dorsal funiculi and components of the lateral funiculi. Dorsal column damage is accompanied by paresthesias of the feet and legs and often of the hands and arms, with sensory ataxia and broad-based gait; by loss of vibratory sensation, joint position sense, and fine discriminatory touch; and by Romberg's sign. Lateral funiculus damage is accompanied by spastic paraparesis with increased tone and muscle stretch reflexes and plantar extensor responses. Early recognition of this condition and treatment with B_{12} can lead to rapid reversal and recovery.

6

VENTRICLES AND THE CEREBROSPINAL FLUID

Ventricles of Brain

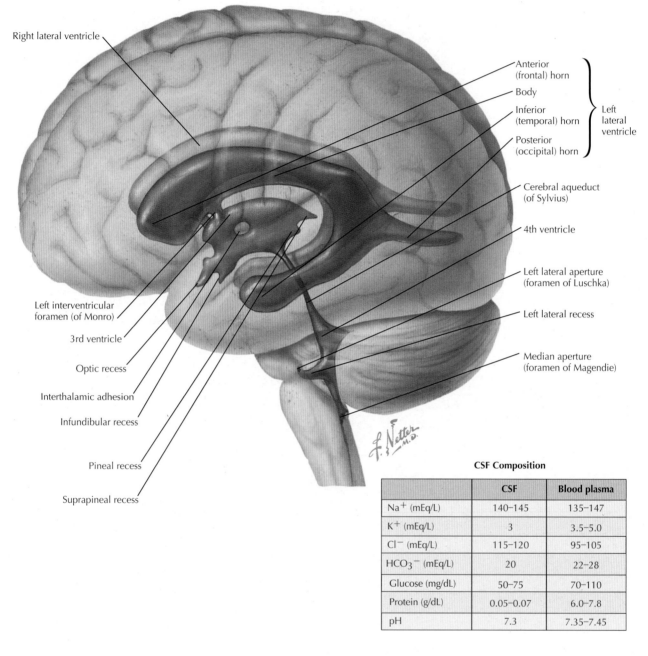

Right lateral ventricle

Anterior (frontal) horn
Body
Inferior (temporal) horn
Posterior (occipital) horn

} Left lateral ventricle

Cerebral aqueduct (of Sylvius)

4th ventricle

Left lateral aperture (foramen of Luschka)

Left lateral recess

Median aperture (foramen of Magendie)

Left interventricular foramen (of Monro)

3rd ventricle

Optic recess

Interthalamic adhesion

Infundibular recess

Pineal recess

Suprapineal recess

CSF Composition

	CSF	Blood plasma
Na$^+$ (mEq/L)	140–145	135–147
K$^+$ (mEq/L)	3	3.5–5.0
Cl$^-$ (mEq/L)	115–120	95–105
HCO$_3$$^-$ (mEq/L)	20	22–28
Glucose (mg/dL)	50–75	70–110
Protein (g/dL)	0.05–0.07	6.0–7.8
pH	7.3	7.35–7.45

6.1 VENTRICULAR ANATOMY

The lateral ventricles are C-shaped, reflecting their association with the developing telencephalon as it sweeps upward, back, and then down and forward as the temporal lobe. The position of the lateral ventricles in relation to the head and body of the caudate nucleus is an important radiological landmark in a variety of conditions, such as hydrocephalus, caudate atrophy in Huntington's disease, and shifting of the midline with a tumor. Cerebrospinal fluid (CSF) flows through the interventricular foramen of Monro into the narrow third ventricle, then into the cerebral aqueduct and the fourth ventricle. Blockage of flow in the aqueduct can precipitate internal hydrocephalus, with swelling of the ventricles rostral to the site of blockage. The escape sites where CSF can flow into expanded regions of the subarachnoid space called cisterns are the medial foramen of Magendie and the lateral foramina of Luschka. These foramina are additional sites where blockage of CSF flow can occur. The choroid plexus, extending into the ventricles, produces the CSF. See Videos 6.1 and 6.2.

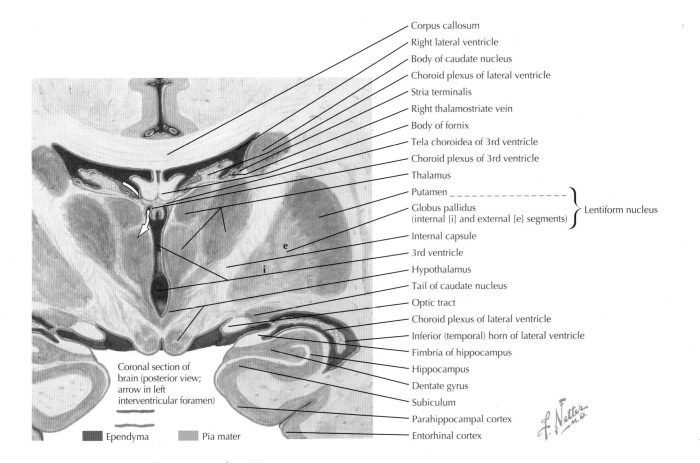

Corpus callosum
Right lateral ventricle
Body of caudate nucleus
Choroid plexus of lateral ventricle
Stria terminalis
Right thalamostriate vein
Body of fornix
Tela choroidea of 3rd ventricle
Choroid plexus of 3rd ventricle
Thalamus
Putamen
Globus pallidus
(internal [i] and external [e] segments)
}Lentiform nucleus
Internal capsule
3rd ventricle
Hypothalamus
Tail of caudate nucleus
Optic tract
Choroid plexus of lateral ventricle
Inferior (temporal) horn of lateral ventricle
Fimbria of hippocampus
Hippocampus
Dentate gyrus
Subiculum
Parahippocampal cortex
Entorhinal cortex

Coronal section of
brain (posterior view;
arrow in left
interventricular foramen)

■ Ependyma　　■ Pia mater

6.2 VENTRICULAR ANATOMY IN CORONAL FOREBRAIN SECTION

A coronal section through the diencephalon shows the bodies of the lateral ventricles, the narrow interventricular foramina of Munro, and the midline third ventricle. The flow of CSF is from the lateral ventricles into the third ventricle. The choroid plexus protrudes into both the lateral and third ventricles and produces CSF. The temporal (inferior) pole of the lateral ventricle and its associated choroid plexus are shown in the temporal lobe.

Posterior View

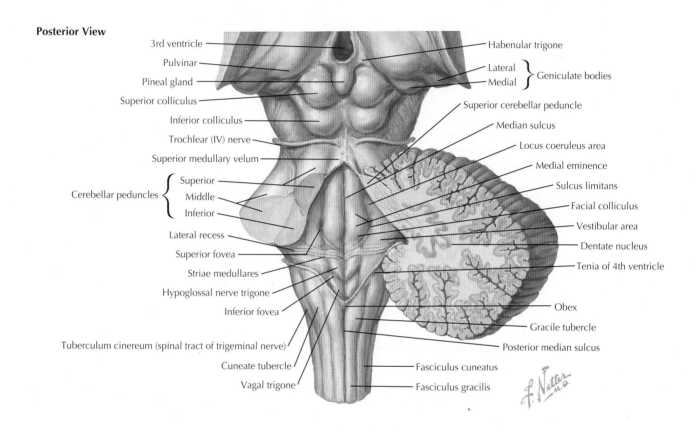

3rd ventricle

Pulvinar

Pineal gland

Superior colliculus

Inferior colliculus

Trochlear (IV) nerve

Superior medullary velum

Cerebellar peduncles { Superior / Middle / Inferior }

Lateral recess

Superior fovea

Striae medullares

Hypoglossal nerve trigone

Inferior fovea

Tuberculum cinereum (spinal tract of trigeminal nerve)

Cuneate tubercle

Vagal trigone

Habenular trigone

Lateral / Medial } Geniculate bodies

Superior cerebellar peduncle

Median sulcus

Locus coeruleus area

Medial eminence

Sulcus limitans

Facial colliculus

Vestibular area

Dentate nucleus

Tenia of 4th ventricle

Obex

Gracile tubercle

Posterior median sulcus

Fasciculus cuneatus

Fasciculus gracilis

6.3 ANATOMY OF THE FOURTH VENTRICLE: POSTERIOR VIEW WITH CEREBELLUM REMOVED

The rhomboid-shaped fourth ventricle extends through the pons and medulla. The foramina of Magendie and Luschka must remain patent for proper flow of the CSF into the cisterns. Bilaterally symmetrical protrusions, depressions, and sulci on the floor of the fourth ventricle define the underlying anatomy of brainstem regions, such as the hypoglossal, vagal, and vestibular areas. Vital brainstem centers for cardiovascular, respiratory, and metabolic functions just below the floor of the fourth ventricle can be damaged by tumors in the region. The lateral margins of the fourth ventricle are embraced by the huge cerebellar peduncles interconnecting the cerebellum with the brainstem and diencephalon. These anatomical relationships are important when interpreting imaging studies in the compact brainstem regions where the diagnosis of tumors and vascular lesions is challenging.

Median Sagittal Section

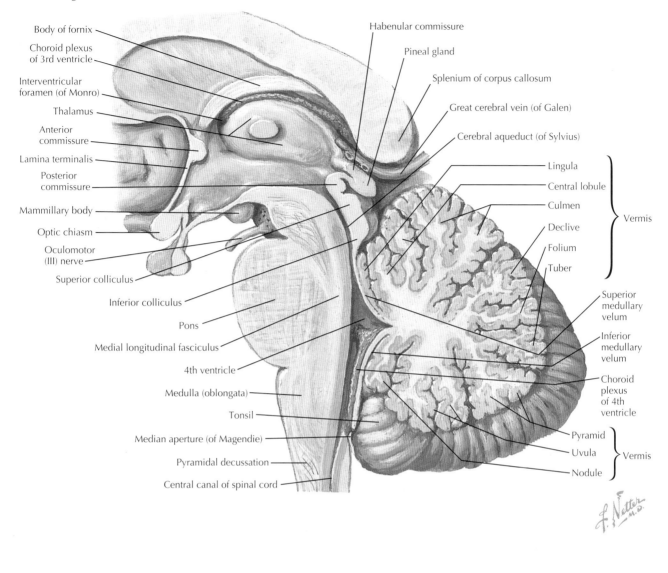

6.4 **ANATOMY OF THE FOURTH VENTRICLE: LATERAL VIEW**

In a midsagittal section, the rhomboid shape of the fourth ventricle is shown. Rostrally, the narrow cerebral aqueduct leads into the fourth ventricle; caudally, the foramen of Magendie provides for escape of CSF into a cistern of the subarachnoid space. CSF normally does not flow through the central canal of the spinal cord. The dorsal surface of the brainstem is on the floor of the fourth ventricle, the cerebral peduncles form the lateral boundaries, and the medullary velum and cerebellum form the roof of the fourth ventricle. The choroid plexus is present in the fourth ventricle. In the diencephalon, the shallow depression of the third ventricle and the interventricular foramen of Munro are shown.

pressure and intracranial pressure. Hydrocephalus is most commonly caused by obstruction of outflow (internal hydrocephalus) or failure of appropriate absorption into the venous sinuses (external hydrocephalus). Occasionally, alterations in CSF production by the choroid plexus may occur. Inflammation of the choroid plexus or a papilloma can lead to hypersecretion hydrocephalus. In contrast, damage to the choroid plexus by radiation, trauma, or meningitis or secondary to lumbar puncture may result in diminished CSF production (hypoliquorrhea), with resultant long-lasting and persistent headache that is responsive to change in posture.

The CSF escapes from the ventricular system from the medial foramen of Magendie and the lateral foramina of Luschka of the fourth ventricle. These apertures must remain unobstructed in order to allow CSF to escape into the subarachnoid space, bathe the CNS, and then be absorbed into the venous sinuses through the arachnoid granulations. The foramen of Magendie is the most important of these apertures; it may become obstructed by tonsillar herniation into the foramen magnum as the result of Arnold-Chiari malformation; by a cerebellar tumor; or by an intraventricular tumor that obstructs the lower portion of the fourth ventricle. Such an obstruction at this lower level results in expansion of the entire ventricular system, including the fourth, third, and lateral ventricles.

CLINICAL POINT

The choroid plexus is the site of production of **CSF in the lateral, third, and fourth ventricles**. Even subtle changes in equilibrium between CSF production and absorption can result in altered intraventricular

A. Clinical appearance
in advanced hydrocephalus

B. Section through brain showing marked dilation of lateral and 3rd ventricles

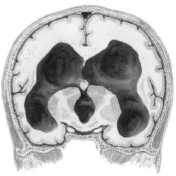

C. Potential lesion sites in obstructive hydrocephalus

1. Interventricular foramina (of Monro)
2. Cerebral aqueduct (of Sylvius)
3. Lateral apertures (of Luschka)
4. Median aperture (of Magendie)

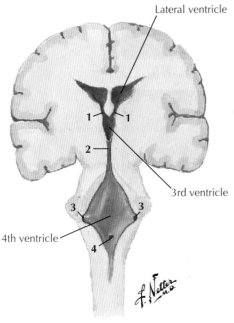

Lateral ventricle

3rd ventricle

4th ventricle

D. Shunt procedure for hydrocephalus

Cannula inserted into anterior horn
of lateral ventricle through trephine
hole in skull

Reservoir at end of cannula implanted
beneath galea permits transcutaneous
needle puncture for withdrawal of
CSF or introduction of antibiotic
medication or dye to test
patency of shunt

One-way, pressure-regulated valve
placed subcutaneously to prevent
reflux of blood or peritoneal fluid
and control CSF pressure

Drainage tube may be introduced into
internal jugular vein and then
into right atrium via neck incision,
or may be continued subcutaneously
to abdomen

Drainage tube is most often introduced
into peritoneal cavity, with extra length to
allow for growth of child

E. Head measurement is of
value in diagnosis, especially in
early cases, and serial measurements will indicate
progression or arrest of hydrocephalus

6.7 HYDROCEPHALUS AND SHUNTING OF THE CEREBROSPINAL FLUID

Hydrocephalus presents as enlargement of the ventricles and increased intracranial pressure. In infants, whose cranial bones have not fused, head size may enlarge, with bulging fontanelles (**A**). Hydrocephalus due to obstruction, which blocks outflow of the CSF and produces enlarged ventricles above the site of obstruction (**B**). **C** shows potential lesion sites in obstructive hydrocephalus. Nonobstructive hydrocephalus occurs because of diminished absorption of CSF into the venous sinuses via the arachnoid granulations; its etiology may be due to infection (e.g., acute purulent meningitis), hemorrhage (intraventricular or subarachnoid), trauma, or tumor spread. A frequent surgical approach to hydrocephalus is the placement of a shunt, draining CSF into the internal jugular vein or the peritoneal cavity (**D**).

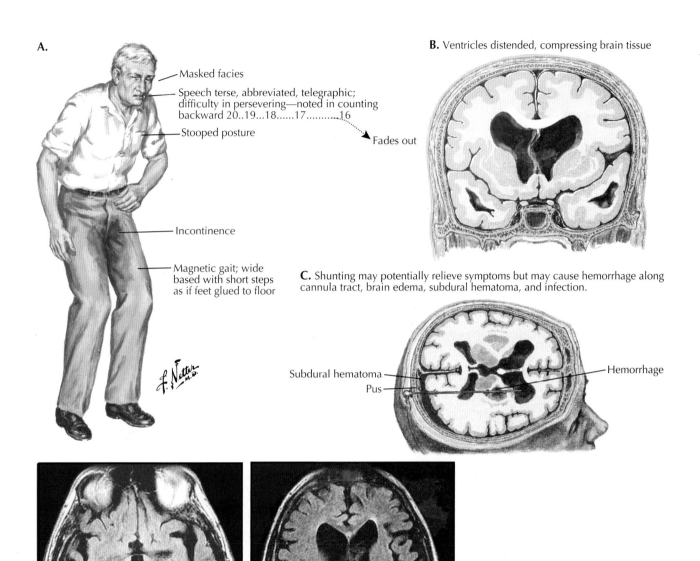

A.

Masked facies

Speech terse, abbreviated, telegraphic; difficulty in persevering—noted in counting backward 20..19...18......17...........16

Stooped posture

Incontinence

Magnetic gait; wide based with short steps as if feet glued to floor

Fades out

B. Ventricles distended, compressing brain tissue

C. Shunting may potentially relieve symptoms but may cause hemorrhage along cannula tract, brain edema, subdural hematoma, and infection.

Subdural hematoma

Pus

Hemorrhage

D. Axial FLAIR images demonstrate moderate enlargement of the third and lateral ventricles, more normal sulcal pattern, and patchy periventricular increased T2 changes.

6.8 NORMAL PRESSURE HYDROCEPHALUS

Normal pressure hydrocephalus is a syndrome in older adults associated with neurological signs and symptoms and enlarged ventricles (**B, C, D**) in the absence of increased intracranial pressure. The increased ventricular size is not attributable to brain atrophy (**B, C, D**). The condition may occur slowly, over the course of a year or more. The enlarged ventricles may compress frontal white matter.

Clinical manifestations of normal pressure hydrocephalus include progressive dementia, stooped posture, "glue-footed gait," and urinary incontinence. Shunting may relieve some of the symptoms but has the risk of infection, bleeds, and brain edema (**C**). The etiology of normal pressure hydrocephalus may be degeneration of arachnoid granulations and diminished CSF absorption.

7

VASCULATURE

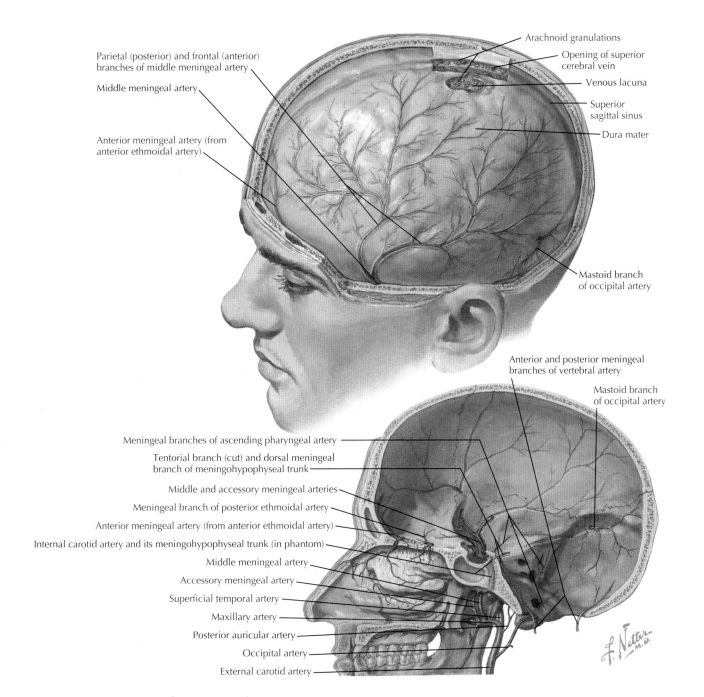

Parietal (posterior) and frontal (anterior) branches of middle meningeal artery

Middle meningeal artery

Anterior meningeal artery (from anterior ethmoidal artery)

Arachnoid granulations

Opening of superior cerebral vein

Venous lacuna

Superior sagittal sinus

Dura mater

Mastoid branch of occipital artery

Anterior and posterior meningeal branches of vertebral artery

Mastoid branch of occipital artery

Meningeal branches of ascending pharyngeal artery

Tentorial branch (cut) and dorsal meningeal branch of meningohypophyseal trunk

Middle and accessory meningeal arteries

Meningeal branch of posterior ethmoidal artery

Anterior meningeal artery (from anterior ethmoidal artery)

Internal carotid artery and its meningohypophyseal trunk (in phantom)

Middle meningeal artery

Accessory meningeal artery

Superficial temporal artery

Maxillary artery

Posterior auricular artery

Occipital artery

External carotid artery

ARTERIAL SYSTEM

7.1 MENINGEAL ARTERIES: RELATIONSHIP TO SKULL AND DURA

Meningeal arteries are found in the outer portion of the dura; they supply it with blood. They also help to supply blood to adjacent skull and have some anastomoses with cerebral arteries. The skull has grooves, or sulci, for the meningeal vessels. This relationship reflects an important functional consequence of skull fractures.

Fractures can rip a meningeal artery (usually the middle meningeal artery) and allow arterial blood to accumulate above the dura. Such an epidural hematoma is a space-occupying mass and can produce increased intracranial pressure and risk for herniation of the brain, particularly across the free edge of the tentorium cerebelli. Even very fine fractures can have this dangerous consequence.

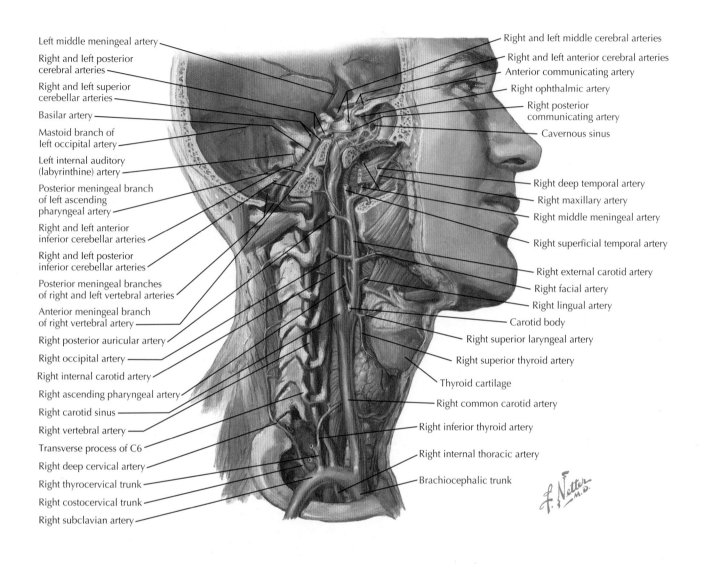

Left middle meningeal artery

Right and left posterior cerebral arteries

Right and left superior cerebellar arteries

Basilar artery

Mastoid branch of left occipital artery

Left internal auditory (labyrinthine) artery

Posterior meningeal branch of left ascending pharyngeal artery

Right and left anterior inferior cerebellar arteries

Right and left posterior inferior cerebellar arteries

Posterior meningeal branches of right and left vertebral arteries

Anterior meningeal branch of right vertebral artery

Right posterior auricular artery

Right occipital artery

Right internal carotid artery

Right ascending pharyngeal artery

Right carotid sinus

Right vertebral artery

Transverse process of C6

Right deep cervical artery

Right thyrocervical trunk

Right costocervical trunk

Right subclavian artery

Right and left middle cerebral arteries

Right and left anterior cerebral arteries

Anterior communicating artery

Right ophthalmic artery

Right posterior communicating artery

Cavernous sinus

Right deep temporal artery

Right maxillary artery

Right middle meningeal artery

Right superficial temporal artery

Right external carotid artery

Right facial artery

Right lingual artery

Carotid body

Right superior laryngeal artery

Right superior thyroid artery

Thyroid cartilage

Right common carotid artery

Right inferior thyroid artery

Right internal thoracic artery

Brachiocephalic trunk

7.2 ARTERIAL SUPPLY TO THE BRAIN AND MENINGES

The internal carotid artery (ICA) and the vertebral artery ascend through the neck and enter the skull to supply the brain with blood. The tortuous bends and sites of branching (such as the bifurcation of the common carotid artery into the internal and external carotids) produce turbulence of blood flow and are sites where atherosclerosis can occur. The bifurcation of the common carotid is particularly vulnerable to plaque formation and occlusion, threatening the major anterior part of the brain with ischemia, which would result in a stroke. The ICA passes through the cavernous sinus, a site where carotid-cavernous fistulae can occur, resulting in damage to the extraocular and trigeminal cranial nerves, which also pass through this sinus. Studies of blood flow through these arteries are important diagnostic tools. Magnetic resonance arteriography and Doppler flow studies have, for most purposes, replaced the older dye studies for performing cerebral angiography.

CLINICAL POINT

The **paired carotid arteries and vertebral arteries** supply the brain and part of the spinal cord with blood. The carotids supply the anterior circulation, including most of the forebrain except for the occipital lobe and inferior surface of the temporal lobe. The bifurcation of the common carotid artery is a common site of plaque formation in atherosclerosis, leading to gradual occlusion of blood flow to the forebrain on the ipsilateral side. Early warnings can be seen in the form of transient ischemic attacks, forerunners of a full-blown stroke. The best treatment is prevention, with exercise, proper diet and weight control, and careful regulation of lipid levels and other contributing factors such as inflammatory mediators. In cases in which severe and symptomatic occlusion has occurred as the result of atherosclerotic plaque, carotid endarterectomy can be performed to remove the plaque and attempt to open up more robust flow to the anterior circulation. Carefully performed controlled studies have established criteria that determine which patients can best benefit from this surgical procedure as opposed to more conservative medical treatment. Current studies are investigating the use of carotid stents to enhance blood flow to the brain.

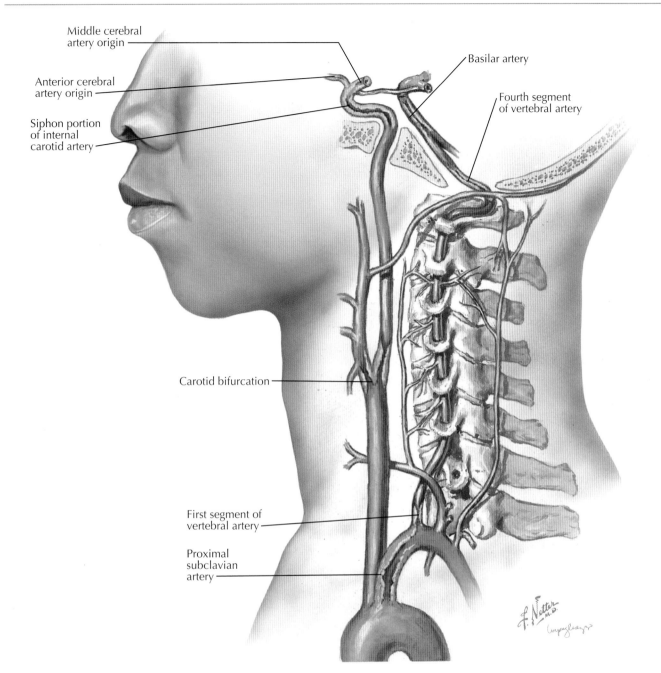

Middle cerebral
artery origin

Anterior cerebral
artery origin

Siphon portion
of internal
carotid artery

Basilar artery

Fourth segment
of vertebral artery

Carotid bifurcation

First segment of
vertebral artery

Proximal
subclavian
artery

7.3 **COMMON SITES OF CEREBROVASCULAR OCCLUSIVE DISEASE**

Atherosclerosis is the most common cause of internal carotid disease, accounting for many cerebral ischemic events, particularly in the elderly. Atherosclerotic plaques are formed by deposition of circulating lipids and the accumulation of fibrous tissue in the subintimal layer of large and medium arteries, exacerbated by the presence of inflammatory mediators and shearing forces from hypertension. Plaque formation particularly occurs at arterial branch points, where turbulence is maximal.

Disruption of the endothelial surface can result in thrombus formation, platelet aggregation, and production of emboli, which are carried upstream into end branches of the vascular system.

In addition to genetic factors, predisposing risks for atherosclerotic plaque formation include smoking, type 2 diabetes, hypertension, and hypercholesterolemia.

Illustrated here are the most common sites for atherosclerosis in the cerebral circulation, including the bifurcation of the common carotid artery and origin of the internal carotid artery, carotid siphon, main stems of the middle and anterior cerebral arteries, proximal subclavian artery, first segment of the vertebral artery, fourth segment of the vertebral artery, and basilar artery.

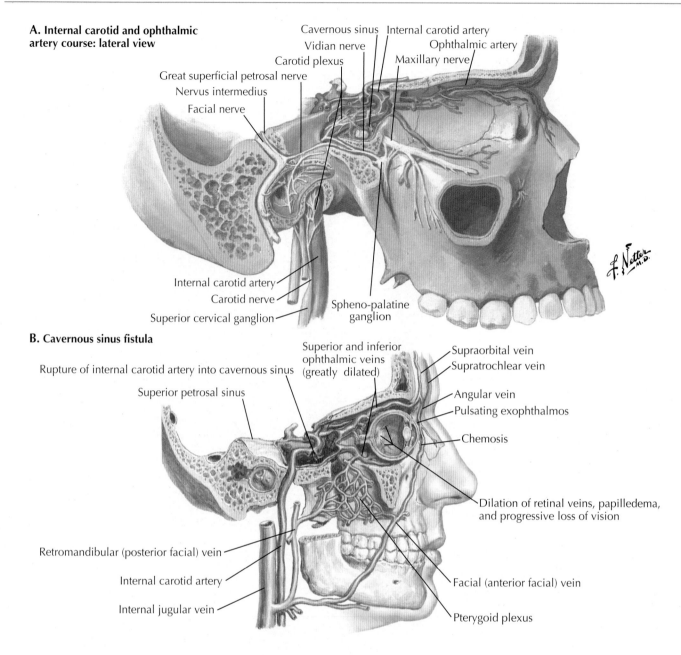

A. Internal carotid and ophthalmic artery course: lateral view

Cavernous sinus   Internal carotid artery
Vidian nerve   Ophthalmic artery
Carotid plexus   Maxillary nerve
Great superficial petrosal nerve
Nervus intermedius
Facial nerve

Internal carotid artery
Carotid nerve
Superior cervical ganglion

Spheno-palatine ganglion

B. Cavernous sinus fistula

Superior and inferior ophthalmic veins (greatly dilated)
Rupture of internal carotid artery into cavernous sinus
Superior petrosal sinus

Supraorbital vein
Supratrochlear vein
Angular vein
Pulsating exophthalmos
Chemosis
Dilation of retinal veins, papilledema, and progressive loss of vision

Retromandibular (posterior facial) vein
Internal carotid artery
Internal jugular vein

Facial (anterior facial) vein
Pterygoid plexus

7.4 INTERNAL CAROTID AND OPHTHALMIC ARTERY COURSE AND CAVERNOUS SINUS FISTULA

The ophthalmic artery is the first major branch of the ICA. It supplies the eyeball, ocular muscles, and adjacent structures with blood. This artery is commonly involved in the first phases of clinical recognition of cerebro-vascular disease. Because of its position as the first branch of the ICA, emboli from atherosclerotic plaques that are found at sites such as the bifurcation of the common carotid artery may travel through the ophthalmic artery, resulting in a transient ischemic attack with the symptom of fleeting blindness (amaurosis fugax) in the affected eye.

The carotid artery may rupture into the cavernous sinus, forming a carotid-cavernous fistula. This occurs mainly from trauma, but also from a ruptured intracavernous aneurysm or an infection. This syndrome is characterized by pulsating exophthalmos from engorged superior and inferior ophthalmic veins, conspicuous diplopia, damage to an extraocular nerve (III, IV, and VI), visual loss from flow changes in the central retinal artery, headache, and chemosis (edema of the conjunctiva). This condition does not resolve spontaneously and requires surgical intervention, usually involving selective occlusion of the fistula with the carotid artery remaining intact.

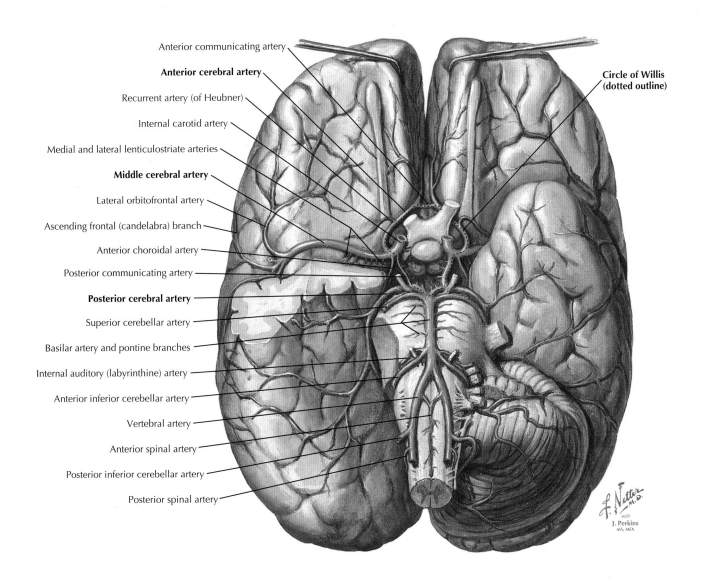

Anterior communicating artery

Anterior cerebral artery

Recurrent artery (of Heubner)

Internal carotid artery

Medial and lateral lenticulostriate arteries

Middle cerebral artery

Lateral orbitofrontal artery

Ascending frontal (candelabra) branch

Anterior choroidal artery

Posterior communicating artery

Posterior cerebral artery

Superior cerebellar artery

Basilar artery and pontine branches

Internal auditory (labyrinthine) artery

Anterior inferior cerebellar artery

Vertebral artery

Anterior spinal artery

Posterior inferior cerebellar artery

Posterior spinal artery

Circle of Willis
(dotted outline)

7.5 ARTERIAL DISTRIBUTION TO THE BRAIN: BASAL VIEW

The anterior circulation (middle and anterior cerebral arteries; MCAs, ACAs) and the posterior circulation (the vertebrobasilar system and its end branch, the posterior cerebral artery; PCA) and their major branches are shown. The right temporal pole is removed to show the course of the MCA through the lateral fissure. The circle of Willis (the paired ACAs, MCAs, and PCAs and the anterior and two posterior communicating arteries) surrounds the basal hypothalamic area. The circle of Willis appears to allow free flow of blood around the anterior and posterior circulation of both sides but usually it is not sufficiently patent to allow bypass of an occluded zone. See Video 7.1.

CLINICAL POINT

The **vertebrobasilar system** supplies blood to the posterior circulation of the brain, including most of the brainstem, part of the diencephalon, and the occipital and inferior temporal lobes of the forebrain. The paired PCAs are the end arteries of the vertebrobasilar system. An infarct in the PCAs (top of the basilar infarct) results in damage to the ipsilateral occipital lobe, including both the upper and lower banks of the calcarine fissure. Functionally, this infarct affecting one side results in contralateral blindness, called contralateral homonymous hemianopia. There may be macular sparing if the MCA has some anastomoses with the posterior cerebral circulation.

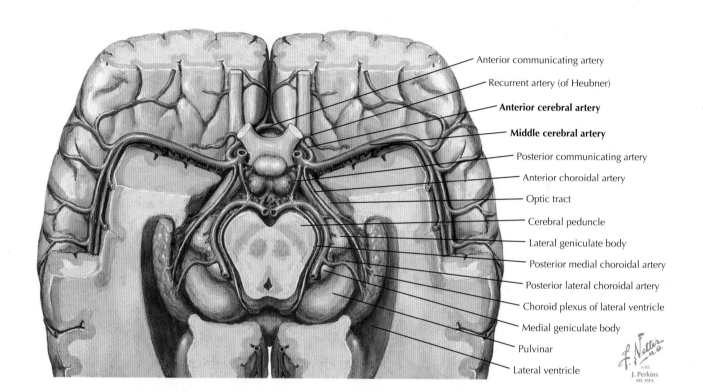

Anterior communicating artery

Recurrent artery (of Heubner)

Anterior cerebral artery

Middle cerebral artery

Posterior communicating artery

Anterior choroidal artery

Optic tract

Cerebral peduncle

Lateral geniculate body

Posterior medial choroidal artery

Posterior lateral choroidal artery

Choroid plexus of lateral ventricle

Medial geniculate body

Pulvinar

Lateral ventricle

7.6 ARTERIAL DISTRIBUTION TO THE BRAIN: CUTAWAY BASAL VIEW SHOWING THE CIRCLE OF WILLIS

The circle of Willis and the course of the choroidal arteries are shown. The arteries supplying the brain are end arteries and do not have sufficient anastomotic channels with other arteries to sustain blood flow in the face of disruption. The occlusion of an artery supplying a specific territory of the brain results in functional damage that affects the performance of structures deprived of adequate blood flow. See Video 7.2.

CLINICAL POINT

Obstruction of the MCA near its origin is relatively unusual compared with obstruction or infarcts in selected branches, but it demonstrates the full range of blood supply of this critical artery. Obstruction near the origin usually results from embolization, not from atherosclerotic or thrombotic lesions. It causes contralateral hemiplegia (resolving to spastic), contralateral central facial palsy (lower face), contralateral hemianesthesia, contralateral homonymous hemianopia, and global aphasia if the left hemisphere is involved. Additional problems with anosognosia (inability to recognize a physical disability), contralateral neglect, and spatial disorientation may occur.

Frontal View with Hemispheres Retracted, Tilted for a View of the Ventral Brainstem

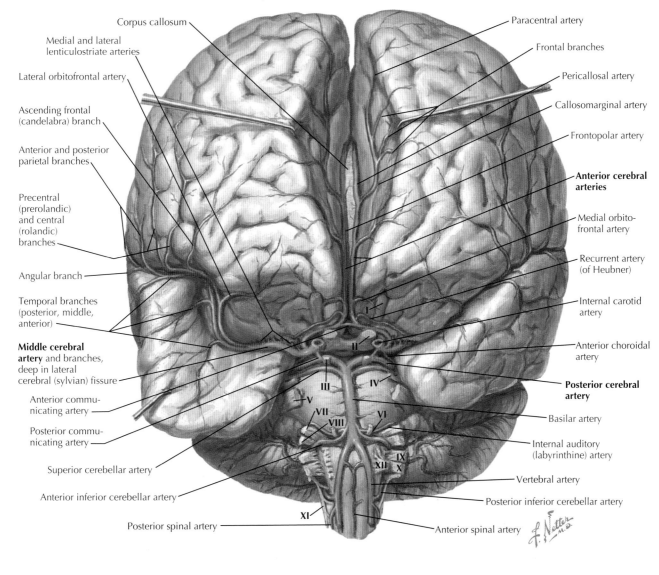

Corpus callosum

Medial and lateral lenticulostriate arteries

Lateral orbitofrontal artery

Ascending frontal (candelabra) branch

Anterior and posterior parietal branches

Precentral (prerolandic) and central (rolandic) branches

Angular branch

Temporal branches (posterior, middle, anterior)

Middle cerebral artery and branches, deep in lateral cerebral (sylvian) fissure

Anterior communicating artery

Posterior communicating artery

Superior cerebellar artery

Anterior inferior cerebellar artery

Posterior spinal artery

Paracentral artery

Frontal branches

Pericallosal artery

Callosomarginal artery

Frontopolar artery

Anterior cerebral arteries

Medial orbito-frontal artery

Recurrent artery (of Heubner)

Internal carotid artery

Anterior choroidal artery

Posterior cerebral artery

Basilar artery

Internal auditory (labyrinthine) artery

Vertebral artery

Posterior inferior cerebellar artery

Anterior spinal artery

7.7 ARTERIAL DISTRIBUTION TO THE BRAIN: FRONTAL VIEW WITH HEMISPHERES RETRACTED

With the hemispheres retracted, the course of the ACAs and their distribution along the midline are visible. This artery supplies blood to the medial zones of the sensory and motor cortex, which are associated with the contralateral lower extremity; an ACA stroke thus affects the contralateral lower limb. With the lateral fissure opened up, the MCA is seen to course laterally and to give branches to the entire convexity of the hemisphere. End-branch infarcts of the MCA affect the contralateral upper extremity and, if on the left, also affect language function. More proximal MCA infarcts affecting the MCA distribution to the internal capsule can cause full contralateral hemiplegia with drooping of the contralateral lower face; this results from damage to corticospinal and other corticomotor fibers traveling in the posterior limb of the internal capsule and damage to corticobulbar fibers traveling in the genu of the internal capsule.

CLINICAL POINT

The **ACA** branches from the internal carotid as it splits from the middle cerebral artery. It supplies a medial strip of the forebrain with blood. ACA occlusion is usually caused by embolization, although an anterior communicating artery aneurysm, vasospasm resulting from a subarachnoid hemorrhage, or subfalcial herniation can occlude this artery. If the ACA is occluded distal to the recurrent artery of Heubner, it results in contralateral spastic paresis and sensory loss in the lower extremity. A more proximal lesion involving the recurrent artery of Heubner may involve the upper body and limb as well. In addition, there may be internal sphincter weakness of the urinary bladder, frontal release signs, and conjugate deviation of the eyes toward the side of the lesion (damage to frontal eye fields with unopposed deviation from the intact side).

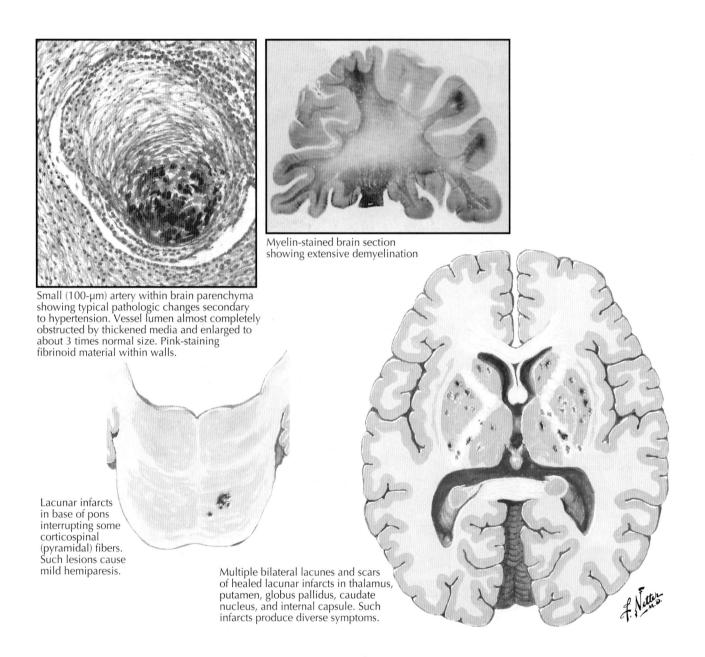

Small (100-μm) artery within brain parenchyma showing typical pathologic changes secondary to hypertension. Vessel lumen almost completely obstructed by thickened media and enlarged to about 3 times normal size. Pink-staining fibrinoid material within walls.

Myelin-stained brain section showing extensive demyelination

Lacunar infarcts in base of pons interrupting some corticospinal (pyramidal) fibers. Such lesions cause mild hemiparesis.

Multiple bilateral lacunes and scars of healed lacunar infarcts in thalamus, putamen, globus pallidus, caudate nucleus, and internal capsule. Such infarcts produce diverse symptoms.

7.10 LACUNAR INFARCTS

Lacunar infarcts are occlusive lesions of small deep arteries, penetrating arteries that arise perpendicular to their main artery of origin. Susceptible arteries include the lenticulostriate penetrating arteries from the middle cerebral artery, branches of the recurrent artery of Heubner (a branch of the anterior cerebral artery), thalamogeniculate branches from the posterior cerebral artery, and penetrating paramedian branches of the basilar artery, especially in the pons. These infarcts are frequently the consequence of hypertension. Lacunar infarcts produce circumscribed areas of ischemic damage of 20 mm or less. The most common sites include the putamen and globus pallidus, the pons, the thalamus, the caudate nucleus, and the internal capsule and corona radiata. Such infarcts do not occur in the cerebral cortex or cerebellum.

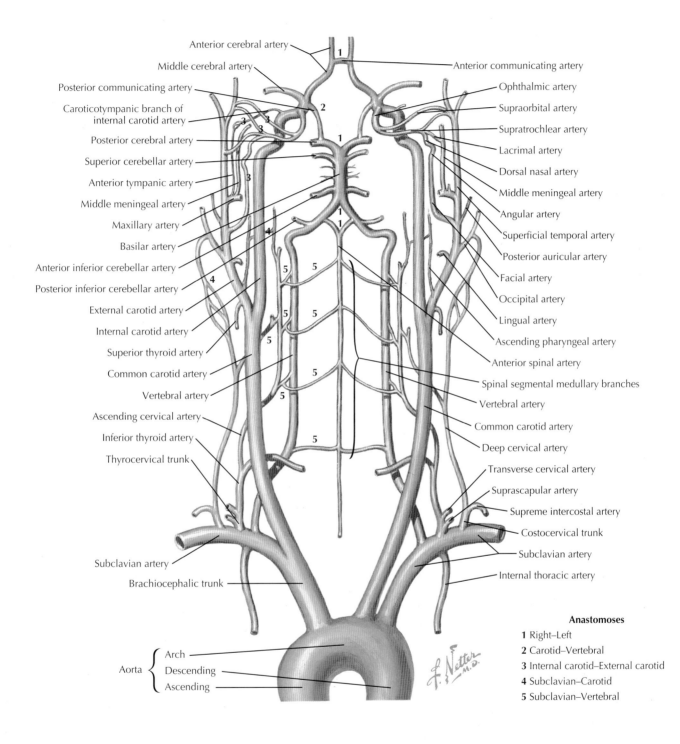

Anterior cerebral artery

Middle cerebral artery

Posterior communicating artery

Caroticotympanic branch of
internal carotid artery

Posterior cerebral artery

Superior cerebellar artery

Anterior tympanic artery

Middle meningeal artery

Maxillary artery

Basilar artery

Anterior inferior cerebellar artery

Posterior inferior cerebellar artery

External carotid artery

Internal carotid artery

Superior thyroid artery

Common carotid artery

Vertebral artery

Ascending cervical artery

Inferior thyroid artery

Thyrocervical trunk

Subclavian artery

Brachiocephalic trunk

Aorta { Arch
Descending
Ascending

Anterior communicating artery

Ophthalmic artery

Supraorbital artery

Supratrochlear artery

Lacrimal artery

Dorsal nasal artery

Middle meningeal artery

Angular artery

Superficial temporal artery

Posterior auricular artery

Facial artery

Occipital artery

Lingual artery

Ascending pharyngeal artery

Anterior spinal artery

Spinal segmental medullary branches

Vertebral artery

Common carotid artery

Deep cervical artery

Transverse cervical artery

Suprascapular artery

Supreme intercostal artery

Costocervical trunk

Subclavian artery

Internal thoracic artery

Anastomoses
1 Right–Left
2 Carotid–Vertebral
3 Internal carotid–External carotid
4 Subclavian–Carotid
5 Subclavian–Vertebral

7.11 SCHEMATIC OF ARTERIES TO THE BRAIN

This schematic diagram shows the entire layout of the arterial blood supply to the brain, including anastomoses. The circle of Willis is present in the upper central portion of this schematic. The relative separation of the anterior (MCA, ACA) and posterior (vertebrobasilar system, PCA) circulation is evident in this diagram. See Videos 7.3 and 7.4.

Vessels Dissected Out: Inferior View

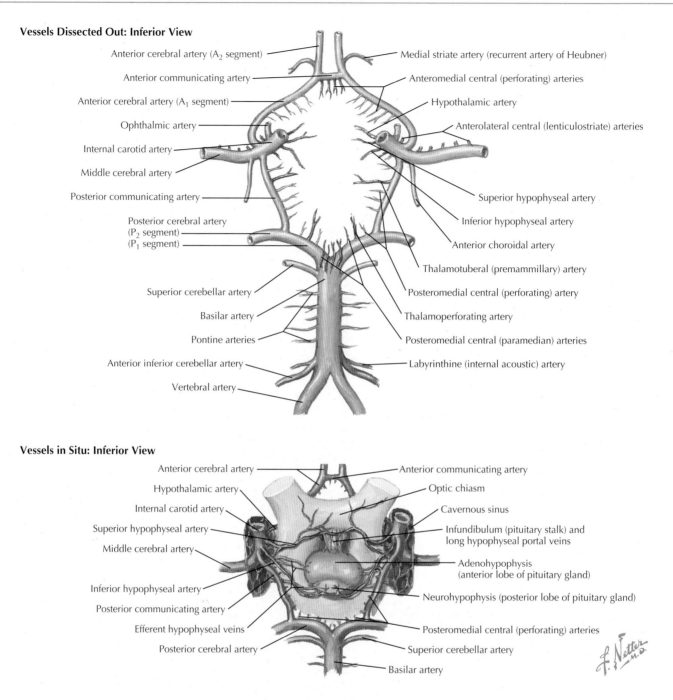

Anterior cerebral artery (A_2 segment)
Anterior communicating artery
Anterior cerebral artery (A_1 segment)
Ophthalmic artery
Internal carotid artery
Middle cerebral artery
Posterior communicating artery
Posterior cerebral artery
(P_2 segment)
(P_1 segment)
Superior cerebellar artery
Basilar artery
Pontine arteries
Anterior inferior cerebellar artery
Vertebral artery

Medial striate artery (recurrent artery of Heubner)
Anteromedial central (perforating) arteries
Hypothalamic artery
Anterolateral central (lenticulostriate) arteries
Superior hypophyseal artery
Inferior hypophyseal artery
Anterior choroidal artery
Thalamotuberal (premammillary) artery
Posteromedial central (perforating) artery
Thalamoperforating artery
Posteromedial central (paramedian) arteries
Labyrinthine (internal acoustic) artery

Vessels in Situ: Inferior View

Anterior cerebral artery
Hypothalamic artery
Internal carotid artery
Superior hypophyseal artery
Middle cerebral artery
Inferior hypophyseal artery
Posterior communicating artery
Efferent hypophyseal veins
Posterior cerebral artery

Anterior communicating artery
Optic chiasm
Cavernous sinus
Infundibulum (pituitary stalk) and
long hypophyseal portal veins
Adenohypophysis
(anterior lobe of pituitary gland)
Neurohypophysis (posterior lobe of pituitary gland)
Posteromedial central (perforating) arteries
Superior cerebellar artery
Basilar artery

7.12 CIRCLE OF WILLIS: SCHEMATIC ILLUSTRATION AND VESSELS IN SITU

The circle of Willis surrounds the optic tracts, pituitary stalk, and basal hypothalamus. It includes the three sets of paired cerebral arteries plus the anterior communicating artery, interconnecting the ACAs, and the posterior communicating arteries, interconnecting the MCAs and PCAs. The free flow of arterial blood through the communicating arteries usually is insufficient to perfuse the brain adequately in the face of an occlusion to a major cerebral artery; the circle of Willis is fully patent and functional for free flow through the communicating arteries in only approximately 20% of individuals. The circle of Willis is the most common site of cerebral aneurysms.

CLINICAL POINT

Saccular, or berry, **aneurysms** account for more than 80% of all intracranial aneurysms; they are outpouchings of cerebral arteries that probably form over a relatively short period of time (days to weeks). The most likely site of these berry aneurysms is at the junctions of arteries in the circle of Willis. Rupture of the aneurysm results in arterial bleeding into the cerebrospinal fluid (**subarachnoid hemorrhage**), which produces an acute, excruciating headache, nausea, vomiting, signs of meningeal irritation, and sometimes loss of consciousness. A sudden subarachnoid hemorrhage may be immediately fatal. Autopsy studies show that most cerebral aneurysms never rupture. Untreated ruptured aneurysms have approximately a one-third likelihood of rebleeding within 2 months, sometimes with fatal results; other sequelae are cerebral infarction and vasospasm of the affected vessel. Treatment sometimes involves clipping the aneurysm or occluding it with coils or balloons.

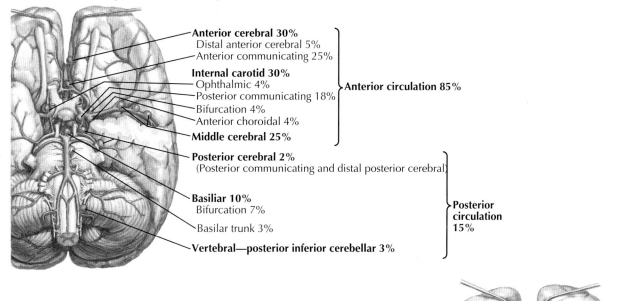

A. Distribution of congenital cerebral aneurysms

Anterior cerebral 30%
Distal anterior cerebral 5%
Anterior communicating 25%

Internal carotid 30%
Ophthalmic 4%
Posterior communicating 18%
Bifurcation 4%
Anterior choroidal 4%

Middle cerebral 25%

⎫ **Anterior circulation 85%**

Posterior cerebral 2%
(Posterior communicating and distal posterior cerebral)

Basiliar 10%
Bifurcation 7%

Basilar trunk 3%

Vertebral—posterior inferior cerebellar 3%

⎫ **Posterior circulation 15%**

B. Aneurysm of middle cerebral artery

C. Aneurysm of anterior cerebral-anterior communicating arteries

D. Aneurysm of posterior inferior cerebellar artery

7.13 INTRACRANIAL ANEURYSMS AND SUBARACHNOID HEMORRHAGE

Saccular (berry) aneurysms are outpouchings of major arteries, often associated with the circle of Willis (85%) or with sites experiencing turbulent blood flow. Many individuals (2–5%) have such aneurysms that never rupture or bleed. The distribution of aneurysms and their clinical manifestations are show in the diagram above.

Ruptured aneurysms are the most common cause of spontaneous subarachnoid hemorrhage. The wall of the berry aneurysm may be thin due to the lack of a second layer of internal elastic lamina, leading to a risk of rupture. An aneurysm may grow in size during adulthood, but the neck of the aneurysm emerging from the parent artery is usually small and does not grow.

Rupture of the aneurysm into the subarachnoid space produces an acute, excruciating headache ("the worst headache of my life"), nausea, vomiting, signs of meningeal irritation, and loss of consciousness. It may be rapidly fatal. Treatment involves clipping the aneurysm to prevent it from bleeding or occluding it with coils or a balloon.

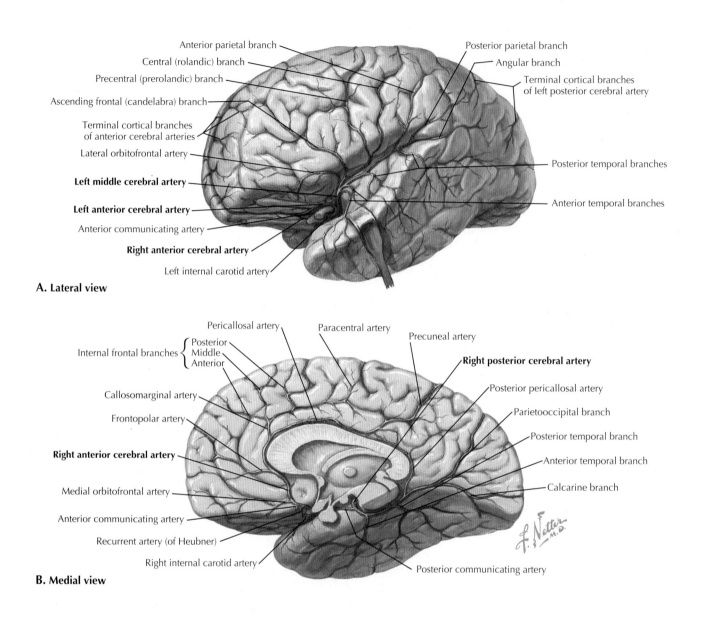

Anterior parietal branch
Central (rolandic) branch
Precentral (prerolandic) branch
Ascending frontal (candelabra) branch
Terminal cortical branches of anterior cerebral arteries
Lateral orbitofrontal artery
Left middle cerebral artery
Left anterior cerebral artery
Anterior communicating artery
Right anterior cerebral artery
Left internal carotid artery

Posterior parietal branch
Angular branch
Terminal cortical branches of left posterior cerebral artery
Posterior temporal branches
Anterior temporal branches

A. Lateral view

Pericallosal artery
Internal frontal branches { Posterior Middle Anterior
Callosomarginal artery
Frontopolar artery
Right anterior cerebral artery
Medial orbitofrontal artery
Anterior communicating artery
Recurrent artery (of Heubner)
Right internal carotid artery

Paracentral artery
Precuneal artery
Right posterior cerebral artery
Posterior pericallosal artery
Parietooccipital branch
Posterior temporal branch
Anterior temporal branch
Calcarine branch
Posterior communicating artery

B. Medial view

7.14 ARTERIAL DISTRIBUTION TO THE BRAIN: LATERAL AND MEDIAL VIEWS

A, The MCA sends named branches along the surface of the hemispheric convexity into the frontal and parietal lobes and into the anterior and middle regions of the temporal lobes. Occlusion disrupts sensory and motor functions in the contralateral body, especially the upper extremity, or in the entire contralateral body if the blood supply to the internal capsule is affected. **B,** The ACA distributes to the midline region of the frontal and parietal lobes. Occlusion disrupts sensory and motor functions in the contralateral lower extremity. The PCA distributes to the occipital lobe and the inferior surface of the temporal lobe. Occlusion disrupts mainly visual functions in the contralateral visual field.

CLINICAL POINT
The **MCA** is a continuation of the ICA, extending through the lateral fissure to supply branches to the convexity of the hemisphere and penetrating branches. Cerebrovascular "strokes" appear in several forms. Approximately one third are atherosclerotic/sclerotic strokes (usually preceded by a transient ischemic attack); about one third are embolic strokes; close to 20% are lacunar (small distal) infarcts; 10% are cerebral hemorrhages; and a small percent are ruptured aneurysms or arteriovenous malformations. **Lacunar infarcts** are small infarcts (between 3 to 4 μm and 2 cm in diameter) in small penetrating vessels supplying the putamen, caudate, internal capsule, thalamus, pons, and cerebral white matter. They occur most commonly as atherosclerosis-related infarcts, particularly in the presence of hypertension or diabetes. Symptoms are determined by which region of the brain is involved; they can include weakness, hemiplegia, contralateral loss of sensation, ataxia, and other symptoms.

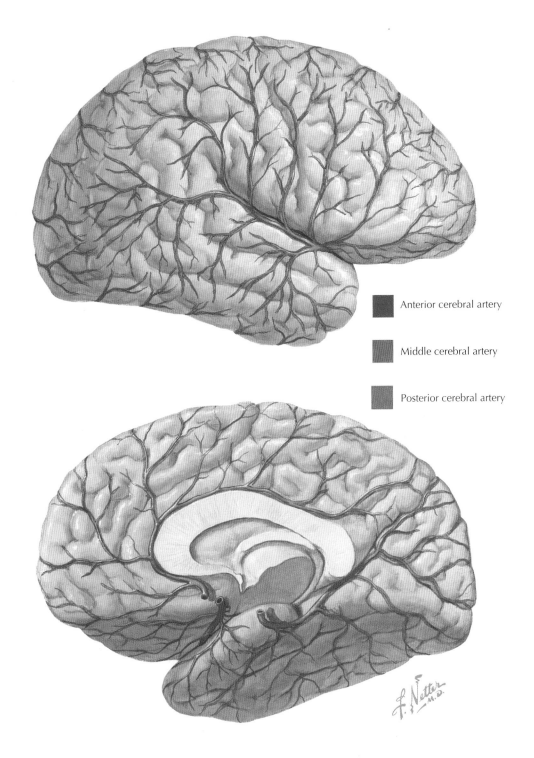

Anterior cerebral artery

Middle cerebral artery

Posterior cerebral artery

7.15 TERRITORIES OF THE CEREBRAL ARTERIES

The specific midline and lateral territories of distribution of the ACA, MCA, and PCA illustrate the exclusive zones supplied by these major arteries and make particularly clear the watershed zones at the junctions of the major cerebral arteries.

Arteries of Posterior Cranial Fossa

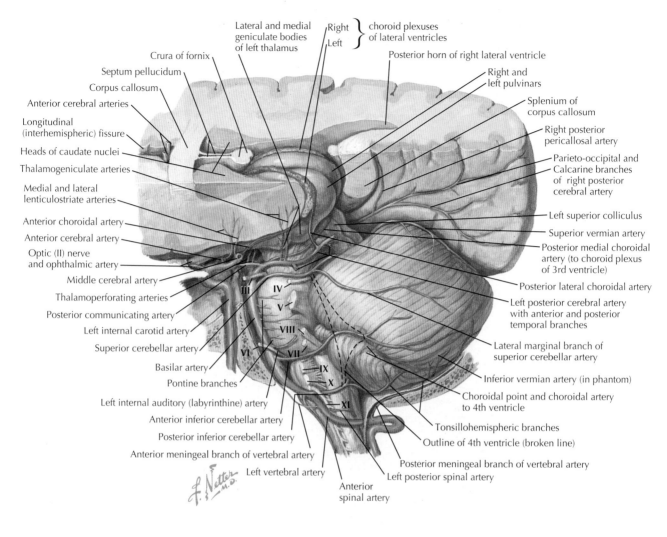

7.18 VERTEBROBASILAR ARTERIAL SYSTEM

The vertebral arteries unite at the midline to form the basilar artery. Medial penetrating branches extend into medial zones of the brainstem, supplying wedgelike territories. Infarcts in these branches can produce "alternating hemiplegias," resulting in contralateral motor deficits (corticospinal system damage above the decussation of the pyramids), and ipsilateral brainstem/cranial nerve signs and symptoms. The vertebral and basilar arteries also give rise to larger short and long circumferential branches, such as the posterior inferior cerebellar artery (PICA), the anterior inferior cerebellar artery (AICA), and the superior cerebellar artery (SCA). Strokes in these arterial territories generally produce a constellation of ipsilateral brainstem sensory, motor, and autonomic symptoms and contralateral somatosensory symptoms. For example, an infarct in the vertebral artery or the PICA can result in loss of pain and temperature sensation on the contralateral body and the ipsilateral face. The end branch of the basilar artery is the PCA, which distributes to the visual cortex and inferior temporal lobe. Occlusion results in contralateral hemianopsia.

CLINICAL POINT

The vertebrobasilar system gives rise to several types of arterial branches. Those located most medially are the **paramedian branches**. An infarct in such a branch commonly involves ipsilateral damage to a cranial nerve and its function as well as contralateral hemiplegia because of involvement of the corticospinal tract before it decussates on its way to the spinal cord. These infarcts are known as alternating hemiplegias. The short and long circumferential arteries distribute into more lateral territories, and infarcts commonly result in a complex mixture of sensory, motor, and autonomic symptoms, as seen in the lateral medullary syndrome resulting from an infarct in the vertebral artery or the PICA on one side.

Arteries of Posterior Cranial Fossa
Vertebral Angiograms: Arterial Phase

A. Lateral projection

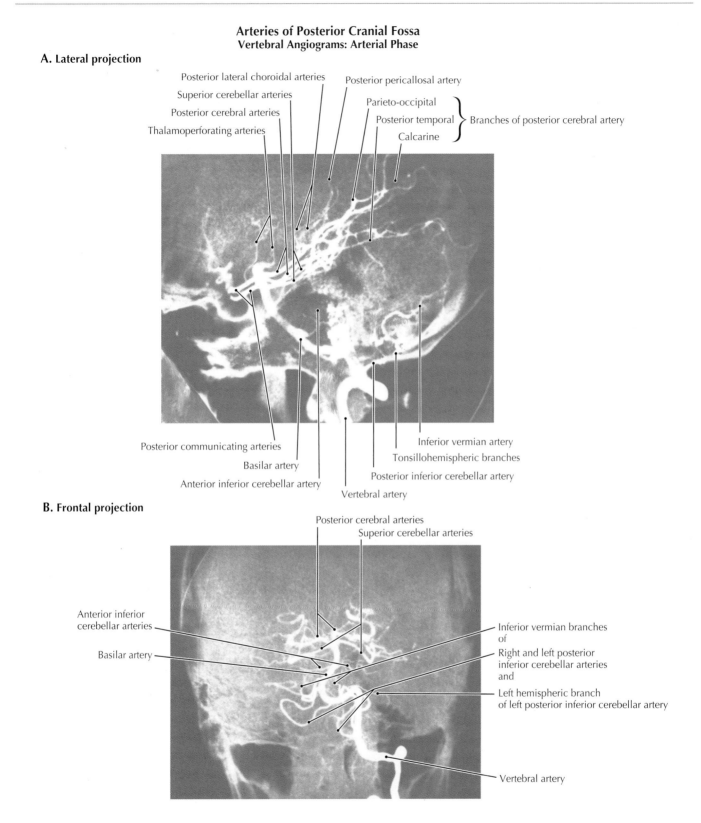

Posterior lateral choroidal arteries

Superior cerebellar arteries

Posterior cerebral arteries

Thalamoperforating arteries

Posterior pericallosal artery

Parieto-occipital

Posterior temporal } Branches of posterior cerebral artery

Calcarine

Posterior communicating arteries

Basilar artery

Anterior inferior cerebellar artery

Vertebral artery

Inferior vermian artery

Tonsillohemispheric branches

Posterior inferior cerebellar artery

B. Frontal projection

Posterior cerebral arteries

Superior cerebellar arteries

Anterior inferior cerebellar arteries

Basilar artery

Inferior vermian branches of

Right and left posterior inferior cerebellar arteries and

Left hemispheric branch of left posterior inferior cerebellar artery

Vertebral artery

7.19 ANGIOGRAPHIC ANATOMY OF THE VERTEBROBASILAR SYSTEM

These figures show angiograms of both lateral and frontal views of the vertebrobasilar (posterior) circulation after injection of a radiopaque contrast agent into the vertebral artery. The major arterial branches of this system are delineated.

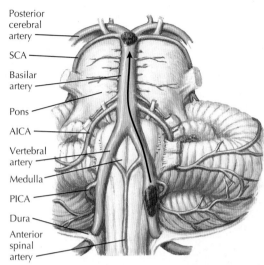

Posterior
cerebral
artery

SCA

Basilar
artery

Pons

AICA

Vertebral
artery

Medulla

PICA

Dura

Anterior
spinal
artery

Internal carotid artery

Middle cerebral artery

Posterior communicating artery

Thalamoperforating arteries
to medial thalamus

Thalamoperforating arteries
to lateral thalamus

Posterior cerebral artery

Superior cerebellar artery

Basilar artery and obstruction

Anterior inferior cerebellar artery

Vertebral artery

Intracranial obstruction of vertebral artery proximal to origin of
posterior inferior cerebellar artery (PICA) may be compensated
by preserved flow from contralateral vertebral artery. If PICA
origin is blocked, lateral medullary syndrome (shown above)
may result. Clot also may extend to block anterior spinal artery
branch, causing hemiplegia, or embolization to basilar
bifurcation may cause "top of basilar" syndrome.

A

C

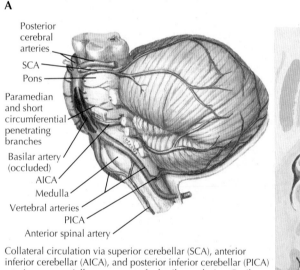

Posterior
cerebral
arteries

SCA

Pons

Paramedian
and short
circumferential
penetrating
branches

Basilar artery
(occluded)

AICA

Medulla

Vertebral arteries

PICA

Anterior spinal artery

Collateral circulation via superior cerebellar (SCA), anterior
inferior cerebellar (AICA), and posterior inferior cerebellar (PICA)
arteries may partially compensate for basilar occlusion. Basilar
artery has paramedian, short circumferential and long circumferential (AICA) and (SCA) penetrating branches. Occlusion of
any or several of these branches may cause pontine infarction.
Occlusion of AICA or PICA may also cause cerebellar infarction.

B

**Areas supplied by posterior
cerebral arteries (blue)
and clinical manifestations
of infarction**

Medial thalamus and midbrain
Hypersomnolence
Small, nonreactive pupils
Bilateral third cranial
 nerve palsy
Behavioral alterations
Hallucinosis

**Lateral thalamus and posterior
limb of internal capsule**
 Hemisensory loss

**Hippocampus and medial
temporal lobes**
 Memory loss

Splenium of corpus callosum
Alexia without agraphia

Calcarine area
Hemianopsia (or bilateral
 blindness if both posterior
 cerebral arteries occluded)

D

7.20 OCCLUSIVE SITES OF THE VERTEBROBASILAR SYSTEM

A, Arteries of the base of the brainstem, illustrating a vertebral
artery/PICA occlusion, and a top of the basilar syndrome. **B,** Arteries of the brainstem in lateral view, showing potential collateral
circulation among paramedian branches and short and long circumferential branches. **C,** Vertebrobasilar arterial system with posterior cerebral artery end branches, illustrating a top of the basilar
occlusion. **D,** The territories of brain supplied by the posterior cerebral arteries and the possible functional consequences of occlusion.

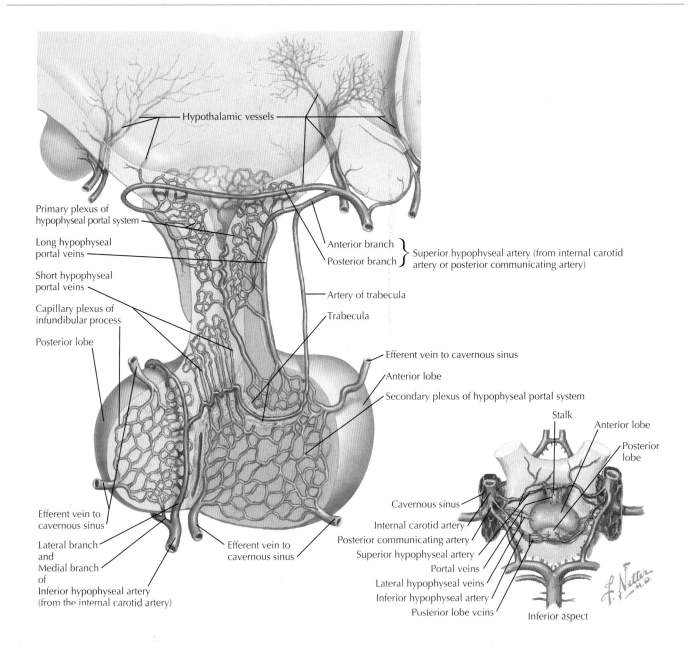

Hypothalamic vessels

Primary plexus of hypophyseal portal system

Long hypophyseal portal veins

Short hypophyseal portal veins

Capillary plexus of infundibular process

Posterior lobe

Efferent vein to cavernous sinus

Lateral branch and Medial branch of Inferior hypophyseal artery (from the internal carotid artery)

Efferent vein to cavernous sinus

Anterior branch
Posterior branch
} Superior hypophyseal artery (from internal carotid artery or posterior communicating artery)

Artery of trabecula

Trabecula

Efferent vein to cavernous sinus

Anterior lobe

Secondary plexus of hypophyseal portal system

Stalk

Anterior lobe

Posterior lobe

Cavernous sinus

Internal carotid artery

Posterior communicating artery

Superior hypophyseal artery

Portal veins

Lateral hypophyseal veins

Inferior hypophyseal artery

Posterior lobe veins

Inferior aspect

7.21 VASCULAR SUPPLY TO THE HYPOTHALAMUS AND THE PITUITARY GLAND

The superior hypophyseal arteries (from the ICA or the posterior communicating artery) supply the hypothalamus and infundibular stalk and anastomose with branches of the inferior hypophyseal artery (from the ICA). A unique aspect of this arterial distribution is the hypophyseal portal system, whose primary plexus derives from small arterioles and capillaries that then send branches into the anterior pituitary gland. This plexus allows neurons producing hypothalamic releasing factors and inhibitory factors to secrete these factors into the hypophyseal portal system, which delivers a very high concentration directly into the secondary plexus in the anterior pituitary. Thus, anterior pituitary cells are bathed in releasing and inhibitory factors in very high concentrations. This private vascular communication channel allows the hypothalamus to exert fine control, both directly and through feedback, over the secretion of anterior pituitary hormones.

CLINICAL POINT

The **primary hypophyseal portal system** coalesces into long hypophyseal portal veins that give rise to a secondary hypophyseal plexus. This arrangement allows the secretion of releasing and inhibitory factors from nerve endings, whose cell bodies are located in the hypothalamus and other structures, into a private vascular portal system, to be delivered to the pituicytes in the anterior pituitary gland in extraordinarily high concentrations. The ultimate CNS control of the releasing and inhibitory factors profoundly influences neuroendocrine secretion and its downstream effects on both target endocrine organs and the entire body. For example, corticotrophin-releasing hormone or factor induces the release of adrenocorticotropic hormone from the anterior pituitary, which is released into the systemic circulation and activates the adrenal cortex to release cortisol and other steroid hormones. This hypothalamo-pituitary-adrenal system helps to regulate glucose metabolism, insulin secretion, immune responses, adipose distribution, and a host of other vital functions. The corticotrophin-releasing hormone neurons are under extensive regulatory control by neural inputs, hormonal feedback, and inflammatory mediators; these neurons help to orchestrate stress reactivity for the organism as a whole.

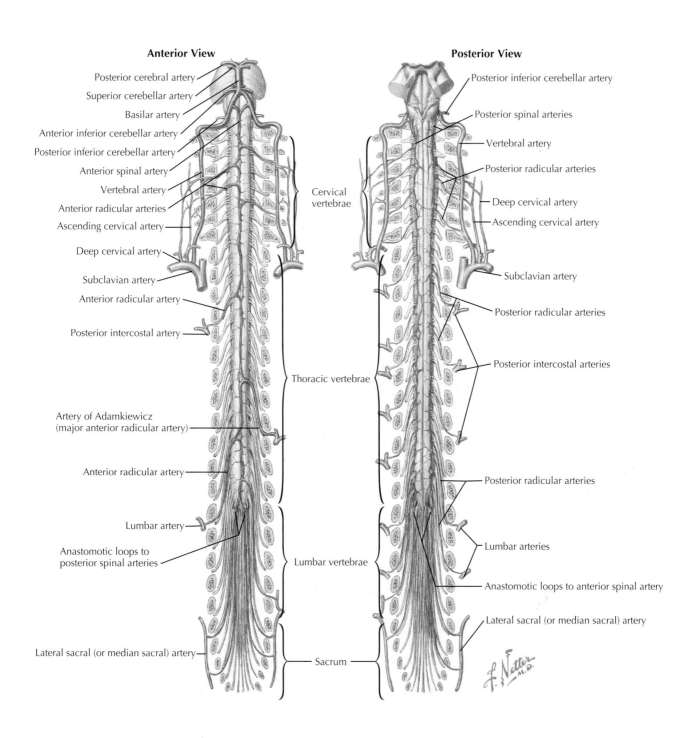

Anterior View

Posterior cerebral artery
Superior cerebellar artery
Basilar artery
Anterior inferior cerebellar artery
Posterior inferior cerebellar artery
Anterior spinal artery
Vertebral artery
Anterior radicular arteries
Ascending cervical artery
Deep cervical artery
Subclavian artery
Anterior radicular artery
Posterior intercostal artery
Artery of Adamkiewicz (major anterior radicular artery)
Anterior radicular artery
Lumbar artery
Anastomotic loops to posterior spinal arteries
Lateral sacral (or median sacral) artery

Cervical vertebrae
Thoracic vertebrae
Lumbar vertebrae
Sacrum

Posterior View

Posterior inferior cerebellar artery
Posterior spinal arteries
Vertebral artery
Posterior radicular arteries
Deep cervical artery
Ascending cervical artery
Subclavian artery
Posterior radicular arteries
Posterior intercostal arteries
Posterior radicular arteries
Lumbar arteries
Anastomotic loops to anterior spinal artery
Lateral sacral (or median sacral) artery

7.22 ARTERIAL BLOOD SUPPLY TO THE SPINAL CORD: LONGITUDINAL VIEW

The major arterial blood supply to the spinal cord derives from the anterior spinal artery and the paired posterior spinal arteries, both branches of the vertebral artery. The actual blood flow through these arteries, derived from the posterior circulation, is inadequate to maintain the spinal cord caudally beyond the cervical segments. Radicular arteries, deriving from the aorta, provide major anastomoses with the anterior and posterior spinal arteries and supplement the blood flow to the spinal cord. The largest of these anterior radicular arteries, often from the L2 region, is the artery of Adamkiewicz. Impaired blood flow through these critical radicular arteries, especially during surgical procedures that involve abrupt disruption of blood flow through the aorta, can result in spinal cord infarct.

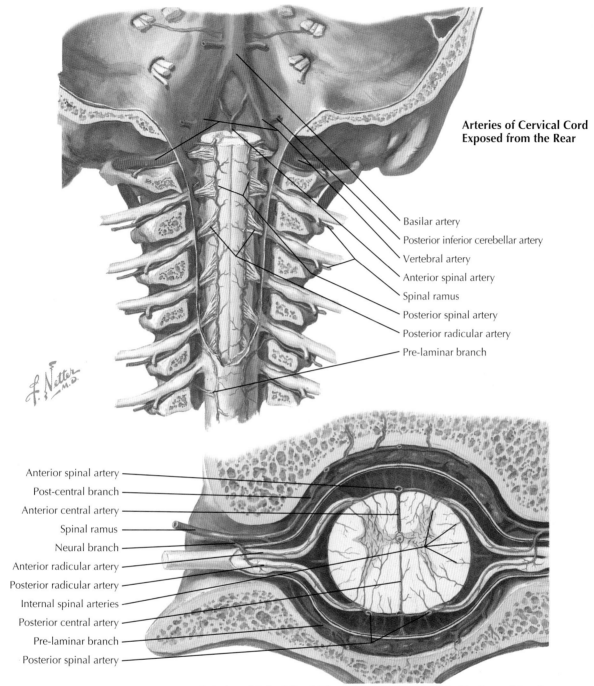

**Arteries of Cervical Cord
Exposed from the Rear**

Basilar artery

Posterior inferior cerebellar artery

Vertebral artery

Anterior spinal artery

Spinal ramus

Posterior spinal artery

Posterior radicular artery

Pre-laminar branch

Anterior spinal artery

Post-central branch

Anterior central artery

Spinal ramus

Neural branch

Anterior radicular artery

Posterior radicular artery

Internal spinal arteries

Posterior central artery

Pre-laminar branch

Posterior spinal artery

Arteries of Spinal Cord Diagrammatically Shown in Horizontal Section

7.23 ANTERIOR AND POSTERIOR SPINAL ARTERIES AND THEIR DISTRIBUTION

The anterior and posterior spinal arteries travel in the subarachnoid space and send branches into the spinal cord. The anterior spinal artery sends alternating branches into the anterior median fissure to supply the anterior two thirds of the spinal cord. Occlusion of one of these branches can result in ipsilateral flaccid paralysis in muscles supplied by the affected segments, ipsilateral spastic paralysis below the affected level (resulting from upper motor neuron axonal damage), and contralateral loss of pain and temperature sensation below the affected level (resulting from damage to the anterolateral spinothalamic/spinoreticular system). The posterior spinal artery branches supply the dorsal third of the spinal cord. Occlusion affects the ipsilateral perception of fine discriminative touch, vibratory sensation, and joint position sense below the level of the lesion (resulting from damage to fasciculi gracilis and cuneatus, the dorsal columns).

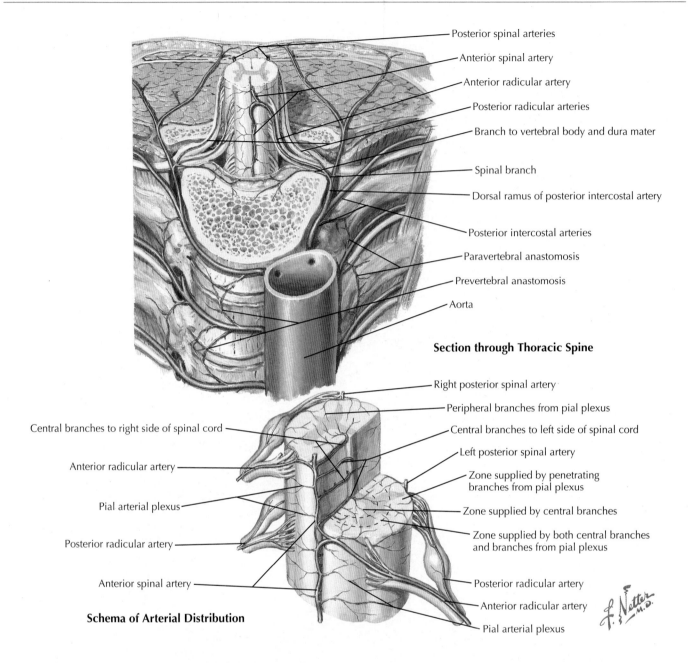

Posterior spinal arteries

Anterior spinal artery

Anterior radicular artery

Posterior radicular arteries

Branch to vertebral body and dura mater

Spinal branch

Dorsal ramus of posterior intercostal artery

Posterior intercostal arteries

Paravertebral anastomosis

Prevertebral anastomosis

Aorta

Section through Thoracic Spine

Right posterior spinal artery

Peripheral branches from pial plexus

Central branches to right side of spinal cord

Central branches to left side of spinal cord

Anterior radicular artery

Left posterior spinal artery

Zone supplied by penetrating branches from pial plexus

Pial arterial plexus

Zone supplied by central branches

Posterior radicular artery

Zone supplied by both central branches and branches from pial plexus

Posterior radicular artery

Anterior radicular artery

Anterior spinal artery

Schema of Arterial Distribution

Pial arterial plexus

7.24 ARTERIAL SUPPLY TO THE SPINAL CORD: CROSS-SECTIONAL VIEW

The major contribution to the arterial blood supply of the spinal cord below the cervical segments derives from the radicular arteries *(top)*. This intercostal blood supply also distributes to adjacent bony and muscular structures. The penetrating vessels supplying the spinal cord derive from central branches of the anterior spinal artery and from a pial plexus of vessels that surround the exterior of the spinal cord.

CLINICAL POINT

Alternating branches arise from the anterior spinal artery into the anterior two thirds of the spinal cord. Following an infarct in the anterior spinal artery, acute radiating leg pain is experienced. Depending on the level of insult, acute flaccid paraparesis or quadraparesis occurs, resolving to spastic paraparesis or quadraparesis with hyperreflexia as the result of the upper motor neuron lesion resulting from damage to the bilateral lateral funiculi. Only at the level of the infarct, where lower motor neurons are lost, does flaccid paralysis remain, along with hyporeflexia. Bilateral plantar extensor responses are seen. Bilateral loss of pain and temperature sensation is seen because of ischemia to the anterolateral territory of the spinothalamic/spinoreticular protopathic system. Descending fibers for control of the bladder and bowel travel in the lateral funiculus and are damaged by an anterior artery infarct. In a lesion of the anterior spinal artery above the T1 level, bilateral damage to descending central sympathetic fibers regulating T1 intermediolateral cell column outflow produces bilateral Horner's syndrome, with bilateral ptosis, myosis, and anhidrosis.

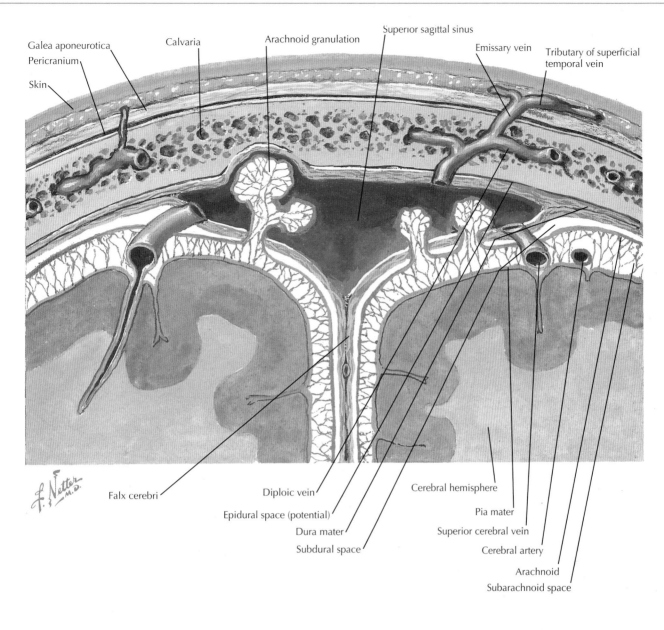

Galea aponeurotica

Pericranium

Skin

Calvaria

Arachnoid granulation

Superior sagittal sinus

Emissary vein

Tributary of superficial temporal vein

Falx cerebri

Diploic vein

Epidural space (potential)

Dura mater

Subdural space

Cerebral hemisphere

Pia mater

Superior cerebral vein

Cerebral artery

Arachnoid

Subarachnoid space

VENOUS SYSTEM

7.25 MENINGES AND SUPERFICIAL CEREBRAL VEINS

The superior sagittal sinus and other dural sinuses receive venous blood from a variety of veins, including superficial cerebral veins draining blood from the cortical surface, meningeal veins draining blood from the meninges, diploic veins draining blood from channels located between the inner and outer tables of the calvaria, and emissary veins, which link the venous sinuses and diploic veins with veins on the surface of the skull. These channels do not have valves and permit free communication between these venous systems and the venous sinuses. This is a significant factor in the possible spread of infections from foci outside the cranium to the venous sinuses. Recent studies demonstrate a lymphatic drainage network for the meningeal system.

CLINICAL POINT

Arachnoid granulations act as one-way valves that convey cerebrospinal fluid into the dural sinus, channeling it back into the venous circulation. The cerebral veins also extend across the subarachnoid space and enter into the superior sagittal sinus. With severe head trauma, these bridging veins can be torn, with resultant venous bleeding into the subdural space; this bleed dissects the dura from the arachnoid and becomes a space-occupying mass. It also brings about cerebral edema and swelling. **Acute subdural hematomas** can be life-threatening, especially in young individuals with head trauma. **Chronic subdural hematomas** often occur in the elderly with relatively minor trauma; the bridging veins tear because of some mild atrophy of the underlying hemisphere, making the course of the bridging veins more extended and more vulnerable to tearing. Slow accumulation of subdural blood eventually can result in increased intracranial pressure with headache, lethargy, confusion, seizures, and focal neurological abnormalities. Surgical drainage is often performed for large subdural hematomas, whereas small hematomas usually regress naturally in the elderly.

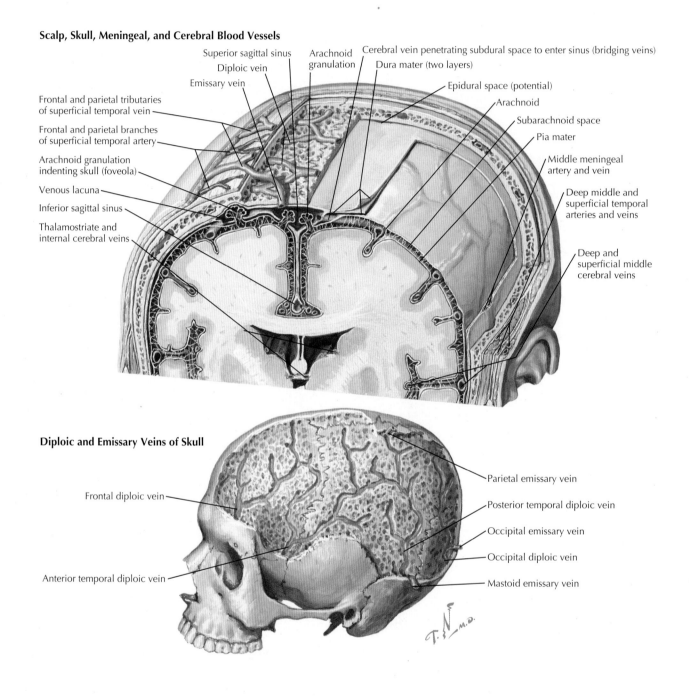

Scalp, Skull, Meningeal, and Cerebral Blood Vessels

Superior sagittal sinus
Diploic vein
Emissary vein
Arachnoid granulation
Cerebral vein penetrating subdural space to enter sinus (bridging veins)
Dura mater (two layers)
Epidural space (potential)
Arachnoid
Subarachnoid space
Pia mater
Middle meningeal artery and vein
Deep middle and superficial temporal arteries and veins
Deep and superficial middle cerebral veins

Frontal and parietal tributaries of superficial temporal vein
Frontal and parietal branches of superficial temporal artery
Arachnoid granulation indenting skull (foveola)
Venous lacuna
Inferior sagittal sinus
Thalamostriate and internal cerebral veins

Diploic and Emissary Veins of Skull

Frontal diploic vein
Anterior temporal diploic vein
Parietal emissary vein
Posterior temporal diploic vein
Occipital emissary vein
Occipital diploic vein
Mastoid emissary vein

7.26 VEINS: SUPERFICIAL CEREBRAL, MENINGEAL, DIPLOIC, AND EMISSARY

Venous blood drains from the skull, the meninges, and the cerebral cortex into the superior sagittal sinus and other dural sinuses. This is a point of vulnerability where potential infections and contamination from the more superficial venous drainage networks can be allowed into the central venous sinus channels.

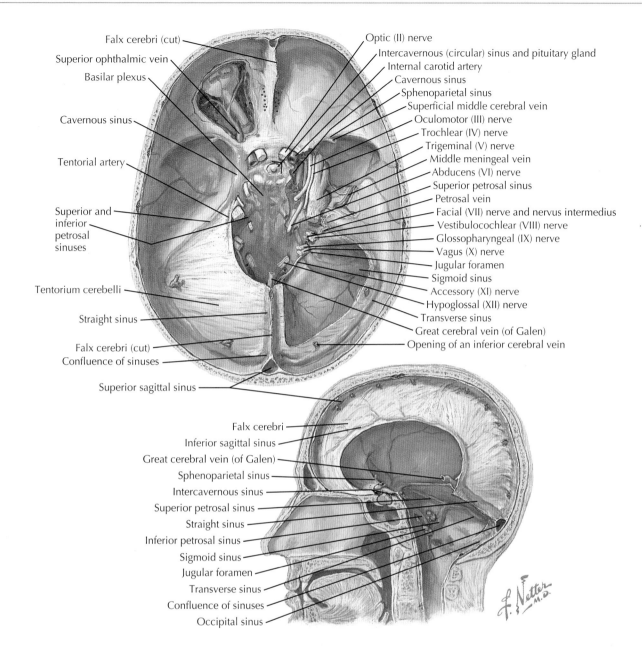

Falx cerebri (cut)
Superior ophthalmic vein
Basilar plexus
Cavernous sinus
Tentorial artery
Superior and inferior petrosal sinuses
Tentorium cerebelli
Straight sinus
Falx cerebri (cut)
Confluence of sinuses
Superior sagittal sinus

Optic (II) nerve
Intercavernous (circular) sinus and pituitary gland
Internal carotid artery
Cavernous sinus
Sphenoparietal sinus
Superficial middle cerebral vein
Oculomotor (III) nerve
Trochlear (IV) nerve
Trigeminal (V) nerve
Middle meningeal vein
Abducens (VI) nerve
Superior petrosal sinus
Petrosal vein
Facial (VII) nerve and nervus intermedius
Vestibulocochlear (VIII) nerve
Glossopharyngeal (IX) nerve
Vagus (X) nerve
Jugular foramen
Sigmoid sinus
Accessory (XI) nerve
Hypoglossal (XII) nerve
Transverse sinus
Great cerebral vein (of Galen)
Opening of an inferior cerebral vein

Falx cerebri
Inferior sagittal sinus
Great cerebral vein (of Galen)
Sphenoparietal sinus
Intercavernous sinus
Superior petrosal sinus
Straight sinus
Inferior petrosal sinus
Sigmoid sinus
Jugular foramen
Transverse sinus
Confluence of sinuses
Occipital sinus

7.27 VENOUS SINUSES

The falx cerebri and tentorium cerebelli, protrusions of fused inner and outer dural membranes, confine the anterior, middle, and posterior fossae of the skull. Outer (superior sagittal) and inner (inferior sagittal) venous channels, found in split layers of the dura, drain blood from the superficial and deep regions of the central nervous system, respectively, into the jugular veins. The great cerebral vein of Galen and the straight sinus merge with the transverse sinus into the confluence of sinuses to drain the deep, more posterior regions of the central nervous system. Infection can be introduced into the cerebral circulation through these sinuses. Venous sinus thrombosis can cause stasis (a backup of the venous pressure), which results in inadequate perfusion of the regions where drainage should occur. The protrusions of dura, such as the tentorium cerebelli and falx cerebri, are tough, rigid membranes through which portions of the brain can herniate when intracranial pressure increases.

CLINICAL POINT

Venous sinus thrombosis commonly occurs with infection. **Cavernous sinus thrombosis** can occur as the result of infection in the paranasal sinuses or middle ear or following a furuncle in the region of the face. Anterior cavernous sinus thrombosis can result in severe pain and headache, ipsilateral visual loss, exophthalmos (protrusion of the eyeball), edema of the eyeball (chemosis), and palsies of the extraocular nerves (III, IV, VI) and V1 (ophthalmic division) that traverse the sinus. This lesion can expand to cause hemiparesis and can involve the interconnected cavernous sinus of the other side, the superior petrosal sinuses, and other venous structures.

The petrosal sinuses can undergo a process of thrombosis caused by the spread of infection in the middle ear. An inferior petrosal sinus thrombosis may cause damage to the VI (abducens) nerve; a superior petrosal sinus thrombosis can result in damage to the semilunar ganglion, producing facial pain. If the transverse sinus is thrombosed, cranial nerve deficits in nerves IX, X, and XI may occur.

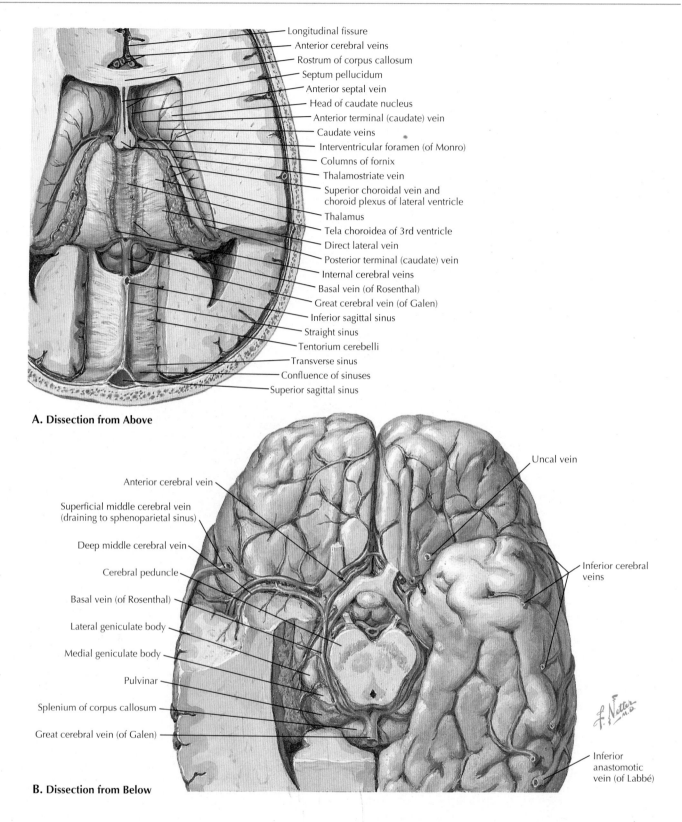

Longitudinal fissure
Anterior cerebral veins
Rostrum of corpus callosum
Septum pellucidum
Anterior septal vein
Head of caudate nucleus
Anterior terminal (caudate) vein
Caudate veins
Interventricular foramen (of Monro)
Columns of fornix
Thalamostriate vein
Superior choroidal vein and choroid plexus of lateral ventricle
Thalamus
Tela choroidea of 3rd ventricle
Direct lateral vein
Posterior terminal (caudate) vein
Internal cerebral veins
Basal vein (of Rosenthal)
Great cerebral vein (of Galen)
Inferior sagittal sinus
Straight sinus
Tentorium cerebelli
Transverse sinus
Confluence of sinuses
Superior sagittal sinus

A. Dissection from Above

Uncal vein

Anterior cerebral vein
Superficial middle cerebral vein (draining to sphenoparietal sinus)
Deep middle cerebral vein
Cerebral peduncle
Basal vein (of Rosenthal)
Lateral geniculate body
Medial geniculate body
Pulvinar
Splenium of corpus callosum
Great cerebral vein (of Galen)

Inferior cerebral veins

Inferior anastomotic vein (of Labbé)

B. Dissection from Below

7.28 DEEP VENOUS DRAINAGE OF THE BRAIN

A, This superior view of the thalamus and basal ganglia reveals the venous drainage of deeper forebrain regions into the posterior venous sinuses. **B,** This basal view of the brain with the brainstem removed illustrates the drainage of forebrain and mesencephalic venous blood into the great cerebral vein of Galen, heading toward the straight sinus.

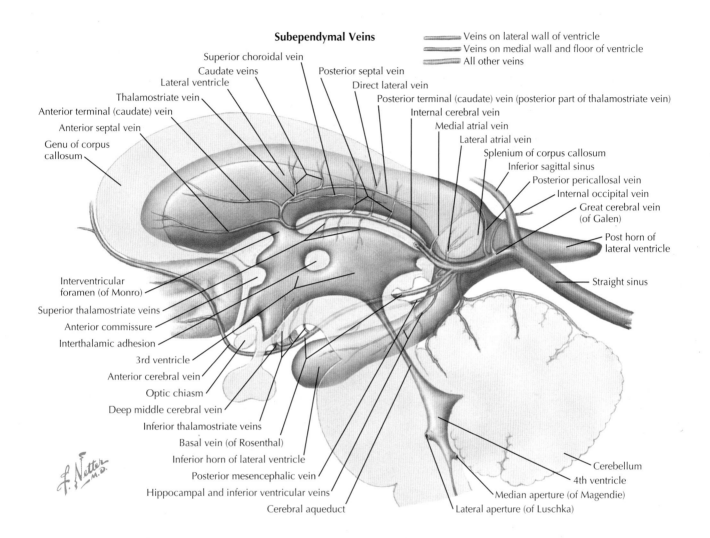

Subependymal Veins

Veins on lateral wall of ventricle
Veins on medial wall and floor of ventricle
All other veins

Superior choroidal vein
Caudate veins
Lateral ventricle
Thalamostriate vein
Anterior terminal (caudate) vein
Anterior septal vein
Genu of corpus callosum
Posterior septal vein
Direct lateral vein
Posterior terminal (caudate) vein (posterior part of thalamostriate vein)
Internal cerebral vein
Medial atrial vein
Lateral atrial vein
Splenium of corpus callosum
Inferior sagittal sinus
Posterior pericallosal vein
Internal occipital vein
Great cerebral vein (of Galen)
Post horn of lateral ventricle
Straight sinus

Interventricular foramen (of Monro)
Superior thalamostriate veins
Anterior commissure
Interthalamic adhesion
3rd ventricle
Anterior cerebral vein
Optic chiasm
Deep middle cerebral vein
Inferior thalamostriate veins
Basal vein (of Rosenthal)
Inferior horn of lateral ventricle
Posterior mesencephalic vein
Hippocampal and inferior ventricular veins
Cerebral aqueduct
Cerebellum
4th ventricle
Median aperture (of Magendie)
Lateral aperture (of Luschka)

7.29 DEEP VENOUS DRAINAGE OF THE BRAIN: RELATIONSHIP TO THE VENTRICLES

Subependymal regions of the central nervous system drain venous blood into the inferior sagittal sinus superiorly or into the great cerebral vein of Galen inferiorly, both of which drain into the straight sinus. Occlusion of a vein in this region causes a blockage of drainage and a backup of perfusion, with resultant ischemia of the tissue in the regions of drainage.

CLINICAL POINT

Venous thrombosis can occur following an infectious process, especially in the nearby sinuses, middle ear, or adjacent facial areas. Noninfectious causes of venous thrombosis include dehydration, cancer, polycythemia vera and other hyperviscosity syndromes, inflammatory conditions, and other disorders. The symptoms vary according to the affected focal territory and the spread of the underlying pathological process; they include severe headache, nausea and vomiting, weakness and sensory losses, sometimes aphasia, and sometimes coma.

Subependymal and Superficial Veins Opacified

A. Lateral projection

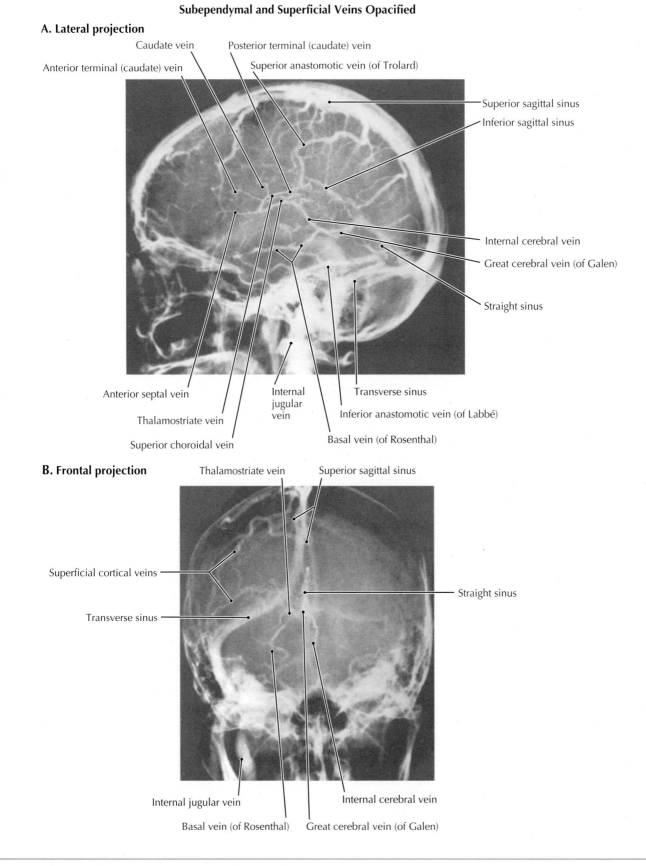

Caudate vein

Posterior terminal (caudate) vein

Anterior terminal (caudate) vein

Superior anastomotic vein (of Trolard)

Superior sagittal sinus

Inferior sagittal sinus

Internal cerebral vein

Great cerebral vein (of Galen)

Straight sinus

Anterior septal vein

Thalamostriate vein

Superior choroidal vein

Internal jugular vein

Transverse sinus

Inferior anastomotic vein (of Labbé)

Basal vein (of Rosenthal)

B. Frontal projection

Thalamostriate vein

Superior sagittal sinus

Superficial cortical veins

Straight sinus

Transverse sinus

Internal jugular vein

Basal vein (of Rosenthal)

Great cerebral vein (of Galen)

Internal cerebral vein

7.30 CAROTID VENOGRAMS: VENOUS PHASE

These lateral and anterior venous-phase angiograms illustrate the superior sagittal sinus, the inferior sagittal sinus, and the great cerebral vein of Galen draining into the straight sinus, the transverse sinus, the basal vein of Rosenthal, and the internal jugular, through which the venous blood of the brain drains back to the heart. See Video 7.5.

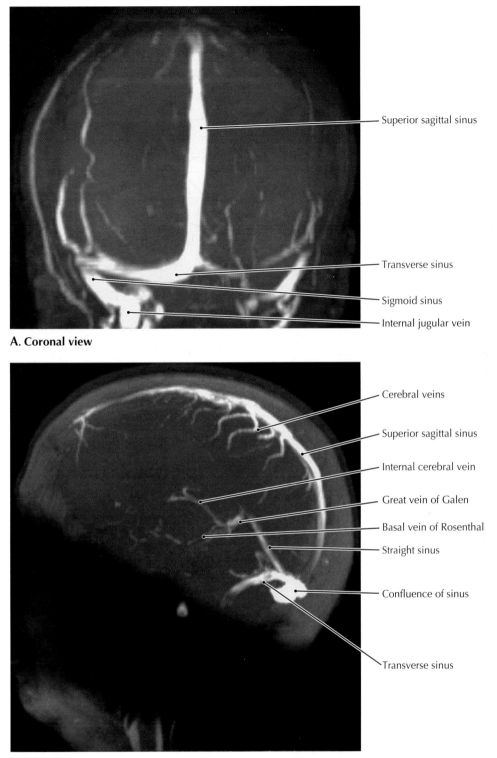

A. Coronal view

— Superior sagittal sinus

— Transverse sinus

— Sigmoid sinus

— Internal jugular vein

— Cerebral veins

— Superior sagittal sinus

— Internal cerebral vein

— Great vein of Galen

— Basal vein of Rosenthal

— Straight sinus

— Confluence of sinus

— Transverse sinus

B. Lateral view

7.31 MAGNETIC RESONANCE VENOGRAPHY: CORONAL AND SAGITTAL VIEWS

Magnetic resonance venography uses the same principles of flow imaging used in MRA (see Fig. 7.16). The flow of venous blood in the brain is relatively slow and steady compared to the flow of arterial blood. Gradient echo sequences are sensitive to flow but are not sensitive to direction of flow. To distinguish arterial flow from venous flow, a presaturation slab must be applied downstream below the heart or upstream above the heart prior to placing imaging slices. In a typical magnetic resonance venography of the head, a saturation slab is placed at the level of the carotid bifurcation, and traveling saturation is placed inferiorly to the slice. Multiple two-dimensional thin slices are placed nearly perpendicular to the vessels. **A,** Coronal view. **B,** Sagittal view. These images illustrate the major cerebral veins and sinuses of the brain. See Video 7.6.

8

DEVELOPMENTAL NEUROSCIENCE

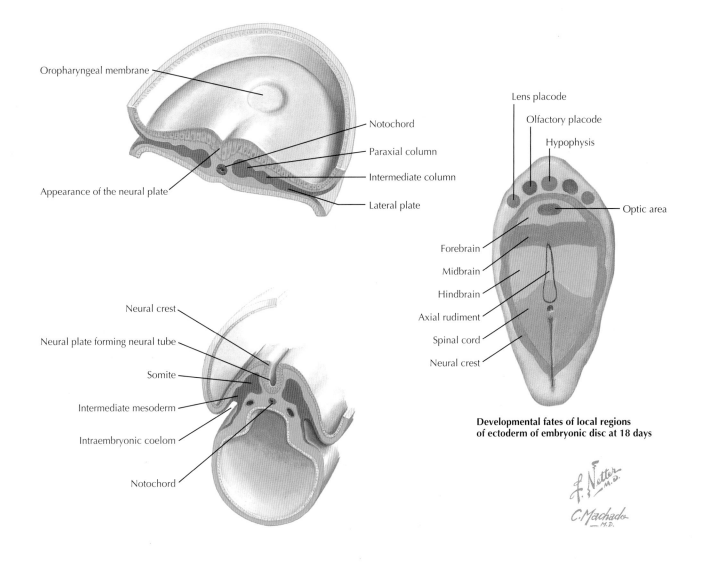

Oropharyngeal membrane

Notochord

Paraxial column

Intermediate column

Lateral plate

Appearance of the neural plate

Neural crest

Neural plate forming neural tube

Somite

Intermediate mesoderm

Intraembryonic coelom

Notochord

Lens placode

Olfactory placode

Hypophysis

Optic area

Forebrain

Midbrain

Hindbrain

Axial rudiment

Spinal cord

Neural crest

**Developmental fates of local regions
of ectoderm of embryonic disc at 18 days**

8.1 FORMATION OF THE NEURAL PLATE, NEURAL TUBE, AND NEURAL CREST

The neural plate, neural tube, and neural crest form at the 18-day stage of embryonic development. The underlying notochord induces the neural plate, and a midline neural groove forms. The elevated lateral margins become the neural folds, tissue destined to become the neural crest with future contributions to many components of the peripheral nervous system (PNS). At this very early stage of embryonic development, these neural precursors are vulnerable to toxic insult and other forms of damage.

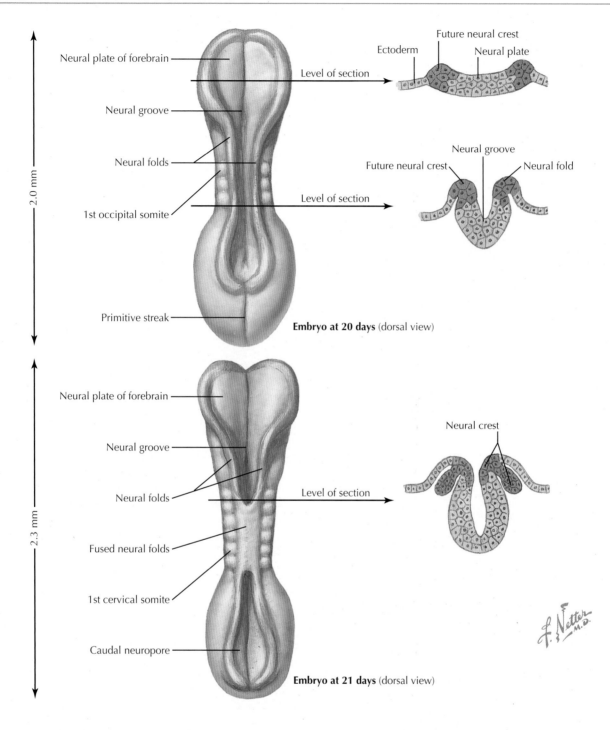

Neural plate of forebrain

Neural groove

Neural folds

1st occipital somite

Primitive streak

2.0 mm

Level of section

Ectoderm — Future neural crest — Neural plate

Level of section

Neural groove — Future neural crest — Neural fold

Embryo at 20 days (dorsal view)

Neural plate of forebrain

Neural groove

Neural folds

Fused neural folds

1st cervical somite

Caudal neuropore

2.3 mm

Level of section

Neural crest

Embryo at 21 days (dorsal view)

8.2 NEURULATION

In the 21- or 22-day-old-embryo, the neural plate, with its midline neural groove, thickens and begins to fold and elevate along either side, allowing the two lateral edges to fuse at the dorsal midline to form the completed neural tube. The central canal, the site of the future development of the ventricular system, is in the center of the neural tube. This process of neurulation continues both caudally and rostrally. Disruption can occur because of failure of full neural tube formation caudally (spina bifida) or rostrally (anencephaly).

CLINICAL POINT
As the neural plate forms into a neural tube, the process of neurulation results in fused neural folds, starting centrally and moving both caudally and rostrally. Failure of the neural tube to close results in dysraphic defects, with altered development of associated muscles, bone, skin, and meninges. If the anterior neuropore fails to form, **anencephaly** results, with failure of the brain to develop, accompanied by facial defects. This condition is lethal. Failure of the posterior (caudal) neuropore to close results in **spina bifida**, with failure of the vertebral arches to fuse. A saccular protrusion from the lumbar region may contain meninges (meningocele) or meninges and spinal cord (meningomyelocele). Meningomyelocele is often accompanied by paraparesis, bowel and bladder dysfunction, sensory disruption at the level of the lesion, motor dysfunction in the lower extremities, and accompanying hydrocephalus or Arnold-Chiari malformation, requiring a ventriculo-peritoneal or ventriculo-jugular shunt.

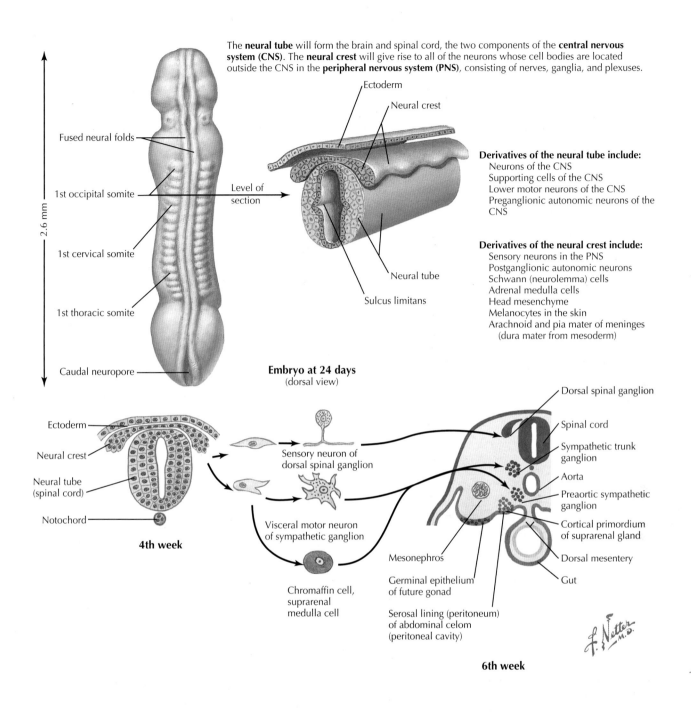

The **neural tube** will form the brain and spinal cord, the two components of the **central nervous system (CNS)**. The **neural crest** will give rise to all of the neurons whose cell bodies are located outside the CNS in the **peripheral nervous system (PNS)**, consisting of nerves, ganglia, and plexuses.

Derivatives of the neural tube include:
Neurons of the CNS
Supporting cells of the CNS
Lower motor neurons of the CNS
Preganglionic autonomic neurons of the CNS

Derivatives of the neural crest include:
Sensory neurons in the PNS
Postganglionic autonomic neurons
Schwann (neurolemma) cells
Adrenal medulla cells
Head mesenchyme
Melanocytes in the skin
Arachnoid and pia mater of meninges
(dura mater from mesoderm)

Embryo at 24 days
(dorsal view)

4th week

6th week

8.3 NEURAL TUBE DEVELOPMENT AND NEURAL CREST FORMATION

The dorsal and ventral halves of the neural tube are separated by the sulcus limitans, an external protrusion from the central canal that demarcates the alar plate above from the basal plate below. This important landmark persists at some sites in the adult ventricular system. The alar plate is the source of generation of many neurons with sensory function. The basal plate is the source of generation of many neurons with motor or autonomic function in the spinal cord and the brainstem. The neural crest cells at the edge of the neural folds unite and become a dorsal crest, with the neural crest above the neural tube. The neural tube and neural crest separate from the originating ectoderm.

CLINICAL POINT

The **neural crest** gives rise to a wide variety of neural elements of the PNS, including primary sensory neurons, postganglionic autonomic neurons, Schwann cells, adrenal medullary chromaffin cells, pia and arachnoid cells, melanocytes, and some mesenchyme of the head. A failure of the neural crest to develop and migrate properly is seen in Hirschsprung's disease (congenital megacolon), in which sensory signals from the colon are absent, and in familial dysautonomia, in which autonomic symptoms (cardiovascular dysfunction, gastrointestinal dysfunction) and sensory deficits (especially pain and temperature sensation) are present.

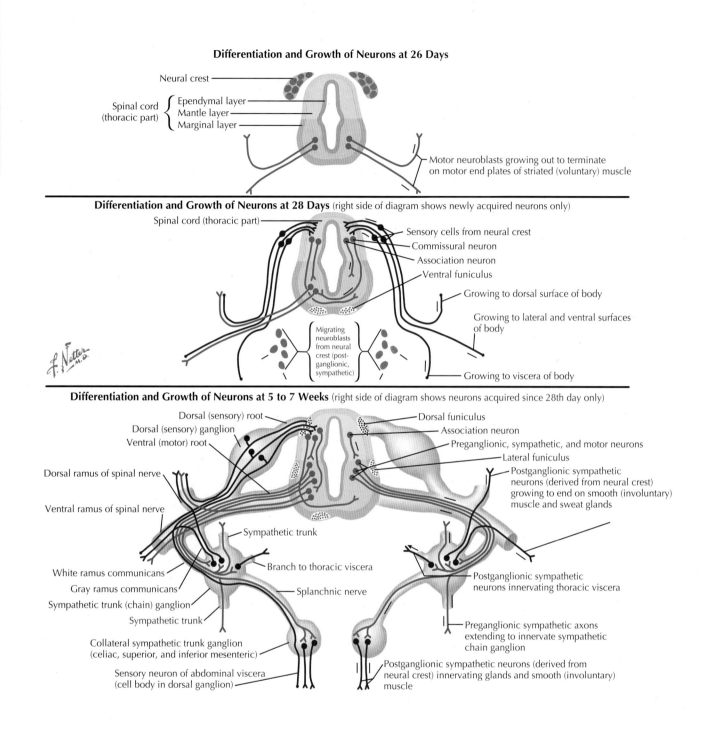

Differentiation and Growth of Neurons at 26 Days

Neural crest

Spinal cord (thoracic part)
- Ependymal layer
- Mantle layer
- Marginal layer

Motor neuroblasts growing out to terminate on motor end plates of striated (voluntary) muscle

Differentiation and Growth of Neurons at 28 Days (right side of diagram shows newly acquired neurons only)

Spinal cord (thoracic part)

Sensory cells from neural crest
Commissural neuron
Association neuron
Ventral funiculus

Growing to dorsal surface of body

Growing to lateral and ventral surfaces of body

Migrating neuroblasts from neural crest (postganglionic, sympathetic)

Growing to viscera of body

Differentiation and Growth of Neurons at 5 to 7 Weeks (right side of diagram shows neurons acquired since 28th day only)

Dorsal (sensory) root
Dorsal (sensory) ganglion
Ventral (motor) root

Dorsal funiculus
Association neuron
Preganglionic, sympathetic, and motor neurons
Lateral funiculus

Dorsal ramus of spinal nerve

Postganglionic sympathetic neurons (derived from neural crest) growing to end on smooth (involuntary) muscle and sweat glands

Ventral ramus of spinal nerve

Sympathetic trunk

White ramus communicans
Gray ramus communicans
Sympathetic trunk (chain) ganglion
Sympathetic trunk

Branch to thoracic viscera

Splanchnic nerve

Postganglionic sympathetic neurons innervating thoracic viscera

Preganglionic sympathetic axons extending to innervate sympathetic chain ganglion

Collateral sympathetic trunk ganglion (celiac, superior, and inferior mesenteric)

Sensory neuron of abdominal viscera (cell body in dorsal ganglion)

Postganglionic sympathetic neurons (derived from neural crest) innervating glands and smooth (involuntary) muscle

8.4 DEVELOPMENT OF PERIPHERAL AXONS

Peripheral axon development is a complex process of central and peripheral neurite extension, trophic and chemotactic factors, and axonal guidance and maintenance by innervated target tissues. Dorsal root ganglion cells are bipolar; a peripheral axonal process is associated with simple or complex sensory receptor cells, and a central axonal process extends into the central nervous system (CNS) to form connections with secondary sensory neurons. The lower motor neurons send motor axons to the developing skeletal muscles through the ventral roots or motor cranial nerves, forming neuromuscular junctions as sites of synaptic connectivity.

Motor neurons that fail to establish such contact with skeletal muscles die. Central preganglionic axons exit in the ventral roots and terminate on sympathetic ganglion cells in the sympathetic chain or collateral ganglia or on parasympathetic intramural ganglia near the organs innervated. Postganglionic axons form connections with target tissues, including smooth muscle, cardiac muscle, secretory glands, some metabolic cells (hepatocytes, fat cells), and cells of the immune system in parenchymal zones of many lymphoid organs. Sensory, motor, and autonomic symptoms can occur in peripheral neuropathies based on disruption of these connections.

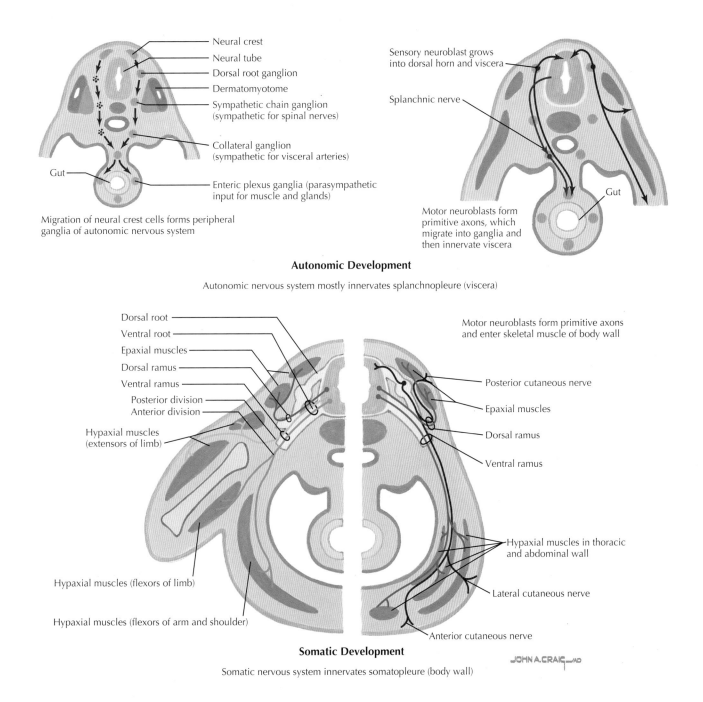

Autonomic Development

Autonomic nervous system mostly innervates splanchnopleure (viscera)

Somatic Development

Somatic nervous system innervates somatopleure (body wall)

JOHN A. CRAIG—AD

8.5 SOMATIC VERSUS SPLANCHNIC NERVE DEVELOPMENT

Somatopleure and splanchnopleure constitute the embryonic basis for the subdivision of the PNS into spinal (somatic) nerves and splanchnic (autonomic) nerves. The somatopleure develops from ectoderm and the somatic portion of lateral plate mesoderm. Somite hypoblasts migrate into somatopleure to form the lateral and ventral aspects of the body wall, including the limbs. Splanchnopleure, derived from endoderm and lateral plate mesoderm, give rise to visceral organs. The ventral rami migrate into somatopleure, and splanchnic nerves grow into splanchnopleure. Thoracic and lumbar splanchnic nerves have sympathetic and visceral sensory axonal components. Pelvic splanchnic nerves (S2–S4) have parasympathetic and visceral sensory axonal components.

Changes in ventral dermatome pattern (cutaneous sensory nerve distribution) during limb development

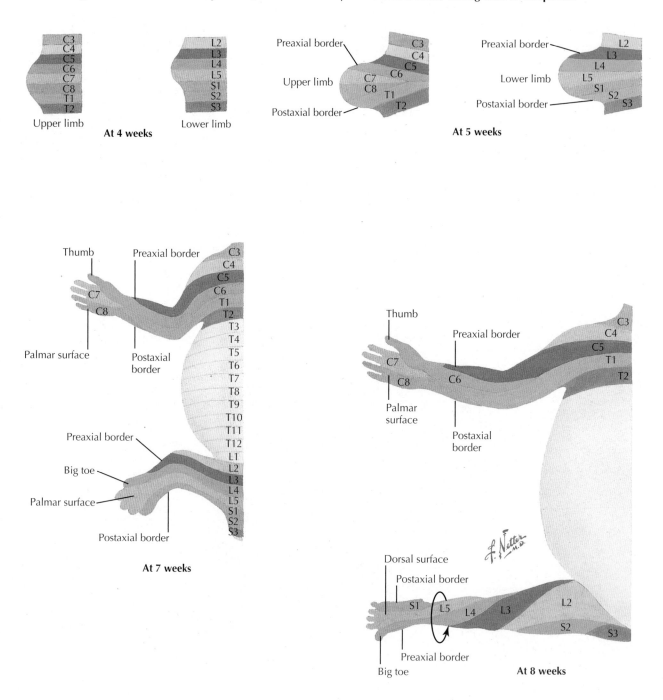

8.6 LIMB ROTATION AND DERMATOMES

Rotation of the lower limb results in a reversal of the preaxial and postaxial borders, producing a spiral arrangement of dermatomes. Spinal nerve segments on the anterior surface of the lower extremity extend medially and inferiorly; the great toe (hallux) is supplied by nerves from a more rostral dermatome (L4) than the little toe (S1). The lower extremity is an extension of the trunk, and the most caudal dermatomes (sacral and coccygeal) supply the perineum, not the foot. Cervical dermatomes maintain a relatively orderly distribution to the upper extremity with minimal rotation.

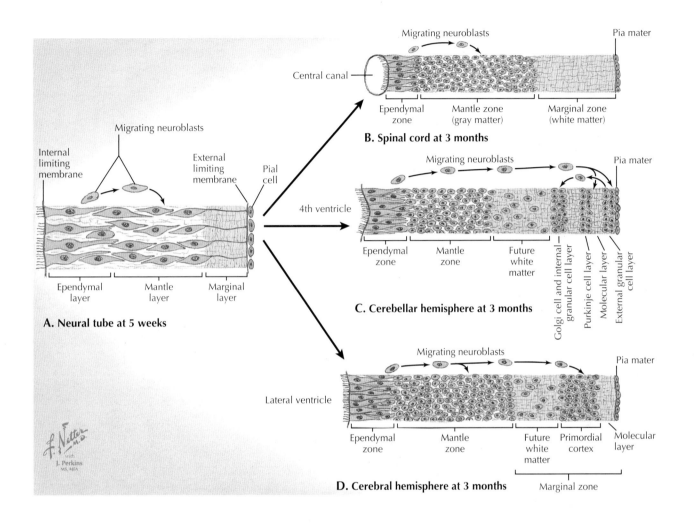

A. Neural tube at 5 weeks

B. Spinal cord at 3 months

C. Cerebellar hemisphere at 3 months

D. Cerebral hemisphere at 3 months

8.7 NEURAL PROLIFERATION AND DIFFERENTIATION: WALLS OF THE NEURAL TUBE

Early in development (5 weeks), neuroblasts in the ependymal layer lining the central canal move back and forth from the ependymal surface to the pial surface, replicating as they go. Neural migration follows distinctive patterns in different regions of the neural tube. In the spinal cord, neurons migrate into the inner mantle zone, leaving the outer marginal zone as a site for axonal pathways. In the cerebellar cortex, some neurons migrate to an outer location on the outer pial surface as an external granular layer, from which granular cells then migrate inward to synapse with other neurons present in deeper layers of the cerebellar cortex. In the cerebral cortex, neurons migrate to the outer zone, where the gray matter (neuronal cell bodies) remains on the surface, external to the white matter (nerve fibers). These developmental patterns reflect the anatomical organization of the mature structures, their blood supply, and their vulnerability to injury by tumors, vascular insults, trauma, and other disorders.

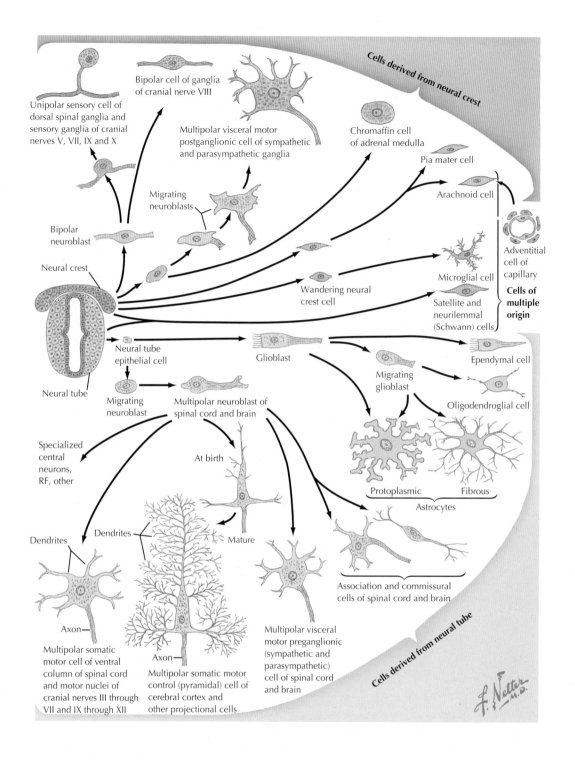

Unipolar sensory cell of dorsal spinal ganglia and sensory ganglia of cranial nerves V, VII, IX and X

Bipolar cell of ganglia of cranial nerve VIII

Multipolar visceral motor postganglionic cell of sympathetic and parasympathetic ganglia

Chromaffin cell of adrenal medulla

Pia mater cell

Arachnoid cell

Cells derived from neural crest

Migrating neuroblasts

Bipolar neuroblast

Neural crest

Wandering neural crest cell

Microglial cell

Adventitial cell of capillary

Cells of multiple origin

Satellite and neurilemmal (Schwann) cells

Neural tube epithelial cell

Glioblast

Migrating glioblast

Ependymal cell

Oligodendroglial cell

Neural tube

Migrating neuroblast

Multipolar neuroblast of spinal cord and brain

Specialized central neurons, RF, other

At birth

Protoplasmic   Fibrous

Astrocytes

Dendrites

Dendrites

Mature

Axon

Association and commissural cells of spinal cord and brain

Multipolar somatic motor cell of ventral column of spinal cord and motor nuclei of cranial nerves III through VII and IX through XII

Axon

Multipolar somatic motor control (pyramidal) cell of cerebral cortex and other projectional cells

Multipolar visceral motor preganglionic (sympathetic and parasympathetic) cell of spinal cord and brain

Cells derived from neural tube

8.8 NEURAL TUBE AND NEURAL CREST DERIVATIVES

Neural tube ependymal cells give rise to neuroblasts, from which the neurons of the CNS are derived. They also give rise to the glioblasts, from which the mature ependymal cells, astrocytes, and oligodendroglia are derived. Microglia, the "scavenger cells" of the CNS, are derived mainly from mesodermal precursors. Cells of glial origin are the predominant cells that give rise to CNS tumors. The neural crest cells give rise to many peripheral neural structures, including primary sensory neurons, postganglionic autonomic neurons of both the sympathetic and parasympathetic systems, adrenal medullary chromaffin cells, pial and arachnoid cells, Schwann cells (the supporting cells of the PNS), and some other specialized cell types. Neural crest cells can be damaged selectively in some disorders (e.g., familial dysautonomias) and also can give rise to specific tumor cell types such as pheochromocytomas. Most microglial cells are derived from specialized mesenchymal cells infiltrating from the yolk sac.

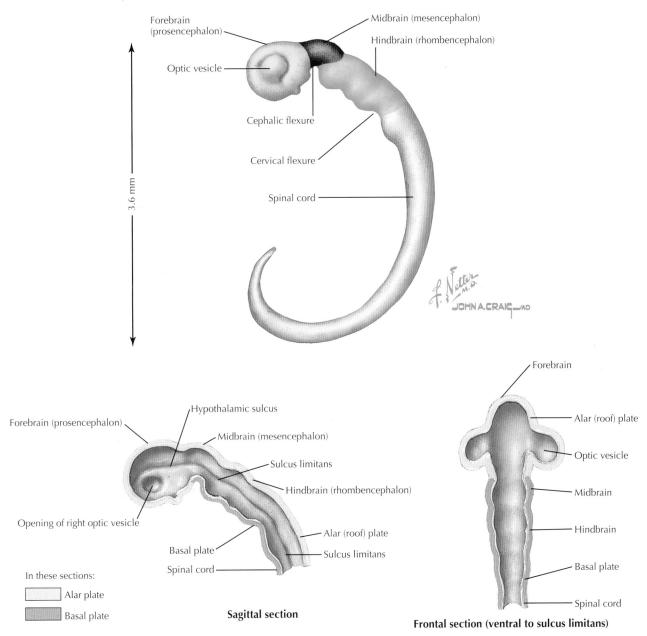

Central nervous system at 28 days

Forebrain (prosencephalon)

Optic vesicle

Midbrain (mesencephalon)

Hindbrain (rhombencephalon)

Cephalic flexure

Cervical flexure

Spinal cord

3.6 mm

Forebrain (prosencephalon)

Hypothalamic sulcus

Midbrain (mesencephalon)

Sulcus limitans

Hindbrain (rhombencephalon)

Opening of right optic vesicle

Basal plate

Spinal cord

Alar (roof) plate

Sulcus limitans

In these sections:

Alar plate

Basal plate

Sagittal section

Forebrain

Alar (roof) plate

Optic vesicle

Midbrain

Hindbrain

Basal plate

Spinal cord

Frontal section (ventral to sulcus limitans)

8.9 EARLY BRAIN DEVELOPMENT: THE 28-DAY-OLD EMBRYO

Some components of the neural tube expand differentially, resulting in bends or flexures that separate the neural tube into caudal to rostral components. The cervical flexure caudally and the cephalic flexure rostrally result from the differential expansion. Three regions of rapid cellular proliferation develop: the forebrain (prosencephalon) rostrally, the mesencephalon (midbrain) in the middle, and the hindbrain (rhombencephalon) caudally. The ventricular system bends and expands to accommodate the increasing neural growth. An outgrowth from the caudal part of the prosencephalon extends from the future diencephalon to become the optic cup, giving rise to the future retina and its central connections.

CLINICAL POINT

The **optic vesicle** develops from the prosencephalon, specifically the future diencephalon. As a consequence, the neuroretina is actually a central neural derivative and not a peripheral neural crest derivative. Therefore, the retina is supplied with CNS vasculature, and the ganglion cells of the retina (projecting into the optic nerve, chiasm, and tract) are actually CNS axons myelinated by oligodendroglia and surrounded by subarachnoid space and its cerebrospinal fluid. As a CNS tract, the optic nerve is subject to central demyelinating lesions as seen in multiple sclerosis. The retinal vasculature is the only CNS vasculature that is directly observable by ophthalmoscopy.

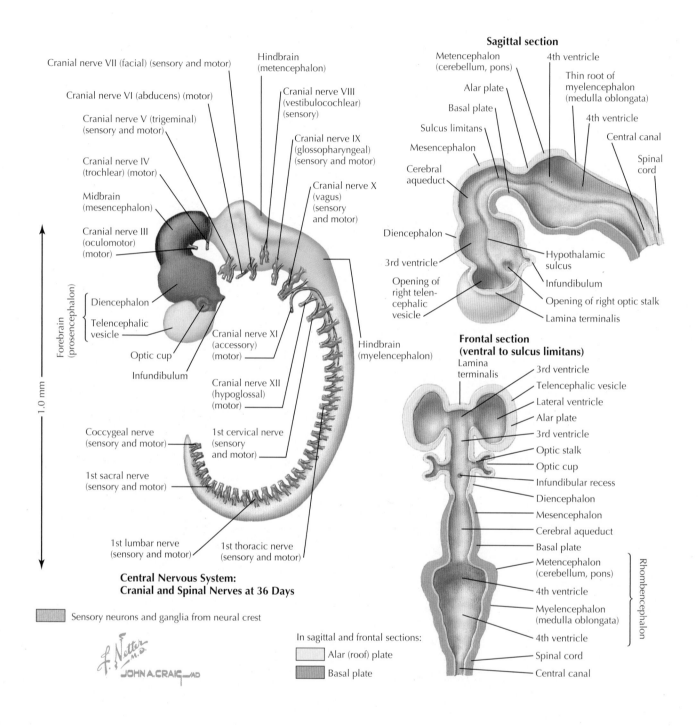

Sagittal section

Metencephalon (cerebellum, pons)
4th ventricle
Thin root of myelencephalon (medulla oblongata)
Alar plate
4th ventricle
Basal plate
Central canal
Sulcus limitans
Spinal cord
Mesencephalon
Cerebral aqueduct
Diencephalon
Hypothalamic sulcus
3rd ventricle
Infundibulum
Opening of right telencephalic vesicle
Opening of right optic stalk
Lamina terminalis

Cranial nerve VII (facial) (sensory and motor)
Hindbrain (metencephalon)
Cranial nerve VI (abducens) (motor)
Cranial nerve VIII (vestibulocochlear) (sensory)
Cranial nerve V (trigeminal) (sensory and motor)
Cranial nerve IX (glossopharyngeal) (sensory and motor)
Cranial nerve IV (trochlear) (motor)
Midbrain (mesencephalon)
Cranial nerve X (vagus) (sensory and motor)
Cranial nerve III (oculomotor) (motor)
Forebrain (prosencephalon)
Diencephalon
Telencephalic vesicle
Optic cup
Infundibulum
Cranial nerve XI (accessory) (motor)
Hindbrain (myelencephalon)
Cranial nerve XII (hypoglossal) (motor)
1.0 mm
Coccygeal nerve (sensory and motor)
1st cervical nerve (sensory and motor)
1st sacral nerve (sensory and motor)
1st lumbar nerve (sensory and motor)
1st thoracic nerve (sensory and motor)

Central Nervous System: Cranial and Spinal Nerves at 36 Days

Sensory neurons and ganglia from neural crest

F. Netter M.D.
JOHN A. CRAIG AD

Frontal section (ventral to sulcus limitans)
Lamina terminalis
3rd ventricle
Telencephalic vesicle
Lateral ventricle
Alar plate
3rd ventricle
Optic stalk
Optic cup
Infundibular recess
Diencephalon
Mesencephalon
Cerebral aqueduct
Basal plate
Metencephalon (cerebellum, pons)
4th ventricle
Myelencephalon (medulla oblongata)
4th ventricle
Spinal cord
Central canal
Rhombencephalon

In sagittal and frontal sections:
Alar (roof) plate
Basal plate

8.10 EARLY BRAIN DEVELOPMENT: THE 36-DAY-OLD EMBRYO

By day 36, the prosencephalon begins to expand rapidly as the future diencephalon (thalamus and hypothalamus) and telencephalon (basal ganglia, limbic forebrain, olfactory system, and cerebral cortex). This rapid growth is accompanied by the formation of the thin third ventricle for the diencephalon and the C-shaped lateral ventricles from the rostral end of the original central canal for the telencephalon. The rhombencephalon further develops into two distinct regions, the metencephalon (future pons and cerebellum) and the myelencephalon (future medulla). Distinct spinal nerves and cranial nerves begin to form as sensory and motor neurons differentiate and begin to connect with their appropriate targets in the periphery.

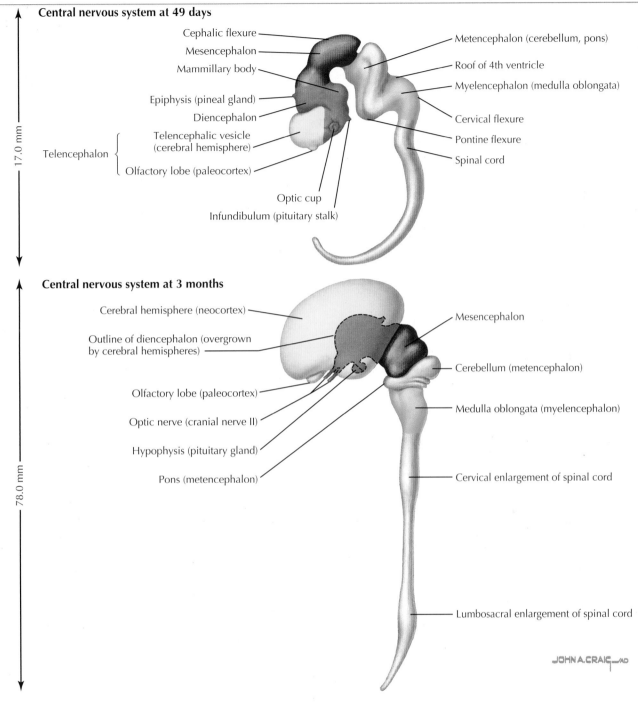

Central nervous system at 49 days

Cephalic flexure
Mesencephalon
Mammillary body
Epiphysis (pineal gland)
Diencephalon
Telencephalon {
Telencephalic vesicle (cerebral hemisphere)
Olfactory lobe (paleocortex)
Optic cup
Infundibulum (pituitary stalk)

Metencephalon (cerebellum, pons)
Roof of 4th ventricle
Myelencephalon (medulla oblongata)
Cervical flexure
Pontine flexure
Spinal cord

17.0 mm

Central nervous system at 3 months

Cerebral hemisphere (neocortex)
Outline of diencephalon (overgrown by cerebral hemispheres)
Olfactory lobe (paleocortex)
Optic nerve (cranial nerve II)
Hypophysis (pituitary gland)
Pons (metencephalon)

Mesencephalon
Cerebellum (metencephalon)
Medulla oblongata (myelencephalon)
Cervical enlargement of spinal cord
Lumbosacral enlargement of spinal cord

78.0 mm

JOHN A. CRAIG—MD

8.11 EARLY BRAIN DEVELOPMENT: THE 49-DAY-OLD EMBRYO AND THE 3-MONTH-OLD EMBRYO

By 49 days of age, the diencephalon and telencephalon differentiate into distinct components: the thalamus dorsally and the hypothalamus ventrally from the diencephalon and the olfactory lobe, basal ganglia, limbic forebrain structures, and cerebral cortex from the telencephalon. The metencephalon (pons) and myelencephalon (medulla) develop further and fold, separated by the pontine flexure. Between 49 days and 3 months, massive development of the telencephalon overrides and covers the diencephalon. The cerebellum forms from the rhombic lips of the metencephalon as neurons travel dorsally to overlie the future pons and eventually most of the brainstem. The mesencephalon expands dorsally, forming the superior and inferior colliculi (quadrigeminal bodies). The continuing growth of the spinal cord as it connects with peripheral tissues in the developing limbs forms the cervical and lumbosacral enlargements.

CLINICAL POINT

The process by which the prosencephalon gives rise to the diencephalon and telencephalon is termed prosencephalization. A failure of this process to form the two hemispheres results in holoprosencephaly, with a single large forebrain ventricle, a poorly developed diencephalon, and aberrant development of telencephalic structures. This severe defect in forebrain formation is also accompanied by severe facial malformations.

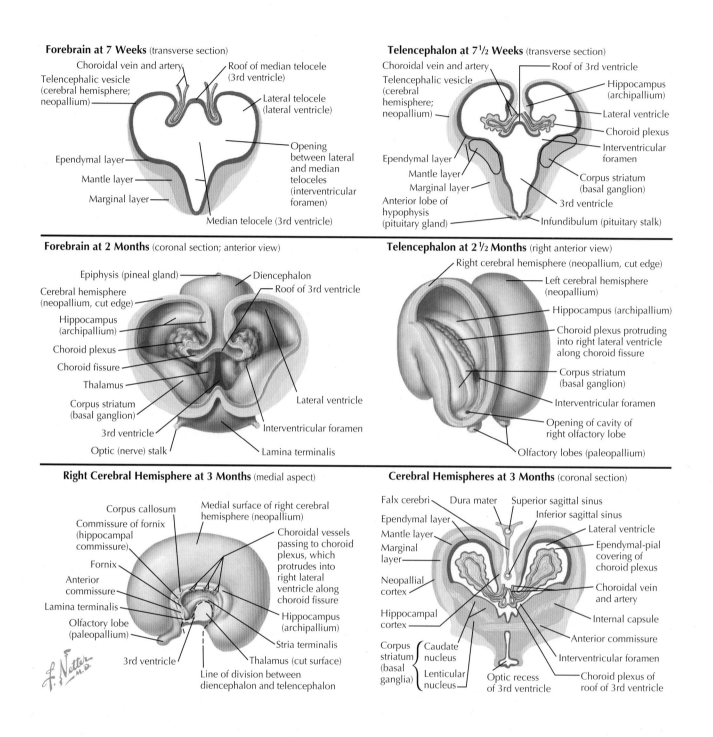

Forebrain at 7 Weeks (transverse section)

Choroidal vein and artery
Telencephalic vesicle (cerebral hemisphere; neopallium)
Roof of median telocele (3rd ventricle)
Lateral telocele (lateral ventricle)
Ependymal layer
Mantle layer
Marginal layer
Opening between lateral and median teloceles (interventricular foramen)
Median telocele (3rd ventricle)

Telencephalon at 7½ Weeks (transverse section)

Choroidal vein and artery
Telencephalic vesicle (cerebral hemisphere; neopallium)
Roof of 3rd ventricle
Hippocampus (archipallium)
Lateral ventricle
Choroid plexus
Interventricular foramen
Ependymal layer
Mantle layer
Marginal layer
Anterior lobe of hypophysis (pituitary gland)
Corpus striatum (basal ganglion)
3rd ventricle
Infundibulum (pituitary stalk)

Forebrain at 2 Months (coronal section; anterior view)

Epiphysis (pineal gland)
Cerebral hemisphere (neopallium, cut edge)
Hippocampus (archipallium)
Choroid plexus
Choroid fissure
Thalamus
Corpus striatum (basal ganglion)
3rd ventricle
Optic (nerve) stalk
Diencephalon
Roof of 3rd ventricle
Lateral ventricle
Interventricular foramen
Lamina terminalis

Telencephalon at 2½ Months (right anterior view)

Right cerebral hemisphere (neopallium, cut edge)
Left cerebral hemisphere (neopallium)
Hippocampus (archipallium)
Choroid plexus protruding into right lateral ventricle along choroid fissure
Corpus striatum (basal ganglion)
Interventricular foramen
Opening of cavity of right olfactory lobe
Olfactory lobes (paleopallium)

Right Cerebral Hemisphere at 3 Months (medial aspect)

Corpus callosum
Commissure of fornix (hippocampal commissure)
Fornix
Anterior commissure
Lamina terminalis
Olfactory lobe (paleopallium)
3rd ventricle
Medial surface of right cerebral hemisphere (neopallium)
Choroidal vessels passing to choroid plexus, which protrudes into right lateral ventricle along choroid fissure
Hippocampus (archipallium)
Stria terminalis
Thalamus (cut surface)
Line of division between diencephalon and telencephalon

Cerebral Hemispheres at 3 Months (coronal section)

Falx cerebri
Dura mater
Superior sagittal sinus
Ependymal layer
Mantle layer
Marginal layer
Inferior sagittal sinus
Lateral ventricle
Ependymal-pial covering of choroid plexus
Neopallial cortex
Hippocampal cortex
Corpus striatum (basal ganglia) { Caudate nucleus / Lenticular nucleus }
Optic recess of 3rd ventricle
Choroidal vein and artery
Internal capsule
Anterior commissure
Interventricular foramen
Choroid plexus of roof of 3rd ventricle

8.12 FOREBRAIN DEVELOPMENT: 7 WEEKS THROUGH 3 MONTHS

Neurons of the developing telencephalon move rostrally, dorsally, and then around the diencephalon in a C shape toward the anterior pole of the temporal lobe. The hippocampal formation forms in a dorsal and anterior position and migrates in a C-shaped course into the anterior temporal lobe. The amygdala develops in a similar manner, giving rise to the stria terminalis pathway in a C shape. The lateral ventricles follow the same C-shaped developmental process anatomically. The caudate nucleus also extends around the telencephalon in a C-shaped pattern, with the large head of the nucleus remaining anterior and the much smaller body and tail following as a thinner C-shaped structure that ends ventrally adjacent to the temporal horn of the lateral ventricle. The corpus callosum and anterior commissure connect the two hemispheres. The internal capsule funnels centrally in the core of the forebrain on either side; the posterior limb continues caudally as the cerebral peduncle.

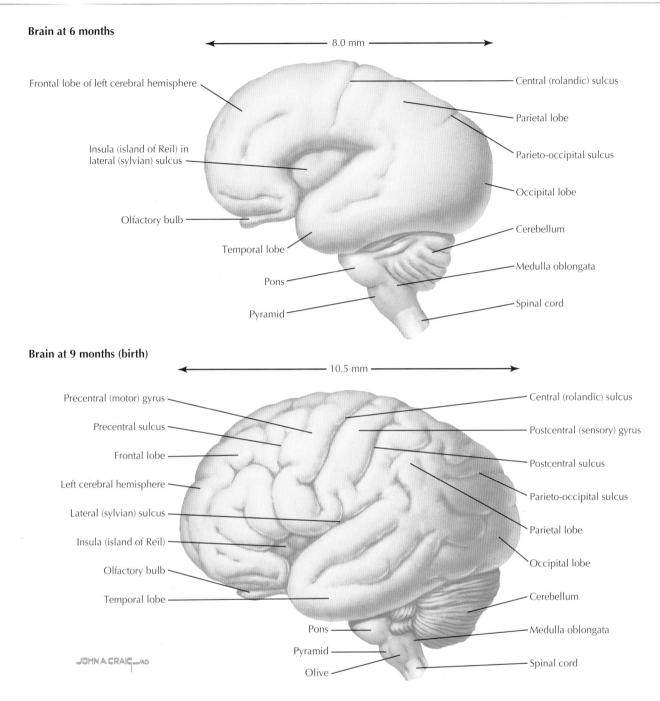

Brain at 6 months

8.0 mm

Frontal lobe of left cerebral hemisphere

Insula (island of Reil) in lateral (sylvian) sulcus

Olfactory bulb

Temporal lobe

Pons

Pyramid

Central (rolandic) sulcus

Parietal lobe

Parieto-occipital sulcus

Occipital lobe

Cerebellum

Medulla oblongata

Spinal cord

Brain at 9 months (birth)

10.5 mm

Precentral (motor) gyrus

Precentral sulcus

Frontal lobe

Left cerebral hemisphere

Lateral (sylvian) sulcus

Insula (island of Reil)

Olfactory bulb

Temporal lobe

Pons

Pyramid

Olive

Central (rolandic) sulcus

Postcentral (sensory) gyrus

Postcentral sulcus

Parieto-occipital sulcus

Parietal lobe

Occipital lobe

Cerebellum

Medulla oblongata

Spinal cord

JOHN A. CRAIG—MD

8.13 THE 6-MONTH AND 9-MONTH CENTRAL NERVOUS SYSTEMS

At 6 months, the brainstem has differentiated into the medulla, pons, and midbrain, with the developing cerebellum overlying them dorsally. Even though the diencephalon is rapidly developing, the overlying telencephalon shows massive growth rostrally, then caudally, downward, and forward into the temporal lobe. From 6 to 9 months of age, the cerebral cortex forms its characteristic convolutions with gyri and sulci, and the cerebellar cortex forms its distinctive folds, the folia. Within the forebrain, the major components of the basal ganglia, the limbic forebrain structures (i.e., the amygdala and hippocampal formation), the olfactory system, and the cerebral cortex develop rapidly. Most neurons are present at birth; some populations of granular cells in the cerebellum, the dentate gyrus of the hippocampus, and the cerebral cortex form postnatally in response to environmental stimuli. The in utero and postnatal environments provide major influences on neural development and function.

CLINICAL POINT

The cerebral cortex develops through an orderly process of cell proliferation from the ventricular zone and then the subventricular zone, with proper cell migration and interconnectivity extending through prenatal life and well into postnatal life. A failure of proper cell proliferation and migration of cortical neurons can result in the failure of proper formation of gyri and sulci, giving a smooth cortical surface appearance called lissencephaly. In some situations, gyri can be unusually small (microgyria) or unusually large (pachygyria). These developmental defects may be accompanied by profound neural deficits and intellectual disability.

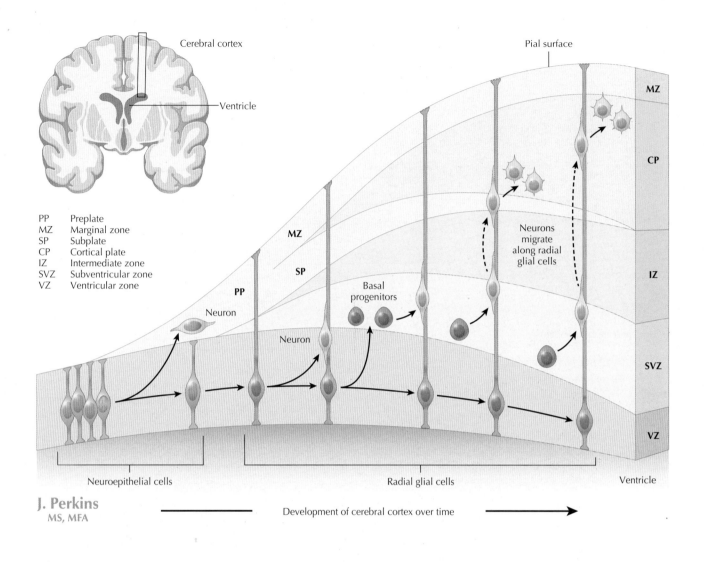

Cerebral cortex

Ventricle

Pial surface

MZ

CP

Neurons migrate along radial glial cells

IZ

SVZ

VZ

Ventricle

PP   Preplate
MZ   Marginal zone
SP   Subplate
CP   Cortical plate
IZ   Intermediate zone
SVZ   Subventricular zone
VZ   Ventricular zone

MZ

SP

PP

Neuron

Neuron

Basal progenitors

Neuroepithelial cells

Radial glial cells

J. Perkins
MS, MFA

Development of cerebral cortex over time

8.14 NEUROGENESIS AND CELL MIGRATION IN THE DEVELOPING NEOCORTEX

During the earliest phases of cortical development, neuroepithelial progenitor cells, with processes extending from the cell body to the inner ventricular surface and the outer pial surface, replicate. They form some neurons that populate the preplate region and also generate the radial glial cells. The radial glial cells maintain their contact with the ventricular and pial surfaces and give rise to postmitotic cortical neurons. These neurons migrate toward the cortical surface along the radial glial processes and populate the cortical plate. Cortical neurons accumulate in the cortical plate region in an inside-out fashion, with earliest generated neurons located deepest and latest generated neurons located more superficially. These neurons differentiate to form association neurons (cortical-cortical connections) and projection neurons (to deeper subcortical structures). Most of the subplate neurons die, although some remain and differentiate into local (interstitial) interneurons. Cortical granule cells proliferate from the subependymal zone and migrate both tangentially and radially into the cortical architecture. These neurons undergo abundant proliferation and migration postnatally in response to environmental stimuli. These complex processes of neurogenesis, proliferation, migration, differentiation,

and integration into complex circuitry (intrinsic, projection, and association), followed by extensive postnatal dendritic and axonal maturation and connectivity, leave cortical development vulnerable to a variety of insults and disruptions.

CLINICAL POINT

The neonatal environment exerts significant influences over postnatal proliferation and migration of granule cells, as well as synaptic connectivity and neuronal maturation. During critical developmental periods, a stressful environment can adversely impact the future reactivity of the major stress axes, the sympathoadrenal system, and the hypothalamo-pituitary-adrenal (HPA) system. In animal models, where careful controls are possible, the stress of maternal separation can lead to heightened reactivity in adulthood in these stress axes with elevated catecholamine and glucocorticoid secretion, elevated inflammatory mediators, and diminished components of immune reactivity. In observations in humans, where carefully controlled environments are not readily achievable, observations of children raised with neglectful or stressful environments also demonstrate greater reactivity of the stress axes, greater likelihood of cardiac disease and type 2 diabetes, and greater incidence of psychosocial disorders in later life. These observations in humans show greater variability than those seen in well-controlled animal models.

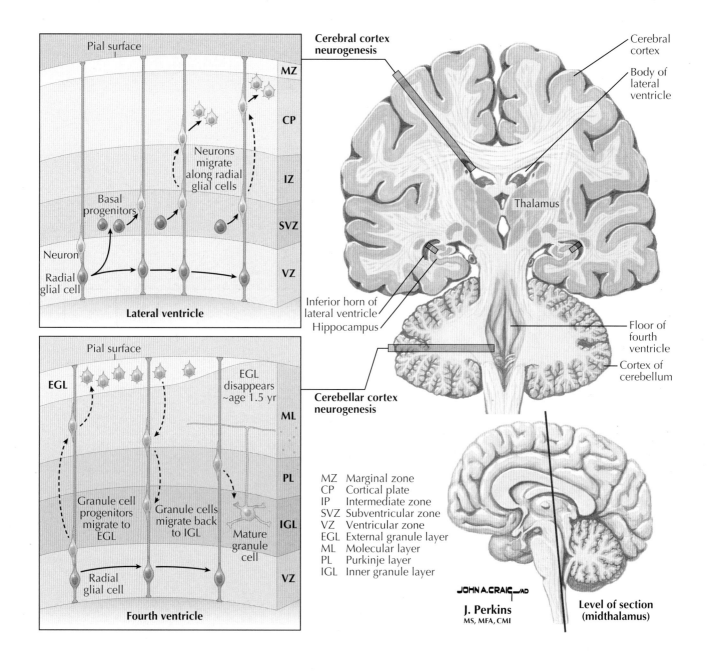

MZ Marginal zone
CP Cortical plate
IP Intermediate zone
SVZ Subventricular zone
VZ Ventricular zone
EGL External granule layer
ML Molecular layer
PL Purkinje layer
IGL Inner granule layer

8.15 **POSTNATAL AND ADULT NEUROGENESIS**

In the neonate, granule cells proliferate and migrate into key neural structures, including the cerebellar cortex, the hippocampus, and the cerebral cortex, in response to postnatal stimuli. Phenomena such as sensory stimuli (external touch) and an enriched environment (affecting balance and cerebellar development, exploratory behavior, maternal interactions) can influence the proliferation, migration, and placement of granule cells into complex synaptic circuitry. This plate illustrates the granule cell process in neonatal cerebellum and cortex. The CNS does not have a full complement of neurons at birth, especially granule cells, and the neonatal environment plays a critical role in brain development, as demonstrated by the early studies of Joseph Altman and Shirley Bayer. More recently, this process of neuronal proliferation, migration, and neuronal replacement has been demonstrated in the adult hippocampus, including in aging. Cells from the subventricular zone of the adjacent ventricle contribute new neurons to the granule cell layer of the hippocampus, a phenomenon of synaptic plasticity that occurs throughout the life span, as shown by Fred "Rusty" Gage of the Salk Institute.

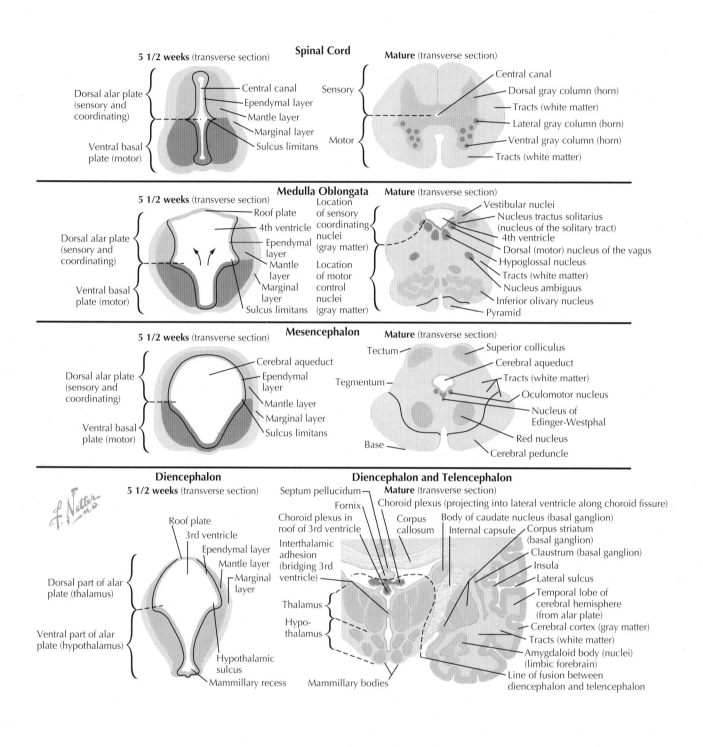

Spinal Cord

5 1/2 weeks (transverse section)

Mature (transverse section)

Dorsal alar plate (sensory and coordinating)

Ventral basal plate (motor)

Central canal
Ependymal layer
Mantle layer
Marginal layer
Sulcus limitans

Sensory

Motor

Central canal
Dorsal gray column (horn)
Tracts (white matter)
Lateral gray column (horn)
Ventral gray column (horn)
Tracts (white matter)

Medulla Oblongata

5 1/2 weeks (transverse section)

Mature (transverse section)

Dorsal alar plate (sensory and coordinating)

Ventral basal plate (motor)

Roof plate
4th ventricle
Ependymal layer
Mantle layer
Marginal layer
Sulcus limitans

Location of sensory coordinating nuclei (gray matter)

Location of motor control nuclei (gray matter)

Vestibular nuclei
Nucleus tractus solitarius (nucleus of the solitary tract)
4th ventricle
Dorsal (motor) nucleus of the vagus
Hypoglossal nucleus
Tracts (white matter)
Nucleus ambiguus
Inferior olivary nucleus
Pyramid

Mesencephalon

5 1/2 weeks (transverse section)

Mature (transverse section)

Dorsal alar plate (sensory and coordinating)

Ventral basal plate (motor)

Cerebral aqueduct
Ependymal layer
Mantle layer
Marginal layer
Sulcus limitans

Tectum
Tegmentum
Base

Superior colliculus
Cerebral aqueduct
Tracts (white matter)
Oculomotor nucleus
Nucleus of Edinger-Westphal
Red nucleus
Cerebral peduncle

Diencephalon

5 1/2 weeks (transverse section)

Diencephalon and Telencephalon

Mature (transverse section)

Dorsal part of alar plate (thalamus)

Ventral part of alar plate (hypothalamus)

Roof plate
3rd ventricle
Ependymal layer
Mantle layer
Marginal layer
Hypothalamic sulcus
Mammillary recess

Septum pellucidum
Fornix
Choroid plexus in roof of 3rd ventricle
Interthalamic adhesion (bridging 3rd ventricle)
Thalamus
Hypo-thalamus
Mammillary bodies

Choroid plexus (projecting into lateral ventricle along choroid fissure)
Corpus callosum
Body of caudate nucleus (basal ganglion)
Internal capsule
Corpus striatum (basal ganglion)
Claustrum (basal ganglion)
Insula
Lateral sulcus
Temporal lobe of cerebral hemisphere (from alar plate)
Cerebral cortex (gray matter)
Tracts (white matter)
Amygdaloid body (nuclei) (limbic forebrain)
Line of fusion between diencephalon and telencephalon

8.16 COMPARISON OF 5½-WEEK AND ADULT CENTRAL NERVOUS SYSTEM REGIONS

The relatively large ventricular system at 5½ weeks becomes comparatively smaller as the process of neuronal growth occurs. In adults, the central canal of the spinal cord becomes virtually obliterated and does not convey cerebrospinal fluid (CSF). The fourth ventricle opens up laterally; the sulcus limitans demarcates motor nuclei (medially) and sensory nuclei (laterally). The cerebral aqueduct remains very small. The third ventricle narrows down to a slit. The lateral ventricles expand massively into a C-shape. The basal plate forms motor and autonomic structures whose axons leave the CNS. The alar plate forms sensory derivatives in the spinal cord and brainstem and structures that migrate ventrally (the inferior olivary complex, the pontine nuclei, and the red nucleus). The rhombic lips, an alar derivative of the metencephalon, give rise to the entire cerebellum. The diencephalon and telencephalon are also alar plate derivatives.

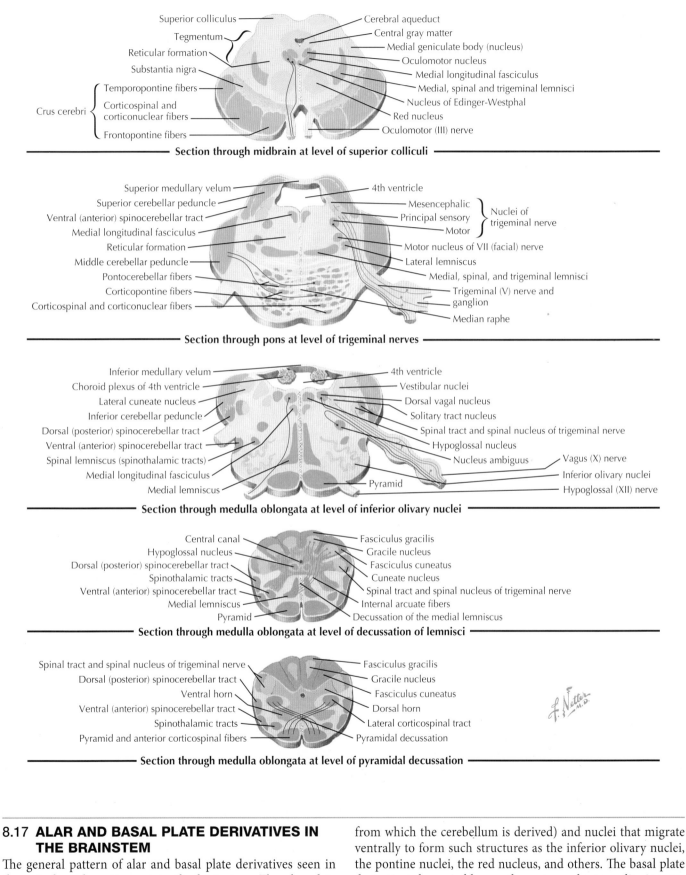

Superior colliculus — Cerebral aqueduct
Tegmentum — Central gray matter
Reticular formation — Medial geniculate body (nucleus)
Substantia nigra — Oculomotor nucleus
Temporopontine fibers — Medial longitudinal fasciculus
Corticospinal and corticonuclear fibers — Medial, spinal and trigeminal lemnisci
Frontopontine fibers — Nucleus of Edinger-Westphal
Crus cerebri — Red nucleus
— Oculomotor (III) nerve

Section through midbrain at level of superior colliculi

Superior medullary velum — 4th ventricle
Superior cerebellar peduncle — Mesencephalic
Ventral (anterior) spinocerebellar tract — Principal sensory } Nuclei of trigeminal nerve
Medial longitudinal fasciculus — Motor
Reticular formation — Motor nucleus of VII (facial) nerve
Middle cerebellar peduncle — Lateral lemniscus
Pontocerebellar fibers — Medial, spinal, and trigeminal lemnisci
Corticopontine fibers — Trigeminal (V) nerve and ganglion
Corticospinal and corticonuclear fibers — Median raphe

Section through pons at level of trigeminal nerves

Inferior medullary velum — 4th ventricle
Choroid plexus of 4th ventricle — Vestibular nuclei
Lateral cuneate nucleus — Dorsal vagal nucleus
Inferior cerebellar peduncle — Solitary tract nucleus
Dorsal (posterior) spinocerebellar tract — Spinal tract and spinal nucleus of trigeminal nerve
Ventral (anterior) spinocerebellar tract — Hypoglossal nucleus
Spinal lemniscus (spinothalamic tracts) — Nucleus ambiguus — Vagus (X) nerve
Medial longitudinal fasciculus — Inferior olivary nuclei
Medial lemniscus — Pyramid — Hypoglossal (XII) nerve

Section through medulla oblongata at level of inferior olivary nuclei

Central canal — Fasciculus gracilis
Hypoglossal nucleus — Gracile nucleus
Dorsal (posterior) spinocerebellar tract — Fasciculus cuneatus
Spinothalamic tracts — Cuneate nucleus
Ventral (anterior) spinocerebellar tract — Spinal tract and spinal nucleus of trigeminal nerve
Medial lemniscus — Internal arcuate fibers
Pyramid — Decussation of the medial lemniscus

Section through medulla oblongata at level of decussation of lemnisci

Spinal tract and spinal nucleus of trigeminal nerve — Fasciculus gracilis
Dorsal (posterior) spinocerebellar tract — Gracile nucleus
Ventral horn — Fasciculus cuneatus
Ventral (anterior) spinocerebellar tract — Dorsal horn
Spinothalamic tracts — Lateral corticospinal tract
Pyramid and anterior corticospinal fibers — Pyramidal decussation

Section through medulla oblongata at level of pyramidal decussation

8.17 ALAR AND BASAL PLATE DERIVATIVES IN THE BRAINSTEM

The general pattern of alar and basal plate derivatives seen in the spinal cord continues into the brainstem. The alar plate derivatives shown in red are the sensory nuclei (the rhombic lip from which the cerebellum is derived) and nuclei that migrate ventrally to form such structures as the inferior olivary nuclei, the pontine nuclei, the red nucleus, and others. The basal plate derivatives shown in blue are the motor and preganglionic autonomic nuclei.

Adult derivatives of brain primordia

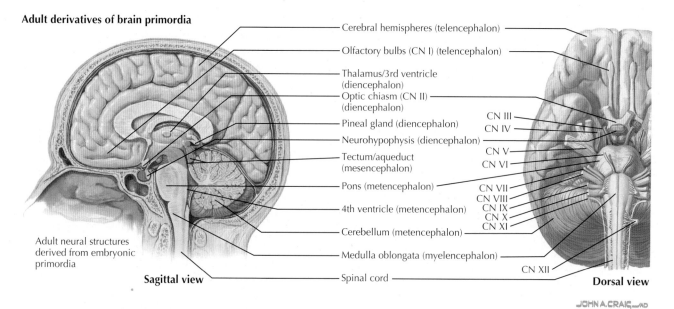

Cerebral hemispheres (telencephalon)

Olfactory bulbs (CN I) (telencephalon)

Thalamus/3rd ventricle
(diencephalon)

Optic chiasm (CN II)
(diencephalon)

Pineal gland (diencephalon)

Neurohypophysis (diencephalon)

Tectum/aqueduct
(mesencephalon)

Pons (metencephalon)

4th ventricle (metencephalon)

Cerebellum (metencephalon)

Medulla oblongata (myelencephalon)

Spinal cord

Adult neural structures
derived from embryonic
primordia

CN III
CN IV
CN V
CN VI
CN VII
CN VIII
CN IX
CN X
CN XI
CN XII

Sagittal view

Dorsal view

JOHN A. CRAIG—AD

Adult derivatives of the forebrain, midbrain, and hindbrain

Forebrain	Telencephalon	Cerebral hemispheres (neocortex) Olfactory cortex (paleocortex) Hippocampus (archicortex) Basal ganglia/corpus striatum Lateral and 3rd ventricles	Nerves: Olfactory (I)
	Diencephalon	Optic cup/nerves Thalamus Hypothalamus Mammillary bodies Part of 3rd ventricle	Optic (II)
Midbrain	Mesencephalon	Tectum (superior, inferior colliculi) Cerebral aqueduct Red nucleus Substantia nigra Crus cerebelli	Oculomotor (III) Trochlear (IV)
Hindbrain	Metencephalon	Pons Cerebellum	Trigeminal (V) Abducens (VI) Facial (VII) Acoustic (VIII) Glossopharyngeal (IX) Vagus (X) Hypoglossal (XI)
	Myelencephalon	Medulla oblongata	

8.18 ADULT DERIVATIVES OF THE FOREBRAIN, MIDBRAIN, AND HINDBRAIN

The telencephalon has four major components: the cerebral cortex, the limbic forebrain structures, the basal ganglia, and the olfactory system. The diencephalon consists of two major structures: the thalamus and hypothalamus and two smaller structures, the epithalamus and subthalamus. The thalamus has extensive interconnections with the cerebral cortex and serves as a gateway to the telencephalon. The hypothalamus receives extensive input from the limbic forebrain and a variety of brainstem and visceral sensory sources and regulates neuroendocrine and visceral autonomic functions. The midbrain consists of the colliculi, the tegmentum, and the cerebral peduncles. The colliculi convey visual (superior) and auditory (inferior) information to higher regions of the brain and to brainstem and reflex pathways. The tegmentum houses important motor, sensory, and autonomic structures and plays a crucial role in consciousness and sleep. The cerebral peduncles are caudal continuations of the posterior limb of the internal capsule and play a particularly important role in motor functions. The cerebellum plays an important role in coordinating movement, posture, locomotion, and equilibrium. The medulla and pons integrate the sensory, motor, and autonomic functions of the body via extensive connections through the cranial nerves, to which the spinal cord inputs contribute.

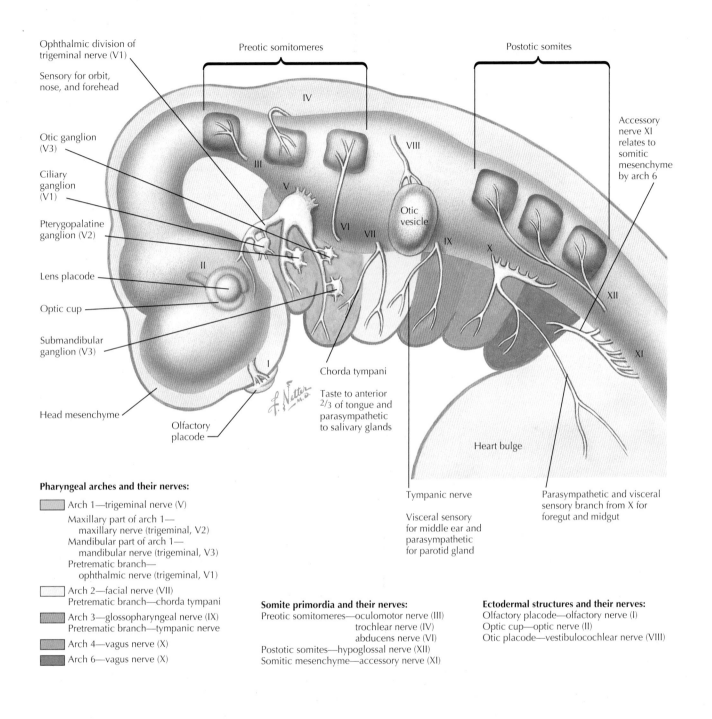

Ophthalmic division of trigeminal nerve (V1)

Sensory for orbit, nose, and forehead

Preotic somitomeres

Postotic somites

Otic ganglion (V3)

Ciliary ganglion (V1)

Pterygopalatine ganglion (V2)

Lens placode

Optic cup

Submandibular ganglion (V3)

Head mesenchyme

Olfactory placode

Accessory nerve XI relates to somitic mesenchyme by arch 6

IV

III

V

VI VII

VIII

Otic vesicle

IX

X

XII

XI

I

II

Chorda tympani

Taste to anterior 2/3 of tongue and parasympathetic to salivary glands

Heart bulge

Tympanic nerve

Visceral sensory for middle ear and parasympathetic for parotid gland

Parasympathetic and visceral sensory branch from X for foregut and midgut

Pharyngeal arches and their nerves:

Arch 1—trigeminal nerve (V)
Maxillary part of arch 1—
maxillary nerve (trigeminal, V2)
Mandibular part of arch 1—
mandibular nerve (trigeminal, V3)
Pretrematic branch—
ophthalmic nerve (trigeminal, V1)

Arch 2—facial nerve (VII)
Pretrematic branch—chorda tympani

Arch 3—glossopharyngeal nerve (IX)
Pretrematic branch—tympanic nerve

Arch 4—vagus nerve (X)

Arch 6—vagus nerve (X)

Somite primordia and their nerves:
Preotic somitomeres—oculomotor nerve (III)
trochlear nerve (IV)
abducens nerve (VI)
Postotic somites—hypoglossal nerve (XII)
Somitic mesenchyme—accessory nerve (XI)

Ectodermal structures and their nerves:
Olfactory placode—olfactory nerve (I)
Optic cup—optic nerve (II)
Otic placode—vestibulocochlear nerve (VIII)

8.19 CRANIAL NERVE PRIMORDIA

The 12 pairs of cranial nerves exit the developing brain in sequence, except for cranial nerve XI, which exits most caudally. Cranial nerves I and II are CNS tracts, not peripheral nerves. The cranial nerves relate to surface placodes, head somites, or the pharyngeal arches, and they innervate all of the structures and tissues that derive from them. The vagus nerve supplies arches 4 and 6. Although the otic, ciliary, pterygopalatine, and submandibular ganglia are associated anatomically with branches of the trigeminal nerve, these ganglia contain postganglionic neurons of the parasympathetic nervous system, receiving inputs from preganglionic neurons whose axons travel with CNs III, VII, and IX.

Special sensory and somatomotor cranial nerve components

Nerve	Primordium innervated	Neuron components
Olfactory (I) Optic (II) Vestibulocochlear (VIII)	Olfactory placode Optic cup Otic placode	Special sensory (olfaction) Special sensory (vision) Special sensory (hearing and balance)

Oculomotor (III)
 	
Trochlear (IV)
Abducens (VI)
Hypoglossal (XII)
Accessory (XI)
	Preotic somitomere
	
	Preotic somitomere
	Preotic somitomere
	Postotic somites
	Somitic mesenchyme
	by arch 6
		Somatomotor to extraocular eye muscles
		Parasympathetics to ciliary ganglion (for pupil
		  constrictor and ciliary muscle)
		Somatomotor to superior oblique muscle
		Somatomotor to lateral rectus muscle
		Somatomotor to tongue muscles
		Somatomotor to sternocleidomastoid and trapezius
		  muscles

Pharyngeal arch cranial nerve components

Nerve	Arch	Neuron components
Trigeminal (V)	1	General sensory (face, orbit, nasal, and oral cavities) Branchiomotor (muscles of mastication, tensor tympani, tensor veli palatini)

Facial (VII)	2	Branchiomotor (muscles of facial expression, stylohyoid, posterior
		  digastric, stapedius)
		Special sensory (taste to anterior two thirds of tongue)
		Parasympathetic to pterygopalatine and submandibular ganglia (for
		  lacrimal glands, nasal mucosa, and salivary glands)

Glossopharyngeal (IX)	3	Visceral sensory to pharynx Branchiomotor to stylopharyngeus Parasympathetic to otic ganglion (for the parotid gland) Special sensory (taste to posterior tongue; carotid body and sinus)
Vagus (X)	4 and 6	Branchiomotor (pharynx and larynx) Visceral sensory (larynx, foregut below pharynx and midgut) General sensory to external acoustic meatus Parasympathetics (enteric ganglia of foregut and midgut) Special sensory (taste in laryngopharynx; carotid body and sinus)

Reprinted with permission from Cochard L. Netter's Atlas of Human Embryology, Updated Edition. Philadelphia: Elsevier, 2012.

8.20 CRANIAL NERVE NEURON COMPONENTS

The pharyngeal arch nerves of the head and neck consist of several neuronal types. Most have branchiomotor neurons for skeletal muscles derived from arch mesenchyme, visceral sensory neurons for the inner endodermal linings of the arches (larynx and pharynx), and general sensory neurons for surface ectoderm or lining of the stomodeum. The somites give rise to extraocular muscles and intrinsic muscles of the tongue. The placodes and optic cup relate to the special sensory organs of the head. Cranial nerves III, VII, IX, and X have preganglionic parasympathetic components that innervate ganglia distant from their nerves of origin.

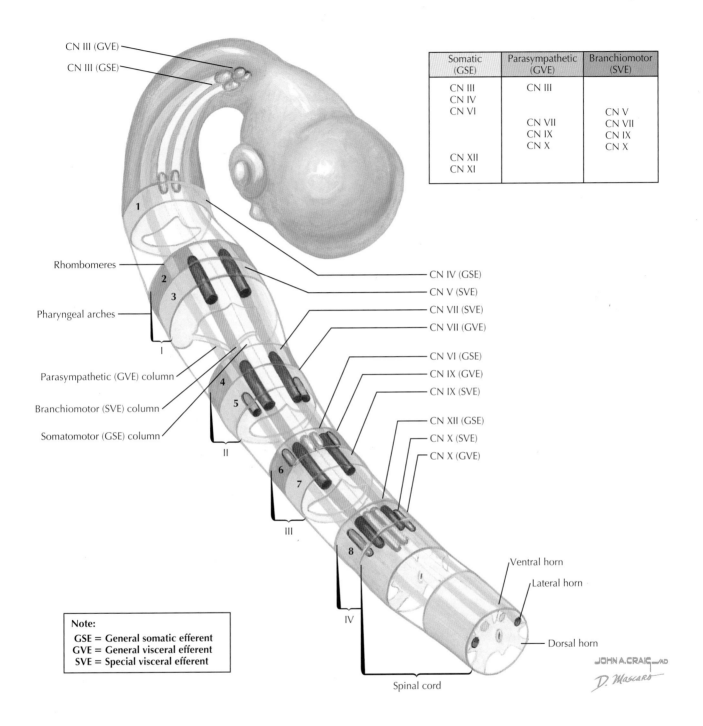

	Somatic (GSE)	Parasympathetic (GVE)	Branchiomotor (SVE)
	CN III	CN III	
	CN IV		
	CN VI		CN V
		CN VII	CN VII
		CN IX	CN IX
		CN X	CN X
	CN XII		
	CN XI		

CN III (GVE)

CN III (GSE)

Rhombomeres

Pharyngeal arches

Parasympathetic (GVE) column

Branchiomotor (SVE) column

Somatomotor (GSE) column

CN IV (GSE)

CN V (SVE)

CN VII (SVE)

CN VII (GVE)

CN VI (GSE)

CN IX (GVE)

CN IX (SVE)

CN XII (GSE)

CN X (SVE)

CN X (GVE)

Ventral horn

Lateral horn

Dorsal horn

Spinal cord

Note:
GSE = General somatic efferent
GVE = General visceral efferent
SVE = Special visceral efferent

JOHN A. CRAIG—MD
D. Mascaro

8.21 DEVELOPMENT OF MOTOR AND PREGANGLIONIC AUTONOMIC NUCLEI IN THE BRAINSTEM AND SPINAL CORD

Gray matter columns develop in the spinal cord for somatic lower motor neurons (ventral horn) and preganglionic autonomic neurons (lateral horn). These columns extend rostrally into the brainstem, maintaining the same general positional relationship to each other but organized into a series of separate but aligned nuclei. A third group of nuclei develops in the rhombencephalon as branchiomotor neurons supplying pharyngeal arch muscles. Both the somatic motor and the branchiomotor neurons are classified as lower motor neurons and have axons exiting the CNS to synapse on skeletal muscle fibers.

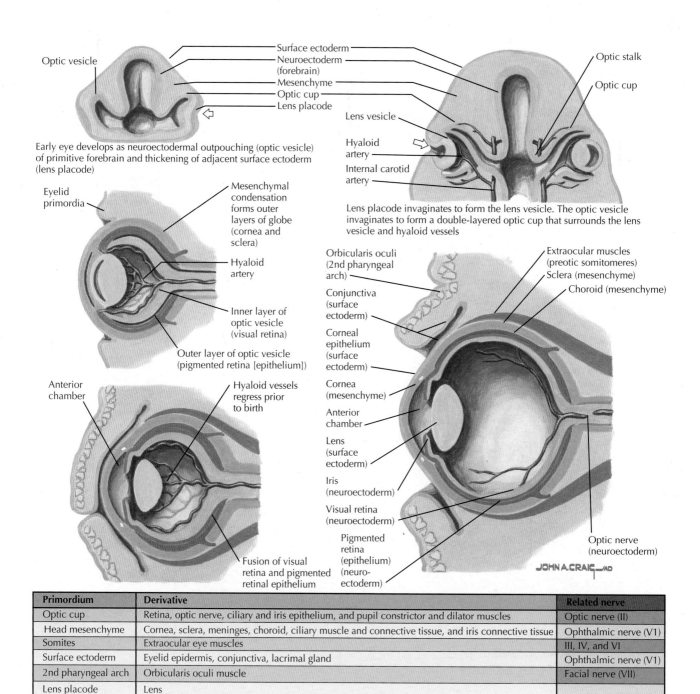

Optic vesicle

Surface ectoderm
Neuroectoderm (forebrain)
Mesenchyme
Optic cup
Lens placode

Optic stalk
Optic cup

Early eye develops as neuroectodermal outpouching (optic vesicle) of primitive forebrain and thickening of adjacent surface ectoderm (lens placode)

Lens vesicle
Hyaloid artery
Internal carotid artery

Lens placode invaginates to form the lens vesicle. The optic vesicle invaginates to form a double-layered optic cup that surrounds the lens vesicle and hyaloid vessels

Eyelid primordia

Mesenchymal condensation forms outer layers of globe (cornea and sclera)
Hyaloid artery
Inner layer of optic vesicle (visual retina)
Outer layer of optic vesicle (pigmented retina [epithelium])

Orbicularis oculi (2nd pharyngeal arch)
Conjunctiva (surface ectoderm)
Corneal epithelium (surface ectoderm)
Cornea (mesenchyme)
Anterior chamber
Lens (surface ectoderm)
Iris (neuroectoderm)
Visual retina (neuroectoderm)
Pigmented retina (epithelium) (neuroectoderm)

Extraocular muscles (preotic somitomeres)
Sclera (mesenchyme)
Choroid (mesenchyme)

Anterior chamber
Hyaloid vessels regress prior to birth
Fusion of visual retina and pigmented retinal epithelium

Optic nerve (neuroectoderm)

JOHN A. CRAIG—AD

Primordium	Derivative	Related nerve
Optic cup	Retina, optic nerve, ciliary and iris epithelium, and pupil constrictor and dilator muscles	Optic nerve (II)
Head mesenchyme	Cornea, sclera, meninges, choroid, ciliary muscle and connective tissue, and iris connective tissue	Ophthalmic nerve (V1)
Somites	Extraocular eye muscles	III, IV, and VI
Surface ectoderm	Eyelid epidermis, conjunctiva, lacrimal gland	Ophthalmic nerve (V1)
2nd pharyngeal arch	Orbicularis oculi muscle	Facial nerve (VII)
Lens placode	Lens	

8.22 DEVELOPMENT OF THE EYE AND ORBIT

The retina and optic nerve develop as a double-layered extension of the neural tube, the optic cup. This extension surrounds the lens vesicle of surface origin and has a ventral groove to accommodate blood vessels. The iris and ciliary body are formed in part from optic cup epithelium. The two layers of the optic cup never fully fuse and can be separated in the case of a retinal detachment. Connective tissues of mesodermal origin include the sclera, cornea, and vascular choroid layer. The extraocular muscles derive from somitomeres. The epidermis of the eyelids develops from surface ectoderm and is continuous with the conjunctiva and corneal epithelium.

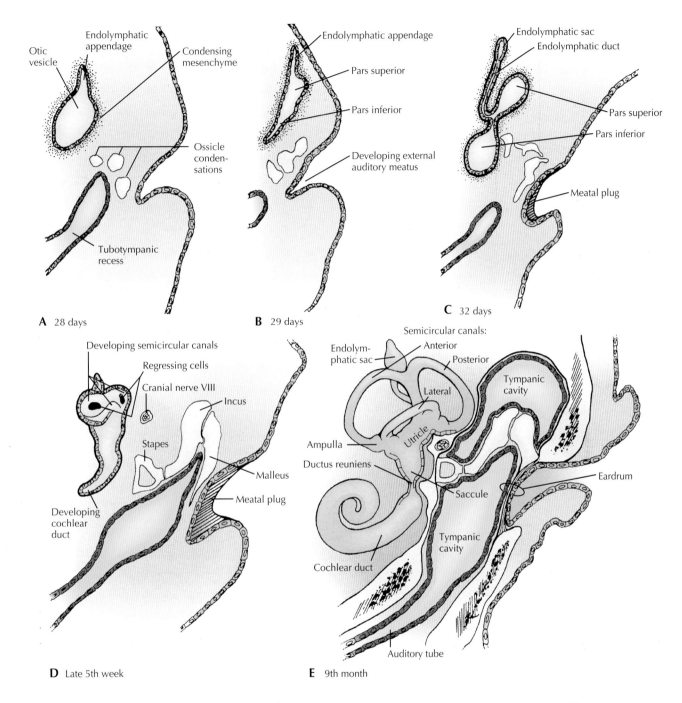

A 28 days

B 29 days

C 32 days

D Late 5th week

E 9th month

8.23 DEVELOPMENT OF THE EAR

The ear consists of the outer component (the auricle, external auditory meatus to the eardrum); the middle component (the ossicles [malleus, incus, stapes]); and the inner component (the bony and membranous labyrinths, the cochlea, and the semicircular canals). The outer ear derives from the first pharyngeal groove, the middle ear from the first pharyngeal pouch, and the inner ear from the otic placode.

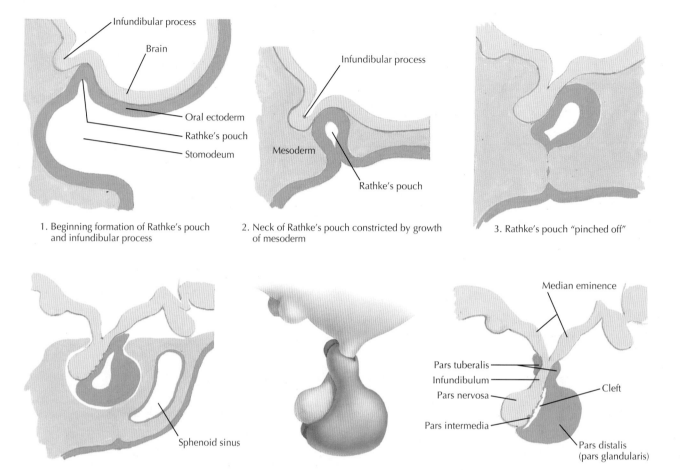

1. Beginning formation of Rathke's pouch and infundibular process

2. Neck of Rathke's pouch constricted by growth of mesoderm

3. Rathke's pouch "pinched off"

4. Pinched-off segment conforms to neural process, forming pars distalis, pars intermedia, and pars tuberalis

5. Pars tuberalis encircles infundibular stalk (lateral surface view)

6. Mature form

Pituitary hormones

From the anterior lobe (pars distalis)		From the posterior lobe (pars nervosa)
Follicle-stimulating hormone (FSH)	Thyroid-stimulating hormone (TSH)	Vasopressin
Luteinizing hormone (LH)	Adrenocorticotropic hormone (ACTH)	Oxytocin
Prolactin	Growth hormone (GH)	

8.24 DEVELOPMENT OF THE PITUITARY GLAND

The pituitary gland develops from outgrowth of two separate primordia. The anterior lobe (adenohypophysis) derives from the roof of the stomodeum and encircles the base of the posterior lobe (neurohypophysis). The posterior lobe derives from the brain and possesses axonal processes from the hypothalamus that secrete oxytocin and vasopressin into the general circulation.

The anterior lobe contains pituicytes that respond to releasing and inhibitory factors from neurons of the brain that are delivered through a private vascular channel, the hypophyseal-portal system, and secreted into this circulation are hormones such as follicle-stimulating hormone, luteinizing hormone, prolactin, thyroid-stimulating hormone, adrenocorticotropic hormone, and growth hormone.

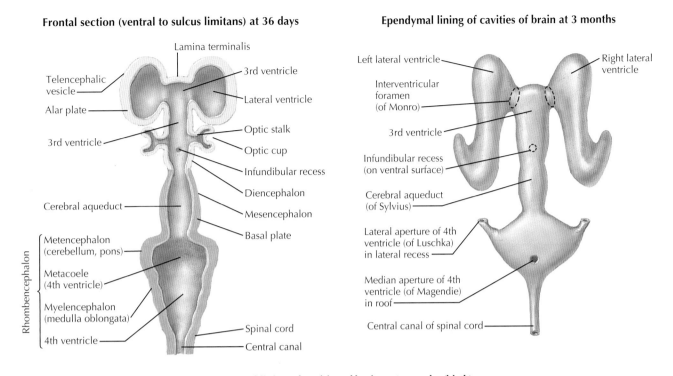

Frontal section (ventral to sulcus limitans) at 36 days

- Lamina terminalis
- Telencephalic vesicle
- 3rd ventricle
- Lateral ventricle
- Alar plate
- Optic stalk
- 3rd ventricle
- Optic cup
- Infundibular recess
- Diencephalon
- Cerebral aqueduct
- Mesencephalon
- Basal plate
- Metencephalon (cerebellum, pons)
- Rhombencephalon
- Metacoele (4th ventricle)
- Myelencephalon (medulla oblongata)
- Spinal cord
- 4th ventricle
- Central canal

Ependymal lining of cavities of brain at 3 months

- Left lateral ventricle
- Right lateral ventricle
- Interventricular foramen (of Monro)
- 3rd ventricle
- Infundibular recess (on ventral surface)
- Cerebral aqueduct (of Sylvius)
- Lateral aperture of 4th ventricle (of Luschka) in lateral recess
- Median aperture of 4th ventricle (of Magendie) in roof
- Central canal of spinal cord

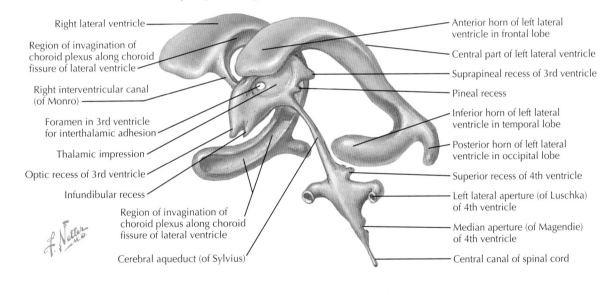

Ependymal lining of cavities of brain at 9 months (birth)

- Right lateral ventricle
- Region of invagination of choroid plexus along choroid fissure of lateral ventricle
- Right interventricular canal (of Monro)
- Foramen in 3rd ventricle for interthalamic adhesion
- Thalamic impression
- Optic recess of 3rd ventricle
- Infundibular recess
- Region of invagination of choroid plexus along choroid fissure of lateral ventricle
- Cerebral aqueduct (of Sylvius)
- Anterior horn of left lateral ventricle in frontal lobe
- Central part of left lateral ventricle
- Suprapineal recess of 3rd ventricle
- Pineal recess
- Inferior horn of left lateral ventricle in temporal lobe
- Posterior horn of left lateral ventricle in occipital lobe
- Superior recess of 4th ventricle
- Left lateral aperture (of Luschka) of 4th ventricle
- Median aperture (of Magendie) of 4th ventricle
- Central canal of spinal cord

8.25 DEVELOPMENT OF THE VENTRICLES

The rapid growth of the brainstem and the forebrain alters the uniform appearance of the ventricles. The C-shaped lateral ventricles follow the growth of the telencephalon, with limited access into the third ventricle through the interventricular foramen of Monro. The narrow cerebral aqueduct remains very small in the upper mesencephalon and opens into the rhomboid-shaped and expanding fourth ventricle. The foramina of Magendie (medial) and Luschka (lateral) in the fourth ventricle allow flow from the ventricular system into the developing cisterns of the subarachnoid space. CSF reenters the venous system through the arachnoid granulations, one-way valves that allow drainage from the subarachnoid space into the dural (venous) sinuses, especially the superior sagittal sinus.

CLINICAL POINT

The C-shaped form of the ventricular system follows from the development of the primary brain vesicles, with the flexures and disproportionate neural development. The lateral ventricles are associated with the telencephalon, the third ventricle with the diencephalon, the cerebral aqueduct with the mesencephalon, and the fourth ventricle with the rhombencephalon (metencephalon [pons] and myelencephalon [medulla]). The foramina of Magendie and Luschka, which allow for the escape of CSF into the subarachnoid space, are already patent at the end of the first trimester. An obstruction of internal CSF flow results in **internal hydrocephalus**. A common site for such an obstruction is atresia of the cerebral aqueduct, with enlarged third and lateral ventricles. Another site of possible obstruction occurs with Dandy-Walker syndrome, a malformation of the fourth ventricle that includes atresia of the foramina of Magendie and Luschka, internal hydrocephalus of the entire ventricular system, hypoplasia of the cerebellum, and posterior fossa cyst formation.

9

PERIPHERAL NERVOUS SYSTEM

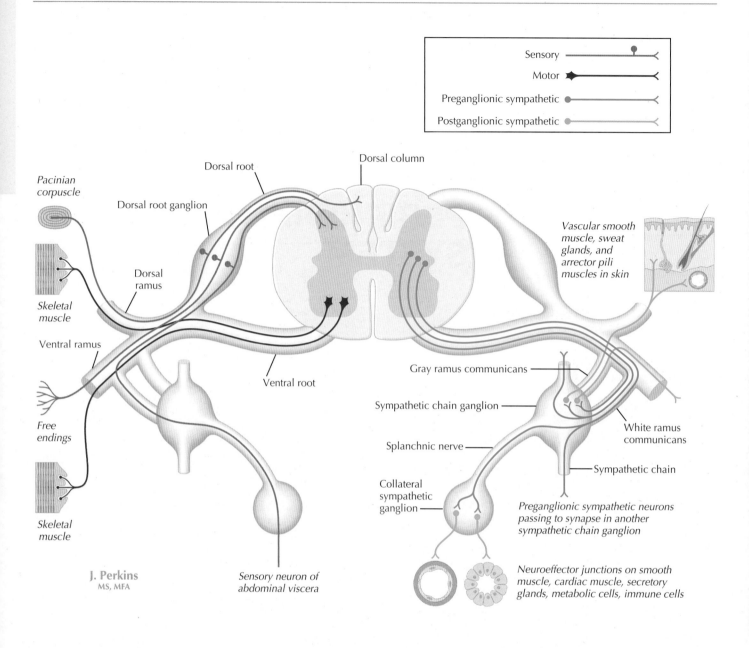

Sensory
Motor
Preganglionic sympathetic
Postganglionic sympathetic

Dorsal column

Dorsal root

Dorsal root ganglion

Pacinian corpuscle

Dorsal ramus

Skeletal muscle

Ventral ramus

Ventral root

Free endings

Skeletal muscle

J. Perkins
MS, MFA

Sensory neuron of abdominal viscera

Vascular smooth muscle, sweat glands, and arrector pili muscles in skin

Gray ramus communicans

Sympathetic chain ganglion

White ramus communicans

Splanchnic nerve

Sympathetic chain

Collateral sympathetic ganglion

Preganglionic sympathetic neurons passing to synapse in another sympathetic chain ganglion

Neuroeffector junctions on smooth muscle, cardiac muscle, secretory glands, metabolic cells, immune cells

INTRODUCTION AND BASIC ORGANIZATION

9.1 SCHEMATIC OF THE SPINAL CORD WITH SENSORY, MOTOR, AND AUTONOMIC COMPONENTS OF PERIPHERAL NERVES

Peripheral nerves consist of axons from primary sensory neurons, lower motor neurons (LMNs), and preganglionic and postganglionic autonomic neurons. The primary sensory axons have sensory receptors (transducing elements) at their peripheral (distal) ends, contiguous with the initial segment of the axon. The proximal portion of the axon enters the central nervous system (CNS) and terminates in secondary sensory nuclei associated with reflex, cerebellar, and lemniscal channels. LMNs in the anterior horn of the spinal cord send axons via the ventral (anterior) roots to travel in peripheral nerves to skeletal muscles, with which they form neuromuscular junctions. The autonomic preganglionic neurons send axons via the ventral roots to terminate in autonomic ganglia or in the adrenal medulla. Postganglionic neurons send axons into splanchnic or peripheral nerves and form neuroeffector junctions

with smooth muscle, cardiac muscle, secretory glands, metabolic cells, and cells of the immune system. Splanchnic nerves convey preganglionic axons to collateral sympathetic ganglia in the abdomen and pelvis viscera, postganglionic axons to the thoracic viscera, and sensory axons from the viscera.

CLINICAL POINT

Peripheral nerves form through the union of dorsal and ventral roots and by subsequent branching, similar to the process that occurs through the brachial plexus. The resultant terminal peripheral nerves contain limited categories of axonal types, including LMN axons (both alpha and gamma), primary sensory axons (both myelinated and unmyelinated), and autonomic axons (mainly postganglionic sympathetic axons). Destructive lesions in peripheral nerves may cause flaccid paralysis of innervated skeletal muscles (with loss of tone and denervation atrophy), loss of some or all aspects of somatic sensation in the innervated territory, and some autonomic dysfunction resulting from loss of sympathetic innervation (e.g., vasodilation and lack of sweating). An irritative lesion of a peripheral nerve is usually manifested as pain radiating to the innervated territory.

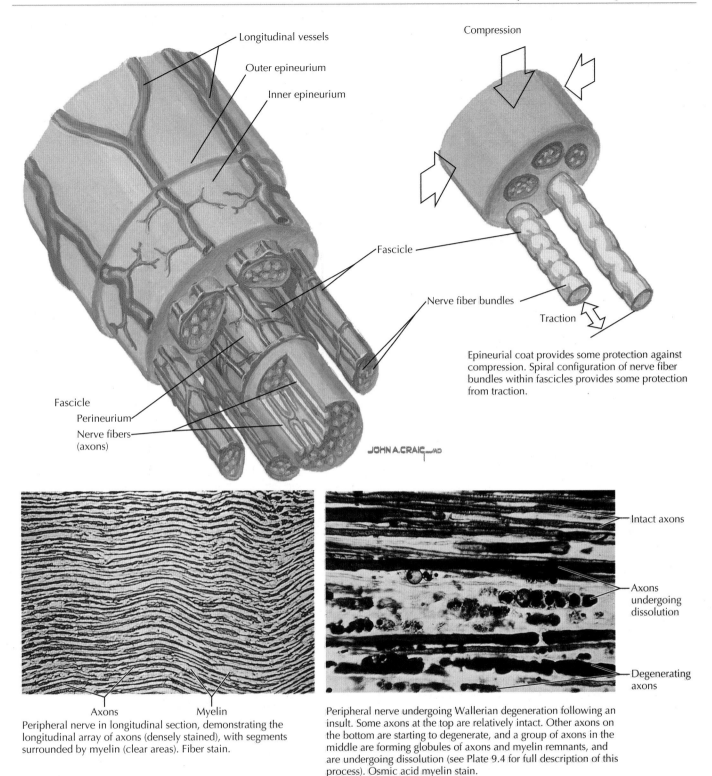

Compression

Longitudinal vessels

Outer epineurium

Inner epineurium

Fascicle

Nerve fiber bundles

Traction

Epineurial coat provides some protection against compression. Spiral configuration of nerve fiber bundles within fascicles provides some protection from traction.

Fascicle
Perineurium
Nerve fibers (axons)

JOHN A. CRAIG—AD

Axons   Myelin

Peripheral nerve in longitudinal section, demonstrating the longitudinal array of axons (densely stained), with segments surrounded by myelin (clear areas). Fiber stain.

Intact axons

Axons undergoing dissolution

Degenerating axons

Peripheral nerve undergoing Wallerian degeneration following an insult. Some axons at the top are relatively intact. Other axons on the bottom are starting to degenerate, and a group of axons in the middle are forming globules of axons and myelin remnants, and are undergoing dissolution (see Plate 9.4 for full description of this process). Osmic acid myelin stain.

9.2 ANATOMY OF A PERIPHERAL NERVE

A peripheral nerve is made up of unmyelinated and myelinated axons, the connective sheaths with which they are associated, and local blood vessels, the vasa nervorum. Unmyelinated axons are surrounded by the cytoplasm of Schwann cells, called Schwann cell sheaths. Each individual segment of a myelinated axon is enwrapped by a myelin sheath, provided by an individual Schwann cell. The bare space between each myelin sheath is called a node of Ranvier and is the site on the membrane where sodium channels are present and is also the site of initiation or reinitiation of the action potential. Endoneurium is loose, supportive, connective tissue that is found between individual axons within a fascicle. Fascicles of multiple axons are enwrapped by a sheath of supportive cells and collagenous connective tissue; this perineurium functions as a blood-nerve barrier and helps to protect the axons from local diffusion of potentially damaging substances. This perineurial barrier can be disrupted in neuropathic conditions such as diabetic neuropathy. The epineurium is the outermost layer of supportive connective tissue that enwraps the entire nerve.

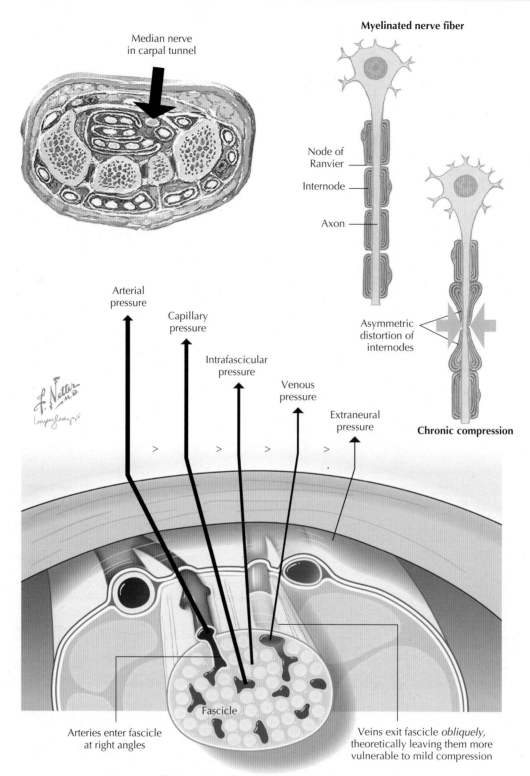

Median nerve
in carpal tunnel

Myelinated nerve fiber

Node of
Ranvier

Internode

Axon

Asymmetric
distortion of
internodes

Chronic compression

Arterial
pressure

Capillary
pressure

Intrafascicular
pressure

Venous
pressure

Extraneural
pressure

Arteries enter fascicle
at right angles

Fascicle

Veins exit fascicle *obliquely,*
theoretically leaving them more
vulnerable to mild compression

Pressure gradient necessary for adequate intrafascicular circulation

9.3 NERVE COMPRESSION AND PRESSURE GRADIENTS

With chronic compression of a nerve, such as median nerve entrapment in carpal tunnel syndrome, internodes of large myelinated axons are distorted (accompanied by repeated demyelination and remyelination), and both ischemia and endoneurial edema occur. Endoneurial edema can induce venous congestion and increase fluid pressure, resulting in metabolic, physiologic, and anatomic damage and dysfunction of the affected peripheral nerves. Affected axons exhibit impaired axoplasmic transport, both anterograde and retrograde. Diabetes increases the susceptibility of peripheral nerves to entrapment, with endoneurial edema and impaired axoplasmic transport. Chronic compression can lead to degeneration of the affected axons.

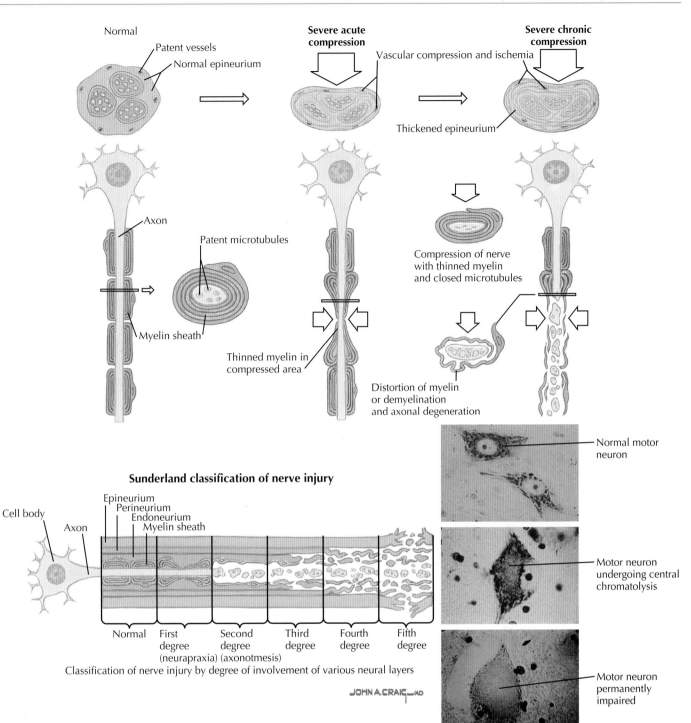

Sunderland classification of nerve injury

Classification of nerve injury by degree of involvement of various neural layers

JOHN A. CRAIG—AD

9.4 PERIPHERAL NERVE INJURY AND DEGENERATION IN A COMPRESSION NEUROPATHY

If a peripheral nerve is compressed or damaged, a series of reactions takes place within the neurons whose axons have been damaged and in the supportive tissue. At the site of the injury, axonal damage and thinning of the myelin or frank demyelination can occur. Distal to the site of the injury, the peripheral portion of the axon can degenerate (called Wallerian degeneration), resulting in the breaking up and dissolution of the peripheral axon. The Schwann cells responsible for myelinating the degenerating axons also break up and degenerate. However, the basement membrane remains intact, providing a scaffold through which future regenerating axons can be directed. The

central (proximal) portion of the neuron can undergo changes called central chromatolysis. The Nissl bodies (endoplasmic reticulum) break up into individual ribosomes, the cell body swells, and the neuron shifts its metabolism to structural and reparative synthetic products that attempt to save the neuron and permit it to try to recover from the injury. If successful, this process gradually reverses, and the neuron begins to sprout a peripheral axonal extension, seeking to reattach to the target from which it was disrupted. The Schwann cells proliferate and generate new myelin sheaths around the regrowing axon, but the intersegmental distances of the new myelin sheath are shorter than the original distances and the myelin sheath is thinner; thus, the regenerated axon shows a slower conduction velocity than the original intact axon.

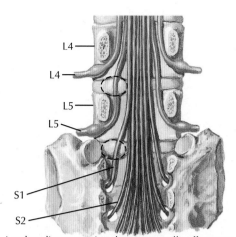

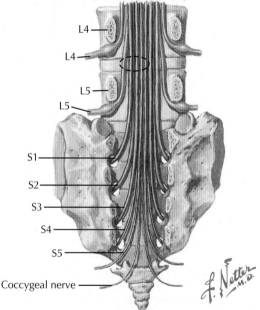

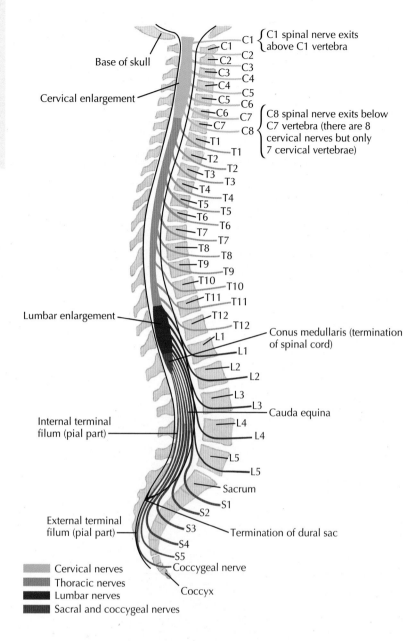

C1 { C1 spinal nerve exits above C1 vertebra

Base of skull

Cervical enlargement

C8 { C8 spinal nerve exits below C7 vertebra (there are 8 cervical nerves but only 7 cervical vertebrae)

Lumbar enlargement

Conus medullaris (termination of spinal cord)

Cauda equina

Internal terminal filum (pial part)

External terminal filum (pial part)

Sacrum

Termination of dural sac

Coccygeal nerve

Coccyx

Cervical nerves
Thoracic nerves
Lumbar nerves
Sacral and coccygeal nerves

Lumbar disc protrusion does not usually affect nerve exiting above disc. Lateral protrusion at disc level L4–5 affects L5 spinal nerve, not L4 spinal nerve. Protrusion at disc level L5–S1 affects S1 spinal nerve, not L5 spinal nerve

Coccygeal nerve

Medial protrusion at disc level L4–5 rarely affects L4 spinal nerve but may affect L5 spinal nerve and sometimes S1–4 spinal nerves.

9.5 RELATIONSHIP OF SPINAL NERVE ROOTS TO VERTEBRAE

The dorsal (posterior) and ventral (anterior) roots of the spinal cord segments extend from the spinal cord as peripheral axons, invested initially with meninges. As the axons enter the peripheral nervous system, they become associated with Schwann cells for myelination and support. The roots exit through the intervertebral foramina, compact openings between the vertebrae where herniated discs (nucleus pulposus) may impinge on the nerve roots and produce sensory or motor symptoms. Sensory and motor axons travel with the dorsal and ventral rami of peripheral nerves. Autonomic preganglionic axons (myelinated) course from the ventral roots into the white (preganglionic) rami communicans and synapse in autonomic ganglia. The ganglion cells give rise to postganglionic axons (unmyelinated) that course through the gray rami communicans and join the peripheral nerves.

CLINICAL POINT

The longitudinal growth of the spinal column outstrips the longitudinal growth of the spinal cord; as a consequence, the spinal cord in adults ends adjacent to the L1 vertebral body. Nerve roots heading for intervertebral foramina below L1 extend caudally through the subarachnoid space in the lumbar cistern, forming the cauda equina. Damage to the cauda equina can occur as the result of tumors, such as ependymomas and lipomas, or of a prolapsed intervertebral disc. It is common for symptoms to occur gradually and be irregular because of the ample room in the lumbar cistern for nerve roots to move. Radicular pain often is experienced in a sciatic distribution, with progressive loss of sensation in radicular patterns. A more caudal location of the obstructing mass may lead to loss of sensation in regions of sacral innervation in the perineal (saddle) zone. Loss of bowel, bladder, and erectile function also may occur. More rostral lesions may result in flaccid paralysis of the legs.

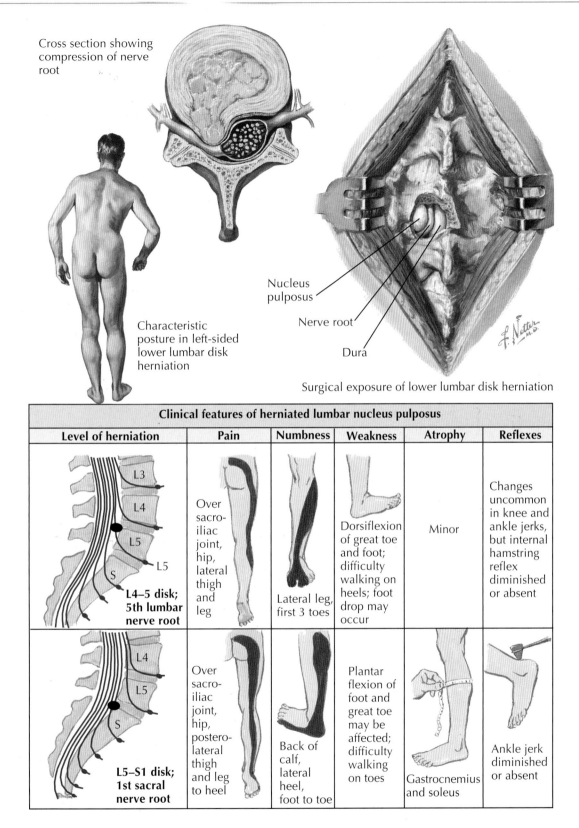

Cross section showing compression of nerve root

Characteristic posture in left-sided lower lumbar disk herniation

Nucleus pulposus

Nerve root

Dura

Surgical exposure of lower lumbar disk herniation

Clinical features of herniated lumbar nucleus pulposus					
Level of herniation	**Pain**	**Numbness**	**Weakness**	**Atrophy**	**Reflexes**
L3 L4 L5 L5 S **L4–5 disk; 5th lumbar nerve root**	Over sacro-iliac joint, hip, lateral thigh and leg	Lateral leg, first 3 toes	Dorsiflexion of great toe and foot; difficulty walking on heels; foot drop may occur	Minor	Changes uncommon in knee and ankle jerks, but internal hamstring reflex diminished or absent
L4 L5 S **L5–S1 disk; 1st sacral nerve root**	Over sacro-iliac joint, hip, postero-lateral thigh and leg to heel	Back of calf, lateral heel, foot to toe	Plantar flexion of foot and great toe may be affected; difficulty walking on toes	Gastrocnemius and soleus	Ankle jerk diminished or absent

9.6 LUMBAR DISC HERNIATION: L4–L5 AND L5–S1

Characteristics and clinical manifestation of lower lumbar disc herniations at L4–L5 and L5–S1.

A. Sensory Channels—Reflex

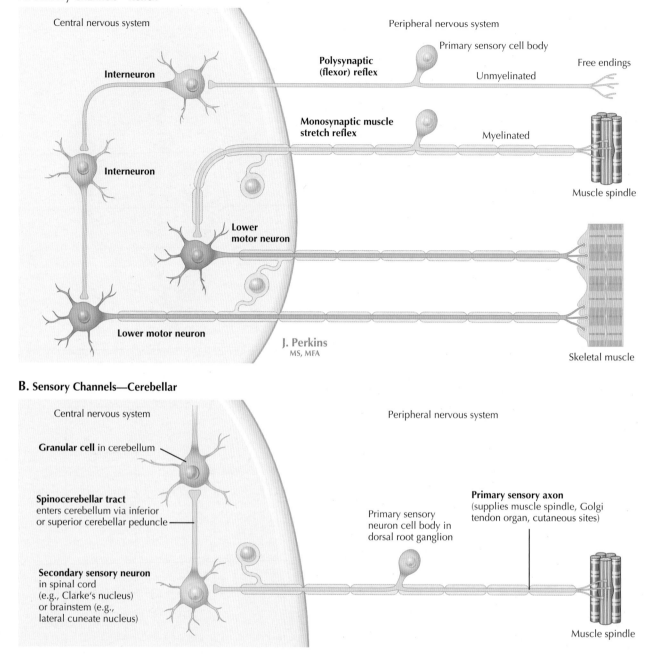

Central nervous system

Peripheral nervous system

Primary sensory cell body

Free endings

Polysynaptic (flexor) reflex

Interneuron

Unmyelinated

Monosynaptic muscle stretch reflex

Myelinated

Interneuron

Muscle spindle

Lower motor neuron

J. Perkins
MS, MFA

Lower motor neuron

Skeletal muscle

B. Sensory Channels—Cerebellar

Central nervous system

Peripheral nervous system

Granular cell in cerebellum

Spinocerebellar tract
enters cerebellum via inferior
or superior cerebellar peduncle

Primary sensory axon
(supplies muscle spindle, Golgi
tendon organ, cutaneous sites)

Primary sensory
neuron cell body in
dorsal root ganglion

Secondary sensory neuron
in spinal cord
(e.g., Clarke's nucleus)
or brainstem (e.g.,
lateral cuneate nucleus)

Muscle spindle

9.7 SENSORY CHANNELS: REFLEX AND CEREBELLAR

Primary sensory axons communicate with secondary sensory neurons in reflex, cerebellar, and lemniscal channels, carrying transduced information from the periphery into the CNS. **A,** The reflex channels interconnect primary sensory axons with anterior horn cells (LMNs) through one or more synapses to achieve unconscious reflex motor responses to sensory input. These responses can be elicited in an isolated spinal cord devoid of connections from the brain. The monosynaptic reflex channels connect primary sensory Ia axons from muscle spindles, via the dorsal roots, directly with LMNs involved in muscle stretch reflex contraction; this is the only monosynaptic reflex seen in the human CNS. Polysynaptic reflex channels are directed particularly toward flexor (withdrawal) responses through one or more interneurons to produce coordinated patterns of muscle activity to remove a portion of the body from a potentially damaging or offending stimulus. This polysynaptic channel can spread ipsilaterally and contralaterally through many segments. **B,** Primary somatosensory axons carrying unconsciously processed information from muscles, joints, tendons, ligaments, and cutaneous sources enter the CNS via dorsal roots and synapse with secondary sensory neurons in the spinal cord or caudal brainstem. These secondary sensory neurons convey information, initially derived from the periphery, to the ipsilateral cerebellum via spinocerebellar pathways. The dorsal and ventral spinocerebellar pathways carry information from the lower body (T6 and below). The rostral spinocerebellar tract and the cuneocerebellar tract carry information from the upper body (above T6). Polysynaptic indirect spinocerebellar pathways (spino-olivocerebellar and spino-reticulo-cerebellar tracts) also are present.

Sensory Channels—Lemniscal

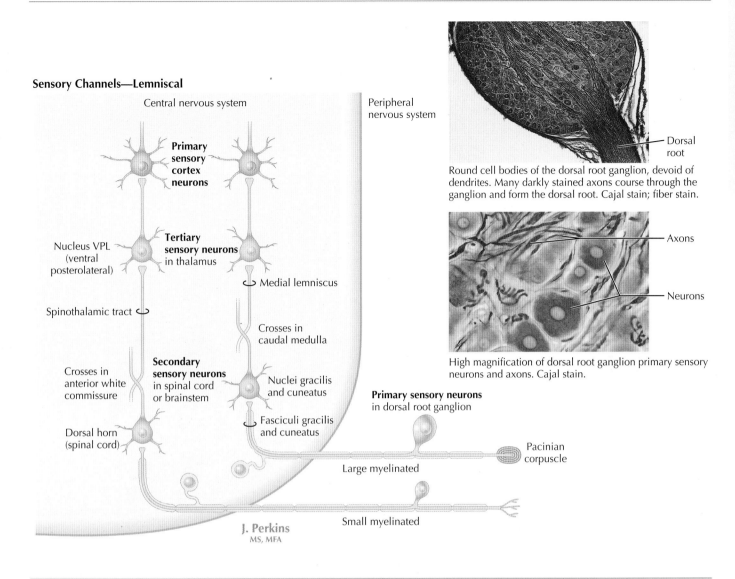

Round cell bodies of the dorsal root ganglion, devoid of dendrites. Many darkly stained axons course through the ganglion and form the dorsal root. Cajal stain; fiber stain.

High magnification of dorsal root ganglion primary sensory neurons and axons. Cajal stain.

J. Perkins
MS, MFA

9.8 SENSORY CHANNELS: LEMNISCAL

Primary sensory axons carrying sensory information destined for conscious perception arise from receptors in superficial and deep tissue. These axons enter the CNS via the dorsal roots and terminate on secondary sensory nuclei in the spinal cord or brainstem. Secondary sensory axons from these nuclei cross the midline (decussate), ascend as lemniscal pathways, and terminate in the contralateral thalamus. These specific thalamic nuclei then project to specific regions of the primary sensory cortex, where fine-grained analysis of incoming, consciously perceived sensory information takes place. Somatosensory information is directed into two sets of channels, protopathic and epicritic. The epicritic information (fine, discriminative sensation; vibratory sensation; joint position sense) is transduced by primary sensory neurons (dorsal root ganglion cells) that send myelinated axons to neurons in the medulla, the nucleus gracilis (lower body, T6 and below), and the nucleus cuneatus (upper body, above T6). Nuclei gracilis and cuneatus give rise to the medial lemniscus, a crossed secondary sensory pathway that terminates in the ventral posterolateral (VPL) nucleus of the thalamus. This thalamic nucleus has reciprocal projections with cortical neurons in the postcentral gyrus (Brodmann's areas 3, 1, and 2). This entire epicritic somatosensory system is highly topographically organized, with each region of the body represented in each nucleus and axonal pathway. The protopathic information (pain, temperature sensation, light moving touch) is transduced by primary sensory neurons (dorsal root ganglion cells) that project mainly via small myelinated and unmyelinated axons to neurons in the dorsal horn of the spinal cord. These spinal cord neurons give rise to the spinothalamic tract (spinal lemniscus), a secondary sensory pathway that terminates in separate neuronal sites in the VPL nucleus of the thalamus. This portion of the VPL nucleus communicates mainly with the primary sensory cortex (SI) and a secondary area of somatosensory cortex (SII) posterior to the lateral postcentral gyrus. Some unmyelinated nociceptive protopathic axons that terminate in the dorsal horn of the spinal cord interconnect with a cascade of spinal cord interneurons that project mainly into the reticular formation of the brainstem (the spinoreticular pathway). This more diffuse pain system is processed through nonspecific thalamic nuclei with projections to somatosensory cortices and more widespread regions of cortex. This system can result in the perception of excruciating, long-lasting pain that may exceed the duration and intensity of direct peripheral stimuli. Chronic activation of this system can result in chronic neuropathic pain, persisting and reinforced by central mechanisms.

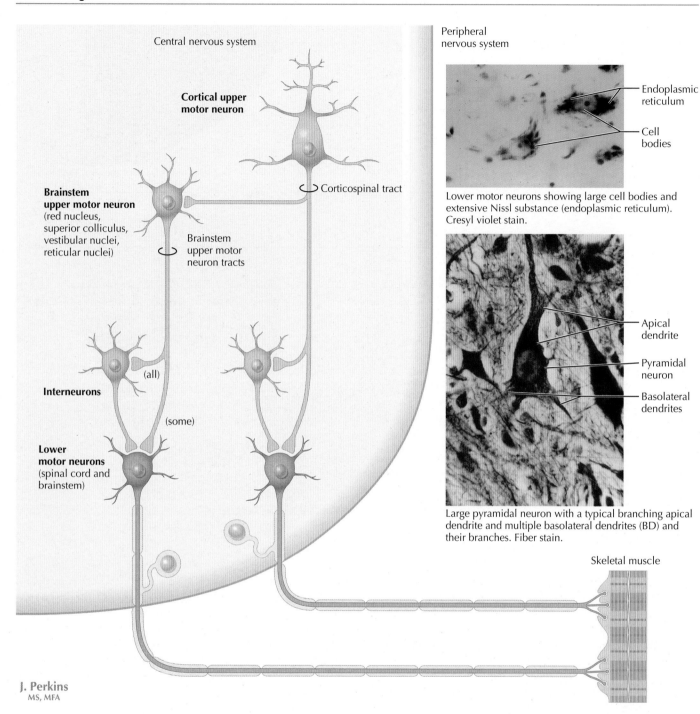

Central nervous system

Cortical upper
motor neuron

Corticospinal tract

Brainstem
upper motor neuron
(red nucleus,
superior colliculus,
vestibular nuclei,
reticular nuclei)

Brainstem
upper motor
neuron tracts

(all)

Interneurons

(some)

Lower
motor neurons
(spinal cord and
brainstem)

J. Perkins
MS, MFA

Peripheral
nervous system

Endoplasmic
reticulum

Cell
bodies

Lower motor neurons showing large cell bodies and
extensive Nissl substance (endoplasmic reticulum).
Cresyl violet stain.

Apical
dendrite

Pyramidal
neuron

Basolateral
dendrites

Large pyramidal neuron with a typical branching apical
dendrite and multiple basolateral dendrites (BD) and
their branches. Fiber stain.

Skeletal muscle

9.9 MOTOR CHANNELS: BASIC ORGANIZATION OF LOWER AND UPPER MOTOR NEURONS

LMNs are found in the anterior horn of the spinal cord and in motor cranial nerve nuclei in the brainstem. Their axons exit via the ventral roots or cranial nerves to supply skeletal muscles. LMN synapses with muscle fibers form neuromuscular junctions and release the neurotransmitter acetylcholine, which acts on nicotinic receptors on the skeletal muscle fibers. A motor unit consists of an LMN, its axon, and the muscle fibers the axon innervates. LMNs are regulated and coordinated by groups of upper motor neurons (UMNs) found in the brain. Brainstem UMNs regulate basic tone and posture. Cortical UMNs (from corticospinal and corticobulbar tracts) regulate consciously directed, or volitional, movements. Cortical UMNs also have extensive connections with brainstem UMNs and may help to coordinate their activities. The cerebellum and basal ganglia aid in the coordination of movement and in pattern selection, respectively, via connections with UMNs; the cerebellum and basal ganglia do not connect with LMNs directly.

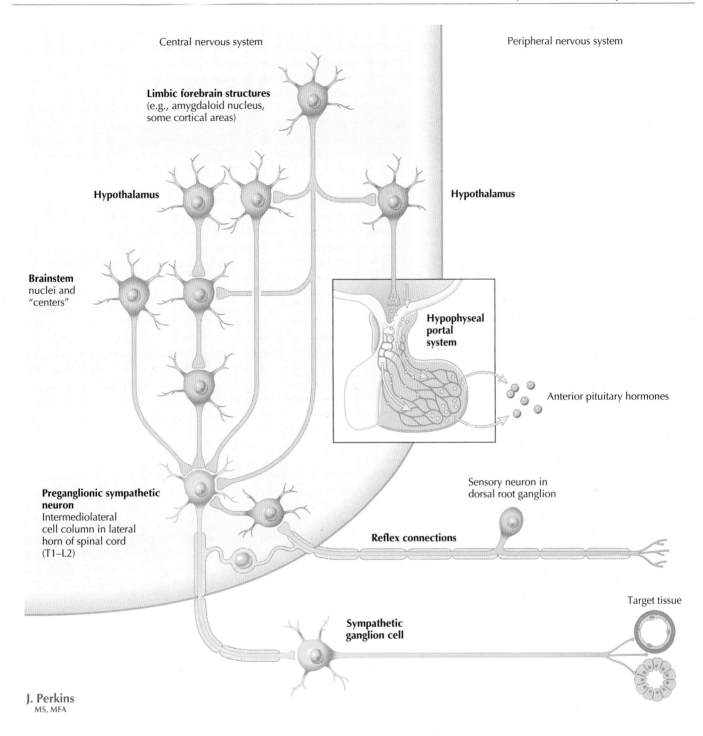

Central nervous system

Peripheral nervous system

Limbic forebrain structures
(e.g., amygdaloid nucleus,
some cortical areas)

Hypothalamus

Hypothalamus

Brainstem
nuclei and
"centers"

**Hypophyseal
portal
system**

Anterior pituitary hormones

Sensory neuron in
dorsal root ganglion

**Preganglionic sympathetic
neuron**
Intermediolateral
cell column in lateral
horn of spinal cord
(T1–L2)

Reflex connections

Target tissue

**Sympathetic
ganglion cell**

J. Perkins
MS, MFA

9.10 **AUTONOMIC CHANNELS**

Preganglionic neurons for the sympathetic nervous system (SNS) are found in the lateral horn (intermediolateral cell column) of the thoracolumbar (T1–L2) spinal cord (thoracolumbar system). Preganglionic neurons for the parasympathetic nervous system (PsNS) are found in nuclei of cranial nerves (CNs) III, VII, IX, and X and in the intermediate gray matter of the spinal cord between S2 and S4 (the craniosacral system). Preganglionic axons exit the CNS via cranial nerves or ventral roots and terminate in chain ganglia or collateral ganglia (the SNS) or in intramural ganglia in or near the organ innervated (the PsNS). Postganglionic autonomic axons innervate smooth muscle, cardiac muscle, secretory glands, metabolic cells (e.g., liver, fat cells), and cells of the immune system. The SNS is a fight-or-flight system that responds to emergency demands. The PsNS is a homeostatic, reparative system active in more quiescent activities and in digestive and eliminative functions. Preganglionic responses are coordinated by autonomic UMN equivalents from the brainstem (autonomic centers), the hypothalamus, and the limbic forebrain structures. Inputs that affect visceral functions or elicit emotional responsiveness, originating from sensory inputs or from the brain (including the cerebral cortex), are conveyed through these central autonomic regulatory systems, which help to coordinate appropriate autonomic responses. These central autonomic regulatory systems coordinate autonomic responses that affect both visceral functions and neuroendocrine outflow from the pituitary gland.

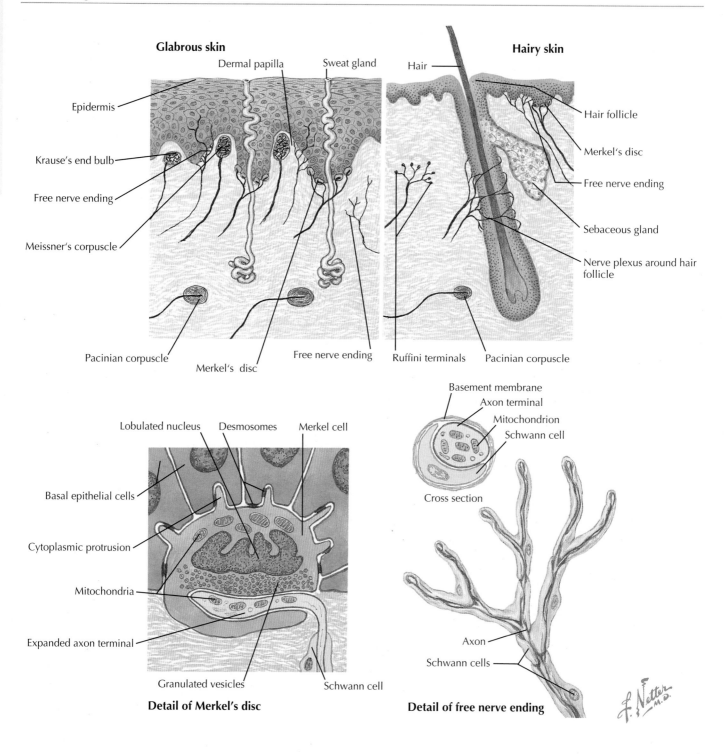

Glabrous skin

Dermal papilla

Sweat gland

Epidermis

Krause's end bulb

Free nerve ending

Meissner's corpuscle

Pacinian corpuscle

Merkel's disc

Free nerve ending

Hairy skin

Hair

Hair follicle

Merkel's disc

Free nerve ending

Sebaceous gland

Nerve plexus around hair follicle

Ruffini terminals

Pacinian corpuscle

Basement membrane

Axon terminal

Mitochondrion

Schwann cell

Cross section

Lobulated nucleus

Desmosomes

Merkel cell

Basal epithelial cells

Cytoplasmic protrusion

Mitochondria

Expanded axon terminal

Granulated vesicles

Schwann cell

Detail of Merkel's disc

Axon

Schwann cells

Detail of free nerve ending

9.11 CUTANEOUS RECEPTORS

Cutaneous receptors are found at the distal ends of the primary sensory axon; they act as dendrites, in which threshold stimuli lead to the firing of an action potential at the initial segment of the primary sensory axon. Although specific types of sensory receptors are thought to code for consciously perceived modalities, there is not an exact correlation. Glabrous skin and hairy skin contain a wide variety of sensory receptors for detecting mechanical, thermal, or nociceptive (consciously perceived as painful) stimuli applied on the body surface. These receptors include bare nerve endings (nociception, thermal sensation) and encapsulated endings. The latter include pacinian corpuscles (rapidly adapting mechanoreceptors for detecting vibration or brief touch), Merkel's discs (slowly adapting mechanoreceptors for detecting maintained deformation or sustained touch on the skin), Meissner's corpuscles (rapidly adapting mechanoreceptors for detecting moving touch), Ruffini endings (slowly adapting mechanoreceptors for detecting steady pressure applied to hairy skin), hair follicle receptors (rapidly adapting), and Krause end bulbs (possibly thermoreceptors). The initial segment of the primary sensory axon is immediately adjacent to the sensory receptor.

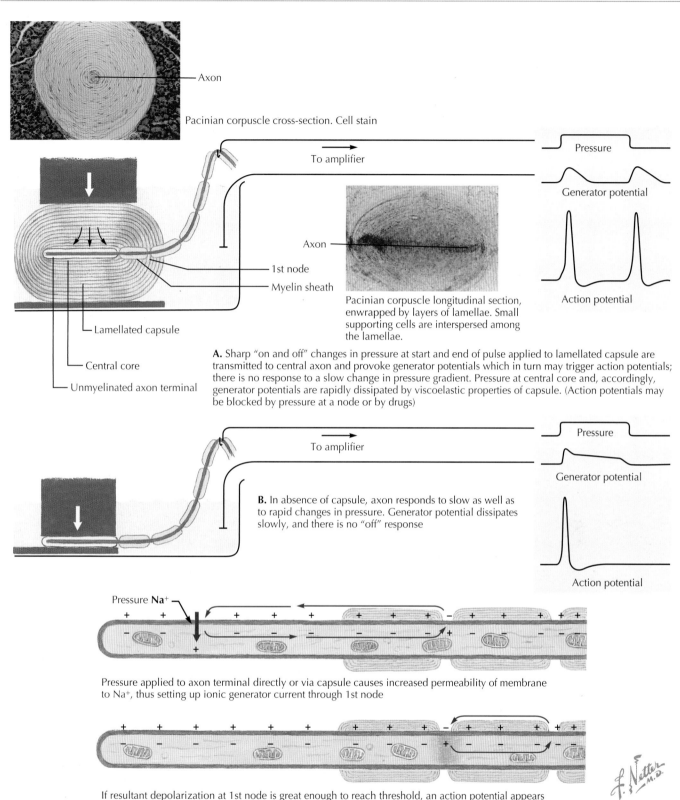

Axon

Pacinian corpuscle cross-section. Cell stain

To amplifier

Pressure

Generator potential

Action potential

1st node

Myelin sheath

Axon

Pacinian corpuscle longitudinal section, enwrapped by layers of lamellae. Small supporting cells are interspersed among the lamellae.

Lamellated capsule

Central core

Unmyelinated axon terminal

A. Sharp "on and off" changes in pressure at start and end of pulse applied to lamellated capsule are transmitted to central axon and provoke generator potentials which in turn may trigger action potentials; there is no response to a slow change in pressure gradient. Pressure at central core and, accordingly, generator potentials are rapidly dissipated by viscoelastic properties of capsule. (Action potentials may be blocked by pressure at a node or by drugs)

To amplifier

Pressure

Generator potential

B. In absence of capsule, axon responds to slow as well as to rapid changes in pressure. Generator potential dissipates slowly, and there is no "off" response

Action potential

Pressure Na$^+$

Pressure applied to axon terminal directly or via capsule causes increased permeability of membrane to Na$^+$, thus setting up ionic generator current through 1st node

If resultant depolarization at 1st node is great enough to reach threshold, an action potential appears which is propagated along nerve fiber

9.12 PACINIAN CORPUSCLES

Pacinian corpuscles are mechanoreceptors that transform mechanical force or displacement into action potentials in large-diameter primary sensory axons. The mechanical stimulus is modified by the viscoelastic properties of the contributing lamellae of the pacinian corpuscle and the associated accessory cells. An action potential results when a generator potential of sufficient magnitude to bring the initial segment of the axon to threshold is elicited. The onset and cessation of mechanical deformation enhance ionic permeability in the axon, optimizing the physiological response of the pacinian corpuscle to vibratory stimuli.

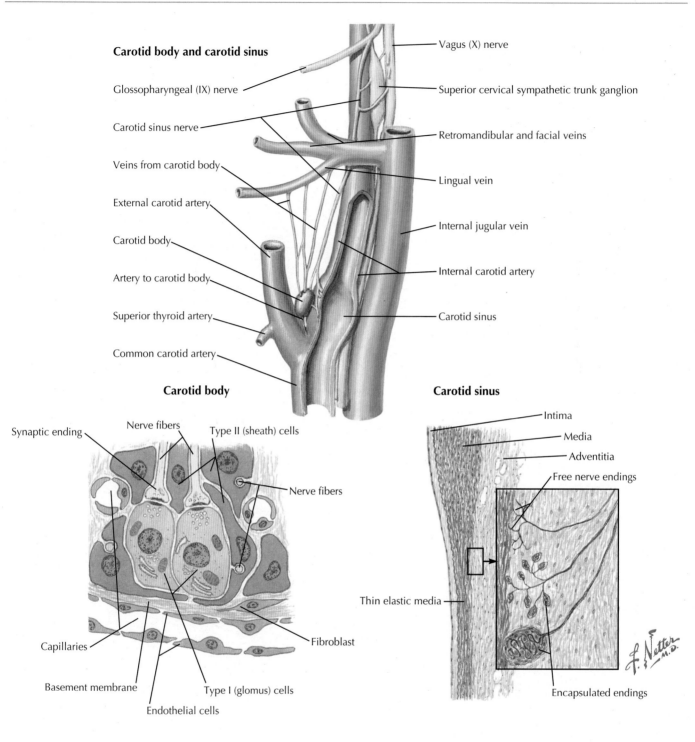

Carotid body and carotid sinus

Vagus (X) nerve

Glossopharyngeal (IX) nerve

Superior cervical sympathetic trunk ganglion

Carotid sinus nerve

Retromandibular and facial veins

Veins from carotid body

Lingual vein

External carotid artery

Carotid body

Internal jugular vein

Artery to carotid body

Internal carotid artery

Superior thyroid artery

Carotid sinus

Common carotid artery

Carotid body

Synaptic ending

Nerve fibers

Type II (sheath) cells

Nerve fibers

Capillaries

Fibroblast

Basement membrane

Type I (glomus) cells

Endothelial cells

Carotid sinus

Intima

Media

Adventitia

Free nerve endings

Thin elastic media

Encapsulated endings

9.13 INTEROCEPTORS

Interoceptors, including internal nociceptors, chemoreceptors, and stretch receptors, inform the CNS about the internal state of the body. The carotid body, a specialized chemoreceptor for detecting carbon dioxide (in a hypoxic state) or, to a lesser extent, low blood pH resulting in increased respiration, is associated with afferent axons of CN IX that project to the caudal nucleus solitarius in the medulla. The carotid sinus, a thin-walled region of the carotid artery, contains encapsulated and bare nerve endings that act as stretch receptors. These stretch receptors respond to increased arterial pressure as baroreceptors, send primary afferents to the caudal nucleus solitarius via CN IX, and elicit reflex bradycardia and a decrease in blood pressure.

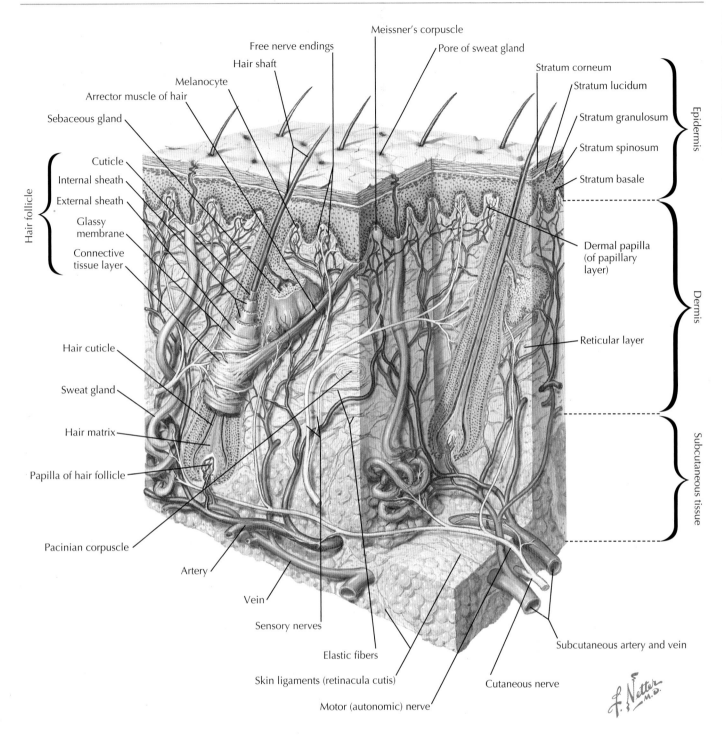

Free nerve endings
Hair shaft
Melanocyte
Arrector muscle of hair
Sebaceous gland
Cuticle
Internal sheath
External sheath
Glassy membrane
Connective tissue layer
Hair follicle
Meissner's corpuscle
Pore of sweat gland
Stratum corneum
Stratum lucidum
Stratum granulosum
Stratum spinosum
Stratum basale
Epidermis
Dermal papilla (of papillary layer)
Hair cuticle
Sweat gland
Hair matrix
Papilla of hair follicle
Pacinian corpuscle
Artery
Vein
Sensory nerves
Elastic fibers
Skin ligaments (retinacula cutis)
Motor (autonomic) nerve
Reticular layer
Dermis
Subcutaneous tissue
Subcutaneous artery and vein
Cutaneous nerve

9.14 SKIN AND ITS NERVES

The skin is supplied with a variety of receptor types (see Fig. 9.11) that transduce slowly and rapidly adapting mechanical stimuli and deformation into electrical impulses in primary afferent fibers. The bare nerve endings are associated mainly with nociceptors, peripheral arborizations of unmyelinated axons. Some nociceptors and thermoreceptors are associated with small myelinated axons. These axons collectively contribute somatosensory information to the spinothalamic/spinoreticular lemniscal system for protopathic sensation. The more complex encapsulated receptors contribute somatosensory information to the dorsal column/medial lemniscal system for epicritic sensation and are associated with larger myelinated axons. Noradrenergic postganglionic sympathetic nerve fibers form dense nerve networks around the hair follicules and can secrete high concentrations of NE during significant stress; the NE can activate beta2-adrenergic receptors. Bing Zhang and colleagues from Harvard recently reported that excessive release of NE can cause melanocyte stem cell depletion, and under extreme conditions may account for graying of hair, or even lead to hair turning white in a short time period of extreme stress.

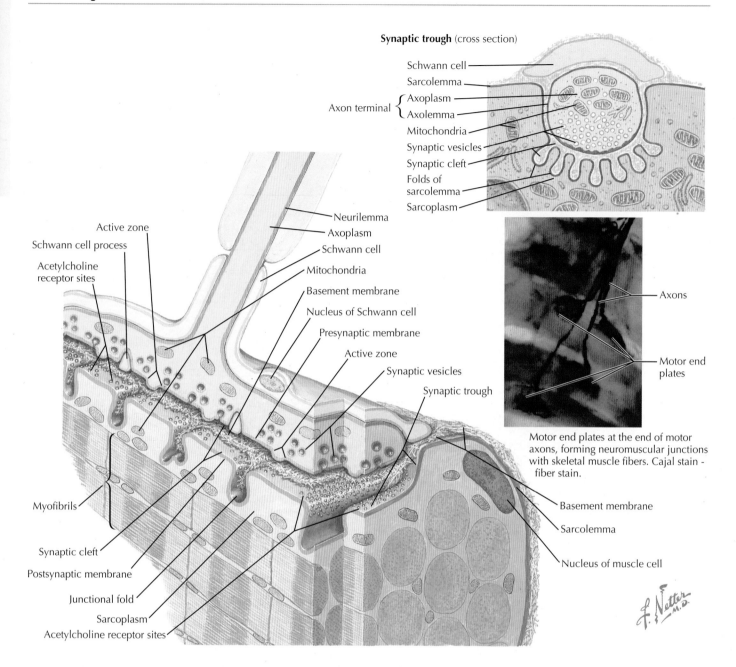

Synaptic trough (cross section)

Schwann cell
Sarcolemma
Axon terminal { Axoplasm / Axolemma
Mitochondria
Synaptic vesicles
Synaptic cleft
Folds of sarcolemma
Sarcoplasm

Active zone
Schwann cell process
Acetylcholine receptor sites

Neurilemma
Axoplasm
Schwann cell
Mitochondria
Basement membrane
Nucleus of Schwann cell
Presynaptic membrane
Active zone
Synaptic vesicles
Synaptic trough

Myofibrils
Synaptic cleft
Postsynaptic membrane
Junctional fold
Sarcoplasm
Acetylcholine receptor sites

Axons
Motor end plates

Motor end plates at the end of motor axons, forming neuromuscular junctions with skeletal muscle fibers. Cajal stain - fiber stain.

Basement membrane
Sarcolemma
Nucleus of muscle cell

9.15 THE NEUROMUSCULAR JUNCTION AND NEUROTRANSMISSION

Axons of LMNs that synapse on skeletal muscle form expanded terminals called neuromuscular junctions (motor end plates). The motor axon loses its myelin sheath and expands into an extended terminal that resides in a trough in the muscle fiber and is covered by a layer of Schwann cell cytoplasm. The postsynaptic membrane is thrown into secondary folds. When an action potential invades the motor terminal, several hundred vesicles simultaneously release their acetylcholine (ACh) into the synaptic cleft. The ACh binds to nicotinic receptors on the muscle sarcolemma, initiating a motor endplate potential, which is normally of sufficient magnitude to result in the firing of a muscle action potential, leading to contraction of the muscle fiber. A single muscle fiber has only one neuromuscular junction, but a motor axon may innervate multiple muscle fibers.

CLINICAL POINT

An action potential that invades the motor end plate results in a calcium-mediated simultaneous release of multiple quanta (vesicles) of ACh. This released ACh acts on nicotinic cholinergic receptors on the postjunctional membrane, normally resulting in a muscle contraction (excitation-contraction coupling). In **myasthenia gravis**, antibodies against the cholinergic nicotinic receptors greatly reduce the number of active receptors available for stimulation by released ACh. The size and number of ACh quanta appear to be normal. As a consequence, there is easy fatigability of involved muscles with repeated attempts at contraction. Ocular, facial, and bulbar muscles are the most likely to be affected by this disease, with resultant ptosis, drooping face, diplopia with strabismus, and dysarthria, dysphonia, and dysphagia. Limb muscles (mainly proximal) are involved only in advanced myasthenia gravis. The muscles do not show wasting and atrophy because they are not denervated; muscle stretch reflexes are elicitable.

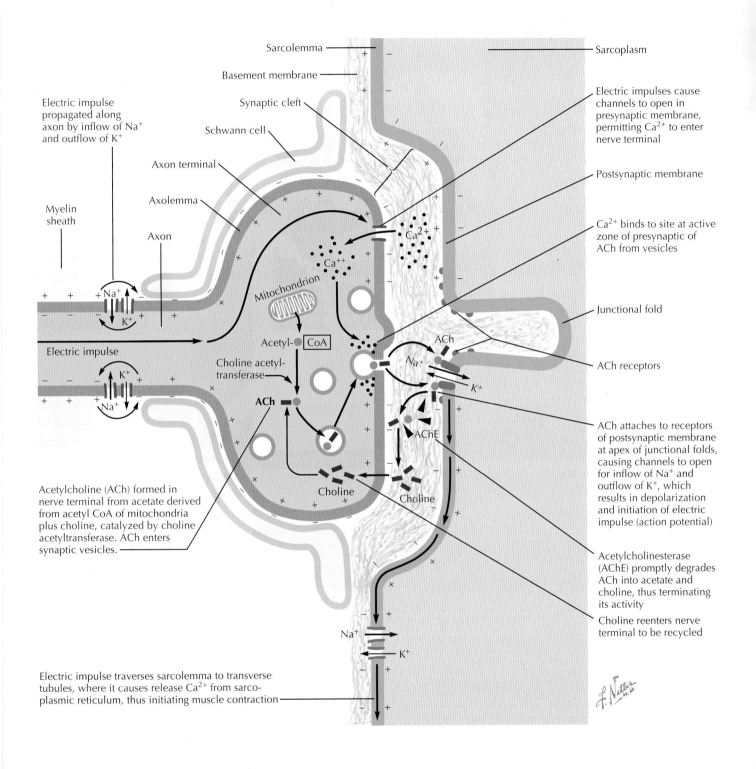

Sarcolemma

Basement membrane

Synaptic cleft

Schwann cell

Axon terminal

Axolemma

Axon

Electric impulse propagated along axon by inflow of Na$^+$ and outflow of K$^+$

Myelin sheath

Electric impulse

Choline acetyl-transferase

Mitochondrion

Acetyl-[CoA]

ACh

Choline

Acetylcholine (ACh) formed in nerve terminal from acetate derived from acetyl CoA of mitochondria plus choline, catalyzed by choline acetyltransferase. ACh enters synaptic vesicles.

Ca^{++}

Ca^{2+}

ACh

Na$^+$

K$^+$

AChE

Choline

Na$^+$

K$^+$

Sarcoplasm

Electric impulses cause channels to open in presynaptic membrane, permitting Ca^{2+} to enter nerve terminal

Postsynaptic membrane

Ca^{2+} binds to site at active zone of presynaptic of ACh from vesicles

Junctional fold

ACh receptors

ACh attaches to receptors of postsynaptic membrane at apex of junctional folds, causing channels to open for inflow of Na$^+$ and outflow of K$^+$, which results in depolarization and initiation of electric impulse (action potential)

Acetylcholinesterase (AChE) promptly degrades ACh into acetate and choline, thus terminating its activity

Choline reenters nerve terminal to be recycled

Electric impulse traverses sarcolemma to transverse tubules, where it causes release Ca^{2+} from sarcoplasmic reticulum, thus initiating muscle contraction

f. Netter

9.16 PHYSIOLOGY OF THE NEUROMUSCULAR JUNCTION

This process is called excitation-contraction coupling; that is, mechanisms by which a motor action potential initiates the release of acetylcholine, activating nicotinic cholinergic receptors on the muscle membrane, initiating muscle contraction.

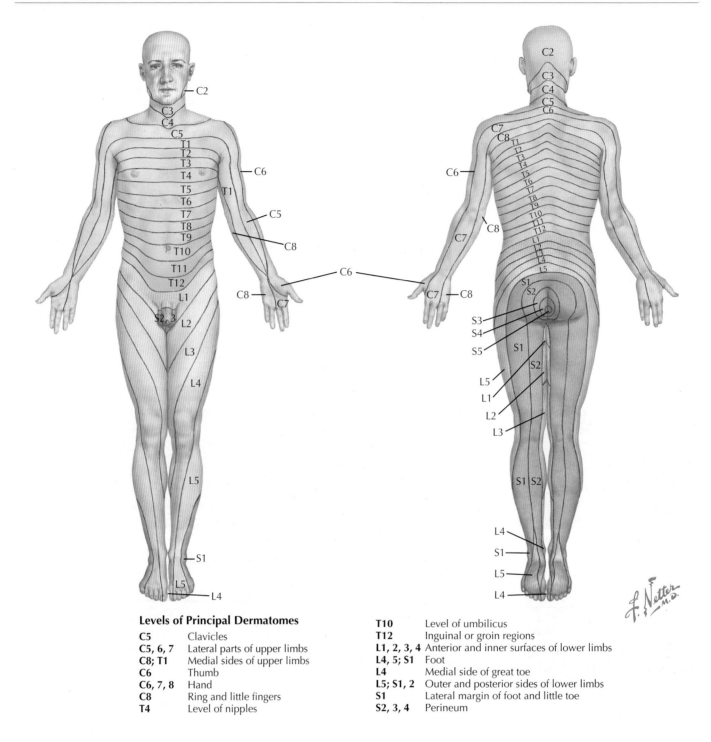

Levels of Principal Dermatomes

C5	Clavicles
C5, 6, 7	Lateral parts of upper limbs
C8; T1	Medial sides of upper limbs
C6	Thumb
C6, 7, 8	Hand
C8	Ring and little fingers
T4	Level of nipples

T10	Level of umbilicus
T12	Inguinal or groin regions
L1, 2, 3, 4	Anterior and inner surfaces of lower limbs
L4, 5; S1	Foot
L4	Medial side of great toe
L5; S1, 2	Outer and posterior sides of lower limbs
S1	Lateral margin of foot and little toe
S2, 3, 4	Perineum

SOMATIC NERVOUS SYSTEM

9.19 DERMATOMAL DISTRIBUTION

A dermatome is the cutaneous area supplied by a single spinal nerve root; the cell bodies are located in dorsal root ganglia. The spinal nerve roots are distributed to structures according to their associations with spinal cord segments. The nerve roots supplying neighboring dermatomes overlap. Thus, sectioning or dysfunction of a single dorsal root produces hypoesthesia (diminished sensation), not anesthesia (total loss of sensation), in the region supplied predominantly by that dermatome, as shown in the figure. Dermatomal anesthesia requires damage to at least three dorsal roots: the central dorsal root and the roots above and below it.

In contrast, an irritative lesion such as a herniated intervertebral disc may produce sharp, radiating pain within the distribution of the affected dermatome. As the limb buds for the lower extremities develop, they draw out the nerve roots that correspond with their mesodermal cores and ectodermal coverings. The developing lower limbs rotate medially around a longitudinal axis, with a resultant oblique orientation of the dermatomes. The L1 and L2 dermatomes can be found in sites adjacent to S2 and S3 dermatomes because of the intervening segments migrating into more distal parts of the lower limbs. Knowledge of dermatomes is important for localizing peripheral nerve root lesions and distinguishing them from peripheral nerve lesions.

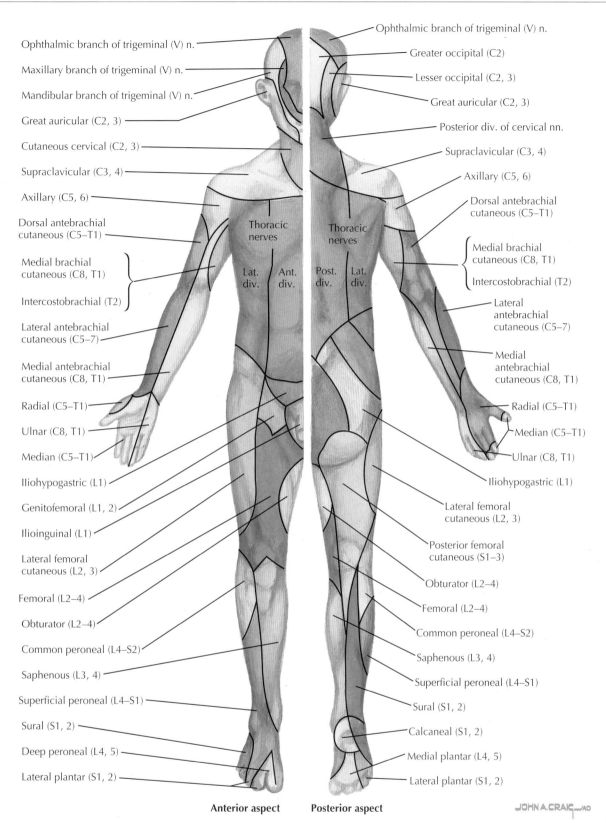

Ophthalmic branch of trigeminal (V) n.

Maxillary branch of trigeminal (V) n.

Mandibular branch of trigeminal (V) n.

Great auricular (C2, 3)

Cutaneous cervical (C2, 3)

Supraclavicular (C3, 4)

Axillary (C5, 6)

Dorsal antebrachial cutaneous (C5–T1)

Medial brachial cutaneous (C8, T1)

Intercostobrachial (T2)

Lateral antebrachial cutaneous (C5–7)

Medial antebrachial cutaneous (C8, T1)

Radial (C5–T1)

Ulnar (C8, T1)

Median (C5–T1)

Iliohypogastric (L1)

Genitofemoral (L1, 2)

Ilioinguinal (L1)

Lateral femoral cutaneous (L2, 3)

Femoral (L2–4)

Obturator (L2–4)

Common peroneal (L4–S2)

Saphenous (L3, 4)

Superficial peroneal (L4–S1)

Sural (S1, 2)

Deep peroneal (L4, 5)

Lateral plantar (S1, 2)

Ophthalmic branch of trigeminal (V) n.

Greater occipital (C2)

Lesser occipital (C2, 3)

Great auricular (C2, 3)

Posterior div. of cervical nn.

Supraclavicular (C3, 4)

Axillary (C5, 6)

Dorsal antebrachial cutaneous (C5–T1)

Medial brachial cutaneous (C8, T1)

Intercostobrachial (T2)

Lateral antebrachial cutaneous (C5–7)

Medial antebrachial cutaneous (C8, T1)

Radial (C5–T1)

Median (C5–T1)

Ulnar (C8, T1)

Iliohypogastric (L1)

Lateral femoral cutaneous (L2, 3)

Posterior femoral cutaneous (S1–3)

Obturator (L2–4)

Femoral (L2–4)

Common peroneal (L4–S2)

Saphenous (L3, 4)

Superficial peroneal (L4–S1)

Sural (S1, 2)

Calcaneal (S1, 2)

Medial plantar (L4, 5)

Lateral plantar (S1, 2)

Thoracic nerves

Lat. div. Ant. div.

Post. div. Lat. div.

Anterior aspect   Posterior aspect

JOHN A. CRAIG—AD

9.20 CUTANEOUS DISTRIBUTION OF PERIPHERAL NERVES

Peripheral nerves distribute sensory processes and endings to specific surface regions of the body. These sites may be innervated by a nerve with contributions from several dermatomes. A nerve lesion can leave the site of cutaneous distribution devoid of all sensation (anesthetic). Sites of innervation by specific nerves vary from person to person.

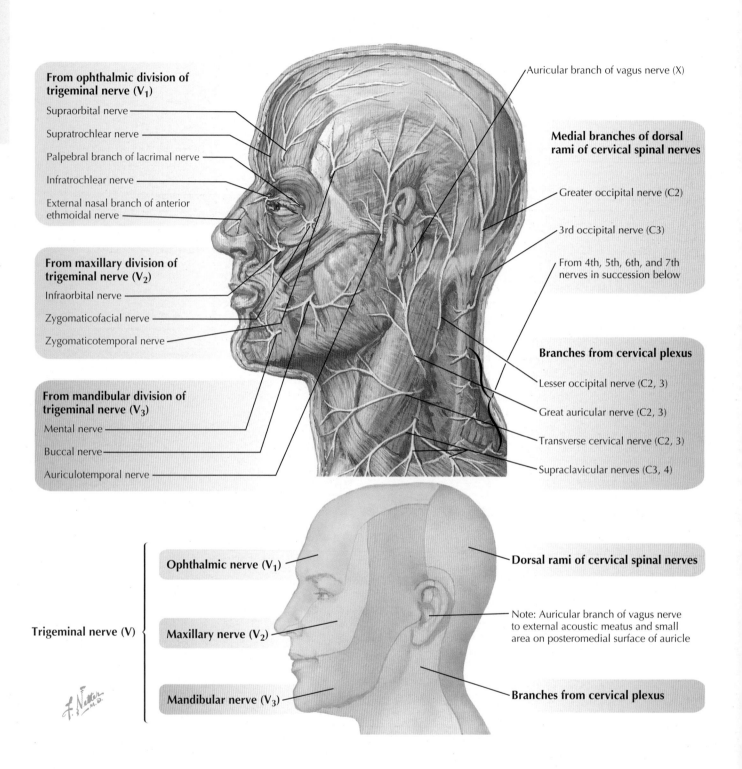

From ophthalmic division of trigeminal nerve (V₁)

Supraorbital nerve

Supratrochlear nerve

Palpebral branch of lacrimal nerve

Infratrochlear nerve

External nasal branch of anterior ethmoidal nerve

From maxillary division of trigeminal nerve (V₂)

Infraorbital nerve

Zygomaticofacial nerve

Zygomaticotemporal nerve

From mandibular division of trigeminal nerve (V₃)

Mental nerve

Buccal nerve

Auriculotemporal nerve

Auricular branch of vagus nerve (X)

Medial branches of dorsal rami of cervical spinal nerves

Greater occipital nerve (C2)

3rd occipital nerve (C3)

From 4th, 5th, 6th, and 7th nerves in succession below

Branches from cervical plexus

Lesser occipital nerve (C2, 3)

Great auricular nerve (C2, 3)

Transverse cervical nerve (C2, 3)

Supraclavicular nerves (C3, 4)

Trigeminal nerve (V)

Ophthalmic nerve (V₁)

Maxillary nerve (V₂)

Mandibular nerve (V₃)

Dorsal rami of cervical spinal nerves

Note: Auricular branch of vagus nerve to external acoustic meatus and small area on posteromedial surface of auricle

Branches from cervical plexus

9.21 CUTANEOUS NERVES OF THE HEAD AND NECK

Cutaneous nerves of the head and neck derive from dorsal rami of cervical spinal nerves, from branches from the cervical plexus, and from all three divisions of the trigeminal nerve (CN V).

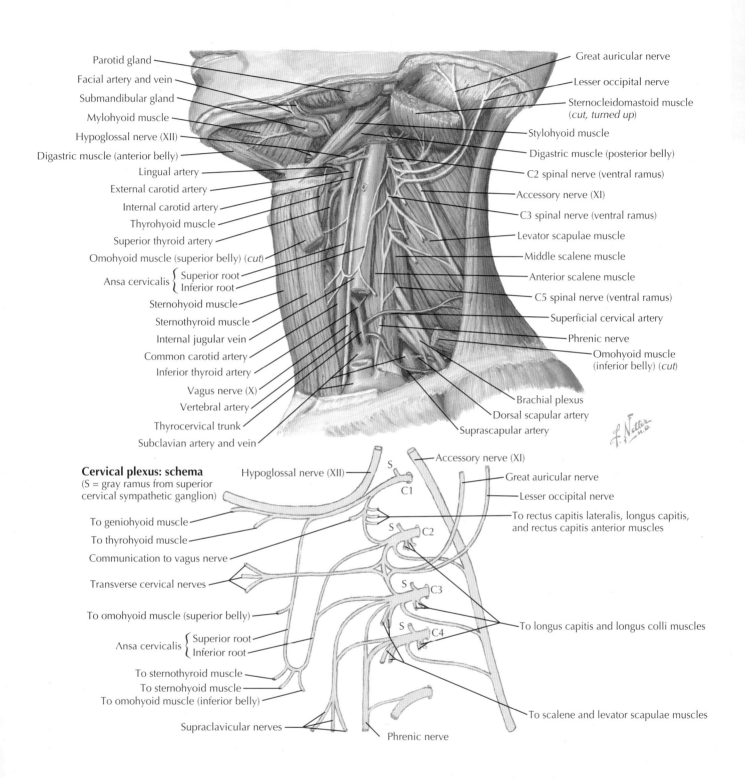

Parotid gland
Facial artery and vein
Submandibular gland
Mylohyoid muscle
Hypoglossal nerve (XII)
Digastric muscle (anterior belly)
Lingual artery
External carotid artery
Internal carotid artery
Thyrohyoid muscle
Superior thyroid artery
Omohyoid muscle (superior belly) (cut)
Ansa cervicalis { Superior root / Inferior root
Sternohyoid muscle
Sternothyroid muscle
Internal jugular vein
Common carotid artery
Inferior thyroid artery
Vagus nerve (X)
Vertebral artery
Thyrocervical trunk
Subclavian artery and vein

Great auricular nerve
Lesser occipital nerve
Sternocleidomastoid muscle (*cut, turned up*)
Stylohyoid muscle
Digastric muscle (posterior belly)
C2 spinal nerve (ventral ramus)
Accessory nerve (XI)
C3 spinal nerve (ventral ramus)
Levator scapulae muscle
Middle scalene muscle
Anterior scalene muscle
C5 spinal nerve (ventral ramus)
Superficial cervical artery
Phrenic nerve
Omohyoid muscle (inferior belly) (*cut*)
Brachial plexus
Dorsal scapular artery
Suprascapular artery

Cervical plexus: schema
(S = gray ramus from superior cervical sympathetic ganglion)

Hypoglossal nerve (XII)
To geniohyoid muscle
To thyrohyoid muscle
Communication to vagus nerve
Transverse cervical nerves
To omohyoid muscle (superior belly)
Ansa cervicalis { Superior root / Inferior root
To sternothyroid muscle
To sternohyoid muscle
To omohyoid muscle (inferior belly)
Supraclavicular nerves

S
C1
S
C2
S
C3
S
C4
Phrenic nerve

Accessory nerve (XI)
Great auricular nerve
Lesser occipital nerve
To rectus capitis lateralis, longus capitis, and rectus capitis anterior muscles
To longus capitis and longus colli muscles
To scalene and levator scapulae muscles

9.22 CERVICAL PLEXUS IN SITU

This diagram of the cervical plexus in situ and the schema below demonstrate the distribution of branches from the C1–C4 nerve roots into the associated peripheral nerves and branches to the innervated muscles.

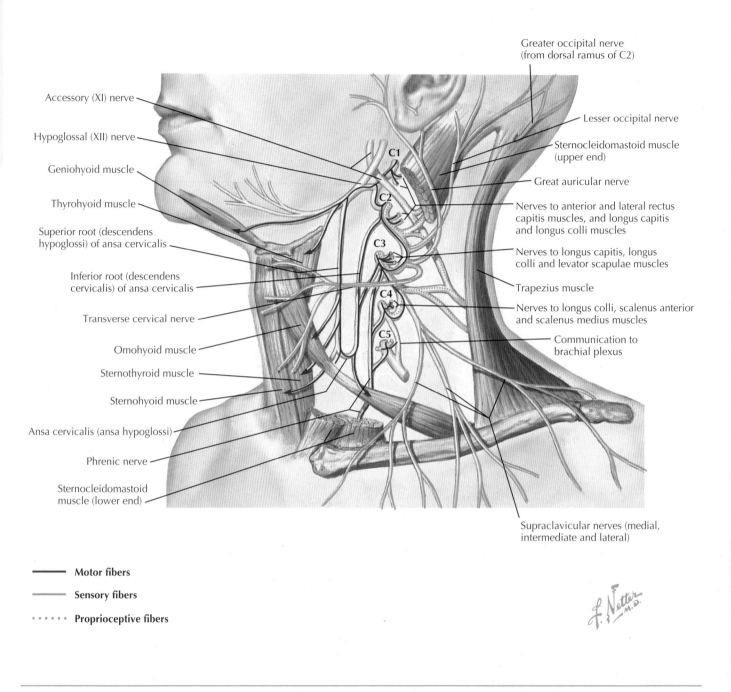

Greater occipital nerve
(from dorsal ramus of C2)

Accessory (XI) nerve

Lesser occipital nerve

Hypoglossal (XII) nerve

Sternocleidomastoid muscle
(upper end)

Geniohyoid muscle

Great auricular nerve

Thyrohyoid muscle

Nerves to anterior and lateral rectus
capitis muscles, and longus capitis
and longus colli muscles

Superior root (descendens
hypoglossi) of ansa cervicalis

Nerves to longus capitis, longus
colli and levator scapulae muscles

Inferior root (descendens
cervicalis) of ansa cervicalis

Trapezius muscle

Transverse cervical nerve

Nerves to longus colli, scalenus anterior
and scalenus medius muscles

Omohyoid muscle

Communication to
brachial plexus

Sternothyroid muscle

Sternohyoid muscle

Ansa cervicalis (ansa hypoglossi)

Phrenic nerve

Sternocleidomastoid
muscle (lower end)

Supraclavicular nerves (medial,
intermediate and lateral)

C1
C2
C3
C4
C5

———— Motor fibers

‒‒‒‒ Sensory fibers

· · · · · Proprioceptive fibers

9.23 CERVICAL PLEXUS

The cervical plexus lies deep to the sternocleidomastoid muscle. Its branches convey motor fibers to many cervical muscles and to the diaphragm. Its sensory fibers convey exteroceptive information from parts of the scalp, neck, and chest as well as proprioceptive information from muscles, tendons, and joints. Sympathetic sudomotor and vasomotor fibers travel with this plexus to blood vessels and glands. The superficial branches perforate the cervical fascia to supply cutaneous structures; the deep branches supply mainly muscles and joints.

CLINICAL POINT

The cervical plexus is formed from the anterior primary rami of C1–C4, deep to the sternocleidomastoid muscle and in front of the scalenus medius and levator scapulae muscles. Sensory branches include the greater and lesser occipital nerves, great auricular nerve, cutaneous cervical nerves, and supraclavicular nerves. The motor branches include the ansa hypoglossi, branches to scalenus medius and levator scapulae muscles, the phrenic nerve, and branches to the spinal accessory nerve. Lesions of the cervical plexus are uncommon, usually resulting from trauma, mass lesions, or as sequelae to surgery such as carotid endartectomy. Involvement of motor branches results in disruption of muscular function, such as shoulder elevation and head rotation and flexion with spinal accessory nerve damage. Involvement of sensory branches results in loss of cutaneous sensation or in pain and paresthesias in regions of the head or neck supplied by these branches.

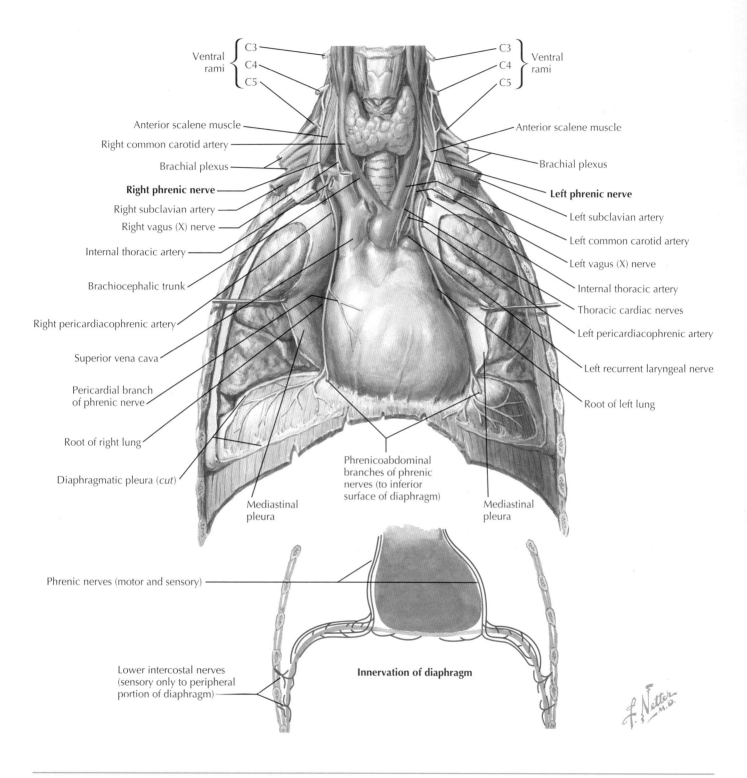

Ventral rami { C3 C4 C5 }

Ventral rami { C3 C4 C5 }

Anterior scalene muscle

Right common carotid artery

Brachial plexus

Right phrenic nerve

Right subclavian artery

Right vagus (X) nerve

Internal thoracic artery

Brachiocephalic trunk

Right pericardiacophrenic artery

Superior vena cava

Pericardial branch of phrenic nerve

Root of right lung

Diaphragmatic pleura (*cut*)

Mediastinal pleura

Anterior scalene muscle

Brachial plexus

Left phrenic nerve

Left subclavian artery

Left common carotid artery

Left vagus (X) nerve

Internal thoracic artery

Thoracic cardiac nerves

Left pericardiacophrenic artery

Left recurrent laryngeal nerve

Root of left lung

Phrenicoabdominal branches of phrenic nerves (to inferior surface of diaphragm)

Mediastinal pleura

Phrenic nerves (motor and sensory)

Lower intercostal nerves (sensory only to peripheral portion of diaphragm)

Innervation of diaphragm

9.24 PHRENIC NERVE

The left and right phrenic nerves are the motor nerves that supply both sides of the diaphragm from the C3, C4, and C5 ventral roots. The phrenic nerve also contains many sensory nerve fibers that supply the fibrous pericardium, the mediastinal pleura, and central areas of the diaphragmatic pleura. Sympathetic postganglionic nerve fibers also travel with this nerve. Coordinated contraction of the diaphragm relies on central control of firing of LMNs through dendrite bundles in the spinal cord.

CLINICAL POINT

The phrenic nerves derive from the C3–C5 ventral roots and provide the motor supply to the diaphragm. Lesions of the phrenic nerve usually occur in the mediastinum, not the cervical plexus. Pathological processes, such as enlarged mediastinal nodes, aortic aneurysms, mediastinal tumors, sequelae of surgery, and demyelination from Guillain-Barré syndrome, can damage these nerves. Unilateral damage to the phrenic nerve results in paralysis of the diaphragm on the ipsilateral side, which can usually be tolerated at rest but not following exertion. Bilateral phrenic nerve damage results in diaphragmatic paralysis with extreme dyspnea and hypoventilation.

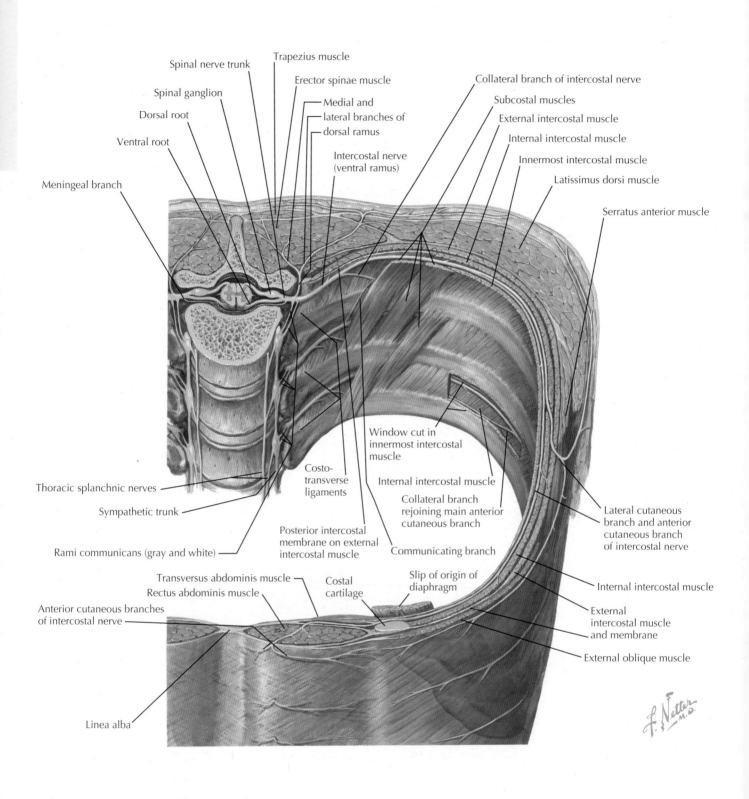

Spinal nerve trunk

Trapezius muscle

Spinal ganglion

Dorsal root

Ventral root

Medial and lateral branches of dorsal ramus

Erector spinae muscle

Intercostal nerve (ventral ramus)

Meningeal branch

Collateral branch of intercostal nerve

Subcostal muscles

External intercostal muscle

Internal intercostal muscle

Innermost intercostal muscle

Latissimus dorsi muscle

Serratus anterior muscle

Thoracic splanchnic nerves

Sympathetic trunk

Costo-transverse ligaments

Window cut in innermost intercostal muscle

Internal intercostal muscle

Collateral branch rejoining main anterior cutaneous branch

Communicating branch

Lateral cutaneous branch and anterior cutaneous branch of intercostal nerve

Rami communicans (gray and white)

Posterior intercostal membrane on external intercostal muscle

Transversus abdominis muscle

Rectus abdominis muscle

Costal cartilage

Slip of origin of diaphragm

Internal intercostal muscle

Anterior cutaneous branches of intercostal nerve

External intercostal muscle and membrane

External oblique muscle

Linea alba

9.25 THORACIC NERVES

The 12 pairs of thoracic nerves are derived from dorsal and ventral roots of their corresponding segments. These nerves do not form plexuses; they distribute cutaneous branches to the thoracic dermatomes and send other sensory fibers to deeper muscular structures, vessels, periosteum, parietal pleura, the peritoneum, and breast tissue. The thoracic nerves also send motor fibers to muscles of the thoracic and abdominal wall and carry preganglionic and postganglionic sympathetic nerve fibers into and out of the sympathetic chain. Muscles of the thoracic and abdominal wall, supplied by these nerves, act as accessory respiratory muscles and may assist in breathing in times of dyspnea or phrenic nerve impairment.

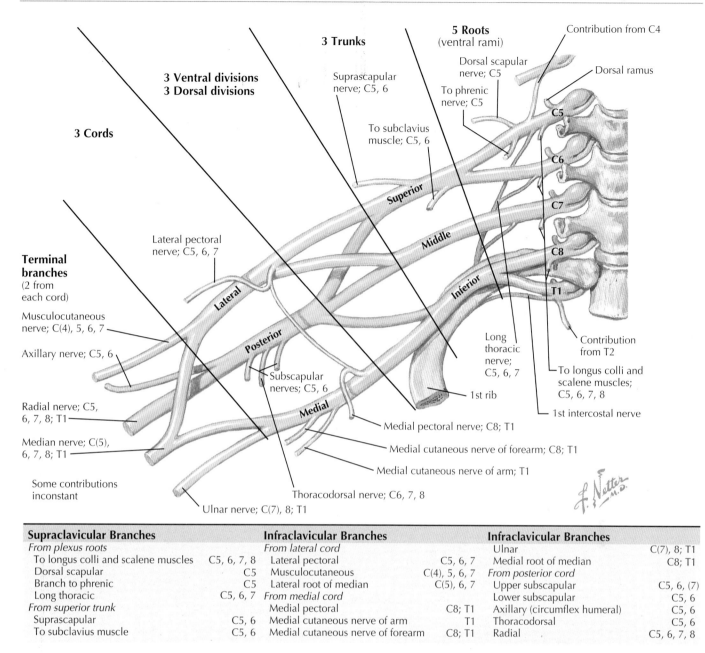

3 Cords

3 Ventral divisions
3 Dorsal divisions

3 Trunks

5 Roots
(ventral rami)

Contribution from C4

Suprascapular
nerve; C5, 6

Dorsal scapular
nerve; C5

Dorsal ramus

To subclavius
muscle; C5, 6

To phrenic
nerve; C5

C5

C6

C7

C8

T1

Superior

Middle

Inferior

Lateral pectoral
nerve; C5, 6, 7

**Terminal
branches**
(2 from
each cord)

Lateral

Posterior

Medial

Musculocutaneous
nerve; C(4), 5, 6, 7

Axillary nerve; C5, 6

Subscapular
nerves; C5, 6

Long
thoracic
nerve;
C5, 6, 7

Contribution
from T2

To longus colli and
scalene muscles;
C5, 6, 7, 8

1st rib

1st intercostal nerve

Radial nerve; C5,
6, 7, 8; T1

Median nerve; C(5),
6, 7, 8; T1

Medial pectoral nerve; C8; T1

Medial cutaneous nerve of forearm; C8; T1

Medial cutaneous nerve of arm; T1

Some contributions
inconstant

Thoracodorsal nerve; C6, 7, 8

Ulnar nerve; C(7), 8; T1

Supraclavicular Branches		Infraclavicular Branches		Infraclavicular Branches	
From plexus roots		*From lateral cord*		Ulnar	C(7), 8; T1
To longus colli and scalene muscles	C5, 6, 7, 8	Lateral pectoral	C5, 6, 7	Medial root of median	C8; T1
Dorsal scapular	C5	Musculocutaneous	C(4), 5, 6, 7	*From posterior cord*	
Branch to phrenic	C5	Lateral root of median	C(5), 6, 7	Upper subscapular	C5, 6, (7)
Long thoracic	C5, 6, 7	*From medial cord*		Lower subscapular	C5, 6
From superior trunk		Medial pectoral	C8; T1	Axillary (circumflex humeral)	C5, 6
Suprascapular	C5, 6	Medial cutaneous nerve of arm	T1	Thoracodorsal	C5, 6
To subclavius muscle	C5, 6	Medial cutaneous nerve of forearm	C8; T1	Radial	C5, 6, 7, 8

9.26 BRACHIAL PLEXUS

The brachial plexus is formed by the union of the ventral roots of C5 through C8 plus T1, with a smaller contribution from C4. Sensory and sympathetic fibers also distribute in the brachial plexus. The roots give rise to three trunks, three ventral and three dorsal divisions, three cords as well as numerous terminal branches, the peripheral nerves. This plexus is vulnerable to birth injury (superior plexus paralysis), which causes paralysis of the deltoid, biceps, brachial, and brachioradialis muscles, with sparing of the hands, and causes sensory loss over the deltoid area and radial aspect of the forearm and hand. Pressure by a cervical rib can cause inferior plexus injury (C8, T1 injury), which results in paralysis of small hand muscles and flexors of the hand, with ulnar sensory loss and possible Horner's syndrome.

CLINICAL POINT

Lesions in the upper brachial plexus, particularly those affecting C5 and C6 contributions, can be caused by traction from a difficult birth, including displacement of the head to the opposite side and depression of the shoulder on the same side (Erb-Duchenne palsy); by radiation damage; from congenital causes; and by tumors. Such lesions may result in paresis of shoulder abduction and external rotation and in paresis of elbow flexion caused by damage to the motor nerve supply to the deltoid, supraspinatus, infraspinatus, biceps, supinator, and brachioradialis muscles. The arm hangs down and is rotated medially; the forearm is pronated. The biceps and brachioradialis muscle stretch reflexes are absent. Sensory loss is experienced over the deltoid region and along the radial side of the forearm.

Lesions of the lower brachial plexus, particularly those affecting C8 and T1 contributions, can result from traction on an abducted arm, a breech delivery (Dejerine-Klumpke paralysis), an apical lung tumor, a cervical rib, radiation damage, or a tumor. These lesions result in paralysis of finger flexion and paralysis of all the small muscles of the hand; a claw hand results. Sensory loss is present along the ulnar surface of the forearm and hand. Ipsilateral Horner's syndrome is sometimes seen due to damage to T1 preganglionic outflow to the superior cervical ganglion, with resultant ptosis, miosis, and hemianhydrosis.

Note: Schematic demarcation of dermatomes shown as
distinct segments. There is actually considerable overlap between adjacent dermatomes.

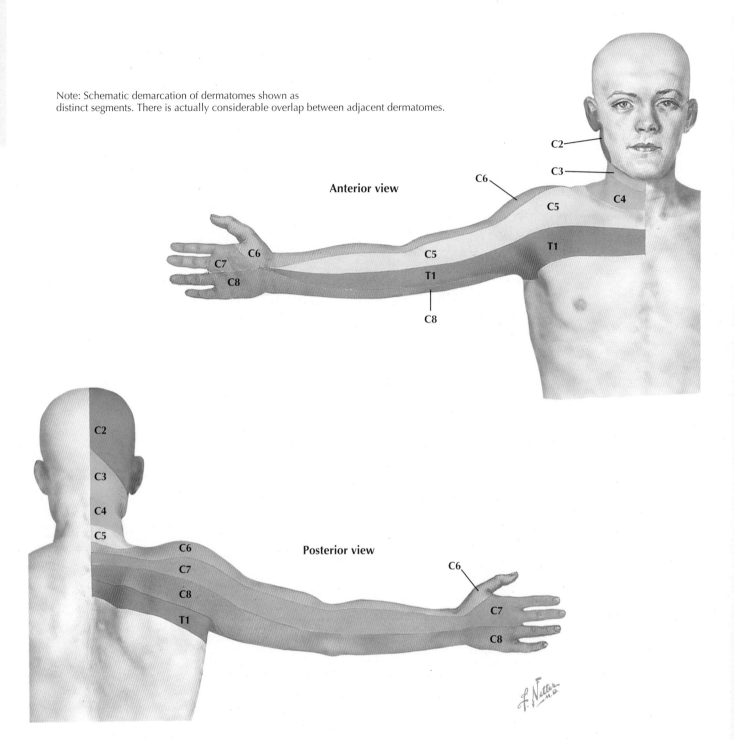

Anterior view

Posterior view

9.27 DERMATOMES OF THE UPPER LIMB

Because of the distribution of nerve fibers in the brachial plexus and the interchange of sensory and motor fibers through the trunks, divisions, and cords, the orderly segmental distribution of cervical dermatomes is obscured to some degree.

However, the arrangement of dermatomes in the upper limb is explicable embryologically as limb buds extend. The more proximal dermatomes are elongated strips located along the outer sides of the limbs, whereas the more distal dermatomes are found medially.

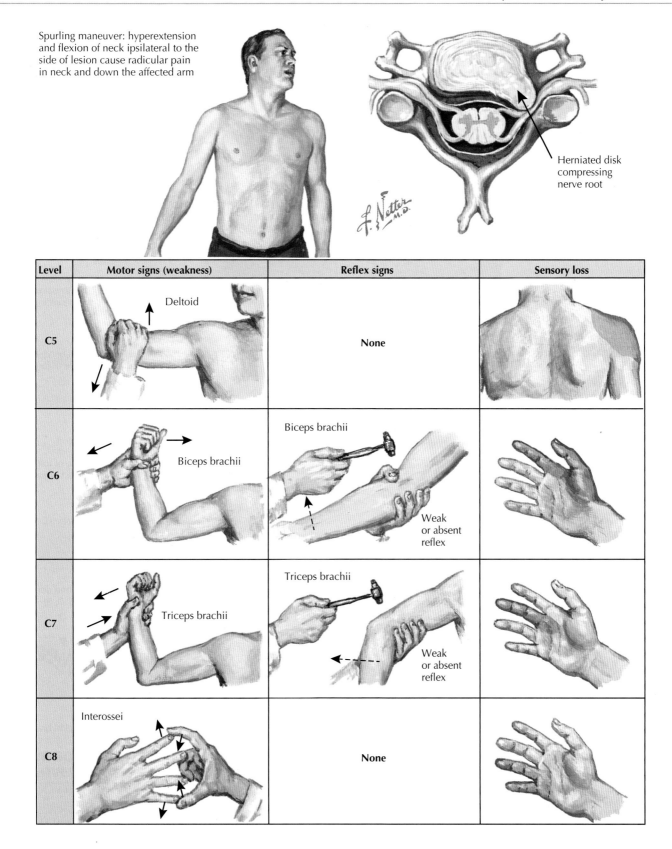

Spurling maneuver: hyperextension and flexion of neck ipsilateral to the side of lesion cause radicular pain in neck and down the affected arm

Herniated disk compressing nerve root

Level	Motor signs (weakness)	Reflex signs	Sensory loss
C5	Deltoid	None	
C6	Biceps brachii	Biceps brachii — Weak or absent reflex	
C7	Triceps brachii	Triceps brachii — Weak or absent reflex	
C8	Interossei	None	

9.28 CERVICAL DISC HERNIATION

Cervical disc herniation is a common neurologic process, often caused by age-related vertebral deterioration and processes other than trauma (a major cause of lumbar disc herniation). The initial manifestation of cervical disc herniation often is radiating pain (radiculopathy). Cervical nerve roots 5, 6, and 7 emerge above their related vertebral body, while cervical nerve root 8 emerges between vertebrae C7 and T1. This plate illustrates characteristics of cervical disc herniation, including motor, sensory, and reflex manifestations.

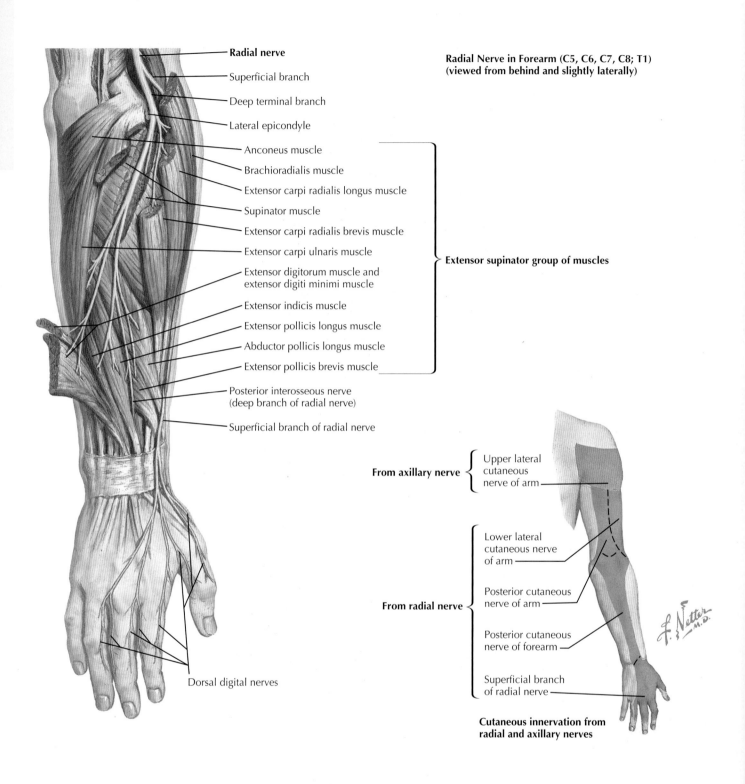

Radial nerve

Superficial branch

Deep terminal branch

Lateral epicondyle

Anconeus muscle

Brachioradialis muscle

Extensor carpi radialis longus muscle

Supinator muscle

Extensor carpi radialis brevis muscle

Extensor carpi ulnaris muscle

Extensor digitorum muscle and extensor digiti minimi muscle

Extensor indicis muscle

Extensor pollicis longus muscle

Abductor pollicis longus muscle

Extensor pollicis brevis muscle

Posterior interosseous nerve (deep branch of radial nerve)

Superficial branch of radial nerve

Dorsal digital nerves

Radial Nerve in Forearm (C5, C6, C7, C8; T1) (viewed from behind and slightly laterally)

Extensor supinator group of muscles

From axillary nerve { Upper lateral cutaneous nerve of arm

From radial nerve { Lower lateral cutaneous nerve of arm

Posterior cutaneous nerve of arm

Posterior cutaneous nerve of forearm

Superficial branch of radial nerve

Cutaneous innervation from radial and axillary nerves

9.31 RADIAL NERVE IN THE FOREARM

In the forearm, the radial nerve (C6–C8) supplies motor fibers to the (1) extensor carpi radialis, (2) extensor digitorum, (3) extensor digiti V, (4) extensor carpi ulnaris, (5) supinator, (6) abductor pollicis longus, (7) extensor pollicis brevis and longus, and (8) extensor indicis proprius muscles. It supplies the posterior upper arm, an elongated zone of the posterior forearm, and the posterior hand, thumb, and lateral 2½ fingers. A lesion results in paralysis of extension and flexion of the elbow, paralysis of supination of the forearm, paralysis of extension of the wrist and fingers, and paralysis of abduction of the thumb, as well as loss of sensation over the radial aspect of the posterior forearm and the dorsum of the hand.

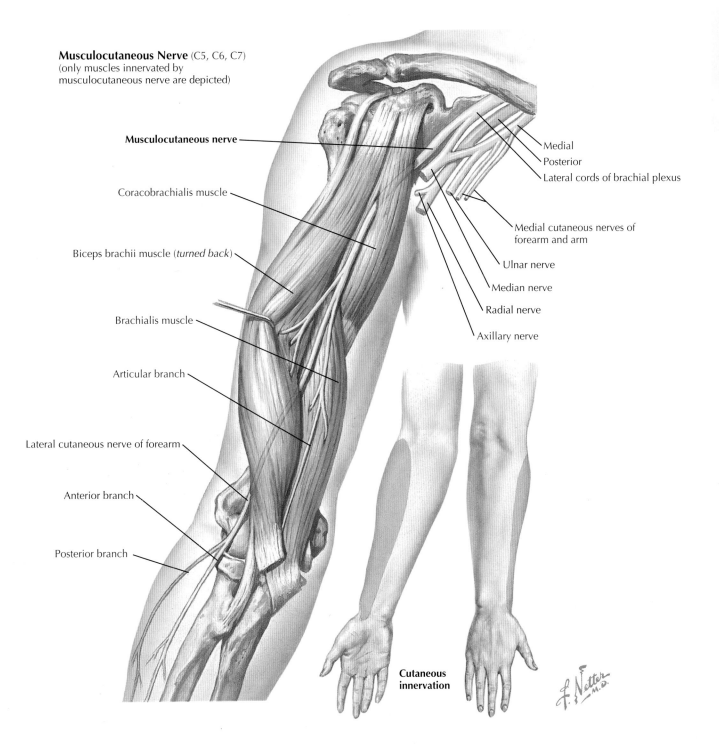

Musculocutaneous Nerve (C5, C6, C7)
(only muscles innervated by
musculocutaneous nerve are depicted)

Musculocutaneous nerve

Coracobrachialis muscle

Biceps brachii muscle (*turned back*)

Brachialis muscle

Articular branch

Lateral cutaneous nerve of forearm

Anterior branch

Posterior branch

Medial
Posterior
Lateral cords of brachial plexus

Medial cutaneous nerves of
forearm and arm

Ulnar nerve

Median nerve

Radial nerve

Axillary nerve

Cutaneous
innervation

9.32 MUSCULOCUTANEOUS NERVE

The musculocutaneous nerve (C5–C6) supplies the biceps bra-chii, coracobrachialis, and brachialis muscles; it aids in flexion of the upper and lower arm, supination of the lower arm, and elevation and adduction of the arm. The nerve supplies sensory innervation to the lateral forearm. A lesion may be caused by a fracture of the humerus and results in the wasting of the muscles supplied, weakness of flexion of the supinated arm, and loss of sensation on the lateral forearm.

Median Nerve (C6, C7, C8; T1)
(only muscles innervated
by median nerve are depicted)

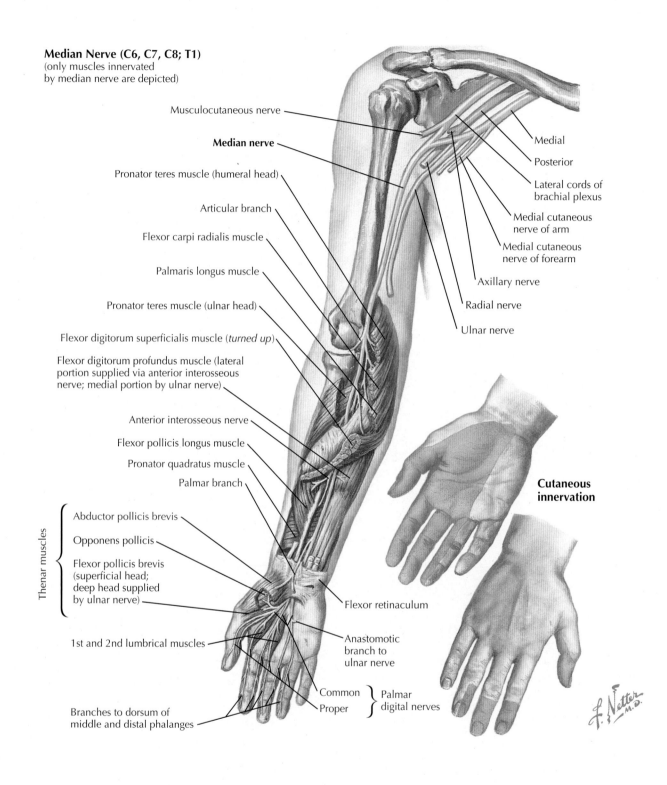

Musculocutaneous nerve

Median nerve

Pronator teres muscle (humeral head)

Articular branch

Flexor carpi radialis muscle

Palmaris longus muscle

Pronator teres muscle (ulnar head)

Flexor digitorum superficialis muscle (*turned up*)

Flexor digitorum profundus muscle (lateral portion supplied via anterior interosseous nerve; medial portion by ulnar nerve)

Anterior interosseous nerve

Flexor pollicis longus muscle

Pronator quadratus muscle

Palmar branch

Thenar muscles

Abductor pollicis brevis

Opponens pollicis

Flexor pollicis brevis (superficial head; deep head supplied by ulnar nerve)

1st and 2nd lumbrical muscles

Branches to dorsum of middle and distal phalanges

Medial

Posterior

Lateral cords of brachial plexus

Medial cutaneous nerve of arm

Medial cutaneous nerve of forearm

Axillary nerve

Radial nerve

Ulnar nerve

Cutaneous innervation

Flexor retinaculum

Anastomotic branch to ulnar nerve

Common
Proper } Palmar digital nerves

9.33 MEDIAN NERVE

The median nerve (C5–T1) supplies motor fibers to the (1) flexor carpiradialis, (2) pronatorteres, (3) palmaris longus, (4) flexor digitorum superficialis and profundus, (5) flexor pollicis longus, (6) abductor pollicis brevis, (7) flexor pollicis brevis, (8) opponens pollicis brevis, and (9) lumbrical muscles of the index and middle fingers. It supplies sensory innervation to the palm and adjacent thumb, the index and middle fingers, and the lateral half of the fourth finger. A lesion (caused by carpal tunnel syndrome) results in weakness in flexion of the fingers, abduction and opposition of the thumb, and loss of sensation or painful sensation in the radial distribution in the hand (thumb, index finger, middle finger, and half of the fourth finger). Pain in that distribution often radiates back to the wrist. A higher lesion also produces weakness in pronation of the forearm.

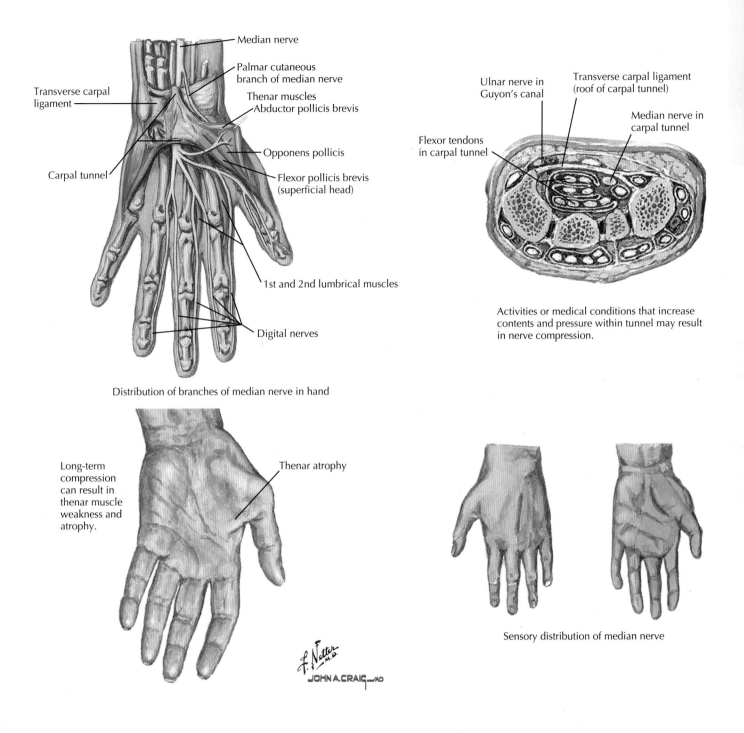

Median nerve

Palmar cutaneous branch of median nerve

Thenar muscles
Abductor pollicis brevis

Transverse carpal ligament

Carpal tunnel

Opponens pollicis

Flexor pollicis brevis (superficial head)

1st and 2nd lumbrical muscles

Digital nerves

Distribution of branches of median nerve in hand

Ulnar nerve in Guyon's canal

Transverse carpal ligament (roof of carpal tunnel)

Median nerve in carpal tunnel

Flexor tendons in carpal tunnel

Activities or medical conditions that increase contents and pressure within tunnel may result in nerve compression.

Long-term compression can result in thenar muscle weakness and atrophy.

Thenar atrophy

Sensory distribution of median nerve

9.34 CARPAL TUNNEL SYNDROME

The median nerve travels through the carpal tunnel in the wrist. The carpal tunnel is a tightly confined space restricted by the presence of the transverse carpal ligament. Repetitive movements of the wrist (e.g., repeated computer activity), chronic extension of the wrist (e.g., bicycling), and even sleeping with the wrist bent can compress the median nerve in the carpal tunnel. The mechanism of damage to the nerve may be direct compression on the nerve and also may involve an accompanying reduction in blood flow to the nerves through the vasa nervorum. This produces a painful neuropathy characterized by tingling and paresthesias or pain (sometimes severe) on the median side of the palm and in the thumb, the index finger, the middle finger, and the adjacent half of the fourth finger, often radiating back to the wrist. The pain is severe enough to awaken the patient. There also may be weakness in the innervated muscles with atrophy in the thenar eminence. Nerve conduction velocity studies show slowing of motor and sensory axons. An electromyogram may show denervation of innervated muscles such as the abductor pollicis brevis.

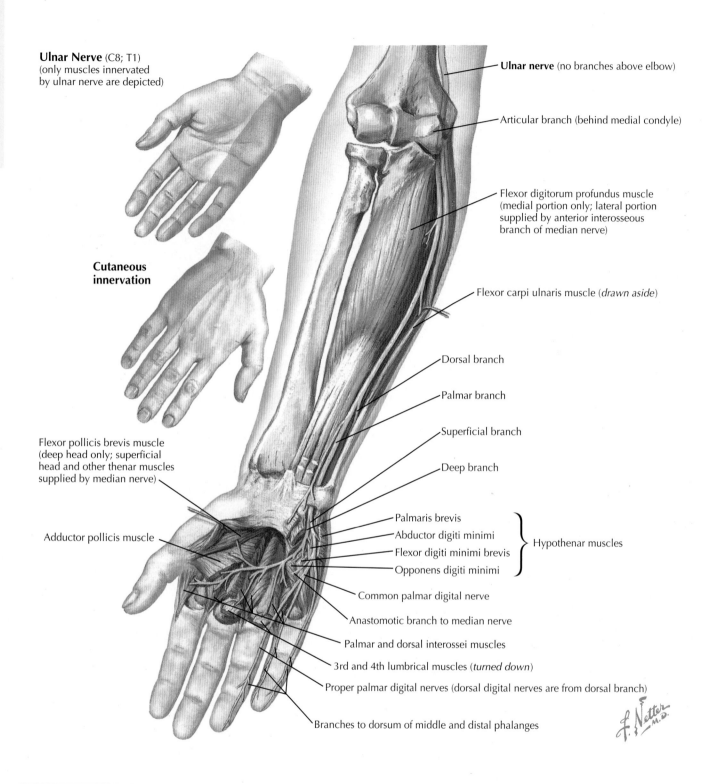

Ulnar Nerve (C8; T1)
(only muscles innervated
by ulnar nerve are depicted)

**Cutaneous
innervation**

Flexor pollicis brevis muscle
(deep head only; superficial
head and other thenar muscles
supplied by median nerve)

Adductor pollicis muscle

Ulnar nerve (no branches above elbow)

Articular branch (behind medial condyle)

Flexor digitorum profundus muscle
(medial portion only; lateral portion
supplied by anterior interosseous
branch of median nerve)

Flexor carpi ulnaris muscle (*drawn aside*)

Dorsal branch

Palmar branch

Superficial branch

Deep branch

Palmaris brevis
Abductor digiti minimi   } Hypothenar muscles
Flexor digiti minimi brevis
Opponens digiti minimi

Common palmar digital nerve

Anastomotic branch to median nerve

Palmar and dorsal interossei muscles

3rd and 4th lumbrical muscles (*turned down*)

Proper palmar digital nerves (dorsal digital nerves are from dorsal branch)

Branches to dorsum of middle and distal phalanges

f. Netter
M.D.

9.35 ULNAR NERVE

The ulnar nerve (C8–T1) supplies motor fibers to the (1) flexor carpi ulnaris, (2) flexor digitorum profundus, (3) adductor pollicis, (4) abductor digiti V, (5) opponens digiti V, (6) flexor digiti brevis V, (7) interosseus dorsal and palmar, and (8) lumbrical muscles of the fourth and little fingers. It supplies sensory innervation to the dorsal and palmar medial surfaces of the hand for the little finger and the medial half of the fourth

finger. A lesion results in wasting of hand muscles; weakness of wrist flexion and ulnar deviation of the hand; weakness of abduction and adduction of fingers, known as claw hand (hyperextension of the fingers at metacarpophalangeal joints and flexion at the interphalangeal joints); and loss of sensation in the ulnar distribution in the hand (dorsal and palmar surfaces of the medial hand, the little finger, and the adjacent half of the fourth finger).

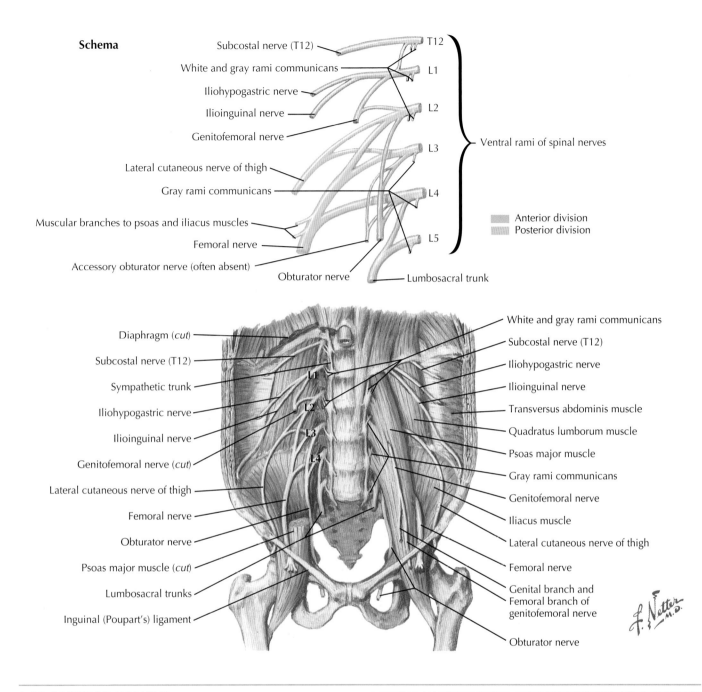

Schema

Subcostal nerve (T12)

White and gray rami communicans

Iliohypogastric nerve

Ilioinguinal nerve

Genitofemoral nerve

Lateral cutaneous nerve of thigh

Gray rami communicans

Muscular branches to psoas and iliacus muscles

Femoral nerve

Accessory obturator nerve (often absent)

Obturator nerve

T12

L1

L2

L3

L4

L5

Ventral rami of spinal nerves

Anterior division
Posterior division

Lumbosacral trunk

Diaphragm (*cut*)

Subcostal nerve (T12)

Sympathetic trunk

Iliohypogastric nerve

Ilioinguinal nerve

Genitofemoral nerve (*cut*)

Lateral cutaneous nerve of thigh

Femoral nerve

Obturator nerve

Psoas major muscle (*cut*)

Lumbosacral trunks

Inguinal (Poupart's) ligament

White and gray rami communicans

Subcostal nerve (T12)

Iliohypogastric nerve

Ilioinguinal nerve

Transversus abdominis muscle

Quadratus lumborum muscle

Psoas major muscle

Gray rami communicans

Genitofemoral nerve

Iliacus muscle

Lateral cutaneous nerve of thigh

Femoral nerve

Genital branch and Femoral branch of genitofemoral nerve

Obturator nerve

9.36 LUMBAR PLEXUS

The lumbar plexus is formed from the anterior primary rami of the L1 through L4 roots within the posterior substance of the psoas muscle. The L1 (and some of L2) root forms the iliohypogastric and ilioinguinal nerves and the genitofemoral nerves. These nerves contribute innervation to the transverse and the oblique abdominal muscles. The remaining roots form the femoral, obturator, and lateral femoral cutaneous nerves. Lesions in the lumbar plexus are unusual because of the protection of the plexus within the psoas muscle. Such lesions result in weakness of hip flexion, weakness of adduction of the thigh and extension of the leg, and decreased sensation on the anterior thigh and leg.

CLINICAL POINT

A **lumbar plexopathy** results in characteristic weakness and sensory losses in nerve roots L2–L4 and involves the distribution of both the obturator and femoral nerves. The most characteristic motor losses are weakness of hip flexion and adduction and weakness of extension of the leg. The motor loss can sometimes occur as the principal finding in a plexopathy but must be distinguished from radiculopathy. Sensory loss over the anterior (and medial) aspect of the thigh may or may not be seen. The patellar reflex usually is diminished. Some lumbar plexopathies present with a patchy motor loss in one or both legs; sometimes the cause is very clear, as in postradiation lumbar plexopathy following treatment of a retroperitoneal tumor or nodes, or in a plexopathy that accompanies pregnancy. And sometimes the cause is not clear and may include an ischemic diabetic plexopathy, a tumor with infiltration, vasculitis, or trauma. Lumbar plexopathies are usually distinguished from radiculopathies because the latter are painful and are accompanied by a nerve root distribution.

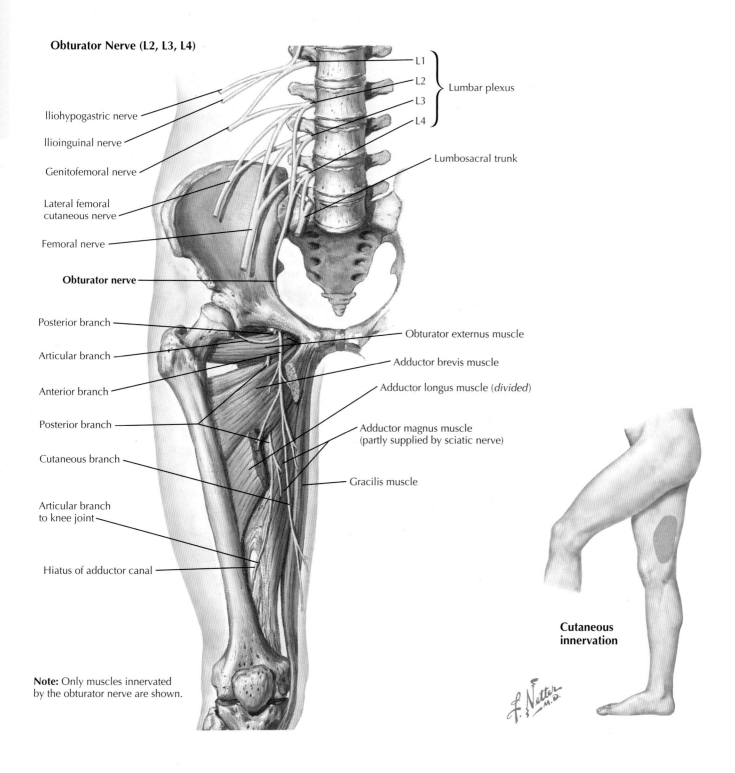

Obturator Nerve (L2, L3, L4)

Iliohypogastric nerve

Ilioinguinal nerve

Genitofemoral nerve

Lateral femoral cutaneous nerve

Femoral nerve

Obturator nerve

Posterior branch

Articular branch

Anterior branch

Posterior branch

Cutaneous branch

Articular branch to knee joint

Hiatus of adductor canal

L1
L2
L3
L4
} Lumbar plexus

Lumbosacral trunk

Obturator externus muscle

Adductor brevis muscle

Adductor longus muscle (*divided*)

Adductor magnus muscle (partly supplied by sciatic nerve)

Gracilis muscle

Note: Only muscles innervated by the obturator nerve are shown.

Cutaneous innervation

9.39 OBTURATOR NERVE

The obturator nerve (L2–L4) supplies the pectineus, adductor (longus, brevis, and magnus), gracilis, and external obturator muscles. This nerve controls adduction and rotation of the thigh. A small cutaneous zone on the internal thigh is supplied by sensory fibers. A lesion of the obturator nerve results in weakness of adduction of the thigh and a tendency to abduct the thigh in walking. There also is weakness of external rotation of the thigh. A small zone of anesthetic skin on the medial thigh is present.

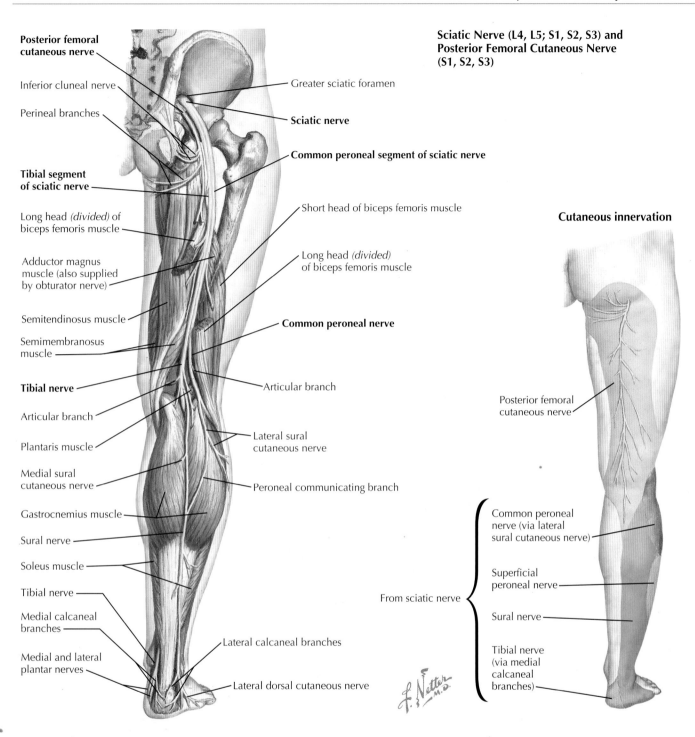

**Posterior femoral
cutaneous nerve**

Inferior cluneal nerve

Perineal branches

**Tibial segment
of sciatic nerve**

Long head *(divided)* of
biceps femoris muscle

Adductor magnus
muscle (also supplied
by obturator nerve)

Semitendinosus muscle

Semimembranosus
muscle

Tibial nerve

Articular branch

Plantaris muscle

Medial sural
cutaneous nerve

Gastrocnemius muscle

Sural nerve

Soleus muscle

Tibial nerve

Medial calcaneal
branches

Medial and lateral
plantar nerves

Greater sciatic foramen

Sciatic nerve

Common peroneal segment of sciatic nerve

Short head of biceps femoris muscle

Long head *(divided)*
of biceps femoris muscle

Common peroneal nerve

Articular branch

Lateral sural
cutaneous nerve

Peroneal communicating branch

Lateral calcaneal branches

Lateral dorsal cutaneous nerve

**Sciatic Nerve (L4, L5; S1, S2, S3) and
Posterior Femoral Cutaneous Nerve
(S1, S2, S3)**

Cutaneous innervation

Posterior femoral
cutaneous nerve

Common peroneal
nerve (via lateral
sural cutaneous nerve)

Superficial
peroneal nerve

From sciatic nerve

Sural nerve

Tibial nerve
(via medial
calcaneal
branches)

*f. Netter
M.D.*

9.40 **SCIATIC AND POSTERIOR FEMORAL CUTANEOUS NERVES**

The sciatic nerve is formed from the roots of the L4–S3 segments. The superior and inferior gluteal nerves branch proximally, just before the sciatic nerve's formation. The superior gluteal nerve (L4–S1) supplies the gluteus medius and minimus, tensor fascia lata, and piriformis muscles. It contributes to abduction and inward rotation and some outward rotation of the thigh, and to flexion of the upper leg at the hip. The inferior gluteal nerve (L4–S1) supplies the gluteus maximus, obturator internus, gemelli, and quadratus muscles. It contributes to extension of the thigh at the hip and to outward rotation of the thigh. A lesion results

in difficulty climbing stairs and rising from a sitting position. The sciatic nerve proper supplies the biceps femoris, semitendinosus, and semimembranosus muscles (hamstrings) and regulates flexion of the lower leg. Because it branches into the tibial and common peroneal nerves, major lesions of the sciatic nerve result in weakness of leg flexion, weakness of all muscles below the knee, and loss of sensation in the posterior thigh, posterior and lateral aspects of the leg, and sole of the foot. Such lesions may result from a fracture of the pelvis or femur, nerve compression, a herniated disc, or diabetes. The posterior femoral cutaneous nerve (S1–S3) supplies sensory innervation to the posterior thigh, lateral part of the perineum, and lower portion of the buttock.

Tibial Nerve (L4, L5; S1, S2, S3)

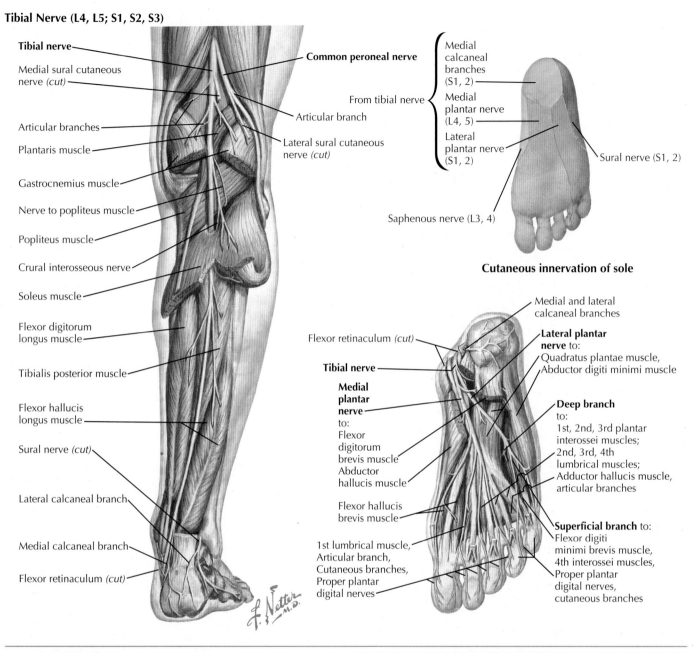

Tibial nerve

Medial sural cutaneous nerve (cut)

Articular branches

Plantaris muscle

Gastrocnemius muscle

Nerve to popliteus muscle

Popliteus muscle

Crural interosseous nerve

Soleus muscle

Flexor digitorum longus muscle

Tibialis posterior muscle

Flexor hallucis longus muscle

Sural nerve (cut)

Lateral calcaneal branch

Medial calcaneal branch

Flexor retinaculum (cut)

Common peroneal nerve

From tibial nerve

Articular branch

Lateral sural cutaneous nerve (cut)

Medial calcaneal branches (S1, 2)

Medial plantar nerve (L4, 5)

Lateral plantar nerve (S1, 2)

Sural nerve (S1, 2)

Saphenous nerve (L3, 4)

Cutaneous innervation of sole

Flexor retinaculum (cut)

Tibial nerve

Medial plantar nerve to: Flexor digitorum brevis muscle Abductor hallucis muscle

Flexor hallucis brevis muscle

1st lumbrical muscle, Articular branch, Cutaneous branches, Proper plantar digital nerves

Medial and lateral calcaneal branches

Lateral plantar nerve to: Quadratus plantae muscle, Abductor digiti minimi muscle

Deep branch to: 1st, 2nd, 3rd plantar interossei muscles; 2nd, 3rd, 4th lumbrical muscles; Adductor hallucis muscle, articular branches

Superficial branch to: Flexor digiti minimi brevis muscle, 4th interossei muscles, Proper plantar digital nerves, cutaneous branches

f. Netter m.d.

9.41 TIBIAL NERVE

The tibial nerve (L4–S2) supplies innervation to (1) the gastrocnemius and soleus muscles (the main plantar flexors of the foot), (2) the tibialis posterior (plantar flexion and inversion), (3) the flexor digitorum longus (plantar flexor and toe flexor), (4) the flexor hallucis longus (plantar flexor and great toe flexor), and (5) the muscles of the foot, including the abductor digiti minimi pedis, flexor digiti minimi, adductor hallucis, interosseous, and third and fourth lumbrical muscles. Sensory branches supply the skin over the lateral calf, foot, heel, and small toe (sural nerve) and the medial aspect of the heel and the sole of the foot (tibial nerve). A lesion can occur because of compression in the tarsal tunnel, a tumor, or diabetes; it results in weakness of plantar flexion and inversion of the foot, weakness of toe flexion, and loss of sensation in the lateral calf and the plantar region of the foot.

CLINICAL POINT

The tibial nerve in the popliteal fossa can be used for **evaluation of conduction velocity** and of specific reflexes. This nerve may be directly stimulated by electrical current. Surface recording electrodes are placed over a distal innervated muscle, and the nerve is stimulated in one or more places, resulting in an indirect evaluation of motor conduction velocity and the muscle response to tibial nerve stimulation. Sensory conduction velocity evaluation is a bit more straightforward; the stimulating electrode is placed at a distal site, and compound action potentials are recorded over at least two proximal sites. A more complex evaluation of reflexes involves evaluation of the muscle stretch (monosynaptic) reflex. With recording electrodes placed over the distal muscle (triceps surae), the tibial nerve is gradually stimulated first by weak and then by stronger electrical current in the popliteal fossa. The first axons that are stimulated are the Ia afferents, which conduct action potentials into the spinal cord and excite the homonymous LMN, whose axon then sends action potentials down to the innervated muscle. This is a long-latency response, called the H wave or H reflex because it involves both the sensory and the motor arms of the muscle stretch reflex. As current strength is increased, the LMN axon is finally stimulated directly, and the muscle response (direct muscle activation) occurs and with a far shorter latency. This H reflex evaluation is useful in assessment of axonal neuropathies and demyelinating neuropathies.

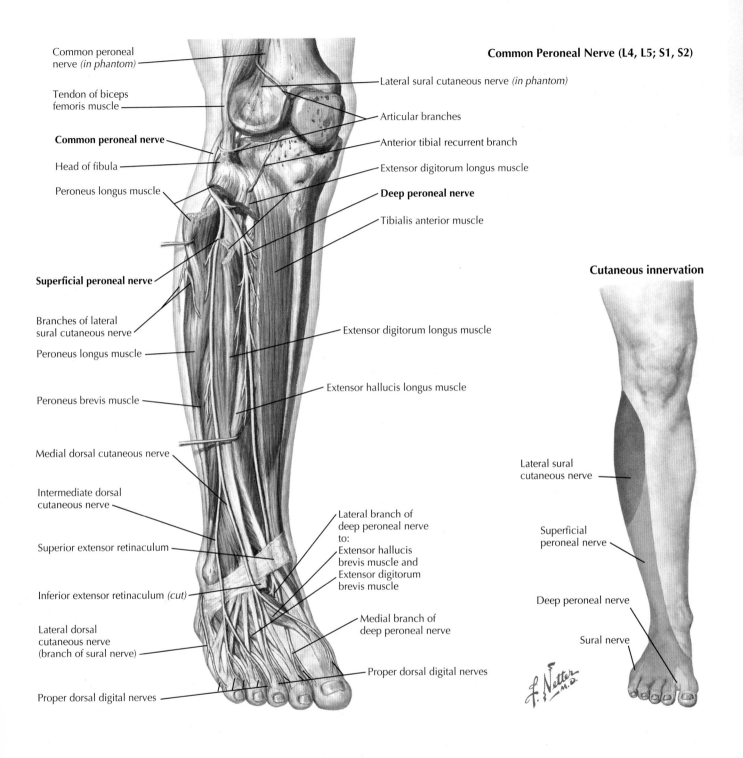

Common peroneal nerve *(in phantom)*

Tendon of biceps femoris muscle

Common peroneal nerve

Head of fibula

Peroneus longus muscle

Superficial peroneal nerve

Branches of lateral sural cutaneous nerve

Peroneus longus muscle

Peroneus brevis muscle

Medial dorsal cutaneous nerve

Intermediate dorsal cutaneous nerve

Superior extensor retinaculum

Inferior extensor retinaculum *(cut)*

Lateral dorsal cutaneous nerve (branch of sural nerve)

Proper dorsal digital nerves

Common Peroneal Nerve (L4, L5; S1, S2)

Lateral sural cutaneous nerve *(in phantom)*

Articular branches

Anterior tibial recurrent branch

Extensor digitorum longus muscle

Deep peroneal nerve

Tibialis anterior muscle

Extensor digitorum longus muscle

Extensor hallucis longus muscle

Lateral branch of deep peroneal nerve to: Extensor hallucis brevis muscle and Extensor digitorum brevis muscle

Medial branch of deep peroneal nerve

Proper dorsal digital nerves

Cutaneous innervation

Lateral sural cutaneous nerve

Superficial peroneal nerve

Deep peroneal nerve

Sural nerve

9.42 COMMON PERONEAL NERVE

The common peroneal nerve (L4–S1) branches into the deep peroneal nerve, supplying (1) the tibialis anterior (foot dorsiflexion and inversion), (2) the extensor hallucis longus (foot dorsiflexion and great toe extension), (3) the extensor digitorum longus (extension of the toes and foot dorsiflexion), and (4) the extensor digitorum brevis muscles (extension of toes) and the superficial peroneal nerve, which supplies the peroneus longus and brevis muscles (plantar flexion and foot eversion). Sensory branches supply the lateral aspect of the leg below the knee and the skin on the dorsal surface of the foot. This nerve may be damaged by compression, a fracture at the head of the fibula, or diabetes, resulting in weakness of dorsiflexion and eversion of the foot, weakness of toe extension (dorsiflexion), and loss of sensation in the lateral aspect of the lower leg and the dorsum of the foot.

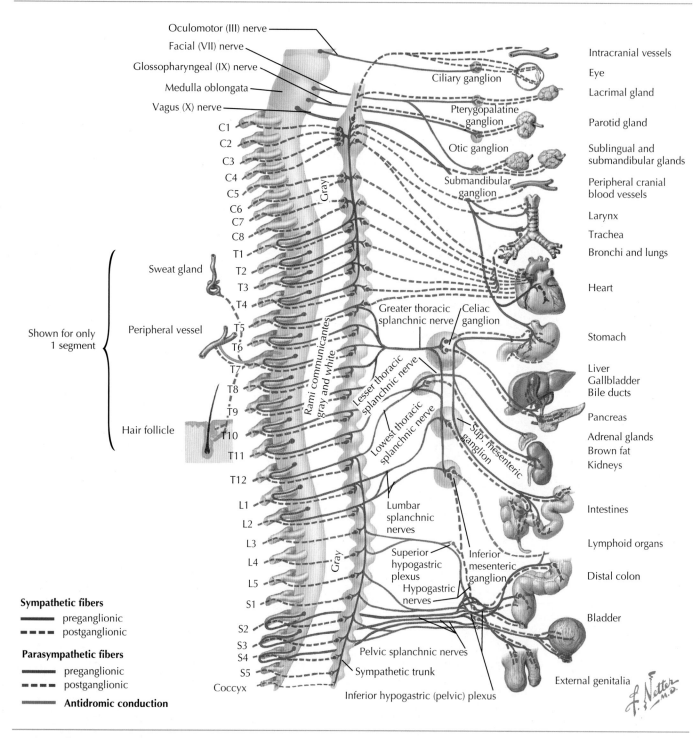

Oculomotor (III) nerve
Facial (VII) nerve
Glossopharyngeal (IX) nerve
Medulla oblongata
Vagus (X) nerve
C1
C2
C3
C4
C5
C6
C7
C8
T1
T2
T3
T4
T5
T6
T7
T8
T9
T10
T11
T12
L1
L2
L3
L4
L5
S1
S2
S3
S4
S5
Coccyx

Gray

Intracranial vessels
Eye
Ciliary ganglion
Lacrimal gland
Pterygopalatine ganglion
Parotid gland
Otic ganglion
Sublingual and submandibular glands
Submandibular ganglion
Peripheral cranial blood vessels
Larynx
Trachea
Bronchi and lungs
Heart
Greater thoracic splanchnic nerve
Celiac ganglion
Stomach
Rami communicantes gray and white
Lesser thoracic splanchnic nerve
Liver Gallbladder Bile ducts
Lowest thoracic splanchnic nerve
Sup. mesenteric ganglion
Pancreas
Adrenal glands Brown fat Kidneys
Lumbar splanchnic nerves
Intestines
Superior hypogastric plexus
Inferior mesenteric ganglion
Lymphoid organs
Hypogastric nerves
Distal colon
Pelvic splanchnic nerves
Bladder
Sympathetic trunk
Inferior hypogastric (pelvic) plexus
External genitalia

Sweat gland
Peripheral vessel
Shown for only 1 segment
Hair follicle

Sympathetic fibers
preganglionic
postganglionic

Parasympathetic fibers
preganglionic
postganglionic
Antidromic conduction

AUTONOMIC NERVOUS SYSTEM

9.43 GENERAL SCHEMA

The autonomic nervous system is a two-neuron chain. The preganglionic neuron arises from the brainstem or spinal cord and synapses on postganglionic neurons in the sympathetic chain or collateral ganglia (sympathetic) or on intramural ganglia (parasympathetic) near the organ innervated. The sympathetic division, derived from neurons in the T1–L2 lateral horn, prepares the body for fight-or-flight mobilization for emergency responses. The parasympathetic division, derived from neurons in the brainstem (CNs III, VII, IX, and X) and the sacral spinal cord (S2–S4 intermediate gray), regulates reparative, homeostatic, and digestive functions. These autonomic systems achieve their actions through innervations of smooth muscle, cardiac muscle, secretory (exocrine) glands, metabolic cells

(hepatocytes, fat cells), and cells of the immune system. Normally, both autonomic divisions work together to regulate visceral activities such as respiration, cardiovascular function, digestion, and some endocrine functions.

CLINICAL POINT

Pure autonomic failure is a gradual deterioration of sympathetic postganglionic neurons; it occurs in middle-aged individuals and is observed more commonly in men than in women. This syndrome includes neurogenic orthostatic hypotension (syncope or dizziness when standing), inability to sweat, urinary tract dysfunction, erectile dysfunction, and retrograde ejaculation. Pure autonomic failure can be present without evidence of involvement of the CNS. Catecholamine challenge results in robust reactivity in target organs caused by denervation hypersensitivity.

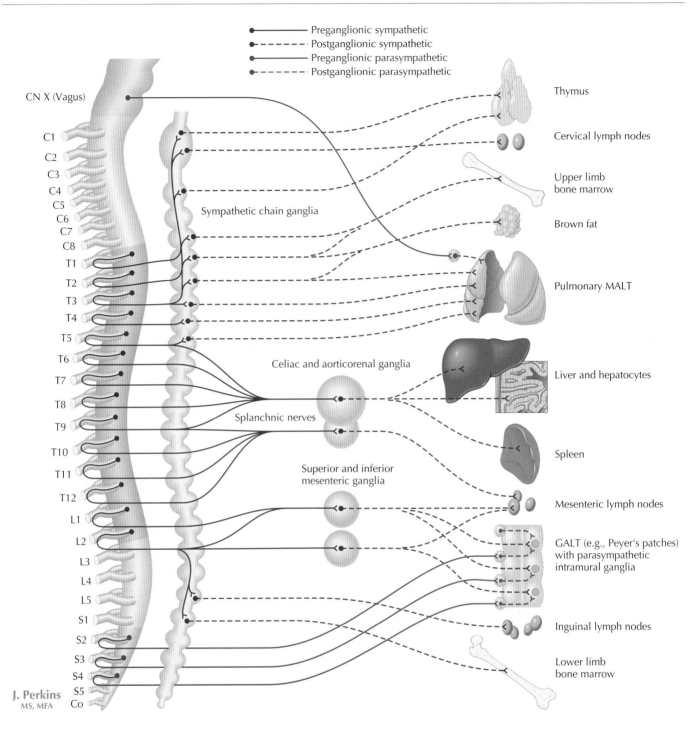

Preganglionic sympathetic
Postganglionic sympathetic
Preganglionic parasympathetic
Postganglionic parasympathetic

CN X (Vagus)

Thymus

Cervical lymph nodes

Upper limb bone marrow

Brown fat

Sympathetic chain ganglia

Pulmonary MALT

Celiac and aorticorenal ganglia

Liver and hepatocytes

Splanchnic nerves

Spleen

Superior and inferior mesenteric ganglia

Mesenteric lymph nodes

GALT (e.g., Peyer's patches) with parasympathetic intramural ganglia

Inguinal lymph nodes

Lower limb bone marrow

J. Perkins
MS, MFA

9.44 AUTONOMIC INNERVATION OF THE IMMUNE SYSTEM AND METABOLIC ORGANS

The autonomic nervous system innervates the vasculature, smooth muscle tissue, and parenchyma of organs of the immune system mainly through the sympathetic division. In the bone marrow and thymus, sympathetic fibers modulate cell proliferation, differentiation, and mobilization. In the spleen and lymph nodes, sympathetic fibers modulate innate immune reactivity and the magnitude and timing of acquired immune responses, particularly the choice of cell-mediated (Th1 cytokines) as opposed to humoral (Th2 cytokines) immunity. Autonomic nerve fibers regulate immune responses and inflammatory responses in the mucosa-associated lymphoid tissue (MALT) in the lungs, the gut-associated lymphoid tissue (GALT), and the skin. Extensive neuropeptidergic innervation, derived from both the autonomic nervous system and the primary sensory neurons, also is present in the parenchyma of lymphoid organs. Many subsets of lymphoid cells express cognate receptors for catecholamines (alpha and beta receptor subsets) and neuropeptides; the expression of these neurotransmitter receptors is highly regulated by both lymphoid and neural molecular signals. Postganglionic sympathetic nerve fibers also directly innervate hepatocytes and fat cells. Th, T helper cells.

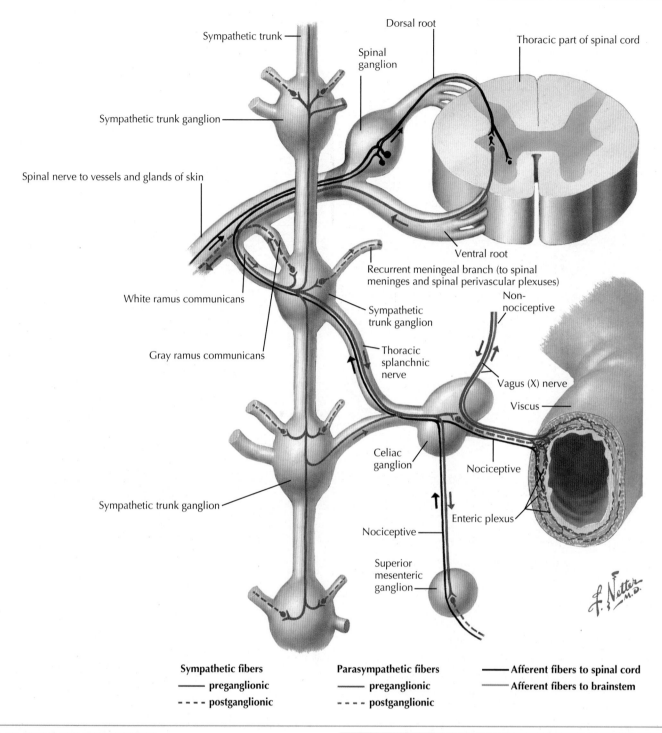

Dorsal root

Thoracic part of spinal cord

Sympathetic trunk

Spinal ganglion

Sympathetic trunk ganglion

Spinal nerve to vessels and glands of skin

White ramus communicans

Gray ramus communicans

Sympathetic trunk ganglion

Ventral root

Recurrent meningeal branch (to spinal meninges and spinal perivascular plexuses)

Sympathetic trunk ganglion

Thoracic splanchnic nerve

Non-nociceptive

Vagus (X) nerve

Viscus

Nociceptive

Celiac ganglion

Enteric plexus

Nociceptive

Superior mesenteric ganglion

Sympathetic fibers
— preganglionic
- - - postganglionic

Parasympathetic fibers
— preganglionic
- - - postganglionic

—— **Afferent fibers to spinal cord**
—— **Afferent fibers to brainstem**

9.45 REFLEX PATHWAYS

Autonomic reflex pathways consist of a sensory (afferent) component, interneurons in the CNS, and autonomic efferent components that innervate the peripheral tissue responding to the afferent stimulus. The afferents can be either autonomic (e.g., from the vagus nerve) and processed by brainstem nuclei such as the nucleus solitarius; or they can be somatic (e.g., nociception) and processed by spinal cord neurons. The preganglionic sympathetic or parasympathetic neurons are activated through interneurons to produce a reflex autonomic response (e.g., contraction of vascular smooth muscle to alter blood pressure and increase heart rate and contractility). The efferent connectivity can be relayed via splanchnic or somatic nerves because of the complexity of autonomic efferent pathways.

CLINICAL POINT

Autonomic reflex pathways are vital for maintenance of homeostasis. Sensory signals associated with standing result in vascular constriction induced by sympathetic neurons to maintain blood pressure, prevent pooling of blood in the lower extremities, and maintain appropriate perfusion of the brain and other vital organs. Nociceptive stimulation may result in reflex elevation of heart rate, blood pressure, and other characteristics of sympathetic activation. Stimulation of the perioral region, particularly in an infant during feeding, activates a parasympathetic state to enhance digestion and diminish sympathetic activation, thereby promoting growth and development. Problems can arise when autonomic reflexes are disrupted, or when hyperactivation of reflex pathways elevates either parasympathetic or sympathetic activity. In such circumstances, there is often a counterpart activation of the other system, as when paradoxical parasympathetic activation leads to compensatory sympathetic activation. This can increase the likelihood of problems such as arrhythmia or even cardiac arrest.

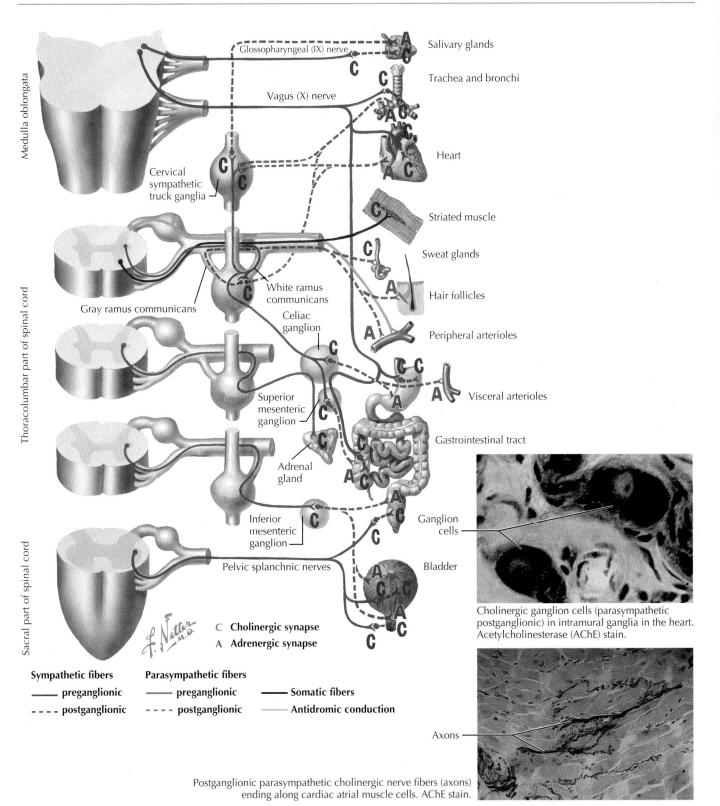

Medulla oblongata

Glossopharyngeal (IX) nerve

Salivary glands

Vagus (X) nerve

Trachea and bronchi

Cervical sympathetic truck ganglia

Heart

Striated muscle

Thoracolumbar part of spinal cord

Gray ramus communicans

White ramus communicans

Celiac ganglion

Sweat glands

Hair follicles

Peripheral arterioles

Superior mesenteric ganglion

Visceral arterioles

Adrenal gland

Gastrointestinal tract

Inferior mesenteric ganglion

Ganglion cells

Sacral part of spinal cord

Pelvic splanchnic nerves

Bladder

C **Cholinergic synapse**
A **Adrenergic synapse**

Sympathetic fibers
—— preganglionic
- - - - postganglionic

Parasympathetic fibers
—— preganglionic
- - - - postganglionic

—— **Somatic fibers**
—— **Antidromic conduction**

Cholinergic ganglion cells (parasympathetic postganglionic) in intramural ganglia in the heart. Acetylcholinesterase (AChE) stain.

Axons

Postganglionic parasympathetic cholinergic nerve fibers (axons) ending along cardiac atrial muscle cells. AChE stain.

9.46 CHOLINERGIC AND ADRENERGIC SYNAPSES

The autonomic nervous system is a two-neuron chain. All preganglionic neurons, sympathetic and parasympathetic, use ACh as the principal neurotransmitter in synapses on ganglion cells. These cholinergic (C) synapses activate mainly nicotinic receptors on the ganglion cells. Postganglionic parasympathetic neurons use ACh at synapses with target tissue, activating mainly muscarinic receptors. Postganglionic sympathetic neurons use mainly norepinephrine (adrenergic responses; A), to activate both alpha and beta receptors on target tissues. Although ACh and norepinephrine are the principal neurotransmitters used by autonomic neurons, many colocalized neuropeptides and other neuromediators are also present, including neuropeptide Y, substance P, somatostatin, enkephalins, histamine, glutamate, and others.

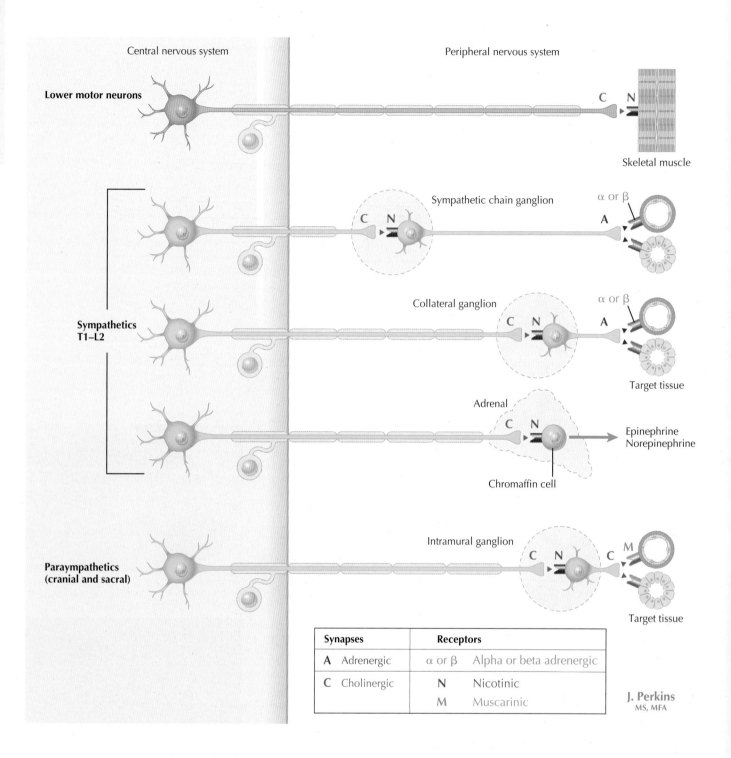

Synapses		Receptors	
A	Adrenergic	α or β	Alpha or beta adrenergic
C	Cholinergic	N	Nicotinic
		M	Muscarinic

J. Perkins
MS, MFA

9.47 SCHEMATIC OF CHOLINERGIC AND ADRENERGIC DISTRIBUTION TO MOTOR AND AUTONOMIC STRUCTURES

All preganglionic neurons of both the SNS and the PsNS use ACh as their neurotransmitter. All ganglion cells possess mainly nicotinic receptors for fast response to cholinergic release from preganglionic axons. However, additional muscarinic receptors and dopamine receptors on ganglion cells help to mediate longer term excitability. The postganglionic sympathetic nerves use mainly norepinephrine as their neurotransmitter and target structures in the periphery possessing different subsets of alpha and beta adrenergic receptors for response to norepinephrine. Some postganglionic nerve fibers to sweat glands use ACh as their neurotransmitter. Postganglionic parasympathetic nerves use ACh as their neurotransmitter and target structures in the periphery possessing mainly muscarinic receptors for response to ACh.

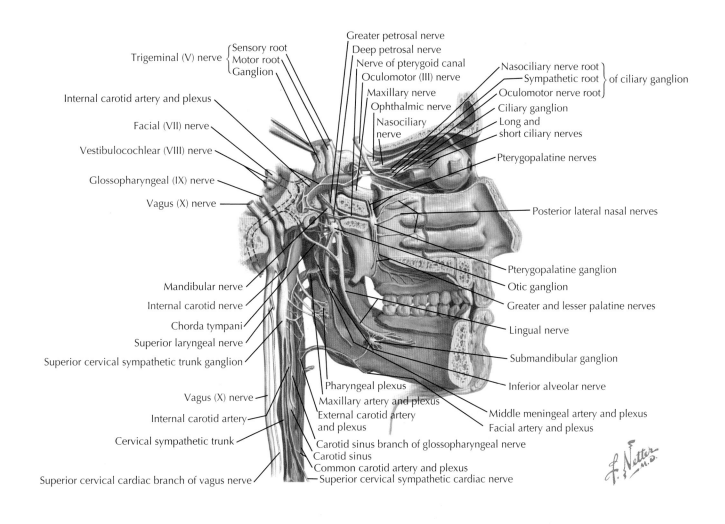

Trigeminal (V) nerve { Sensory root / Motor root / Ganglion }

Internal carotid artery and plexus

Facial (VII) nerve

Vestibulocochlear (VIII) nerve

Glossopharyngeal (IX) nerve

Vagus (X) nerve

Greater petrosal nerve
Deep petrosal nerve
Nerve of pterygoid canal
Oculomotor (III) nerve
Maxillary nerve
Ophthalmic nerve
Nasociliary nerve

Nasociliary nerve root
Sympathetic root } of ciliary ganglion
Oculomotor nerve root
Ciliary ganglion
Long and short ciliary nerves
Pterygopalatine nerves

Posterior lateral nasal nerves

Mandibular nerve
Internal carotid nerve
Chorda tympani
Superior laryngeal nerve
Superior cervical sympathetic trunk ganglion

Vagus (X) nerve
Internal carotid artery
Cervical sympathetic trunk

Superior cervical cardiac branch of vagus nerve

Pharyngeal plexus
Maxillary artery and plexus
External carotid artery and plexus
Carotid sinus branch of glossopharyngeal nerve
Carotid sinus
Common carotid artery and plexus
Superior cervical sympathetic cardiac nerve

Pterygopalatine ganglion
Otic ganglion
Greater and lesser palatine nerves
Lingual nerve
Submandibular ganglion
Inferior alveolar nerve
Middle meningeal artery and plexus
Facial artery and plexus

f. Netter M.D.

9.48 AUTONOMIC DISTRIBUTION TO THE HEAD AND NECK: MEDIAL VIEW

Autonomic nerve distribution to the head and neck includes components of both the SNS and the PsNS. The parasympathetic components are associated with CNs III (ciliary ganglion), VII (pterygopalatine, submandibular ganglia), and IX (otic ganglion). The vagus nerve and its associated ganglia do not innervate effector tissue in the head and neck, although they are present in the neck. Sympathetic components are associated with the superior cervical ganglion and, to a lesser extent, the middle cervical ganglion. The geniculate ganglion (CN VII), petrosal ganglion (CN IX), and nodose ganglion (CN X) process taste information. They are sometimes thought of as autonomic afferents, but they are not components of the autonomic efferent nervous system.

CLINICAL POINT

The oculomotor (III nerve) parasympathetic distribution to the eye forms a vital link in one of the most important reflexes in neurology, the **pupillary light reflex**. Light shone into one eye provides an afferent signal that is processed by the retina, resulting in ganglion cell activation and axonal projections to the pretectum on both sides. The pretectum, through direct and contralateral connections via the posterior commissure, stimulates the nucleus of Edinger-Westphal bilaterally.

This system, via connections in the ciliary ganglion, distributes to the pupillary constrictor muscle, resulting in constriction of the ipsilateral (direct) and contralateral (consensual) pupils. The pupillary light reflex is particularly important in someone with a head injury, intracranial bleed, or space-occupying mass in whom possible brain herniation is suspected. The third nerve may be trapped and compressed against the free edge of the tentorium cerebelli, resulting in failure of the ipsilateral pupil to constrict and disruption of the pupillary light reflex

The superior cervical ganglion (SCG) is the most rostral component of the sympathetic chain. It supplies structures in the head and neck, including the pupillary dilator muscle, blood vessels, sweat glands, pineal gland, thymus gland, and superior tarsal (Müller's) muscle. The T1–T2 intermediolateral cell column in the spinal cord (preganglionic sympathetic neurons) innervates the SCG; this ganglion then distributes noradrenergic fibers to the pupillary dilator muscle, resulting in dilation of the pupil. When CN III is damaged (e.g., by compression during transtentorial herniation), the actions of the sympathetic SCG are unopposed, resulting in a fixed (unresponsive to the pupillary light reflex), dilated pupil. In circumstances in which the SCG or its central innervation is damaged (e.g., apical lung tumor, Horner's syndrome), the ipsilateral pupil cannot dilate and the pupil is constricted (miotic).

A pupil that constricts when light is shone into one eye and paradoxically appears to dilate when light is shone into the other eye (swinging flashlight test) indicates an afferent (CN II) defect, with the paradoxical dilation occurring as the result of recovery from the initial constriction because of the unresponsiveness of the damaged CN II.

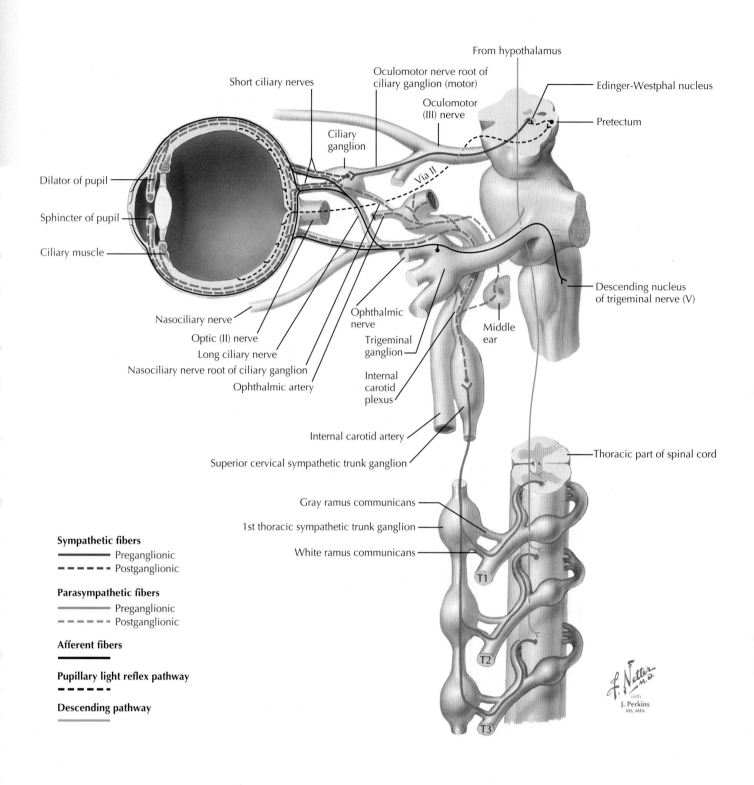

From hypothalamus

Short ciliary nerves

Oculomotor nerve root of
ciliary ganglion (motor)

Edinger-Westphal nucleus

Oculomotor
(III) nerve

Pretectum

Ciliary
ganglion

Via II

Dilator of pupil

Sphincter of pupil

Ciliary muscle

Descending nucleus
of trigeminal nerve (V)

Nasociliary nerve

Ophthalmic
nerve

Optic (II) nerve

Middle
ear

Trigeminal
ganglion

Long ciliary nerve

Nasociliary nerve root of ciliary ganglion

Ophthalmic artery

Internal
carotid
plexus

Internal carotid artery

Superior cervical sympathetic trunk ganglion

Thoracic part of spinal cord

Gray ramus communicans

1st thoracic sympathetic trunk ganglion

White ramus communicans

T1

T2

T3

Sympathetic fibers
———————— Preganglionic
– – – – – – Postganglionic

Parasympathetic fibers
▬▬▬▬▬▬▬ Preganglionic
– – – – – – Postganglionic

Afferent fibers

Pupillary light reflex pathway
▬ ▬ ▬ ▬ ▬

Descending pathway

9.51 AUTONOMIC DISTRIBUTION TO THE EYE

Parasympathetic preganglionic nerve fibers from the Edinger-Westphal nucleus innervate the ciliary ganglion, which supplies the ciliary muscle (aiding in accommodation to near vision) and the pupillary constrictor muscle (constricting the pupil). Sympathetic preganglionic nerve fibers from the T1–T2 intermediolateral cell column innervate the superior cervical ganglion, which supplies the dilator muscle of the pupil.

The pupillary light reflex is a major reflex in neurological testing. The afferent limb is activated by light shone in either eye via CN II and processed through the pretectum to the Edinger-Westphal nucleus on both sides (via the posterior commissure); the efferent limb consists of autonomic parasympathetic outflow to the pupillary constrictor muscles of both sides.

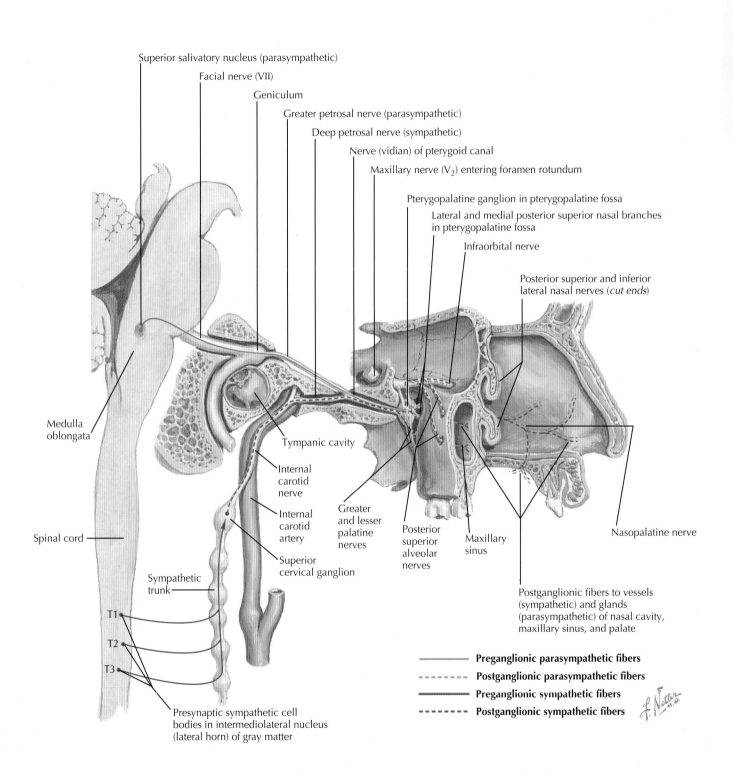

Superior salivatory nucleus (parasympathetic)

Facial nerve (VII)

Geniculum

Greater petrosal nerve (parasympathetic)

Deep petrosal nerve (sympathetic)

Nerve (vidian) of pterygoid canal

Maxillary nerve (V_2) entering foramen rotundum

Pterygopalatine ganglion in pterygopalatine fossa

Lateral and medial posterior superior nasal branches in pterygopalatine fossa

Infraorbital nerve

Posterior superior and inferior lateral nasal nerves (*cut ends*)

Medulla oblongata

Tympanic cavity

Internal carotid nerve

Internal carotid artery

Greater and lesser palatine nerves

Posterior superior alveolar nerves

Maxillary sinus

Nasopalatine nerve

Spinal cord

Superior cervical ganglion

Sympathetic trunk

T1

T2

T3

Presynaptic sympathetic cell bodies in intermediolateral nucleus (lateral horn) of gray matter

Postganglionic fibers to vessels (sympathetic) and glands (parasympathetic) of nasal cavity, maxillary sinus, and palate

———— Preganglionic parasympathetic fibers
------ Postganglionic parasympathetic fibers
———— Preganglionic sympathetic fibers
------ Postganglionic sympathetic fibers

9.52 **AUTONOMIC INNERVATION OF THE NASAL CAVITY**

Parasympathetic preganglionic neurons in the superior salivatory nucleus innervate the pterygopalatine ganglion. Sympathetic preganglionic neurons from the T1–T2 intermediolateral cell column innervate the SCG. The pterygopalatine ganglion supplies secretory glands, and the SCG supplies blood vessels with postganglionic nerve fibers in the nasal cavity, maxillary sinus, and palate.

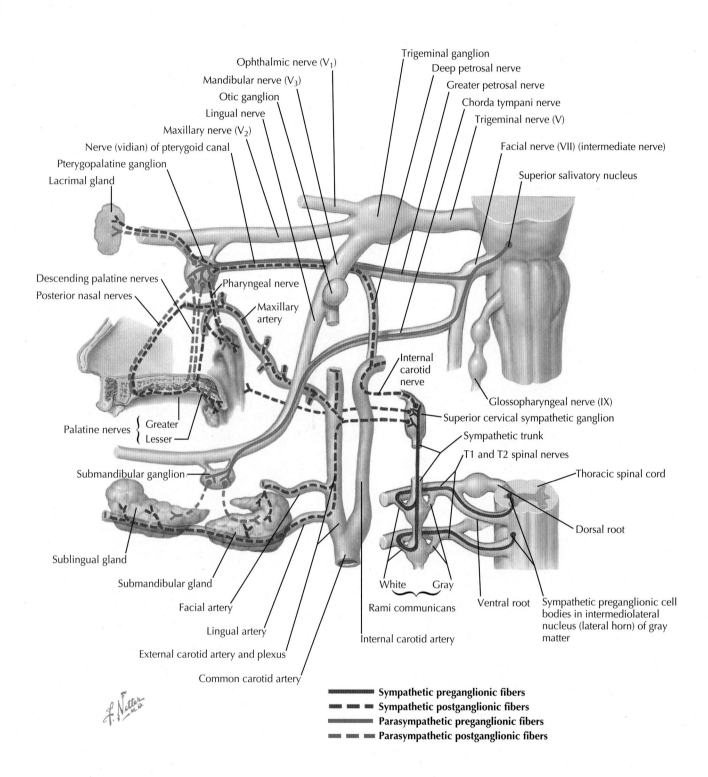

Ophthalmic nerve (V₁)

Mandibular nerve (V₃)

Otic ganglion

Lingual nerve

Maxillary nerve (V₂)

Nerve (vidian) of pterygoid canal

Pterygopalatine ganglion

Lacrimal gland

Trigeminal ganglion

Deep petrosal nerve

Greater petrosal nerve

Chorda tympani nerve

Trigeminal nerve (V)

Facial nerve (VII) (intermediate nerve)

Superior salivatory nucleus

Descending palatine nerves

Posterior nasal nerves

Pharyngeal nerve

Maxillary artery

Palatine nerves { Greater Lesser

Submandibular ganglion

Internal carotid nerve

Glossopharyngeal nerve (IX)

Superior cervical sympathetic ganglion

Sympathetic trunk

T1 and T2 spinal nerves

Thoracic spinal cord

Dorsal root

Sublingual gland

Submandibular gland

Facial artery

Lingual artery

External carotid artery and plexus

Common carotid artery

White   Gray

Rami communicans

Internal carotid artery

Ventral root

Sympathetic preganglionic cell bodies in intermediolateral nucleus (lateral horn) of gray matter

▬▬▬▬▬ **Sympathetic preganglionic fibers**

▬ ▬ ▬ **Sympathetic postganglionic fibers**

▬▬▬▬ **Parasympathetic preganglionic fibers**

▬ ▬ ▬ **Parasympathetic postganglionic fibers**

9.53 SCHEMATIC OF THE PTERYGOPALATINE AND SUBMANDIBULAR GANGLIA

The pterygopalatine and submandibular ganglia, innervated by the superior salivatory nucleus via CN VII, supply the lacrimal glands and nasal mucosal glands as well as the submandibular and sublingual salivary glands, respectively, with postganglionic parasympathetic cholinergic nerve fibers.

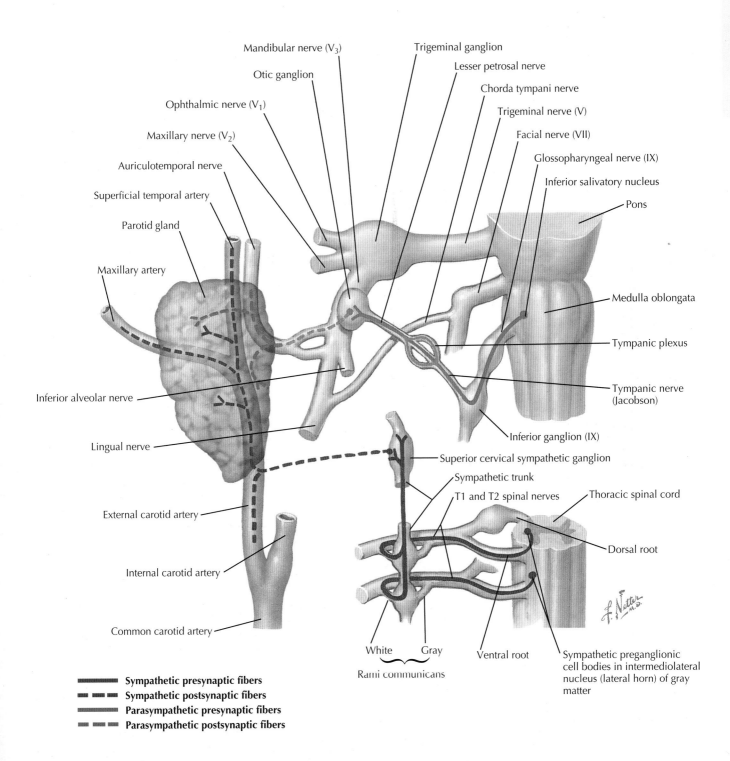

Mandibular nerve (V₃)

Trigeminal ganglion

Otic ganglion

Lesser petrosal nerve

Chorda tympani nerve

Ophthalmic nerve (V₁)

Trigeminal nerve (V)

Maxillary nerve (V₂)

Facial nerve (VII)

Auriculotemporal nerve

Glossopharyngeal nerve (IX)

Superficial temporal artery

Inferior salivatory nucleus

Parotid gland

Pons

Maxillary artery

Medulla oblongata

Tympanic plexus

Inferior alveolar nerve

Tympanic nerve (Jacobson)

Lingual nerve

Inferior ganglion (IX)

Superior cervical sympathetic ganglion

Sympathetic trunk

T1 and T2 spinal nerves

Thoracic spinal cord

External carotid artery

Dorsal root

Internal carotid artery

Common carotid artery

White   Gray

Rami communicans

Ventral root

Sympathetic preganglionic cell bodies in intermediolateral nucleus (lateral horn) of gray matter

▬▬▬▬ **Sympathetic presynaptic fibers**
▬ ▬ ▬ **Sympathetic postsynaptic fibers**
▬▬▬▬ **Parasympathetic presynaptic fibers**
▬ ▬ ▬ **Parasympathetic postsynaptic fibers**

9.54 SCHEMATIC OF THE OTIC GANGLION

The otic ganglion, innervated by the inferior salivatory nucleus via CN IX, supplies the parotid salivary gland with postganglionic parasympathetic cholinergic nerve fibers.

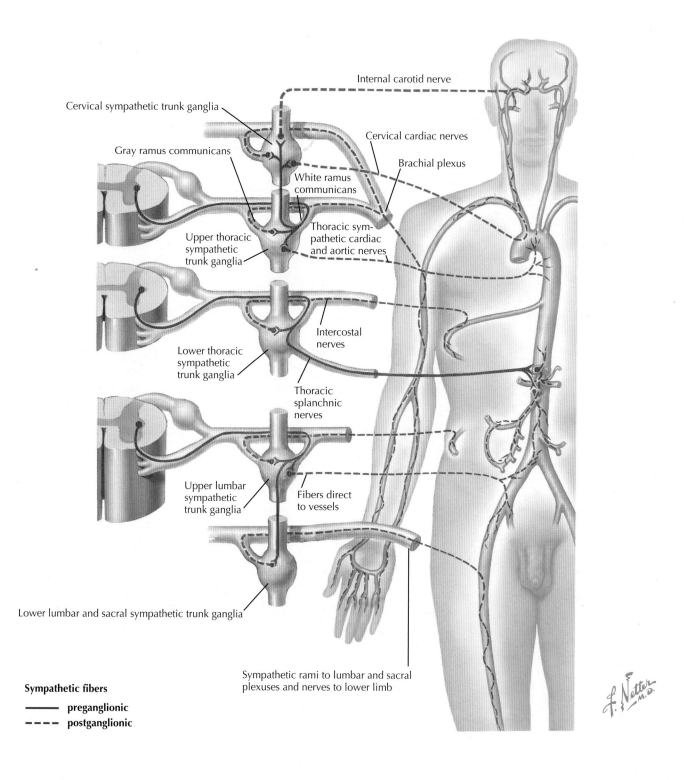

Internal carotid nerve

Cervical sympathetic trunk ganglia

Cervical cardiac nerves

Gray ramus communicans

Brachial plexus

White ramus communicans

Upper thoracic sympathetic trunk ganglia

Thoracic sympathetic cardiac and aortic nerves

Intercostal nerves

Lower thoracic sympathetic trunk ganglia

Thoracic splanchnic nerves

Upper lumbar sympathetic trunk ganglia

Fibers direct to vessels

Lower lumbar and sacral sympathetic trunk ganglia

Sympathetic rami to lumbar and sacral plexuses and nerves to lower limb

Sympathetic fibers

—— **preganglionic**

- - - - **postganglionic**

9.55 INNERVATION OF THE LIMBS

Autonomic innervation to the limbs derives from the SNS. Preganglionic sympathetic nerve fibers from the thoracolumbar intermediolateral cell column supply sympathetic chain ganglia. These ganglia send postganglionic noradrenergic nerve fibers through the gray rami communicans into the peripheral nerves to supply vascular smooth muscle (vasomotor fibers), sweat glands (sudomotor fibers), and arrector pili muscles associated with hair follicles (pilomotor fibers). Smooth muscle fibers of blood vessels in the viscera also are supplied with postganglionic sympathetic nerve fibers.

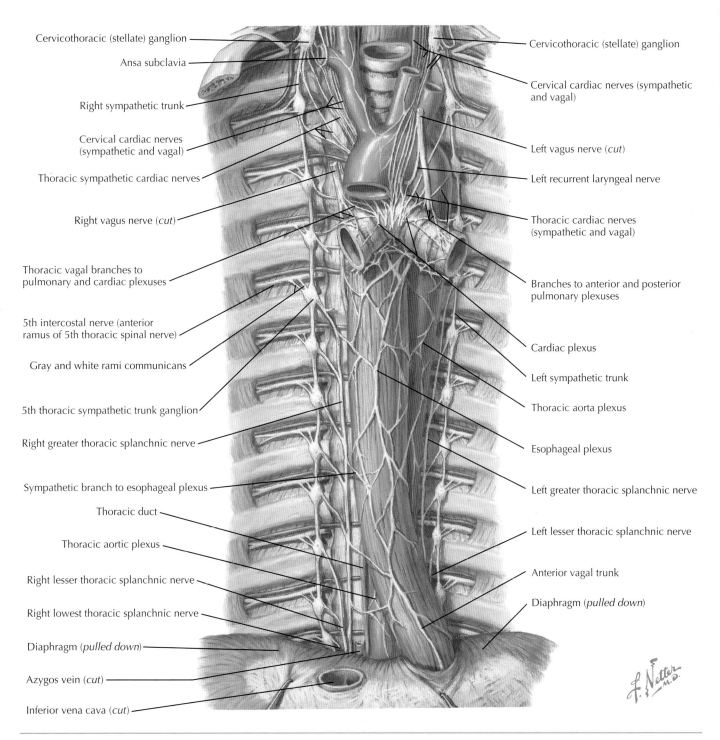

Cervicothoracic (stellate) ganglion

Ansa subclavia

Right sympathetic trunk

Cervical cardiac nerves
(sympathetic and vagal)

Thoracic sympathetic cardiac nerves

Right vagus nerve (cut)

Thoracic vagal branches to
pulmonary and cardiac plexuses

5th intercostal nerve (anterior
ramus of 5th thoracic spinal nerve)

Gray and white rami communicans

5th thoracic sympathetic trunk ganglion

Right greater thoracic splanchnic nerve

Sympathetic branch to esophageal plexus

Thoracic duct

Thoracic aortic plexus

Right lesser thoracic splanchnic nerve

Right lowest thoracic splanchnic nerve

Diaphragm (pulled down)

Azygos vein (cut)

Inferior vena cava (cut)

Cervicothoracic (stellate) ganglion

Cervical cardiac nerves (sympathetic
and vagal)

Left vagus nerve (cut)

Left recurrent laryngeal nerve

Thoracic cardiac nerves
(sympathetic and vagal)

Branches to anterior and posterior
pulmonary plexuses

Cardiac plexus

Left sympathetic trunk

Thoracic aorta plexus

Esophageal plexus

Left greater thoracic splanchnic nerve

Left lesser thoracic splanchnic nerve

Anterior vagal trunk

Diaphragm (pulled down)

9.56 THORACIC SYMPATHETIC CHAIN AND SPLANCHNIC NERVES

The sympathetic chain is a collection of sympathetic ganglia that receive input from the thoracolumbar preganglionic nerve fibers derived from the spinal cord. The ganglia, interconnected by nerve trunks, are located in a paravertebral array from the neck to the coccygeal region. Postganglionic noradrenergic nerve fibers from the sympathetic chain supply effector tissue in the periphery. Some preganglionic nerve fibers do not synapse as they travel through the sympathetic chain. They continue along the splanchnic nerves to synapse in collateral ganglia, which supply noradrenergic innervation to effector tissue in the viscera.

CLINICAL POINT

The sympathetic chain (paravertebral ganglia) extends from the neck to the pelvis, whereas collateral (prevertebral) ganglia are present along the great vessels and distribute to internal target organs. These ganglia are supplied by preganglionic cholinergic fibers from the T1–L2 intermediolateral cell column (lateral horn), the chain ganglia via white rami communicans, and the collateral ganglia via splanchnic nerves. A **spinal cord crush injury above the T1 level** damages the central regulation of the sympathetic preganglionic neurons and the parasympathetic S2–S4 preganglionic neurons. Initially the patient experiences a spinal shock syndrome, with hypotension (worse on standing), loss of sweating, loss of piloerection, paralysis of bladder function (neurogenic bladder), gastric dilation, and paralytic ileus. As the process of spinal cord injury resolves to a permanent state and spinal shock recedes, the autonomic equivalent of spasticity (hyperresponsiveness) may result, accompanied by spikes in blood pressure and a spastic bladder.

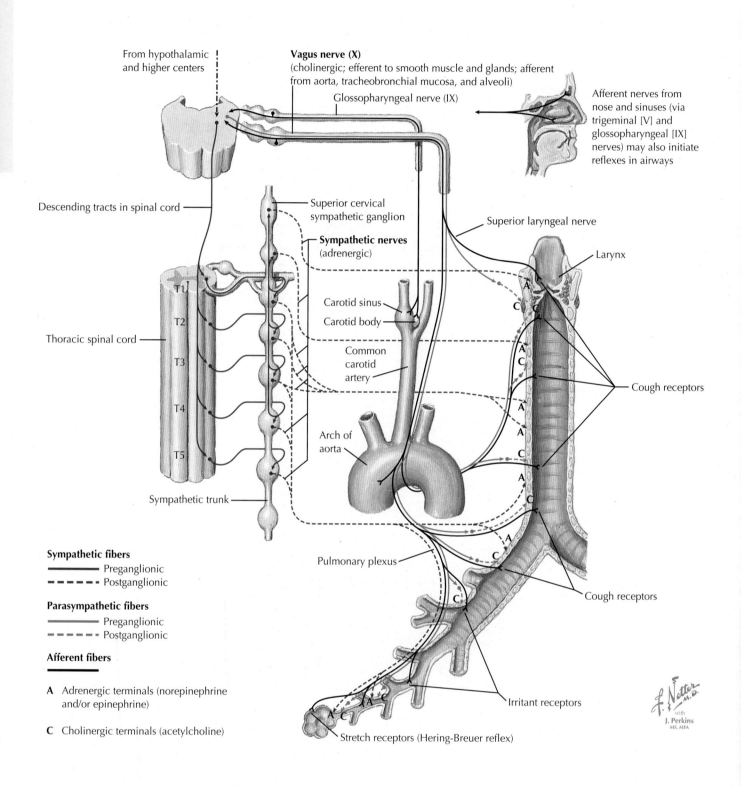

From hypothalamic and higher centers

Vagus nerve (X)
(cholinergic; efferent to smooth muscle and glands; afferent from aorta, tracheobronchial mucosa, and alveoli)

Glossopharyngeal nerve (IX)

Afferent nerves from nose and sinuses (via trigeminal [V] and glossopharyngeal [IX] nerves) may also initiate reflexes in airways

Descending tracts in spinal cord

Superior cervical sympathetic ganglion

Sympathetic nerves (adrenergic)

Superior laryngeal nerve

Larynx

Thoracic spinal cord

T1
T2
T3
T4
T5

Carotid sinus

Carotid body

Common carotid artery

Arch of aorta

Sympathetic trunk

Cough receptors

Sympathetic fibers
——————— Preganglionic
- - - - - - - Postganglionic

Parasympathetic fibers
——————— Preganglionic
- - - - - - - Postganglionic

Afferent fibers

A Adrenergic terminals (norepinephrine and/or epinephrine)

C Cholinergic terminals (acetylcholine)

Pulmonary plexus

Cough receptors

Irritant receptors

Stretch receptors (Hering-Breuer reflex)

9.57 INNERVATION OF THE TRACHEOBRONCHIAL TREE

Both sympathetic (noradrenergic) and parasympathetic (cholinergic) innervation supplies smooth muscle of the tracheobronchial tree. Sympathetics derive from the sympathetic chain, and parasympathetics derive from vagal autonomic input to local intramural ganglia. Sympathetic influences result in bronchodilation and parasympathetic influences result in bronchoconstriction. Some

medications for asthma use a sympathomimetic compound; others use a parasympathetic blocker. Additional neuropeptidergic innervation, some as colocalized or independent autonomic fibers and some as primary afferent fibers, also distributes along the epithelium and among the alveoli, where they can influence innate immune reactivity and the production of inflammatory mediators.

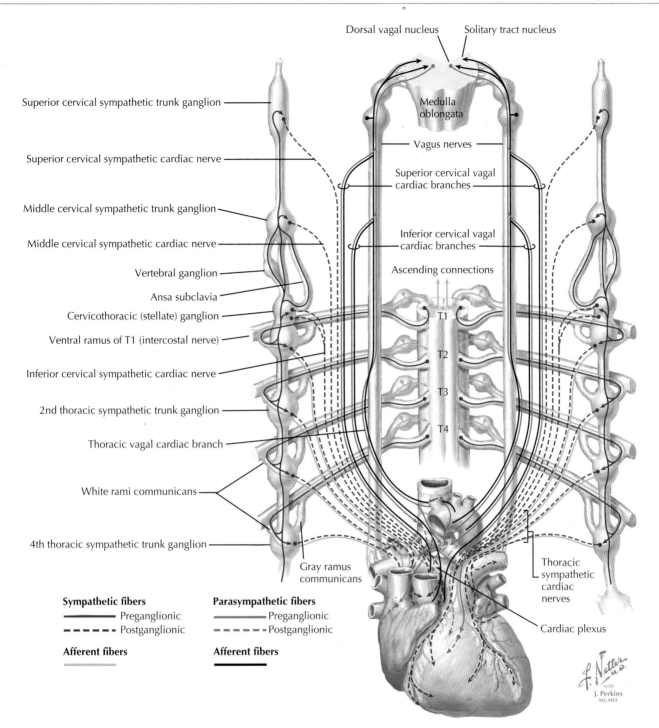

Dorsal vagal nucleus · Solitary tract nucleus

Medulla oblongata

Superior cervical sympathetic trunk ganglion

Superior cervical sympathetic cardiac nerve

Middle cervical sympathetic trunk ganglion

Middle cervical sympathetic cardiac nerve

Vertebral ganglion

Ansa subclavia

Cervicothoracic (stellate) ganglion

Ventral ramus of T1 (intercostal nerve)

Inferior cervical sympathetic cardiac nerve

2nd thoracic sympathetic trunk ganglion

Thoracic vagal cardiac branch

White rami communicans

4th thoracic sympathetic trunk ganglion

Vagus nerves

Superior cervical vagal cardiac branches

Inferior cervical vagal cardiac branches

Ascending connections

T1

T2

T3

T4

Thoracic sympathetic cardiac nerves

Cardiac plexus

Gray ramus communicans

Sympathetic fibers
——————— Preganglionic
– – – – – · Postganglionic

Afferent fibers
———————

Parasympathetic fibers
——————— Preganglionic
– – – – – · Postganglionic

Afferent fibers
———————

9.58 INNERVATION OF THE HEART

Sympathetic noradrenergic nerve fibers (derived from chain ganglia) and parasympathetic cholinergic nerve fibers (derived from cardiac intramural ganglia innervated by the vagus nerve) supply the atria, ventricles, sinoatrial node, and atrioventricular node and bundle. Sympathetic noradrenergic nerve fibers also distribute along the great vessels and the coronary arteries. Sympathetic fibers increase the force and rate of cardiac contraction, increase cardiac output, and dilate the coronary arteries. Parasympathetic fibers decrease the force and rate of cardiac contraction and decrease cardiac output.

CLINICAL POINT
Both sympathetic noradrenergic and parasympathetic cholinergic vagal postganglionic fibers innervate the heart. **Cardiovascular autonomic**

neuropathies sometimes occur in diabetes and other disorders. Vagal nerve damage can result in sustained tachycardia; excessive vagal activity can provoke bradycardia, atrial fibrillation or flutter, ventricular fibrillation, or paroxysmal tachycardia. Loss of sympathetic innervation of the heart results in severe exercise intolerance, painless myocardial ischemia, cardiomyopathy, and possibly sudden death. In studies of cardiac failure, the increased reflex drive on sympathetic cardiac nerves in an attempt to increase cardiac output results in accelerated release of norepinephrine, which produces highly toxic oxidative metabolites (free radicals) that are taken up by the noradrenergic nerve endings (through the high-affinity uptake carriers) and produce a dying-back sympathetic neuropathy, leaving the heart further denervated. In experimental models in dogs, either a norepinephrine-specific uptake inhibitor (desmethylimipramine) or potent antioxidants (vitamins C and E) can prevent this free radical autodestructive process.

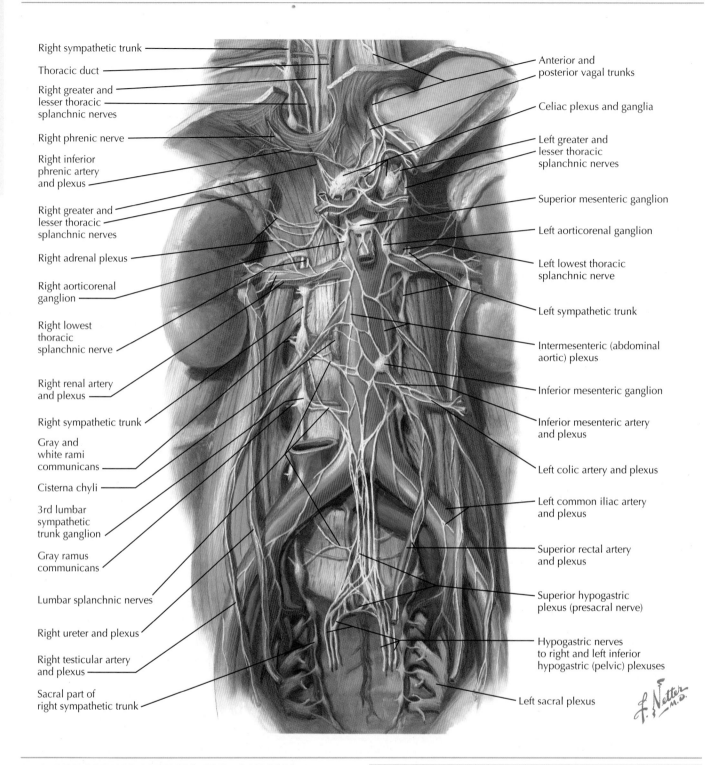

Right sympathetic trunk

Thoracic duct

Right greater and
lesser thoracic
splanchnic nerves

Right phrenic nerve

Right inferior
phrenic artery
and plexus

Right greater and
lesser thoracic
splanchnic nerves

Right adrenal plexus

Right aorticorenal
ganglion

Right lowest
thoracic
splanchnic nerve

Right renal artery
and plexus

Right sympathetic trunk

Gray and
white rami
communicans

Cisterna chyli

3rd lumbar
sympathetic
trunk ganglion

Gray ramus
communicans

Lumbar splanchnic nerves

Right ureter and plexus

Right testicular artery
and plexus

Sacral part of
right sympathetic trunk

Anterior and
posterior vagal trunks

Celiac plexus and ganglia

Left greater and
lesser thoracic
splanchnic nerves

Superior mesenteric ganglion

Left aorticorenal ganglion

Left lowest thoracic
splanchnic nerve

Left sympathetic trunk

Intermesenteric (abdominal
aortic) plexus

Inferior mesenteric ganglion

Inferior mesenteric artery
and plexus

Left colic artery and plexus

Left common iliac artery
and plexus

Superior rectal artery
and plexus

Superior hypogastric
plexus (presacral nerve)

Hypogastric nerves
to right and left inferior
hypogastric (pelvic) plexuses

Left sacral plexus

9.59 ABDOMINAL NERVES AND GANGLIA

Abundant sympathetic nerves are present in the abdomen and pelvis and are associated with innervation of the gastrointestinal and urogenital systems, associated vessels, the peritoneum, and the adrenal gland. The lumbar portion of the sympathetic chain and its branches and the splanchnic nerves and their collateral ganglia (celiac, superior and inferior mesenteric, hepatic, aorticorenal, adrenal, superior hypogastric, and others) innervate smooth muscle, glands, lymphoid tissue, and metabolic cells in the abdomen and pelvis. Most of the collateral ganglia (plexuses) also contain parasympathetic contributions from the vagus nerve and associated ganglia.

CLINICAL POINT

The collateral ganglia (celiac, superior and inferior mesenteric, hepatic, aorticorenal, adrenal, superior hypogastric) and the lumbar sympathetic chain supply sympathetic innervation to the abdomen and pelvis. Parasympathetic vagal fibers and their associated intramural ganglia provide parasympathetic innervation. The importance of this innervation is illustrated by the relatively unusual disorder known as dysautonomic polyneuropathy, which is a postganglionic polyneuropathy of both sympathetic and parasympathetic nerves, most likely the result of autoimmune reactivity. The affected individual develops orthostatic hypotension, unresponsive pupillary light reflexes, paralytic ileus and constipation, bladder dysfunction, and diminished sweating, peripheral vasoconstriction, and piloerection.

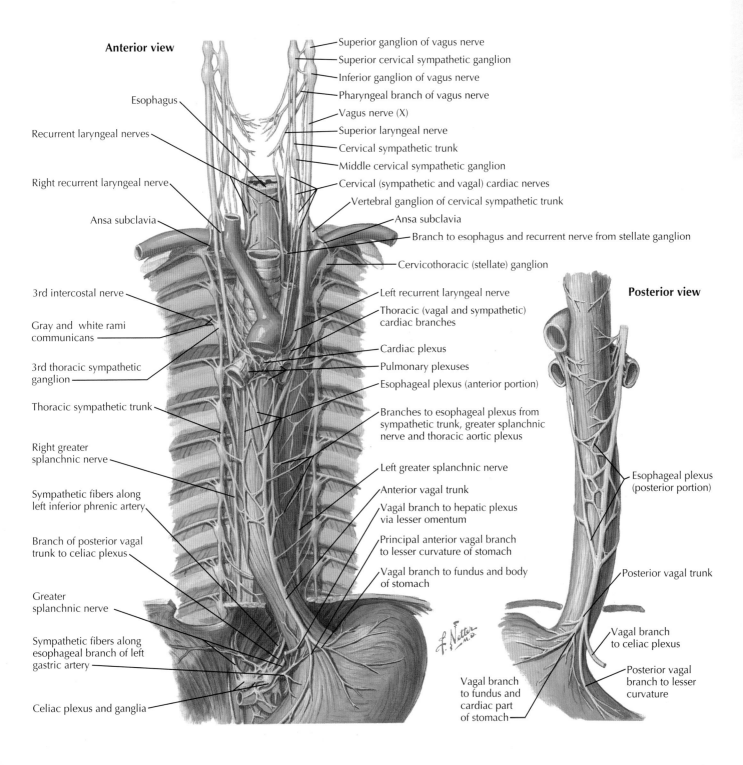

Anterior view

Esophagus

Recurrent laryngeal nerves

Right recurrent laryngeal nerve

Ansa subclavia

3rd intercostal nerve

Gray and white rami communicans

3rd thoracic sympathetic ganglion

Thoracic sympathetic trunk

Right greater splanchnic nerve

Sympathetic fibers along left inferior phrenic artery

Branch of posterior vagal trunk to celiac plexus

Greater splanchnic nerve

Sympathetic fibers along esophageal branch of left gastric artery

Celiac plexus and ganglia

Superior ganglion of vagus nerve

Superior cervical sympathetic ganglion

Inferior ganglion of vagus nerve

Pharyngeal branch of vagus nerve

Vagus nerve (X)

Superior laryngeal nerve

Cervical sympathetic trunk

Middle cervical sympathetic ganglion

Cervical (sympathetic and vagal) cardiac nerves

Vertebral ganglion of cervical sympathetic trunk

Ansa subclavia

Branch to esophagus and recurrent nerve from stellate ganglion

Cervicothoracic (stellate) ganglion

Left recurrent laryngeal nerve

Thoracic (vagal and sympathetic) cardiac branches

Cardiac plexus

Pulmonary plexuses

Esophageal plexus (anterior portion)

Branches to esophageal plexus from sympathetic trunk, greater splanchnic nerve and thoracic aortic plexus

Left greater splanchnic nerve

Anterior vagal trunk

Vagal branch to hepatic plexus via lesser omentum

Principal anterior vagal branch to lesser curvature of stomach

Vagal branch to fundus and body of stomach

Posterior view

Esophageal plexus (posterior portion)

Posterior vagal trunk

Vagal branch to celiac plexus

Posterior vagal branch to lesser curvature

Vagal branch to fundus and cardiac part of stomach

9.60 NERVES OF THE ESOPHAGUS

The sensory stimuli that initiate swallowing derive mainly from CN IX (some also from CNs V and X) and are mediated through nucleus solitarius in the medulla. Food passes through the crico-pharyngeal sphincter at the proximal esophagus; this sphincter is controlled by the vagal nerve fibers derived from the dorsal motor nucleus of CN X. Movement of food through the esophagus is regulated by vagal nerve fibers derived from the dorsal motor nucleus of CN X, which synapse on neurons within the myenteric plexus of the esophagus. This plexus directly controls peristalsis through the esophagus by alternately relaxing and then contracting the muscles of the esophagus. Food then moves into the stomach through the lower esophageal sphincter, which relaxes when nitric oxide and VIP are released from some neurons of the myenteric plexus.

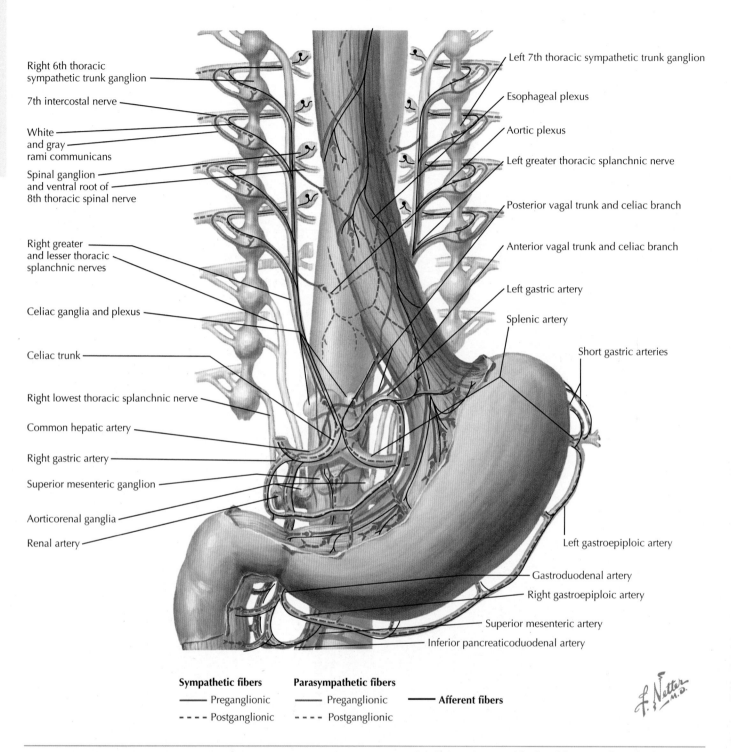

Right 6th thoracic sympathetic trunk ganglion

7th intercostal nerve

White and gray rami communicans

Spinal ganglion and ventral root of 8th thoracic spinal nerve

Right greater and lesser thoracic splanchnic nerves

Celiac ganglia and plexus

Celiac trunk

Right lowest thoracic splanchnic nerve

Common hepatic artery

Right gastric artery

Superior mesenteric ganglion

Aorticorenal ganglia

Renal artery

Left 7th thoracic sympathetic trunk ganglion

Esophageal plexus

Aortic plexus

Left greater thoracic splanchnic nerve

Posterior vagal trunk and celiac branch

Anterior vagal trunk and celiac branch

Left gastric artery

Splenic artery

Short gastric arteries

Left gastroepiploic artery

Gastroduodenal artery

Right gastroepiploic artery

Superior mesenteric artery

Inferior pancreaticoduodenal artery

Sympathetic fibers	Parasympathetic fibers	
—— Preganglionic	—— Preganglionic	**—— Afferent fibers**
- - - Postganglionic	- - - Postganglionic	

9.61 INNERVATION OF THE STOMACH AND PROXIMAL DUODENUM

The stomach and proximal duodenum receive abundant sympathetic innervation from the celiac and superior mesenteric ganglia and, to a lesser extent, from the thoracic sympathetic trunk ganglia. The celiac and superior mesenteric ganglia receive their preganglionic input from the greater and lesser thoracic splanchnic nerves. Parasympathetic fibers distribute to the stomach and proximal duodenum from the celiac branches of the vagus nerve. Sympathetic fibers decrease peristalsis and secretomotor activities. Parasympathetic fibers increase peristalsis and secretomotor

activity (such as gastrin and hydrochloric acid) and relax associated sphincters.

CLINICAL POINT

Diabetic neuropathy may be accompanied by delayed gastric emptying. The patient may experience nausea and vomiting, premature satiety, and large fluctuations in blood glucose. Weight loss may be noted. Approaches for treatment include parasympathetic agonists that stimulate gastric emptying and dopamine antagonists that remove the dopaminergic inhibition of gastric emptying. Delayed gastric emptying may also be accompanied by dysfunction of esophageal motility, resulting in dysphagia.

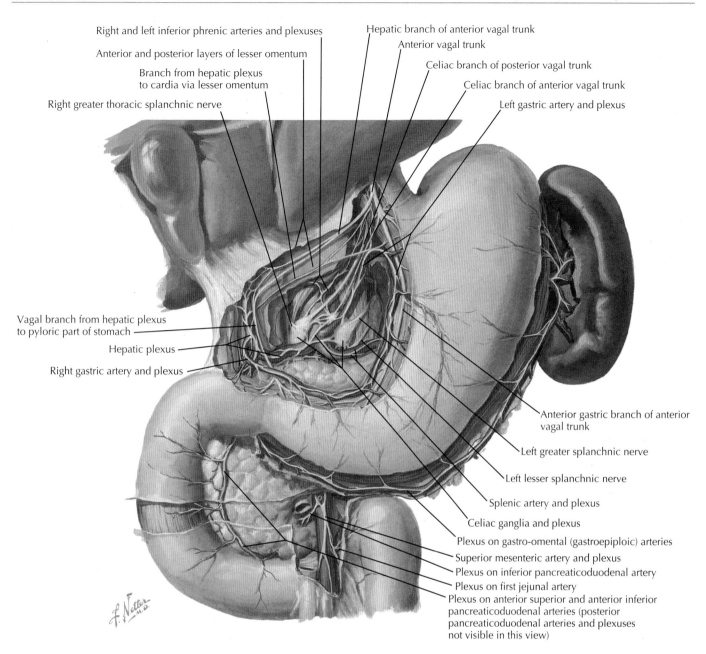

Right and left inferior phrenic arteries and plexuses

Anterior and posterior layers of lesser omentum

Branch from hepatic plexus to cardia via lesser omentum

Right greater thoracic splanchnic nerve

Hepatic branch of anterior vagal trunk

Anterior vagal trunk

Celiac branch of posterior vagal trunk

Celiac branch of anterior vagal trunk

Left gastric artery and plexus

Vagal branch from hepatic plexus to pyloric part of stomach

Hepatic plexus

Right gastric artery and plexus

Anterior gastric branch of anterior vagal trunk

Left greater splanchnic nerve

Left lesser splanchnic nerve

Splenic artery and plexus

Celiac ganglia and plexus

Plexus on gastro-omental (gastroepiploic) arteries

Superior mesenteric artery and plexus

Plexus on inferior pancreaticoduodenal artery

Plexus on first jejunal artery

Plexus on anterior superior and anterior inferior pancreaticoduodenal arteries (posterior pancreaticoduodenal arteries and plexuses not visible in this view)

9.62 NERVES OF THE STOMACH AND DUODENUM

Parasympathetic and sympathetic nerve fibers distribute to the stomach and proximal duodenum through specific splanchnic nerves and branches of the vagus nerve. Sympathetic fibers decrease peristalsis and secretomotor activities. Parasympathetic fibers increase peristalsis and secretomotor activity (such as gastrin and hydrochloric acid) and relax associated sphincters.

CLINICAL POINT

Obesity may occur for a variety of reasons. The stomach expands, neural satiety signals do not provide effective feedback to the brain, and compulsive eating can overcome normal appetitive control mechanisms. In situations in which diet and exercise are ineffective for weight control and when diabetes and other serious comorbidities are life-threatening for a morbidly obese individual, **bariatric surgery** is an option. The Roux-en-Y gastric bypass procedure takes the distal

90% of the stomach, the duodenum, and approximately 20 cm of the proximal jejunum off-line; the digestive tract then consists of the esophagus and a very small proximal stomach pouch that is connected with the remaining jejunum (the off-line jejunum is anastomosed farther downstream). This procedure markedly reduces the stomach's capacity, slows gastric emptying, and produces deliberate partial malabsorption. Long-term data indicate extensive and permanent weight loss in many subjects (more than 70% of needed weight loss) and common reversal of diabetes, hypertension, sleep apnea, and many of the comorbid conditions that accompany morbid obesity. In addition, a striking alteration in the secretion of a variety of gastrointestinal hormones, inflammatory mediators, and other mediators has been noted. Autonomic and somatic neural signals are altered, central setpoints related to appetitive behavior are reset, and changes in morbidity and mortality rates have been observed. The Roux-en-Y procedure is not without risks and complications, and chronic supplementation of nutrients such as calcium, iron, and B vitamins is required. Underlying psychopathology may lead to circumvention of the effectiveness of the procedure.

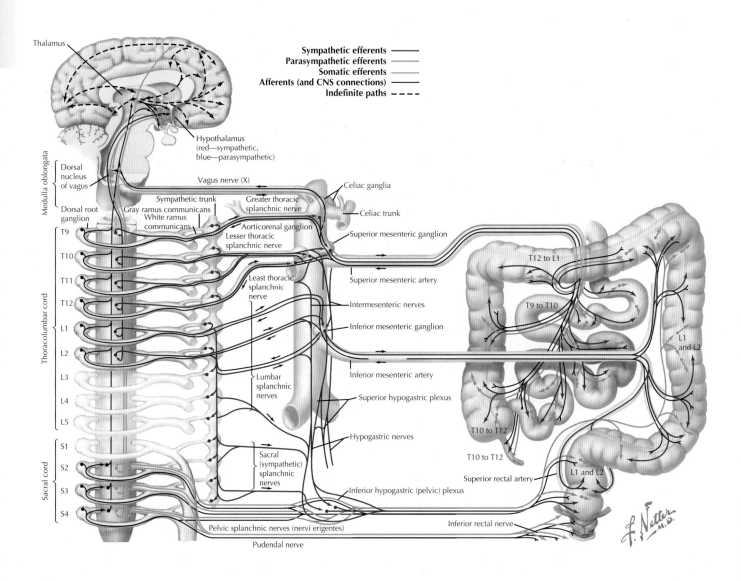

9.63 INNERVATION OF THE SMALL AND LARGE INTESTINES

Autonomic innervation of the small and large intestines is supplied by extrinsic sympathetic and parasympathetic fibers. Sympathetic innervation derives from the T5–L2 intermediolateral cell column of the spinal cord and distributes to collateral ganglia (superior and inferior mesenteric, celiac). Parasympathetic innervation derives from the vagus nerve and from the S2–S4 intermediate gray of the spinal cord; it distributes to intramural ganglia and plexuses via CN X and pelvis splanchnic nerves. Sympathetic nerve fibers generally decrease peristalsis and secretomotor functions (i.e., decreased fluid secretion). Parasympathetic nerve fibers generally increase peristalsis, relax involuntary sphincters, and increase secretomotor activities. The extrinsic innervation of the intestines is integrated with the intrinsic (enteric) innervation. Autonomic gastrointestinal neuropathies such as those seen in diabetes most commonly result in constipation, requiring treatment with pharmacological agents and high-fiber agents. However, diabetic diarrhea also is common and may require treatment to slow secretomotor function.

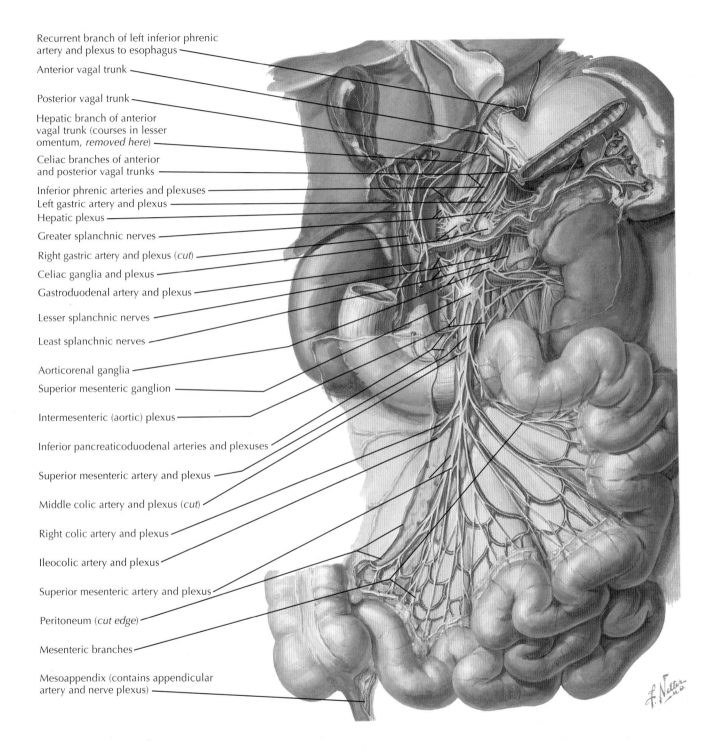

Recurrent branch of left inferior phrenic artery and plexus to esophagus

Anterior vagal trunk

Posterior vagal trunk

Hepatic branch of anterior vagal trunk (courses in lesser omentum, *removed here*)

Celiac branches of anterior and posterior vagal trunks

Inferior phrenic arteries and plexuses

Left gastric artery and plexus

Hepatic plexus

Greater splanchnic nerves

Right gastric artery and plexus (*cut*)

Celiac ganglia and plexus

Gastroduodenal artery and plexus

Lesser splanchnic nerves

Least splanchnic nerves

Aorticorenal ganglia

Superior mesenteric ganglion

Intermesenteric (aortic) plexus

Inferior pancreaticoduodenal arteries and plexuses

Superior mesenteric artery and plexus

Middle colic artery and plexus (*cut*)

Right colic artery and plexus

Ileocolic artery and plexus

Superior mesenteric artery and plexus

Peritoneum (*cut edge*)

Mesenteric branches

Mesoappendix (contains appendicular artery and nerve plexus)

9.64 NERVES OF THE SMALL INTESTINE

This figure shows the anatomy of the extrinsic innervation of the small intestine by the splanchnic and vagal nerves and their associated plexuses.

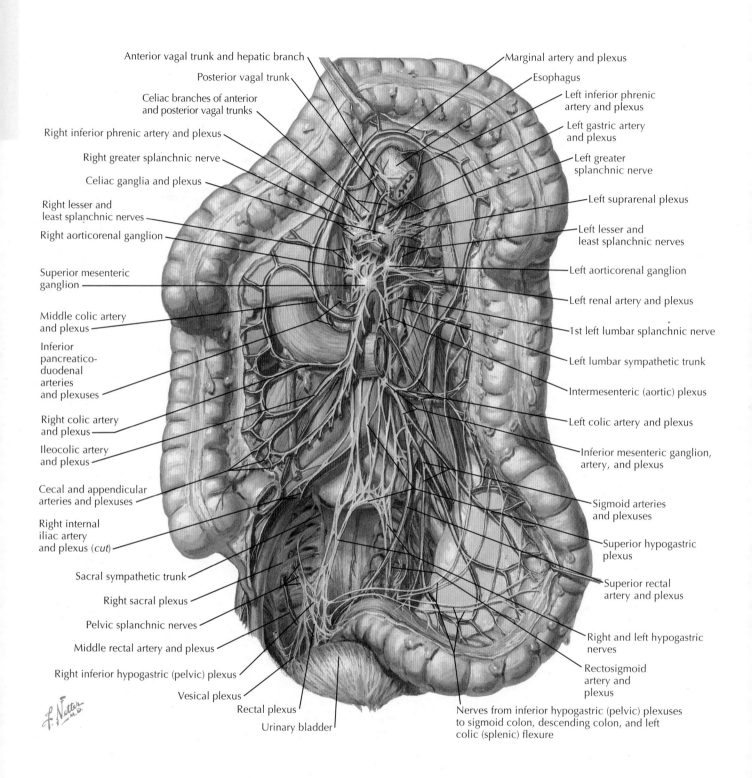

Anterior vagal trunk and hepatic branch

Posterior vagal trunk

Celiac branches of anterior
and posterior vagal trunks

Right inferior phrenic artery and plexus

Right greater splanchnic nerve

Celiac ganglia and plexus

Right lesser and
least splanchnic nerves

Right aorticorenal ganglion

Superior mesenteric
ganglion

Middle colic artery
and plexus

Inferior
pancreatico-
duodenal
arteries
and plexuses

Right colic artery
and plexus

Ileocolic artery
and plexus

Cecal and appendicular
arteries and plexuses

Right internal
iliac artery
and plexus (cut)

Sacral sympathetic trunk

Right sacral plexus

Pelvic splanchnic nerves

Middle rectal artery and plexus

Right inferior hypogastric (pelvic) plexus

Vesical plexus

Rectal plexus

Urinary bladder

Marginal artery and plexus

Esophagus

Left inferior phrenic
artery and plexus

Left gastric artery
and plexus

Left greater
splanchnic nerve

Left suprarenal plexus

Left lesser and
least splanchnic nerves

Left aorticorenal ganglion

Left renal artery and plexus

1st left lumbar splanchnic nerve

Left lumbar sympathetic trunk

Intermesenteric (aortic) plexus

Left colic artery and plexus

Inferior mesenteric ganglion,
artery, and plexus

Sigmoid arteries
and plexuses

Superior hypogastric
plexus

Superior rectal
artery and plexus

Right and left hypogastric
nerves

Rectosigmoid
artery and
plexus

Nerves from inferior hypogastric (pelvic) plexuses
to sigmoid colon, descending colon, and left
colic (splenic) flexure

9.65 NERVES OF THE LARGE INTESTINE

This figure shows the anatomy of the extrinsic innervation of the
large intestine by the splanchnic and vagal nerves and their associated plexuses.

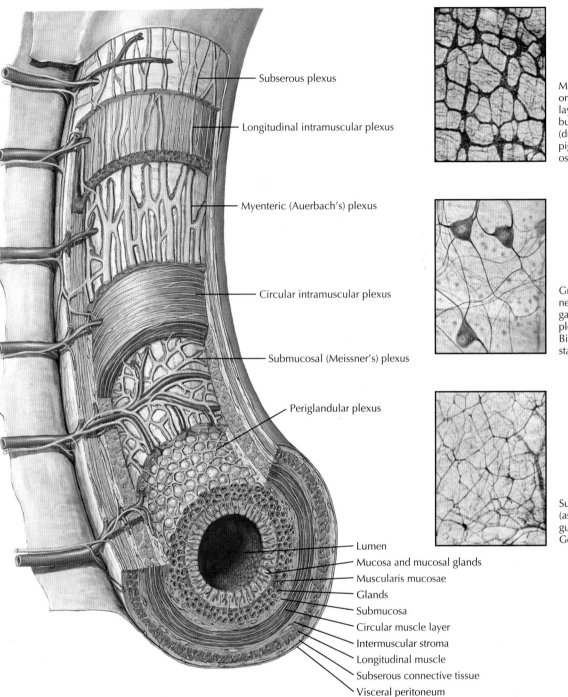

Subserous plexus

Longitudinal intramuscular plexus

Myenteric (Auerbach's) plexus

Circular intramuscular plexus

Submucosal (Meissner's) plexus

Periglandular plexus

Lumen
Mucosa and mucosal glands
Muscularis mucosae
Glands
Submucosa
Circular muscle layer
Intermuscular stroma
Longitudinal muscle
Subserous connective tissue
Visceral peritoneum

Myenteric plexus lying on longitudinal muscular layer. Fine secondary bundles crossing meshes (duodenum of guinea pig, Champy-Coujard, osmic stain, × 20)

Group of multipolar neurons, type II, in ganglion of myenteric plexus (ileum of cat, Bielschowsky, silver stain, × 200)

Submucous plexus (ascending colon of guinea pig, stained by Golgi impregnation, × 20)

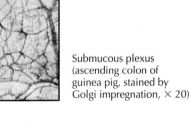

9.66 ENTERIC NERVOUS SYSTEM: LONGITUDINAL VIEW

The enteric nervous system is made up of approximately 100 million neurons arranged principally in submucosal (Meissner's) and myenteric (Auerbach's) plexuses; it provides intrinsic innervation to the small and large intestines. Neurons of this system interconnect with one another and with neuronal processes of the autonomic nervous system, although most neuronal components of this network are free of autonomic influence. The enteric plexuses regulate peristaltic responses (which can proceed without extrinsic innervation), pacemaker activity, and other automated secretory processes. The myenteric plexus controls primarily motility;

the submucosal plexus controls primarily fluid secretion and absorption. More than 20 distinct neurotransmitters have been identified in enteric neurons (e.g., ACh, substance P, serotonin, VIP, somatostatin, nitric oxide). ACh and substance P are excitatory to smooth muscle, whereas VIP and nitric oxide are inhibitory. Extrinsic autonomic innervation helps to coordinate these enteric plexuses and circuits; optimal functioning of the gastrointestinal tract requires coordinated interactions among endocrine, paracrine, and neurocrine mediators. Disturbance of extrinsic innervation by a neuropathy can result in disorders of motility such as constipation or diarrhea.

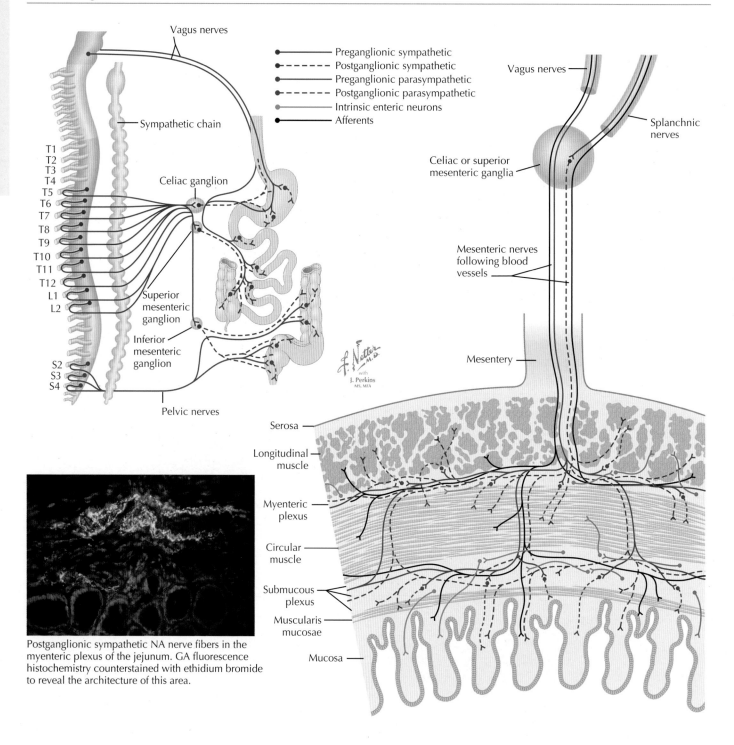

Postganglionic sympathetic NA nerve fibers in the myenteric plexus of the jejunum. GA fluorescence histochemistry counterstained with ethidium bromide to reveal the architecture of this area.

9.67 ENTERIC NERVOUS SYSTEM: CROSS-SECTIONAL VIEW

In the myenteric and the submucosal plexuses, some neurons are innervated by sympathetic nerve fibers from the sympathetic chain and collateral ganglia and by vagal or pelvic splanchnic parasympathetic nerve fibers; other neurons are independent of autonomic regulation. Autonomic postganglionic nerve fibers and intrinsic neuropeptidergic nerve fibers also supply macrophages, T lymphocytes, plasma cells, and other cells of the immune system with innervation. This provides a regulatory network that modulates the host defenses of the gastrointestinal tract and the immune reactivity of gut-associated lymphoid tissue.

CLINICAL POINT

The intrinsic neuronal clusters that form the enteric nervous system derive from the neural crest. If these neural crest derivatives fail to migrate properly into the colon, as occurs in a developmental abnormality called Hirschsprung's disease (chronic megacolon), the intrinsic circuitry for peristalsis, pacemaker activity, and other gut functions cannot occur. The vagus nerve and sympathetic innervation from the pelvic splanchnic nerves cannot coordinate the activity of the colon in the absence of its enteric components. Therefore, megacolon (intestinal obstruction) results from absent peristalsis and loss of smooth muscle tone of the colon. Distention and hypertrophy of the colon may ensue.

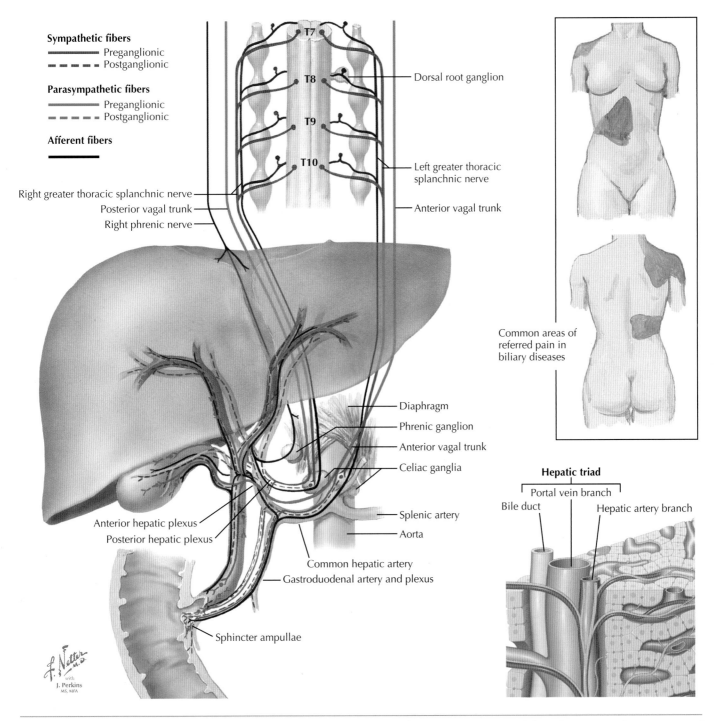

Sympathetic fibers
—————— Preganglionic
– – – – – Postganglionic

Parasympathetic fibers
—————— Preganglionic
– – – – – Postganglionic

Afferent fibers
——————

T7
T8
T9
T10

Dorsal root ganglion

Left greater thoracic splanchnic nerve

Right greater thoracic splanchnic nerve
Posterior vagal trunk
Right phrenic nerve

Anterior vagal trunk

Diaphragm
Phrenic ganglion
Anterior vagal trunk
Celiac ganglia

Anterior hepatic plexus
Posterior hepatic plexus

Splenic artery
Aorta

Common hepatic artery
Gastroduodenal artery and plexus

Sphincter ampullae

Common areas of referred pain in biliary diseases

Hepatic triad
Portal vein branch
Bile duct
Hepatic artery branch

9.68 AUTONOMIC INNERVATION OF THE LIVER AND BILIARY TRACT

Sympathetic nerve fibers to the liver derive from T7–T10 of the spinal cord and distribute mainly via the celiac ganglion and its associated plexus. Parasympathetic nerve fibers to the liver derive from the abdominal vagus nerve. Postganglionic noradrenergic sympathetic nerve fibers end directly adjacent to hepatocytes; norepinephrine released from these nerve fibers initiates glycogenolysis and hyperglycemia for fight-or-flight responses and induces gluconeogenesis. Autonomic innervation helps to regulate vascular, secretory, and phagocytic processes in the liver. The gallbladder, especially the sphincter ampullae and the sphincter of the choledochal duct, is also supplied by autonomic nerve fibers. The sympathetic nerve fibers cause contraction of the sphincters and dilation of the gallbladder; the parasympathetic nerve fibers cause opening of the sphincters and contraction of the gallbladder.

CLINICAL POINT

Postganglionic sympathetic noradrenergic nerves to the liver can trigger glycogenolysis and gluconeogenesis, providing glucose as fuel for sympathetic arousal. Chronic activation of the SNS, with increased secretion of norepinephrine, can drive glucose levels, provoke insulin secretion, increase free radical formation, increase platelet aggregation, and initiate other actions that are beneficial in an emergency but problematic when present chronically. These connections may be one route by which chronic stressors intersect with metabolic syndrome, diminish antiviral and antitumor immunity, and increase the risk for a variety of chronic diseases, including hypertension, cardiovascular disease and stroke, some cancers, and type II diabetes. Autonomic neuropathy to the gallbladder can result in atonic smooth muscle responses, with the development of gallstones (especially in individuals with hypercholesterolemia) and diarrhea.

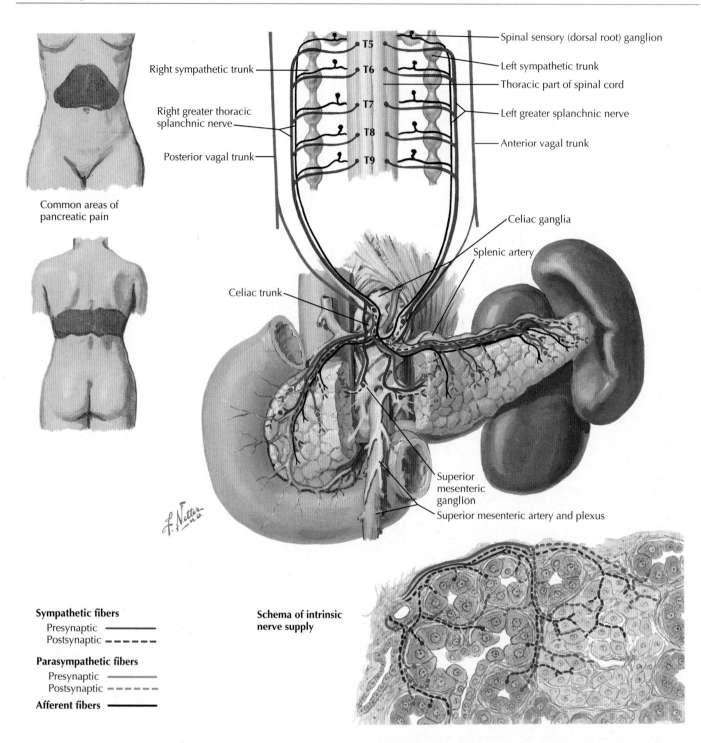

Common areas of pancreatic pain

Right sympathetic trunk

Right greater thoracic splanchnic nerve

Posterior vagal trunk

T5
T6
T7
T8
T9

Spinal sensory (dorsal root) ganglion

Left sympathetic trunk

Thoracic part of spinal cord

Left greater splanchnic nerve

Anterior vagal trunk

Celiac ganglia

Splenic artery

Celiac trunk

Superior mesenteric ganglion

Superior mesenteric artery and plexus

Sympathetic fibers
Presynaptic ———
Postsynaptic – – – –

Parasympathetic fibers
Presynaptic ———
Postsynaptic – – – –

Afferent fibers ———

Schema of intrinsic nerve supply

9.69 AUTONOMIC INNERVATION OF THE PANCREAS

Secretion by the pancreas is under both neural and endocrine control. Pancreatic exocrine glands and endocrine cells (islets of Langerhans) are innervated by parasympathetic subdiaphragmatic vagal nerve fibers via intramural ganglia and by sympathetic nerve fibers derived from T5–T9 intermediolateral spinal cord gray via the celiac ganglion. Although only a small anatomical component of the pancreas (1%), the endocrine pancreas secretes several vital endocrine products, including glucagon (a fuel-mobilizing hormone), insulin (a fuel-storing hormone), somatostatin (a suppressor of glucagons and insulin secretion),

and pancreatic polypeptide (an inhibitor of the secretion of enzymes and HCO_3^-, the bicarbonate ion, by the exocrine pancreas). ACh supplied by the parasympathetic fibers stimulates insulin secretion by islet cells, and norepinephrine secretion by the sympathetic fibers (as well as epinephrine by the adrenal medulla) inhibits insulin secretion from the islet cells. ACh stimulates a variety of hormones. Secretin acts on ductal cells of the pancreas to stimulate secretion of fluid with a high HCO_3^- content. Cholecystokinin is secreted by I cells in response to fats in the duodenum and upper jejunum and acts on acinar cells to stimulate the secretion of enzymes.

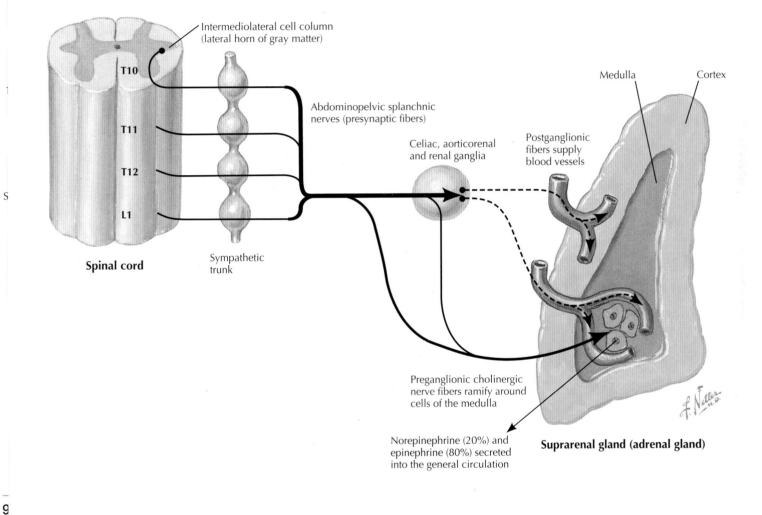

Intermediolateral cell column
(lateral horn of gray matter)

T10

Abdominopelvic splanchnic
nerves (presynaptic fibers)

T11

T12

L1

Spinal cord

Sympathetic
trunk

Celiac, aorticorenal
and renal ganglia

Medulla   Cortex

Postganglionic
fibers supply
blood vessels

Preganglionic cholinergic
nerve fibers ramify around
cells of the medulla

Norepinephrine (20%) and
epinephrine (80%) secreted
into the general circulation

Suprarenal gland (adrenal gland)

9.70 SCHEMATIC OF INNERVATION OF THE ADRENAL GLAND

Sympathetic preganglionic nerve fibers from neurons in the T10–L1 intermediolateral cell column pass through the sympathetic chain, travel in splanchnic nerves, and directly innervate adrenal medullary chromaffin cells. These chromaffin cells are of neural crest origin and function as sympathetic ganglion cells.

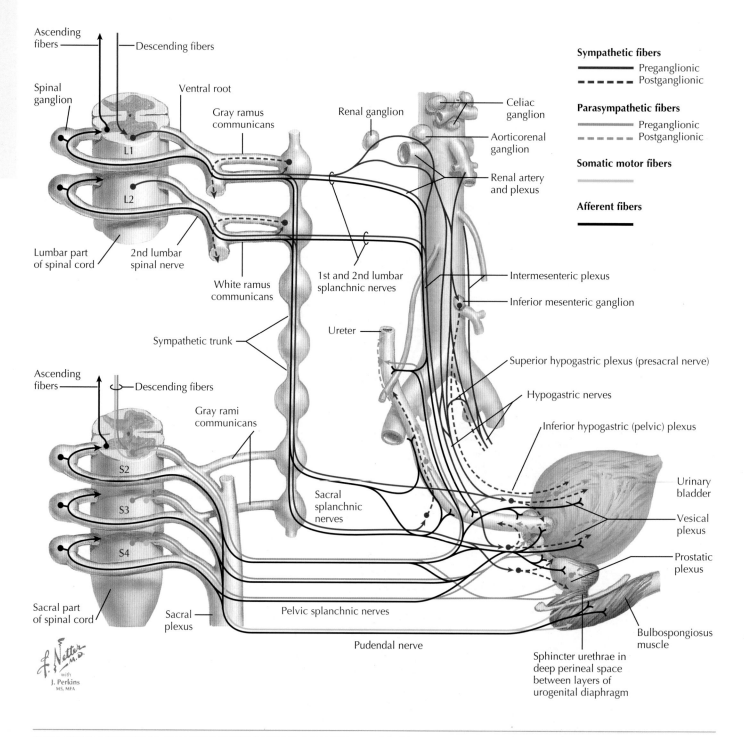

Ascending fibers

Descending fibers

Spinal ganglion

Ventral root

Gray ramus communicans

Renal ganglion

Celiac ganglion

Aorticorenal ganglion

Renal artery and plexus

L1

L2

Lumbar part of spinal cord

2nd lumbar spinal nerve

White ramus communicans

1st and 2nd lumbar splanchnic nerves

Intermesenteric plexus

Inferior mesenteric ganglion

Sympathetic trunk

Ureter

Superior hypogastric plexus (presacral nerve)

Ascending fibers

Descending fibers

Gray rami communicans

Hypogastric nerves

Inferior hypogastric (pelvic) plexus

S2

S3

S4

Urinary bladder

Vesical plexus

Prostatic plexus

Sacral splanchnic nerves

Sacral part of spinal cord

Sacral plexus

Pelvic splanchnic nerves

Pudendal nerve

Bulbospongiosus muscle

Sphincter urethrae in deep perineal space between layers of urogenital diaphragm

Sympathetic fibers
—— Preganglionic
- - - - Postganglionic

Parasympathetic fibers
—— Preganglionic
- - - - Postganglionic

Somatic motor fibers

Afferent fibers

f. Netter M.D.

with
J. Perkins
MS, MFA

9.75 INNERVATION OF THE URINARY BLADDER AND LOWER URETER

The sympathetic innervation of the bladder and lower ureter derives mainly from the L1–L2 preganglionic neurons in the spinal cord and travels through sacral splanchnic nerves to the hypogastric plexus. Parasympathetic innervation derives from the S2–S4 intermediate gray of the spinal cord and distributes to intramural ganglia in the wall of the bladder via pelvic splanchnic nerves. Sympathetic nerve fibers relax the detrusor muscle and contract the trigone and the internal sphincter. Parasympathetic nerve fibers contract the detrusor muscle and relax the trigone and the internal sphincter, thus stimulating emptying of the

bladder. Sensory nerves also are present in the bladder; when the bladder is stretched because it is full, these nerves can initiate the sensation of the need to empty the bladder.

CLINICAL POINT

Parasympathetic nerve damage, particularly in diabetic neuropathy, results in initial problems of incomplete emptying of the bladder, dribbling, and urinary stasis sufficient to increase the likelihood of infection. Later in the course of parasympathetic damage, a flaccid bladder with incomplete emptying and incontinence can occur. Sensory neuropathy also can result in an enlarged bladder caused by incomplete emptying because of the inability of the patient to sense fullness and by the decreased sense of urgency for urination.

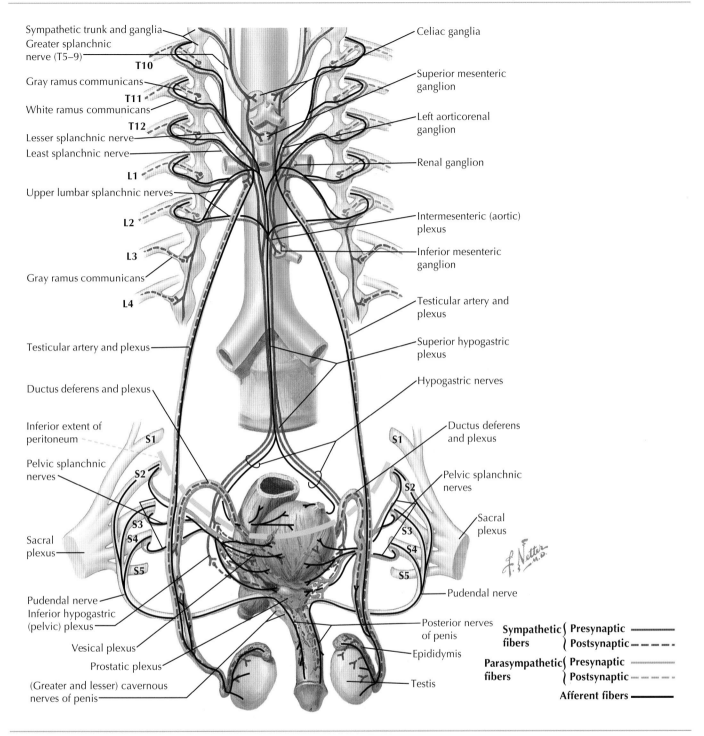

Sympathetic trunk and ganglia
Greater splanchnic nerve (T5–9)

T10

Gray ramus communicans

T11

White ramus communicans

T12

Lesser splanchnic nerve
Least splanchnic nerve

L1

Upper lumbar splanchnic nerves

L2

L3

Gray ramus communicans

L4

Testicular artery and plexus

Ductus deferens and plexus

Inferior extent of peritoneum   **S1**

Pelvic splanchnic nerves   **S2**

S3
S4

Sacral plexus   **S5**

Pudendal nerve
Inferior hypogastric (pelvic) plexus

Vesical plexus

Prostatic plexus

(Greater and lesser) cavernous nerves of penis

Celiac ganglia

Superior mesenteric ganglion

Left aorticorenal ganglion

Renal ganglion

Intermesenteric (aortic) plexus

Inferior mesenteric ganglion

Testicular artery and plexus

Superior hypogastric plexus

Hypogastric nerves

Ductus deferens and plexus   **S1**

Pelvic splanchnic nerves   **S2**

Sacral plexus   **S3**

S4

S5

Pudendal nerve

Posterior nerves of penis

Epididymis

Testis

Sympathetic fibers	Presynaptic ——— Postsynaptic -----
Parasympathetic fibers	Presynaptic ········· Postsynaptic -----
	Afferent fibers ———

9.76 INNERVATION OF THE MALE REPRODUCTIVE ORGANS

Sympathetic innervation to the male reproductive organs derives from T10–L2 intermediolateral cell column neurons and reaches the hypogastric plexus via thoracic and upper lumbar splanchnic nerves. Parasympathetic innervation derives from the S2–S4 intermediate gray of the spinal cord and travels to the inferior hypogastric plexus via pelvic splanchnic nerves. Sympathetic nerve fibers cause contraction of the vas deferens and prostatic capsule and contract the sphincter to the bladder, which prevents retrograde ejaculation. Sympathetic nerve fibers also contribute to vascular responses in the penile corpora cavernosa that are related to erection; beta-receptor blockade can result in erectile dysfunction. Parasympathetic nerve fibers regulate the vascular dilation that initiates and maintains penile erection. Sympathetic and parasympathetic nerve fibers must work together to optimize sexual and reproductive function.

CLINICAL POINT

Parasympathetic nerve damage may lead to autonomic erectile dysfunction. Some individuals taking beta blockers might have similar responses. However, erectile function also depends extensively on psychological, perceptive, and sensory factors in addition to the need for coordinated autonomic function. Pharmacological compounds that enhance erectile function influence vascular responses through the production of nitric oxide to promote erection; these drugs may interact adversely with alpha blockers used to treat benign prostatic hypertrophy and other conditions, resulting in hypotensive responses that are potentially fatal.

Nuclear cell columns   **Laminae of Rexed**

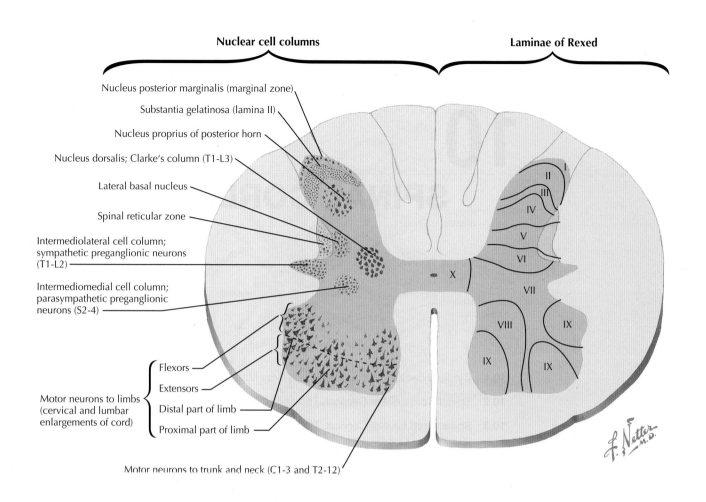

Nucleus posterior marginalis (marginal zone)

Substantia gelatinosa (lamina II)

Nucleus proprius of posterior horn

Nucleus dorsalis; Clarke's column (T1–L3)

Lateral basal nucleus

Spinal reticular zone

Intermediolateral cell column; sympathetic preganglionic neurons (T1–L2)

Intermediomedial cell column; parasympathetic preganglionic neurons (S2–4)

Motor neurons to limbs (cervical and lumbar enlargements of cord)
- Flexors
- Extensors
- Distal part of limb
- Proximal part of limb

Motor neurons to trunk and neck (C1–3 and T2–12)

10.1 CYTOARCHITECTURE OF THE SPINAL CORD GRAY MATTER

The spinal cord gray matter is located centrally in the interior of the spinal cord in a butterfly pattern. The gray matter is subdivided into three horns: (1) the dorsal horn, a site of major sensory processing; (2) the intermediate gray with a lateral horn, a site where preganglionic sympathetic (thoracolumbar) and parasympathetic (sacral) neurons reside and where interneuronal processing occurs; and (3) the ventral horn, a site where lower motor neurons (LMNs) reside and where converging reflex and descending control of LMNs occurs. Neuronal cell groups appear homogeneous in some regions of gray matter, intermixed with a presence of some discrete nuclei (e.g., Clarke's nucleus, substantia gelatinosa). Laminae of Rexed, an alternative system of cytoarchitectural classification established in the 1950s, subdivides the spinal cord gray matter into 10 laminae. This system is used extensively for the dorsal horn and the intermediate gray, laminae I–VII, particularly in conjunction with anatomical details of nociceptive processing and for some reflex and cerebellar processing. Although these laminae have distinctive characteristics at each segmental level, they show some similarities across segmental levels. The absolute amount of spinal cord gray is more extensive in the cervical and lumbosacral enlargements of the spinal cord, which correspond to zones associated with limb innervation, than it is in upper cervical, thoracic, and sacral regions.

CLINICAL POINT

Classical descriptions of **secondary sensory processing** in the spinal cord describe neurons of lamina I (marginal zone) and lamina V of the dorsal horn as cells of origin for crossed projections into the spinothalamic/anterolateral system for the processing of pain and temperature sensation (protopathic modalities). Primary sensory large-diameter axons, carrying information about fine discriminative touch, vibratory sensation, and joint position sense (epicritic modalities), enter through the dorsal root entry zone and travel rostrally into the dorsal column system, bypassing synapses in the spinal cord; these axons terminate in their secondary sensory nuclei, gracilis and cuneatus, in the caudal medulla. According to this scheme, pure dorsal column lesions should result in the total loss of epicritic sensation on the ipsilateral side of the body below the level of the lesion. However, such lesions result in diminution of these epicritic sensations or in the inability to discriminate vibratory sensations of different frequencies, but not in the total loss of these modalities. Only with additional damage to the dorsolateral part of the lateral funiculus is profound loss of epicritic sensation observed. This is because additional dorsal horn neurons receive primary sensory input related to epicritic sensation and send ipsilateral projections into the dorsolateral funiculus, providing additional contributions to lemniscal processing of fine discriminative modalities. In addition, some large-diameter primary axons of the epicritic dorsal column system send collaterals into nociceptive processing zones in the spinal cord, where they can alter pain thresholds and dampen nociception. These collaterals are activated by rubbing an area of the body that has just sustained a potentially painful injury and also are a major mechanism of pain control from dorsal column stimulation.

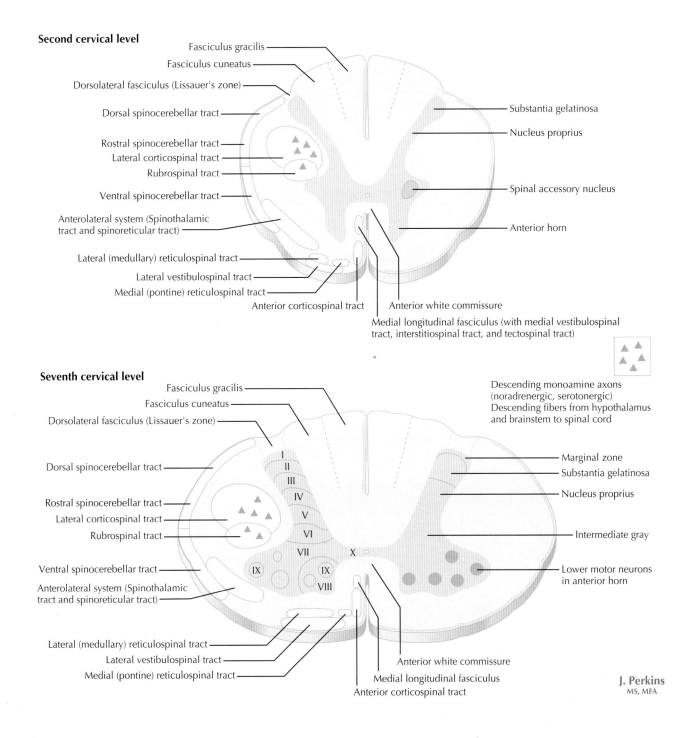

Second cervical level

Fasciculus gracilis
Fasciculus cuneatus
Dorsolateral fasciculus (Lissauer's zone)
Dorsal spinocerebellar tract
Rostral spinocerebellar tract
Lateral corticospinal tract
Rubrospinal tract
Ventral spinocerebellar tract
Anterolateral system (Spinothalamic tract and spinoreticular tract)
Lateral (medullary) reticulospinal tract
Lateral vestibulospinal tract
Medial (pontine) reticulospinal tract
Anterior corticospinal tract

Substantia gelatinosa
Nucleus proprius
Spinal accessory nucleus
Anterior horn
Anterior white commissure
Medial longitudinal fasciculus (with medial vestibulospinal tract, interstitiospinal tract, and tectospinal tract)

Seventh cervical level

Fasciculus gracilis
Fasciculus cuneatus
Dorsolateral fasciculus (Lissauer's zone)
Dorsal spinocerebellar tract
Rostral spinocerebellar tract
Lateral corticospinal tract
Rubrospinal tract
Ventral spinocerebellar tract
Anterolateral system (Spinothalamic tract and spinoreticular tract)
Lateral (medullary) reticulospinal tract
Lateral vestibulospinal tract
Medial (pontine) reticulospinal tract
Anterior corticospinal tract

Descending monoamine axons (noradrenergic, serotonergic) Descending fibers from hypothalamus and brainstem to spinal cord
Marginal zone
Substantia gelatinosa
Nucleus proprius
Intermediate gray
Lower motor neurons in anterior horn
Anterior white commissure
Medial longitudinal fasciculus

I, II, III, IV, V, VI, VII, VIII, IX, IX, X

J. Perkins
MS, MFA

10.2 SPINAL CORD LEVELS: CERVICAL, THORACIC, LUMBAR, AND SACRAL

The organization of the gray matter into laminae of Rexed is retained throughout the spinal cord. The dorsal and ventral horns are larger and wider at levels of the cervical and lumbosacral enlargements. The lateral horn is present from L1 to T2. Some nuclei are found only in circumscribed regions, such as the intermediolateral cell column with preganglionic sympathetic neurons (T1–L2 lateral horn), Clarke's nucleus (C8–L2), and the parasympathetic preganglionic nucleus (S2–S4).

The white matter increases in absolute amount from caudal to rostral. The dorsal columns contain only fasciculus gracilis below T6; fasciculus cuneatus is added laterally above T6. The spinothalamic/spinoreticular anterolateral system increases from caudal to rostral. The descending upper motor neuron (UMN) pathways diminish from rostral to caudal. The lateral corticospinal pathway loses more than half of its axons as they synapse in the cervical segments; this tract then diminishes in size as it extends caudally.

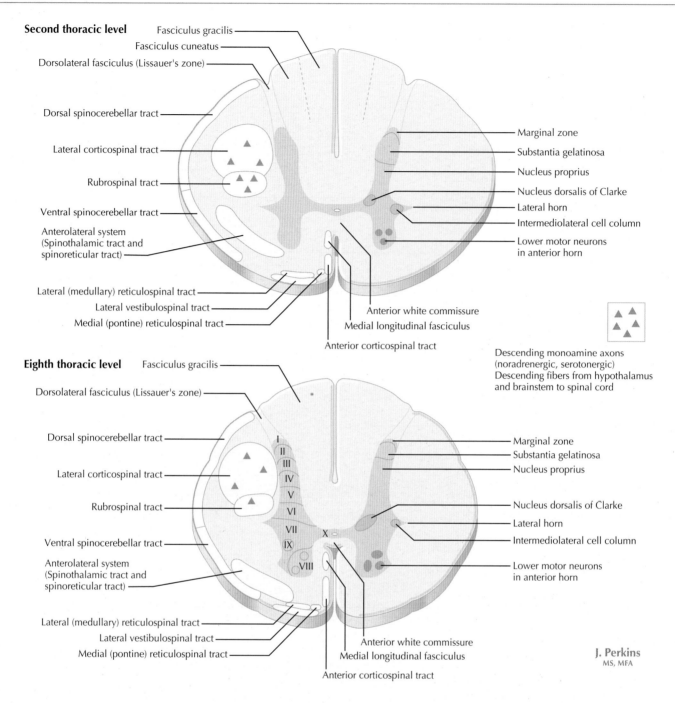

Second thoracic level

Fasciculus gracilis
Fasciculus cuneatus
Dorsolateral fasciculus (Lissauer's zone)
Dorsal spinocerebellar tract
Lateral corticospinal tract
Rubrospinal tract
Ventral spinocerebellar tract
Anterolateral system
(Spinothalamic tract and
spinoreticular tract)
Lateral (medullary) reticulospinal tract
Lateral vestibulospinal tract
Medial (pontine) reticulospinal tract
Anterior corticospinal tract

Marginal zone
Substantia gelatinosa
Nucleus proprius
Nucleus dorsalis of Clarke
Lateral horn
Intermediolateral cell column
Lower motor neurons
in anterior horn
Anterior white commissure
Medial longitudinal fasciculus

Descending monoamine axons
(noradrenergic, serotonergic)
Descending fibers from hypothalamus
and brainstem to spinal cord

Eighth thoracic level

Fasciculus gracilis
Dorsolateral fasciculus (Lissauer's zone)
Dorsal spinocerebellar tract
Lateral corticospinal tract
Rubrospinal tract
Ventral spinocerebellar tract
Anterolateral system
(Spinothalamic tract and
spinoreticular tract)
Lateral (medullary) reticulospinal tract
Lateral vestibulospinal tract
Medial (pontine) reticulospinal tract
Anterior corticospinal tract

Marginal zone
Substantia gelatinosa
Nucleus proprius
Nucleus dorsalis of Clarke
Lateral horn
Intermediolateral cell column
Lower motor neurons
in anterior horn
Anterior white commissure
Medial longitudinal fasciculus

J. Perkins
MS, MFA

10.3 SPINAL CORD LEVELS: CERVICAL, THORACIC, LUMBAR, AND SACRAL (CONTINUED)

CLINICAL POINT

Damage to the lateral funiculus of the cervical spinal cord caused by demyelination, trauma, ischemia, or other causes can lead to disruption of (1) the descending lateral corticospinal tract and rubrospinal tract, resulting in ipsilateral spastic (long-term result) hemiplegia below the level of the lesion, and (2) the descending axons from the hypothalamus to the preganglionic sympathetic neurons in the intermediolateral cell column at the T1 and T2 segments of the cord. These preganglionic neurons supply the superior cervical ganglion, which provides postganglionic noradrenergic sympathetic innervation to the ipsilateral head. Disruption of these descending axons in the lateral

funiculus or at any point distal in the sympathetic pathway can result in Horner's syndrome, which consists of ipsilateral ptosis (because of effects on the superior tarsal muscle), miosis (because of effects on the pupillary dilator muscle), and anhidrosis (less sweat gland activity). Trauma that damages one entire side of the spinal cord at the cervical level produces the same symptoms (ipsilateral spastic paralysis with brisk reflexes and ipsilateral Horner's syndrome) and also causes (1) flaccid paralysis of ipsilateral muscles innervated by LMNs damaged by the trauma, (2) loss of epicritic sensation (fine discriminative touch, vibratory sensation, joint position sense) ipsilaterally below the level of the trauma because of damage to the dorsal column and dorsolateral funiculus axons, and (3) loss of pain and temperature sensation contralaterally below the level of the lesion because of damage to the anterolateral system (spinothalamic/spinoreticular system). This collection of neurological deficits resulting from a hemisection lesion to the spinal cord is called a **Brown-Séquard lesion**.

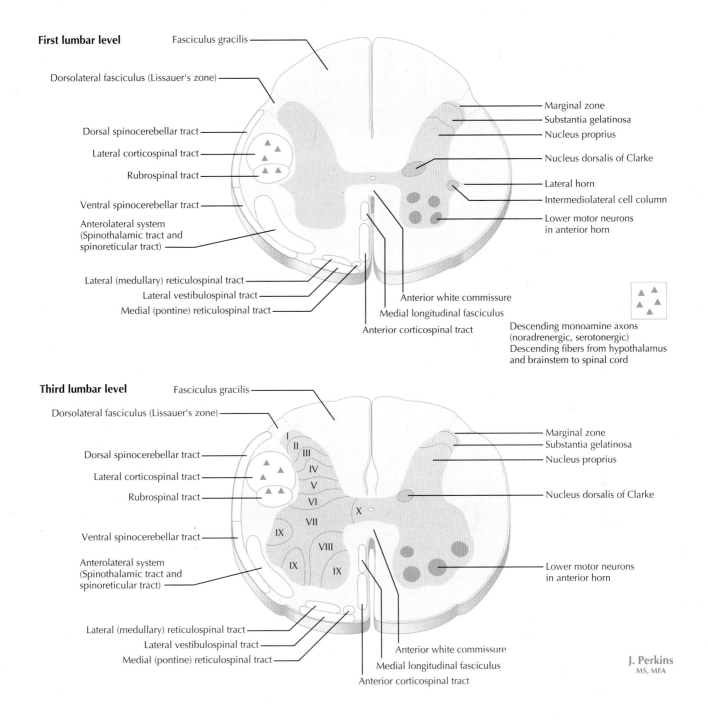

First lumbar level

Fasciculus gracilis

Dorsolateral fasciculus (Lissauer's zone)

Dorsal spinocerebellar tract

Lateral corticospinal tract

Rubrospinal tract

Ventral spinocerebellar tract

Anterolateral system
(Spinothalamic tract and
spinoreticular tract)

Lateral (medullary) reticulospinal tract

Lateral vestibulospinal tract

Medial (pontine) reticulospinal tract

Marginal zone

Substantia gelatinosa

Nucleus proprius

Nucleus dorsalis of Clarke

Lateral horn

Intermediolateral cell column

Lower motor neurons
in anterior horn

Anterior white commissure

Medial longitudinal fasciculus

Anterior corticospinal tract

Descending monoamine axons
(noradrenergic, serotonergic)
Descending fibers from hypothalamus
and brainstem to spinal cord

Third lumbar level

Fasciculus gracilis

Dorsolateral fasciculus (Lissauer's zone)

Dorsal spinocerebellar tract

Lateral corticospinal tract

Rubrospinal tract

Ventral spinocerebellar tract

Anterolateral system
(Spinothalamic tract and
spinoreticular tract)

Lateral (medullary) reticulospinal tract

Lateral vestibulospinal tract

Medial (pontine) reticulospinal tract

Marginal zone

Substantia gelatinosa

Nucleus proprius

Nucleus dorsalis of Clarke

Lower motor neurons
in anterior horn

Anterior white commissure

Medial longitudinal fasciculus

Anterior corticospinal tract

J. Perkins
MS, MFA

10.4 SPINAL CORD LEVELS: CERVICAL, THORACIC, LUMBAR, AND SACRAL (CONTINUED)

CLINICAL POINT

The central canal of the spinal cord is ordinarily a closed remnant of former neural tube development and in the adult does not convey or produce cerebrospinal fluid. However, a developmental defect may result in the formation of a syrinx in the central canal region of the spinal cord, either alone or in the presence of an obstruction of the foramen magnum (with Arnold-Chiari malformation). This condition, called **syringomyelia,** occurs mainly at a lower cervical or a thoracic level. The distinguishing feature is destruction of the axons in the anterior white commissure, resulting in a dissociated sensory loss of pain and temperature sensation at the levels of the syrinx, with preservation of epicritic sensation (dorsal columns and the dorsolateral funiculus are usually preserved). If the syrinx extends laterally, it most likely will involve adjacent LMNs; this manifests as segmental weakness and muscle atrophy. Larger lesions may extend into the lateral funiculus and damage the descending UMN systems (the corticospinal and rubrospinal tracts), causing ipsilateral spastic paresis below the level of the lesion. Syringomyelia is sometimes accompanied by kyphoscoliosis and pain in the region of the neck and arms. The syrinx may extend to the brainstem (**syringobulbia**) and produce damage to lower brainstem structures.

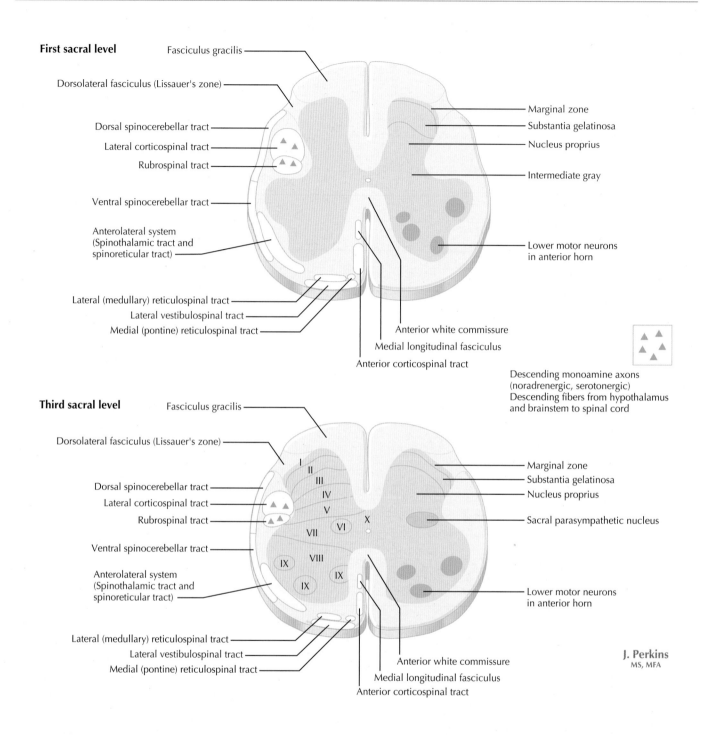

First sacral level

Fasciculus gracilis

Dorsolateral fasciculus (Lissauer's zone)

Dorsal spinocerebellar tract

Lateral corticospinal tract

Rubrospinal tract

Ventral spinocerebellar tract

Anterolateral system (Spinothalamic tract and spinoreticular tract)

Lateral (medullary) reticulospinal tract

Lateral vestibulospinal tract

Medial (pontine) reticulospinal tract

Marginal zone

Substantia gelatinosa

Nucleus proprius

Intermediate gray

Lower motor neurons in anterior horn

Anterior white commissure

Medial longitudinal fasciculus

Anterior corticospinal tract

Descending monoamine axons (noradrenergic, serotonergic) Descending fibers from hypothalamus and brainstem to spinal cord

Third sacral level

Fasciculus gracilis

Dorsolateral fasciculus (Lissauer's zone)

Dorsal spinocerebellar tract

Lateral corticospinal tract

Rubrospinal tract

Ventral spinocerebellar tract

Anterolateral system (Spinothalamic tract and spinoreticular tract)

Lateral (medullary) reticulospinal tract

Lateral vestibulospinal tract

Medial (pontine) reticulospinal tract

Marginal zone

Substantia gelatinosa

Nucleus proprius

Sacral parasympathetic nucleus

Lower motor neurons in anterior horn

Anterior white commissure

Medial longitudinal fasciculus

Anterior corticospinal tract

J. Perkins
MS, MFA

10.5 SPINAL CORD LEVELS: CERVICAL, THORACIC, LUMBAR, AND SACRAL (CONTINUED)

CLINICAL POINT

A **severe spinal cord crush injury** damages local neurons and disrupts both the ascending and the descending tracts. Such a lesion at the lumbar level causes flaccid paralysis of muscles (with loss of tone and muscle stretch reflexes) at the damaged levels as the result of LMN injury and spastic paralysis of muscles (with increased tone and muscle stretch reflexes, possible clonus, and extensor plantar responses) in muscles supplied by LMNs below the level of the lesion as the result of damage to the UMN axons in the lateral funiculus. All sensation is lost below the level of the lesion because of disruption of both dorsal column and anterolateral axons, although some protopathic sensation may remain present, even in the case of a very extensive lesion. A severe crush injury also damages descending axons in both lateral funiculi that help to regulate bowel function, bladder function, and sexual function. The patient initially shows spinal shock syndrome, with unresponsive bowel and bladder; after recovery from spinal shock, a spastic bladder (small, stimulated to empty by reflex, with incontinence) occurs. In addition, voluntary control over erectile function in males is lost, but reflex erection caused by specific sensory stimuli may occur. Severe crush injury at higher levels (cervical) also can disrupt descending axons that regulate sympathetic outflow, resulting in dysregulated blood pressure, Horner's syndrome, and other autonomic symptoms.

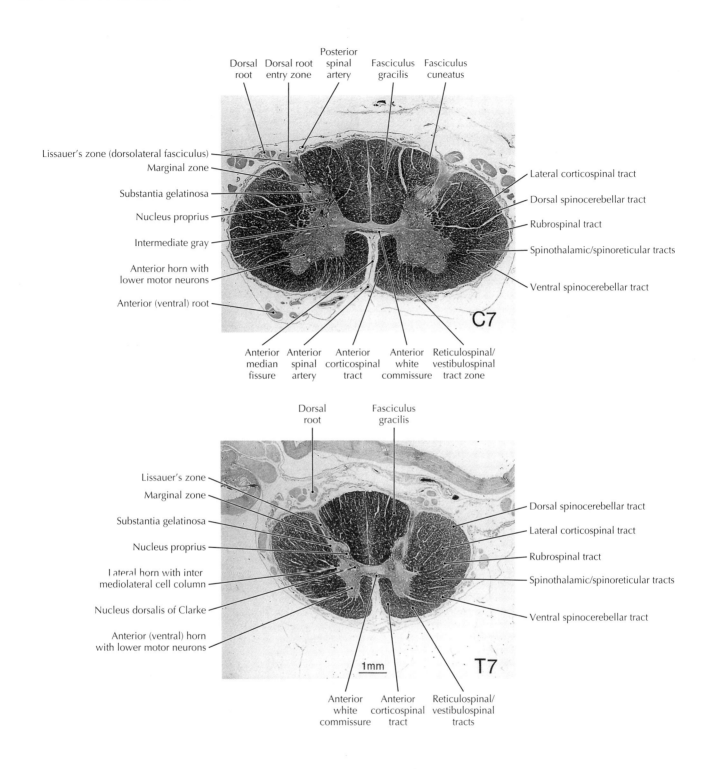

Dorsal root
Dorsal root entry zone
Posterior spinal artery
Fasciculus gracilis
Fasciculus cuneatus

Lissauer's zone (dorsolateral fasciculus)
Marginal zone
Substantia gelatinosa
Nucleus proprius
Intermediate gray
Anterior horn with lower motor neurons
Anterior (ventral) root

Lateral corticospinal tract
Dorsal spinocerebellar tract
Rubrospinal tract
Spinothalamic/spinoreticular tracts
Ventral spinocerebellar tract

C7

Anterior median fissure
Anterior spinal artery
Anterior corticospinal tract
Anterior white commissure
Reticulospinal/vestibulospinal tract zone

Dorsal root
Fasciculus gracilis

Lissauer's zone
Marginal zone
Substantia gelatinosa
Nucleus proprius
Lateral horn with inter mediolateral cell column
Nucleus dorsalis of Clarke
Anterior (ventral) horn with lower motor neurons

Dorsal spinocerebellar tract
Lateral corticospinal tract
Rubrospinal tract
Spinothalamic/spinoreticular tracts
Ventral spinocerebellar tract

1mm
T7

Anterior white commissure
Anterior corticospinal tract
Reticulospinal/vestibulospinal tracts

10.6 SPINAL CORD HISTOLOGICAL CROSS SECTIONS

Cross sections through the spinal cord at levels C7 and T7 prepared with a Weigert stain. Major gray matter and white matter zones are labeled.

CLINICAL POINT

Combined systems degeneration (subacute combined degeneration) is a degeneration of the dorsal columns and lateral funiculi, frequently in the lower cervical and thoracic cord. Demyelination is the hallmark of this disorder followed by axonal degeneration. The syndrome occurs with prolonged vitamin B_{12} deficiency, Crohn disease, Roux-en-Y gastric bypass or, less frequently, copper deficiency. Initial symptoms include fatigue, irritability, depression, or mental disabilities such as dementia. Neurological symptoms include (1) numbness and paresthesias of the distal extremities (then the full extremities) from dorsal column damage, (2) stiffness of the extremities leading to spastic paraplegia, (3) possible bowel and bladder dysfunction, and (4) sensory ataxia from dorsal column and spinocerebellar damage. Some symptoms may resolve with full restoration of vitamin B_{12} stores.

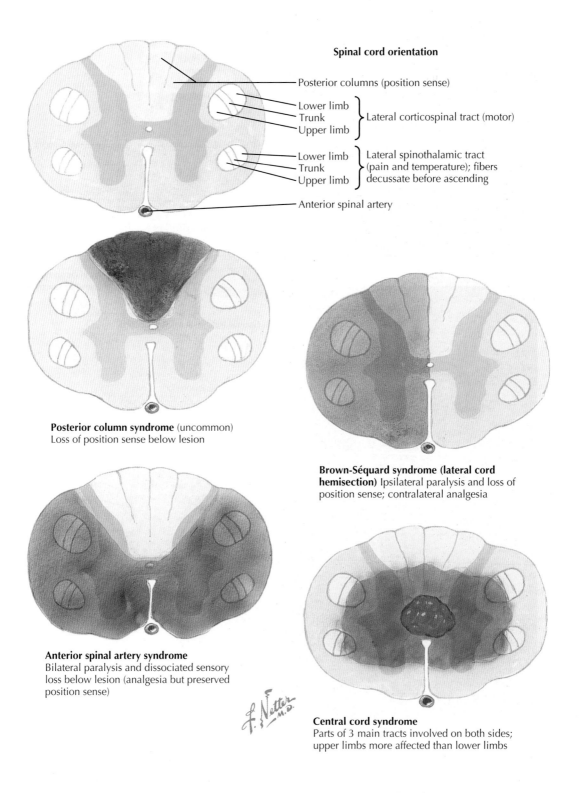

Spinal cord orientation

Posterior columns (position sense)

Lower limb
Trunk
Upper limb } Lateral corticospinal tract (motor)

Lower limb
Trunk
Upper limb } Lateral spinothalamic tract (pain and temperature); fibers decussate before ascending

Anterior spinal artery

Posterior column syndrome (uncommon)
Loss of position sense below lesion

Brown-Séquard syndrome (lateral cord hemisection) Ipsilateral paralysis and loss of position sense; contralateral analgesia

Anterior spinal artery syndrome
Bilateral paralysis and dissociated sensory loss below lesion (analgesia but preserved position sense)

Central cord syndrome
Parts of 3 main tracts involved on both sides; upper limbs more affected than lower limbs

10.9 SPINAL CORD SYNDROMES

These illustrations demonstrate a summary of normal spinal cord tract locations nend the sites and consequences of incomplete spinal cord lesions, including posterior (dorsal) column syndrome, Brown-Séquard lesion (lateral cord hemisection), anterior spinal artery syndrome, and central cord syndrome. The clinical points for 10.3 and 10.5 provide further details of the anatomical basis for the classical consequences of some of these syndromes.

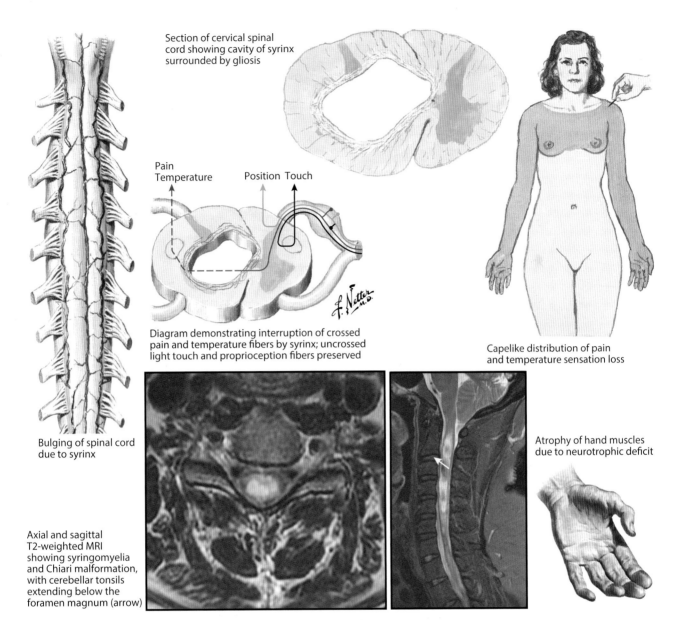

Section of cervical spinal cord showing cavity of syrinx surrounded by gliosis

Pain
Temperature
Position Touch

Diagram demonstrating interruption of crossed pain and temperature fibers by syrinx; uncrossed light touch and proprioception fibers preserved

Capelike distribution of pain and temperature sensation loss

Bulging of spinal cord due to syrinx

Axial and sagittal T2-weighted MRI showing syringomyelia and Chiari malformation, with cerebellar tonsils extending below the foramen magnum (arrow)

Atrophy of hand muscles due to neurotrophic deficit

10.10 SYRINGOMYELIA

Syringomyelia involves the development of a central cavity in the vicinity of the central canal of the spinal cord that expands to involve both neuronal pathways and neuronal cell groups. If congenital, syringomyelia is accompanied by Arnold-Chiari malformation, type 1, with cerebellar tonsillar herniation and possible compression of caudal medullary or upper cervical cord structures. Pressure on the CSF from Arnold-Chiari malformation, type 1, may contribute to the expansion of the syrinx.

Syringomyelia is a rare disorder, and some cases are asymptomatic, found coincidentally in imaging studies. However, the clinical manifestations are reflective of the anatomical organization of the spinal cord. The principal finding is dissociated sensory loss, with bilateral loss of pain and temperature sensation, but not fine, discriminative modalities, due to destruction of the anterior white commissure in the affected region of the syrinx. The syrinx may expand to involve the anterior horn (trophic changes, LMN-associated weakness and atrophy), the lateral funiculus (spastic weakness below the level of the lesion on the affected side due to corticospinal and rubrospinal tract damage), and further pain and temperature sensation loss due to anterolateral damage. For further anatomical and clinical discussion, see the Clinical Point for 10.4.

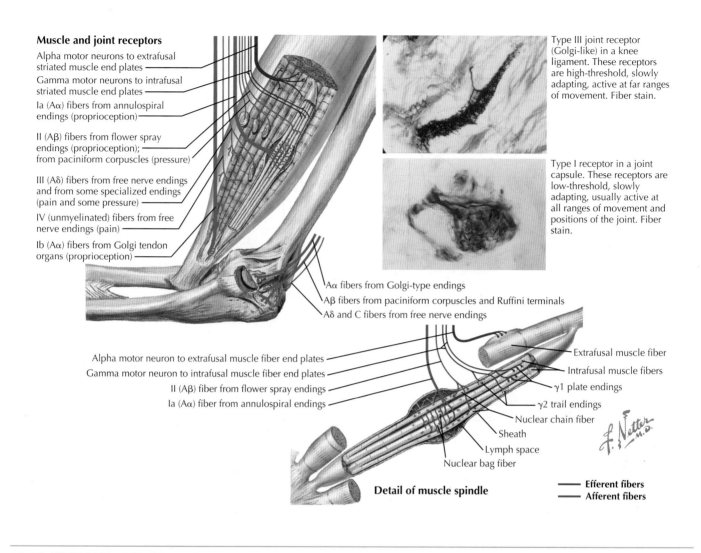

Muscle and joint receptors

Alpha motor neurons to extrafusal striated muscle end plates

Gamma motor neurons to intrafusal striated muscle end plates

Ia (Aα) fibers from annulospiral endings (proprioception)

II (Aβ) fibers from flower spray endings (proprioception); from paciniform corpuscles (pressure)

III (Aδ) fibers from free nerve endings and from some specialized endings (pain and some pressure)

IV (unmyelinated) fibers from free nerve endings (pain)

Ib (Aα) fibers from Golgi tendon organs (proprioception)

Type III joint receptor (Golgi-like) in a knee ligament. These receptors are high-threshold, slowly adapting, active at far ranges of movement. Fiber stain.

Type I receptor in a joint capsule. These receptors are low-threshold, slowly adapting, usually active at all ranges of movement and positions of the joint. Fiber stain.

Aα fibers from Golgi-type endings
Aβ fibers from paciniform corpuscles and Ruffini terminals
Aδ and C fibers from free nerve endings

Alpha motor neuron to extrafusal muscle fiber end plates
Gamma motor neuron to intrafusal muscle fiber end plates
II (Aβ) fiber from flower spray endings
Ia (Aα) fiber from annulospiral endings

Extrafusal muscle fiber
Intrafusal muscle fibers
γ1 plate endings
γ2 trail endings
Nuclear chain fiber
Sheath
Lymph space
Nuclear bag fiber

Detail of muscle spindle

— Efferent fibers
— Afferent fibers

10.13 MUSCLE AND JOINT RECEPTORS AND MUSCLE SPINDLES

Joints are innervated by a host of afferent receptors, including bare nerve endings, Golgi-type endings, paciniform endings, Ruffini-like endings, and other encapsulated endings. Golgi tendon organs innervate tendons and respond to stretch with increased discharge, causing disynaptic inhibition of the LMNs that contract the homonymous muscles at high-threshold activation. Muscle spindles are complex sensory receptors within muscles; they are arranged in parallel with the extrafusal (skeletal) muscle fibers. These receptors contain small intrafusal muscle fibers that are stretched when the skeletal muscle is stretched. The Ia afferent from the muscle spindle excites the homonymous LMN pool monosynaptically and responds to both the length and the velocity (change in length with respect to time) of the extrafusal muscle fiber. These muscle reflexes assist in maintaining homeostasis during contraction and help to regulate muscle tone during movement.

CLINICAL POINT

Skeletal muscles are supplied by both afferent (sensory) and efferent (motor) nerves and receptors. The sensory fibers are associated mainly with specialized sensory receptors, the **muscle spindles**.

Muscle spindles are small, encapsulated sensory receptors that lie in parallel with the skeletal muscle fibers (extrafusal fibers). Each spindle contains nuclear bag fibers (innervated mainly by group Ia afferents) and nuclear chain fibers (innervated mainly by group II afferents). These afferents are responsive to the tension on the muscle spindle. The group II afferents report mainly the lengths of the extrafusal fibers with which they are associated, whereas the Ia afferents report both the lengths and the velocities (dL/dt). In conjunction with the Ib afferents associated with Golgi tendon organs that report the force exerted on the tendon, Ia and group II muscle afferents provide continuous information to the CNS about the current state of the muscle and the projected changes occurring, based on the velocity response. The skeletal muscle fibers are supplied by motor axons derived from the alpha motor neurons in the ventral horn of the spinal cord. The muscle spindle's nuclear bag and chain fibers have small contractile fibers on either end by which they are anchored into the spindle. These contractile fibers (intrafusal fibers) are innervated by gamma (γ) LMNs whose cell bodies also are found in the ventral horn of the spinal cord. Descending UMN pathways generally activate both alpha and gamma LMNs (alpha-gamma coactivation), thereby achieving the shortening of the muscle spindle by the gamma LMNs in parallel with the shortening of the extrafusal fibers, keeping the muscle spindle in its dynamic range of sensory activity. Without such coactivation, the muscle spindle afferents would be silent in most ranges of extrafusal muscle contraction.

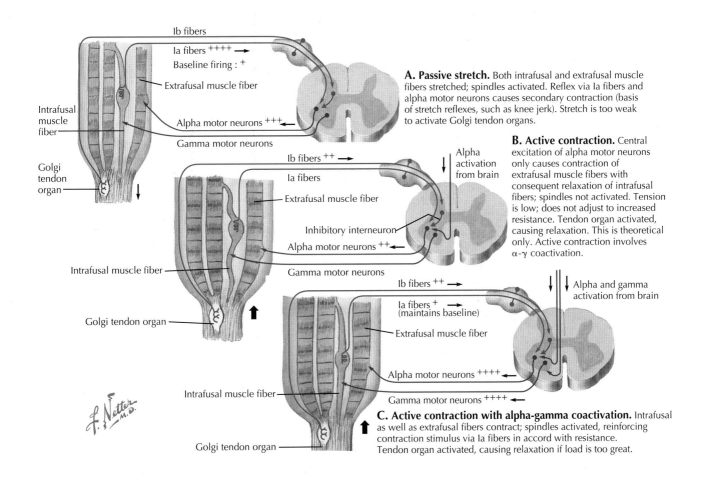

A. Passive stretch. Both intrafusal and extrafusal muscle fibers stretched; spindles activated. Reflex via Ia fibers and alpha motor neurons causes secondary contraction (basis of stretch reflexes, such as knee jerk). Stretch is too weak to activate Golgi tendon organs.

B. Active contraction. Central excitation of alpha motor neurons only causes contraction of extrafusal muscle fibers with consequent relaxation of intrafusal fibers; spindles not activated. Tension is low; does not adjust to increased resistance. Tendon organ activated, causing relaxation. This is theoretical only. Active contraction involves α-γ coactivation.

C. Active contraction with alpha-gamma coactivation. Intrafusal as well as extrafusal fibers contract; spindles activated, reinforcing contraction stimulus via Ia fibers in accord with resistance. Tendon organ activated, causing relaxation if load is too great.

10.14 THE MUSCLE STRETCH REFLEX AND ITS CENTRAL CONTROL VIA GAMMA MOTOR NEURONS

During passive stretch, a muscle stretch reflex excites homonymous LMNs, which results in muscle contraction to restore homeostasis. If active skeletal muscle contraction occurs without the activation of gamma LMNs (theoretical), the muscle spindle "unloads" and the tension on the intrafusal fibers is reduced, resulting in diminished firing of both Ia and II afferents. However, when LMNs contract because of activity in the brainstem's UMNs or because of voluntary corticospinal activity, both alpha LMNs and gamma LMNs are activated together. This process, alpha-gamma coactivation, ensures that the tension on the muscle spindle (through the intrafusal innervation by gamma fibers) adjusts immediately, that is, as the extrafusal muscle contraction occurs (through alpha fiber innervation). Although alpha and gamma LMNs can be modulated separately by specific central neuronal circuits, in normal physiological circumstances they are coactivated. If gamma LMNs are differentially activated in pathological circumstances, increased muscle tone and spasticity may ensue.

CLINICAL POINT

The **muscle stretch reflex**, a mainstay of neurological diagnosis, depends upon the activity of afferents and efferents associated with the muscle spindle and the skeletal muscle (extrafusal) fibers. When a tendon is tapped with a reflex hammer (e.g., the patellar tendon), the skeletal muscle is briefly stretched, as are the muscle spindles lying in parallel with them. The stretch of the muscle spindle puts tension on the equatorial region of the nuclear bag fibers, resulting in a burst of action potentials from the associated Ia afferents. The Ia afferents synapse directly with alpha LMNs in the spinal cord ventral horn, resulting in contraction of the homonymous muscle (quadriceps) and restoration of homeostasis. The Ia afferents also synapse on Ia inhibitory interneurons in the spinal cord, producing reciprocal inhibition of the antagonist muscles (hamstrings). The excitability of the muscle spindles can determine the robustness of the Ia afferent response to stretch. If the muscle spindle is floppy (unloaded), no Ia afferent response is forthcoming when the related tendon is tapped, and no muscle contraction occurs (areflexia or hyporeflexia); if the muscle spindle is on a hair-trigger of heightened responsiveness, as happens when the gamma LMNs are excessively activated, then a very brisk muscle contraction occurs when the related tendon is tapped (hyperreflexia). The latter situation may occur in cases of lesions in the UMNs of the spinal cord and brain, which may produce disinhibition of the dynamic gamma LMNs accompanied by hyperreflexia of the muscle stretch reflexes and spasticity of the involved muscles.

11

BRAINSTEM AND CEREBELLUM

Medulla–Spinal Cord Transition—Decussation of the Pyramids

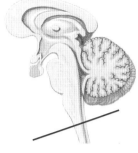

Level of section

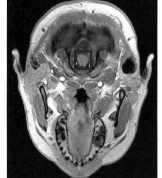

Labeled image available as eFig. 11.1.

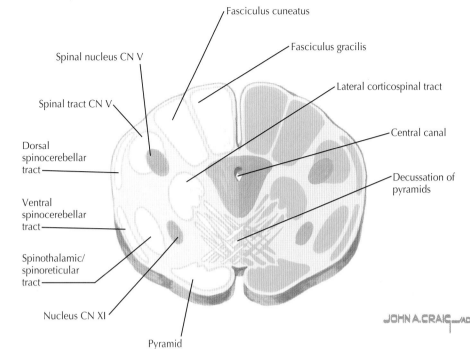

Spinal nucleus CN V

Spinal tract CN V

Dorsal spinocerebellar tract

Ventral spinocerebellar tract

Spinothalamic/ spinoreticular tract

Nucleus CN XI

Pyramid

Fasciculus cuneatus

Fasciculus gracilis

Lateral corticospinal tract

Central canal

Decussation of pyramids

JOHN A. CRAIG_AD

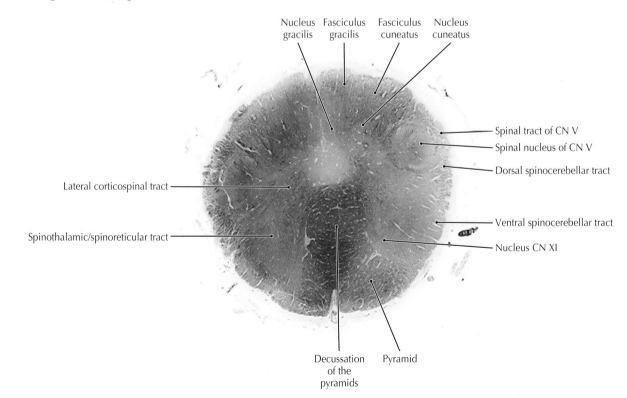

Nucleus gracilis   Fasciculus gracilis   Fasciculus cuneatus   Nucleus cuneatus

Lateral corticospinal tract

Spinothalamic/spinoreticular tract

Spinal tract of CN V

Spinal nucleus of CN V

Dorsal spinocerebellar tract

Ventral spinocerebellar tract

Nucleus CN XI

Decussation of the pyramids

Pyramid

BRAINSTEM CROSS-SECTIONAL ANATOMY

11.1 BRAINSTEM CROSS-SECTIONAL ANATOMY: SECTION 1

Illustrations of brainstem cross sections (Figs. 11.1–11.4) are arranged from caudal to rostral, from the spinal-medullary junction to the rostral mesencephalon-diencephalon junction; T1-weighted magnetic resonance images of the brainstem and surrounding tissue are provided for each level. Corresponding histology cross sections, stained with a fiber stain, are provided of each level. CN, cranial nerve.

Medulla—Level of the Inferior Olive

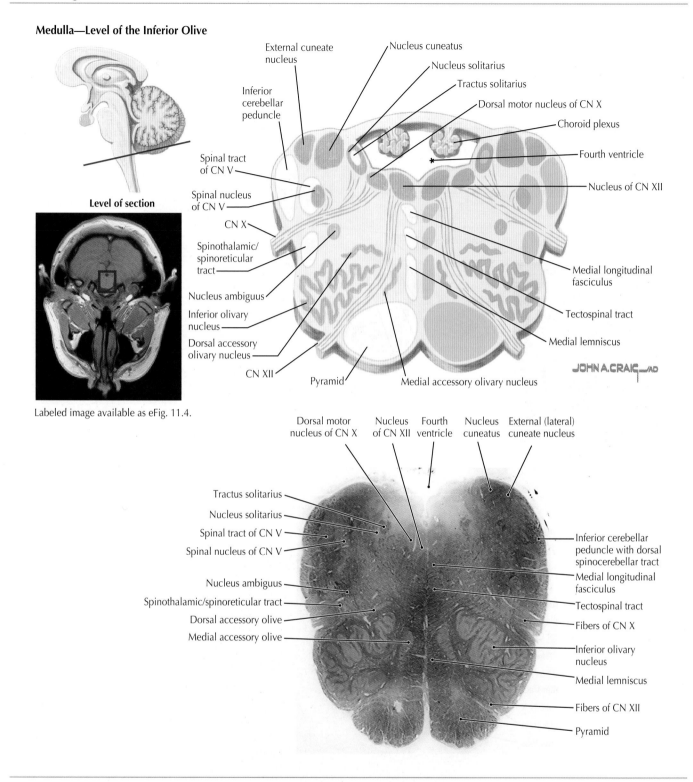

Level of section

Labeled image available as eFig. 11.4.

External cuneate nucleus
Nucleus cuneatus
Nucleus solitarius
Tractus solitarius
Inferior cerebellar peduncle
Dorsal motor nucleus of CN X
Choroid plexus
Spinal tract of CN V
Fourth ventricle
Spinal nucleus of CN V
Nucleus of CN XII
CN X
Spinothalamic/ spinoreticular tract
Medial longitudinal fasciculus
Nucleus ambiguus
Tectospinal tract
Inferior olivary nucleus
Medial lemniscus
Dorsal accessory olivary nucleus
CN XII
Pyramid
Medial accessory olivary nucleus

JOHN A. CRAIG—AD

Dorsal motor nucleus of CN X
Nucleus of CN XII
Fourth ventricle
Nucleus cuneatus
External (lateral) cuneate nucleus
Tractus solitarius
Nucleus solitarius
Spinal tract of CN V
Spinal nucleus of CN V
Inferior cerebellar peduncle with dorsal spinocerebellar tract
Medial longitudinal fasciculus
Nucleus ambiguus
Tectospinal tract
Spinothalamic/spinoreticular tract
Fibers of CN X
Dorsal accessory olive
Inferior olivary nucleus
Medial accessory olive
Medial lemniscus
Fibers of CN XII
Pyramid

11.4 BRAINSTEM CROSS-SECTIONAL ANATOMY: SECTION 4

CLINICAL POINT

The medulla is supplied with blood by the paramedian and circumferential branches of the anterior spinal artery and the vertebral arteries. A major circumferential branch of the vertebral artery, the posterior inferior cerebellar artery (PICA), supplies a lateral wedge of medulla with blood. A brainstem stroke or an infarct in a vertebral artery or in the PICA produces a complex of symptoms called the **lateral medullary syndrome** (Wallenberg syndrome), which is caused by damage to an array of nuclei and tracts. The patient can demonstrate (1) loss of pain and temperature sensation on the ipsilateral side of the face (descending nucleus and tract of V) and the contralateral side of the body (spinothalamic/spinoreticular system); (2) dysphagia and dysarthria (paralysis of ipsilateral pharyngeal and laryngeal muscles resulting from damage to the ipsilateral nucleus ambiguus); (3) ataxia of the limbs and falling to the ipsilateral side (inferior cerebellar peduncle and its afferent tracts); (4) vertigo with nausea, vomiting, and nystagmus (vestibular nuclei); and (5) ipsilateral Horner's syndrome, with ptosis, miosis, and anhidrosis (descending axons from the hypothalamus to the T1–T2 intermediolateral cell column of the spinal cord).

Medulla—Level of the CN X and the Vestibular Nuclei

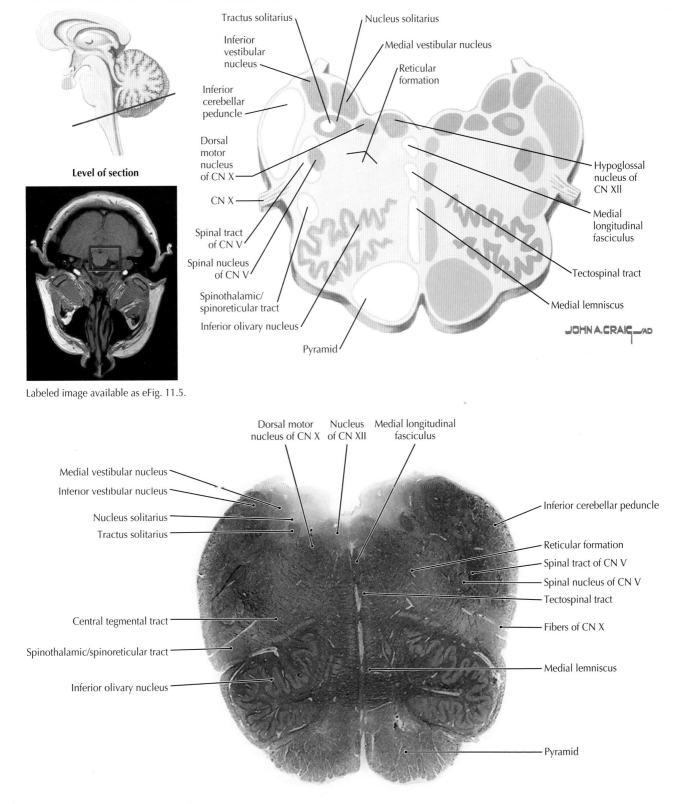

Level of section

Tractus solitarius

Nucleus solitarius

Inferior vestibular nucleus

Medial vestibular nucleus

Reticular formation

Inferior cerebellar peduncle

Dorsal motor nucleus of CN X

CN X

Spinal tract of CN V

Spinal nucleus of CN V

Spinothalamic/ spinoreticular tract

Inferior olivary nucleus

Pyramid

Hypoglossal nucleus of CN XII

Medial longitudinal fasciculus

Tectospinal tract

Medial lemniscus

JOHN A. CRAIG—AD

Labeled image available as eFig. 11.5.

Dorsal motor nucleus of CN X

Nucleus of CN XII

Medial longitudinal fasciculus

Medial vestibular nucleus

Inferior vestibular nucleus

Nucleus solitarius

Tractus solitarius

Central tegmental tract

Spinothalamic/spinoreticular tract

Inferior olivary nucleus

Inferior cerebellar peduncle

Reticular formation

Spinal tract of CN V

Spinal nucleus of CN V

Tectospinal tract

Fibers of CN X

Medial lemniscus

Pyramid

11.5 BRAINSTEM CROSS-SECTIONAL ANATOMY: SECTION 5

Pons—Level of the Genu of the Facial Nerve

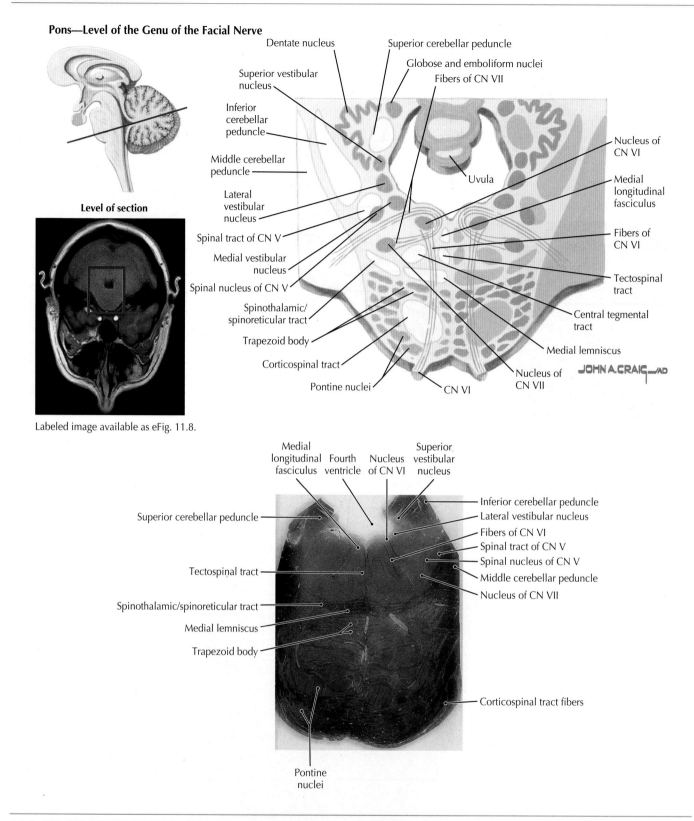

Level of section

Labeled image available as eFig. 11.8.

JOHN A. CRAIG—AD

11.8 BRAINSTEM CROSS-SECTIONAL ANATOMY: SECTION 8

CLINICAL POINT

The pons is a common site for a hemorrhagic stroke. A **pontine hemorrhage** is commonly large and lethal. When not fatal, such a hemorrhage may result in the rapid progression of (1) total paralysis (quadriplegia); (2) decerebrate posturing (extensor posturing) caused by UMN damage to the corticospinal and rubrospinal systems, thereby disinhibiting the lateral vestibular nuclei; (3) coma; (4) paralysis of ocular movements; and (5) small but reactive pupils. A pontine hemorrhage that results in coma is commonly lethal. A large infarct in the basilar artery may produce the same clinical picture. Some small, lacunar infarcts also may occur in the pons; these infarcts may produce purely motor symptoms (contralateral UMN paresis at base of pons), ataxia, or both (cerebellar peduncles, pontine nuclei).

Pons—Level of Trigeminal Motor and Main Sensory Nuclei

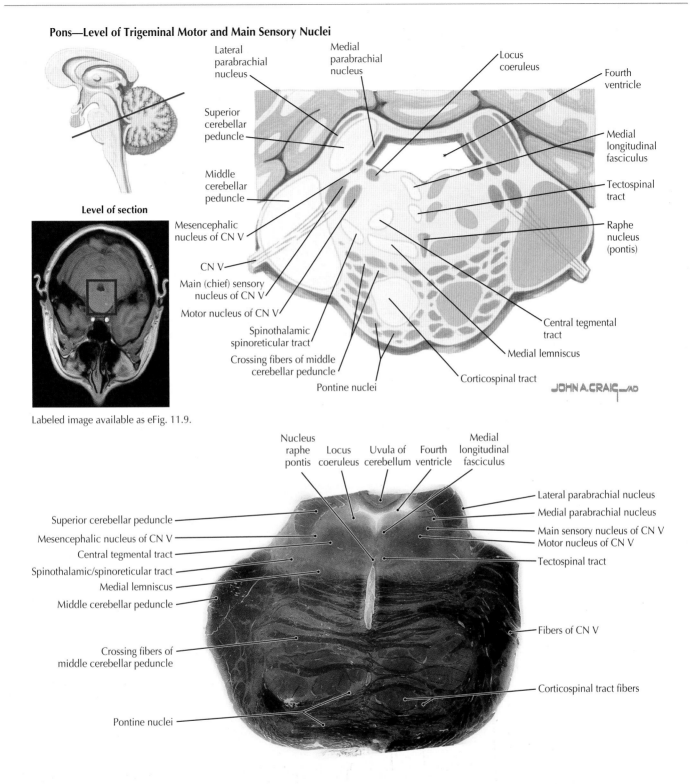

Level of section

Labeled image available as eFig. 11.9.

Labels (top illustration):
Lateral parabrachial nucleus
Medial parabrachial nucleus
Locus coeruleus
Fourth ventricle
Superior cerebellar peduncle
Medial longitudinal fasciculus
Middle cerebellar peduncle
Tectospinal tract
Mesencephalic nucleus of CN V
Raphe nucleus (pontis)
CN V
Main (chief) sensory nucleus of CN V
Motor nucleus of CN V
Spinothalamic spinoreticular tract
Central tegmental tract
Crossing fibers of middle cerebellar peduncle
Medial lemniscus
Pontine nuclei
Corticospinal tract
JOHN A. CRAIG_AD

Labels (bottom specimen):
Nucleus raphe pontis
Locus coeruleus
Uvula of cerebellum
Fourth ventricle
Medial longitudinal fasciculus
Superior cerebellar peduncle
Lateral parabrachial nucleus
Mesencephalic nucleus of CN V
Medial parabrachial nucleus
Central tegmental tract
Main sensory nucleus of CN V
Spinothalamic/spinoreticular tract
Motor nucleus of CN V
Medial lemniscus
Tectospinal tract
Middle cerebellar peduncle
Crossing fibers of middle cerebellar peduncle
Fibers of CN V
Pontine nuclei
Corticospinal tract fibers

11.9 BRAINSTEM CROSS-SECTIONAL ANATOMY: SECTION 9

CLINICAL POINT

A vascular lesion of circumferential branches of the basilar artery or the anterior inferior cerebellar artery can cause **lateral pontine syndrome**, which is characterized by (1) contralateral loss of sensation in the body, both epicritic and protopathic (medial lemniscus and anterolateral system); (2) loss of pain and temperature sensation on the contralateral face (ventral trigeminal lemniscus, located on dorsal surface of the medial lemniscus); (3) loss of fine, discriminative touch (main sensory nucleus of CN V) or impaired general sensation (CN V fibers) on the ipsilateral face; (4) ipsilateral paralysis of muscles of mastication (motor nucleus of CN V); (5) limb ataxia (middle and superior cerebellar peduncles); (6) paralysis of conjugate gaze to the ipsilateral side (parapontine reticular formation and its connections); and (7) other possible ipsilateral brainstem problems, depending on the extent of the vascular involvement, such as deafness or tinnitus (auditory nuclei or nerve fibers), vertigo and nystagmus (vestibular nuclei or nerve fibers), facial palsy (CN VII nucleus or nerve fibers), and Horner's syndrome (descending hypothalamo-spinal sympathetic connections).

Pons-Midbrain Junction—Level of CN IV and Locus Coeruleus

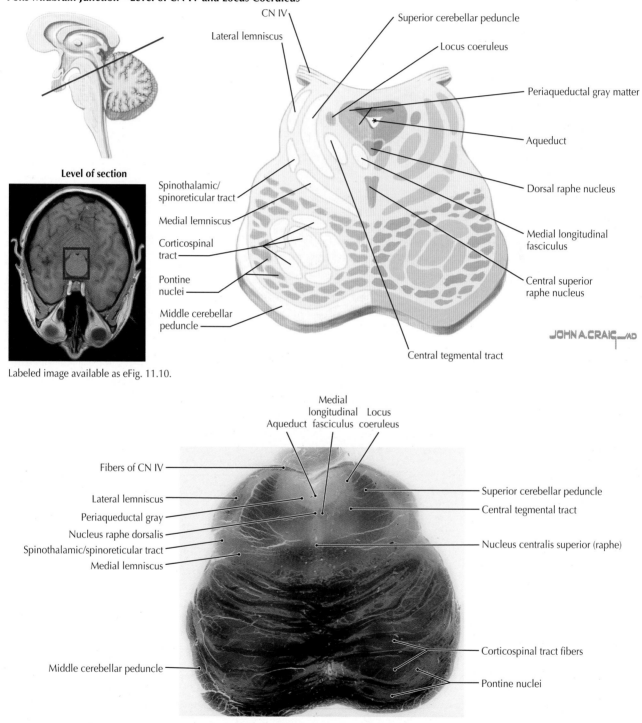

Level of section

Labeled image available as eFig. 11.10.

Labels (upper illustration):
- CN IV
- Lateral lemniscus
- Superior cerebellar peduncle
- Locus coeruleus
- Periaqueductal gray matter
- Aqueduct
- Dorsal raphe nucleus
- Medial longitudinal fasciculus
- Central superior raphe nucleus
- Central tegmental tract
- Middle cerebellar peduncle
- Pontine nuclei
- Corticospinal tract
- Medial lemniscus
- Spinothalamic/spinoreticular tract

JOHN A. CRAIG—AD

Labels (lower photograph):
- Aqueduct
- Medial longitudinal fasciculus
- Locus coeruleus
- Fibers of CN IV
- Lateral lemniscus
- Periaqueductal gray
- Nucleus raphe dorsalis
- Spinothalamic/spinoreticular tract
- Medial lemniscus
- Superior cerebellar peduncle
- Central tegmental tract
- Nucleus centralis superior (raphe)
- Middle cerebellar peduncle
- Corticospinal tract fibers
- Pontine nuclei

11.10 BRAINSTEM CROSS-SECTIONAL ANATOMY: SECTION 10

Midbrain—Level of the Inferior Colliculus

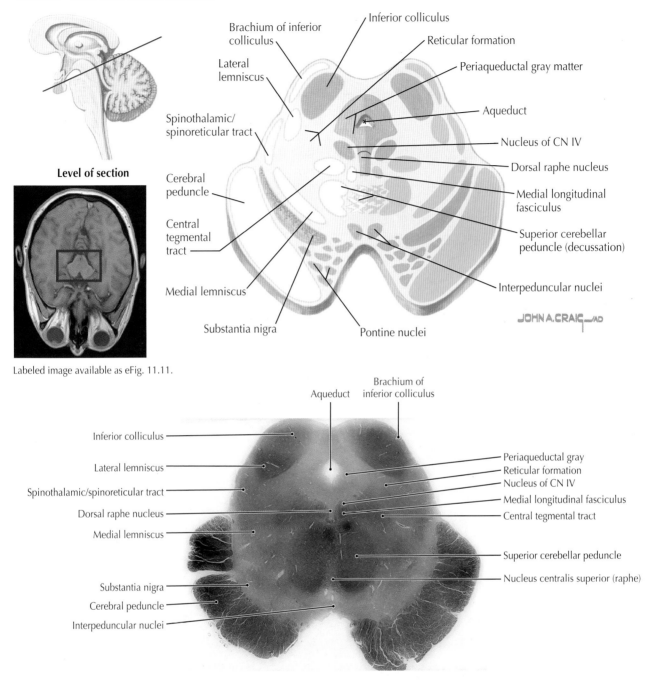

Level of section

Labeled image available as eFig. 11.11.

JOHN A. CRAIG—AD

11.11 BRAINSTEM CROSS-SECTIONAL ANATOMY: SECTION 11

CLINICAL POINT

A space-occupying lesion in the forebrain, such as a bleed (epidural or subdural hematoma), a tumor, or increased intracranial pressure resulting from a variety of causes, can cause herniation of the forebrain through the tentorium cerebelli. This **transtentorial herniation** displaces the thalamus and upper midbrain in a downward direction and causes a variety of changes in brain function. These changes are characterized by functions attributable to the remaining intact lower midbrain and more caudal structures, with loss of function of the upper midbrain and more rostral structures. Most conspicuous is a progressive deterioration of the state of consciousness, rapidly going from drowsiness to stupor to an unarousable state of coma; consciousness requires an intact brainstem reticular formation and at least one functioning cerebral hemisphere. When both hemispheres are nonfunctional, coma ensues. With the loss of activity in the corticospinal system and the rubrospinal system and removal of cortical influence on the other UMN pathways, a state of decerebration occurs (called decerebrate rigidity, although it is really spasticity, not true rigidity). The neck is extended (opisthotonus), the arms and legs are extended and rotated inward, and the hands, fingers, feet, and toes are flexed. Plantar responses are extensor. Cheyne-Stokes respiration is seen (crescendo-decrescendo breathing), followed at a slightly later stage of damage by shallow hyperventilation. The pupils are midsized and usually unresponsive because of compression of the third nerves against the free edge of the tentorium. Caloric testing or the doll's-eye maneuver shows no vertical eye movements (visual tectal damage), and the eyes do not move in a conjugate fashion.

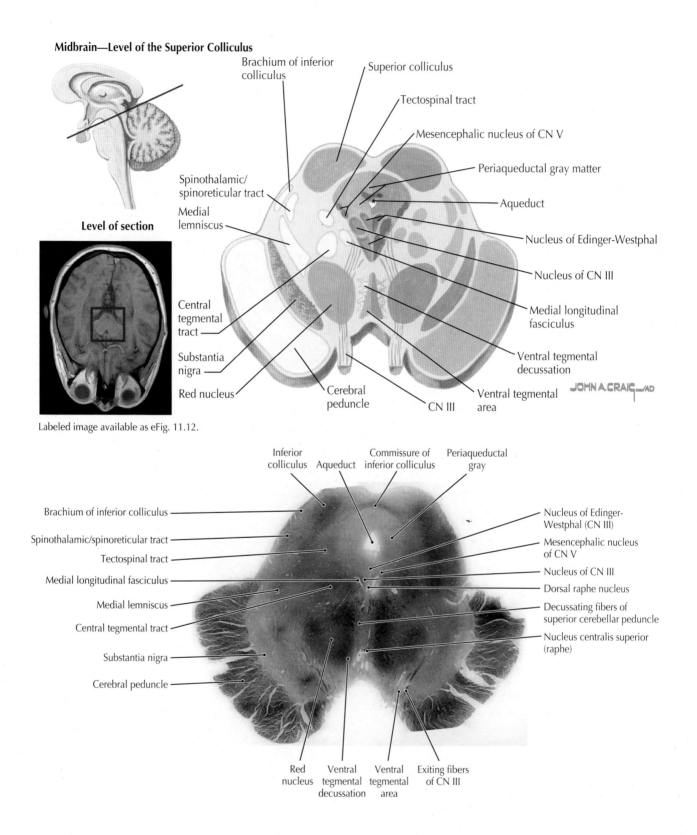

Midbrain—Level of the Superior Colliculus

Brachium of inferior colliculus

Superior colliculus

Tectospinal tract

Mesencephalic nucleus of CN V

Periaqueductal gray matter

Level of section

Aqueduct

Spinothalamic/spinoreticular tract

Nucleus of Edinger-Westphal

Medial lemniscus

Nucleus of CN III

Medial longitudinal fasciculus

Central tegmental tract

Ventral tegmental decussation

Substantia nigra

Ventral tegmental area

Red nucleus

Cerebral peduncle

CN III

JOHN A. CRAIG—AD

Labeled image available as eFig. 11.12.

Inferior colliculus　Aqueduct　Commissure of inferior colliculus　Periaqueductal gray

Brachium of inferior colliculus

Nucleus of Edinger-Westphal (CN III)

Spinothalamic/spinoreticular tract

Mesencephalic nucleus of CN V

Tectospinal tract

Nucleus of CN III

Medial longitudinal fasciculus

Dorsal raphe nucleus

Medial lemniscus

Decussating fibers of superior cerebellar peduncle

Central tegmental tract

Nucleus centralis superior (raphe)

Substantia nigra

Cerebral peduncle

Red nucleus　Ventral tegmental decussation　Ventral tegmental area　Exiting fibers of CN III

11.12　BRAINSTEM CROSS-SECTIONAL ANATOMY: SECTION 12

Midbrain—Level of the Medial Geniculate Body

Level of section

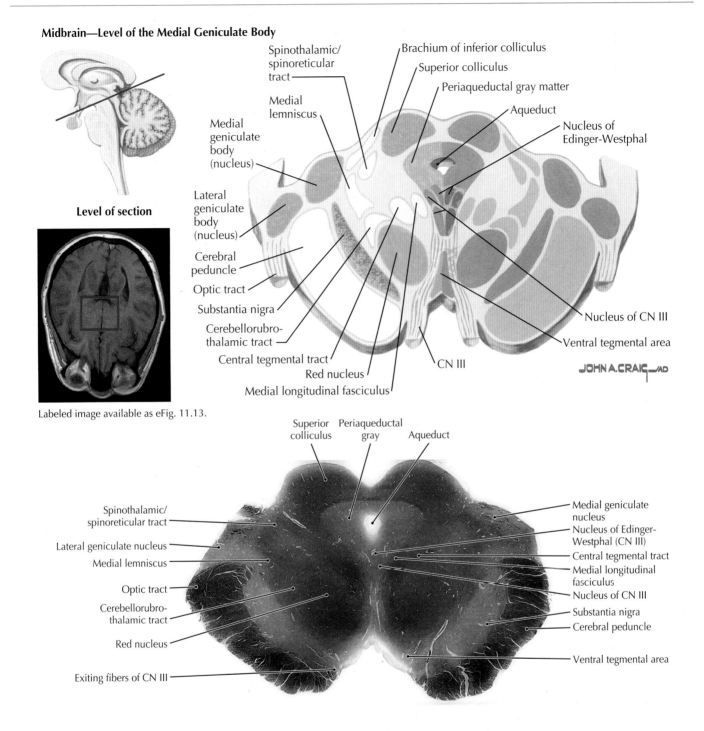

Labeled image available as eFig. 11.13.

11.13 BRAINSTEM CROSS-SECTIONAL ANATOMY: SECTION 13

CLINICAL POINT

Paramedian regions of the upper midbrain receive their blood supply mainly from branches of the posterior cerebral and posterior communicating arteries. A vascular lesion at this level (**Weber's syndrome**) results in damage to the exiting third nerve fibers, the medial and central portions of the cerebral peduncle, and some passing tracts.

A supratentorial mass lesion also can cause lateral and downward compression of one cerebral peduncle and the third nerve against the free edge of the tentorium cerebelli, presenting a similar clinical picture. Compression of the cerebral peduncle with possible involvement of the red nucleus on the affected side produces contralateral hemiplegia, rapidly evolving to a spastic state with a plantar extensor response.

A central (lower) facial palsy occurs because of damage to corticobulbar fibers, which travel in the cerebral peduncle. An ipsilateral oculomotor palsy also occurs, with the ipsilateral eye deviated laterally and the ipsilateral pupil fixed (unresponsive to light) and dilated because of unopposed actions of the sympathetics. If the lesion involves the substantia nigra, red nucleus, pallidothalamic fibers, or dentatorubral and dentatothalamic fibers, contralateral movement problems may occur, including akinesia, intention tremor, or choreoathetoid movements. Damage to these later structures, with their accompanying contralateral problems, may occur in isolation along with third nerve damage caused by more distal vascular involvement of the paramedian branches to the upper midbrain (**Benedikt's syndrome**).

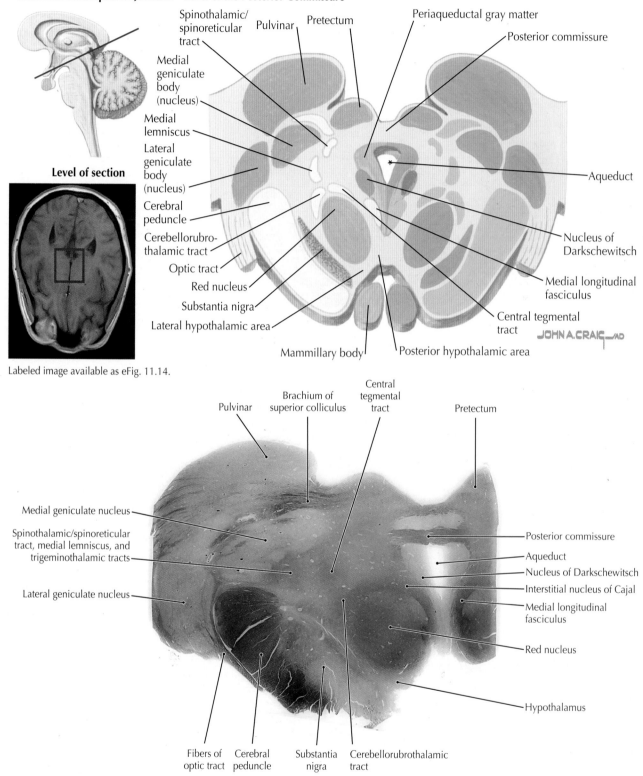

Midbrain-Diencephalon Junction—Level of the Posterior Commissure

Spinothalamic/spinoreticular tract
Pulvinar
Pretectum
Periaqueductal gray matter
Posterior commissure
Medial geniculate body (nucleus)
Medial lemniscus
Lateral geniculate body (nucleus)
Cerebral peduncle
Cerebellorubrothalamic tract
Optic tract
Red nucleus
Substantia nigra
Lateral hypothalamic area
Aqueduct
Nucleus of Darkschewitsch
Medial longitudinal fasciculus
Central tegmental tract
Mammillary body
Posterior hypothalamic area

Level of section

Labeled image available as eFig. 11.14.

JOHN A.CRAIG_AD

Pulvinar
Brachium of superior colliculus
Central tegmental tract
Pretectum

Medial geniculate nucleus
Spinothalamic/spinoreticular tract, medial lemniscus, and trigeminothalamic tracts
Lateral geniculate nucleus
Posterior commissure
Aqueduct
Nucleus of Darkschewitsch
Interstitial nucleus of Cajal
Medial longitudinal fasciculus
Red nucleus
Hypothalamus

Fibers of optic tract
Cerebral peduncle
Substantia nigra
Cerebellorubrothalamic tract

11.14 BRAINSTEM CROSS-SECTIONAL ANATOMY: SECTION 14

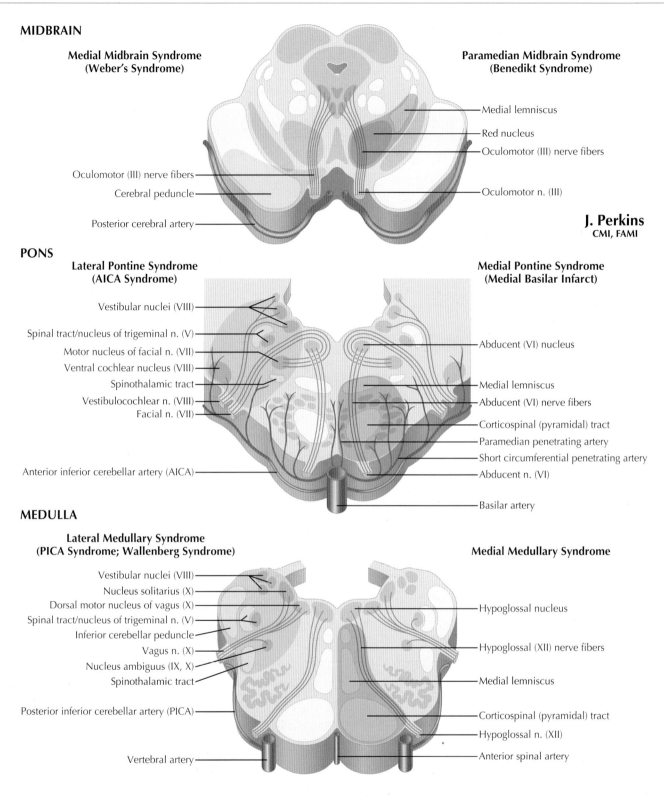

MIDBRAIN

Medial Midbrain Syndrome
(Weber's Syndrome)

Paramedian Midbrain Syndrome
(Benedikt Syndrome)

Medial lemniscus

Red nucleus

Oculomotor (III) nerve fibers

Oculomotor n. (III)

Oculomotor (III) nerve fibers

Cerebral peduncle

Posterior cerebral artery

J. Perkins
CMI, FAMI

PONS

Lateral Pontine Syndrome
(AICA Syndrome)

Medial Pontine Syndrome
(Medial Basilar Infarct)

Vestibular nuclei (VIII)

Spinal tract/nucleus of trigeminal n. (V)

Motor nucleus of facial n. (VII)

Ventral cochlear nucleus (VIII)

Spinothalamic tract

Vestibulocochlear n. (VIII)

Facial n. (VII)

Abducent (VI) nucleus

Medial lemniscus

Abducent (VI) nerve fibers

Corticospinal (pyramidal) tract

Paramedian penetrating artery

Short circumferential penetrating artery

Abducent n. (VI)

Anterior inferior cerebellar artery (AICA)

Basilar artery

MEDULLA

Lateral Medullary Syndrome
(PICA Syndrome; Wallenberg Syndrome)

Medial Medullary Syndrome

Vestibular nuclei (VIII)

Nucleus solitarius (X)

Dorsal motor nucleus of vagus (X)

Spinal tract/nucleus of trigeminal n. (V)

Inferior cerebellar peduncle

Vagus n. (X)

Nucleus ambiguus (IX, X)

Spinothalamic tract

Hypoglossal nucleus

Hypoglossal (XII) nerve fibers

Medial lemniscus

Posterior inferior cerebellar artery (PICA)

Corticospinal (pyramidal) tract

Hypoglossal n. (XII)

Vertebral artery

Anterior spinal artery

11.15 **BRAINSTEM ARTERIAL SYNDROMES**

These brainstem cross sections demonstrate major regions of vascular infarcts affecting the medulla, pons, and midbrain. Thorough knowledge of the nuclei and tracts in each territory is necessary to understand the resultant symptoms. In the medulla the main syndromes are lateral medullary syndrome (see Plate 11.4 Clinical Point) and medial medullary syndrome (see Plate 4.2 Clinical Point). In the pons the main syndromes are lateral pontine syndrome (see Plate 11.9 Clinical Point) and medial pontine syndrome (see Plate 11.6). In the midbrain the main syndromes are Weber's syndrome and Benedikt's syndrome (see Plate 11.13 Clinical Point).

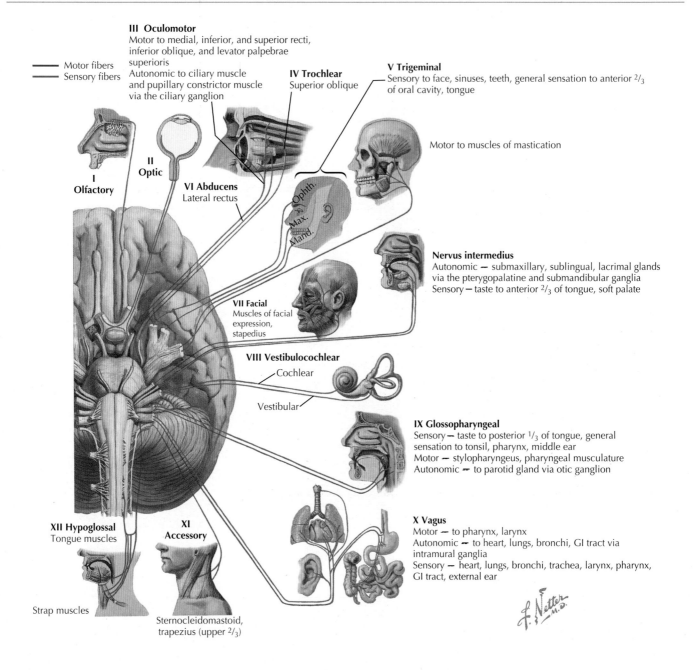

Motor fibers
Sensory fibers

III Oculomotor
Motor to medial, inferior, and superior recti, inferior oblique, and levator palpebrae superioris
Autonomic to ciliary muscle and pupillary constrictor muscle via the ciliary ganglion

II Optic

I Olfactory

IV Trochlear
Superior oblique

VI Abducens
Lateral rectus

Ophth.
Max.
Mand.

V Trigeminal
Sensory to face, sinuses, teeth, general sensation to anterior ⅔ of oral cavity, tongue

Motor to muscles of mastication

Nervus intermedius
Autonomic — submaxillary, sublingual, lacrimal glands via the pterygopalatine and submandibular ganglia
Sensory — taste to anterior ⅔ of tongue, soft palate

VII Facial
Muscles of facial expression, stapedius

VIII Vestibulocochlear
Cochlear
Vestibular

IX Glossopharyngeal
Sensory — taste to posterior ⅓ of tongue, general sensation to tonsil, pharynx, middle ear
Motor — stylopharyngeus, pharyngeal musculature
Autonomic — to parotid gland via otic ganglion

XII Hypoglossal
Tongue muscles

XI Accessory

Strap muscles

Sternocleidomastoid, trapezius (upper ⅔)

X Vagus
Motor — to pharynx, larynx
Autonomic — to heart, lungs, bronchi, GI tract via intramural ganglia
Sensory — heart, lungs, bronchi, trachea, larynx, pharynx, GI tract, external ear

CRANIAL NERVES AND CRANIAL NERVE NUCLEI

11.16 CRANIAL NERVES: SCHEMATIC OF DISTRIBUTION OF SENSORY, MOTOR, AND AUTONOMIC FIBERS

CNs I and II, both sensory, are tracts of the central nervous system (CNS) that are derived from the neural tube and myelinated by oligodendroglia. CNs III–XII emerge from the brainstem and supply sensory (CNs V, VII–X), motor (CNs III—VII and IX–XII), and autonomic (CNs III, VII, IX, X) nerve fibers to structures in the head, neck, and body (autonomic). All of the CNs that emerge from the brainstem distribute ipsilaterally to their target structures. With the exception of CN nucleus IV (trochlear) and some motor components of CN nucleus III (oculomotor), the CN nuclei are located ipsilateral to the point of emergence of the CN. The spinal accessory portion of CN XI emerges from motor neurons in the rostral spinal cord; it ascends through the foramen magnum and then exits with CNs IX and X; thus it is considered a CN.

CLINICAL POINT
Multiple CNs can be affected by some pathological conditions, such as tumors and granulomas, brainstem infarcts, leptomeningeal carcinomatosis, and aneurysms. Extramedullary pathology affects mainly the sensory, motor, and autonomic components of the involved CNs; internal pathology in the brainstem also involves the long tracts. An aneurysm in the cavernous sinus may involve CNs III–VI. A large tumor in the middle cranial fossa in the retrosphenoid space may affect cranial nerves III–VI. A large tumor in the cerebellopontine angle involves CNs VII and VIII and sometimes expands to involve V and IX. Tumors and aneurysms in the jugular foramen may involve CNs IX, X, and XI. Granulomatous lesions such as sarcoids in the posterior retroparotid space may affect cranial nerves IX–XII as well as the sympathetic nerves to the head.

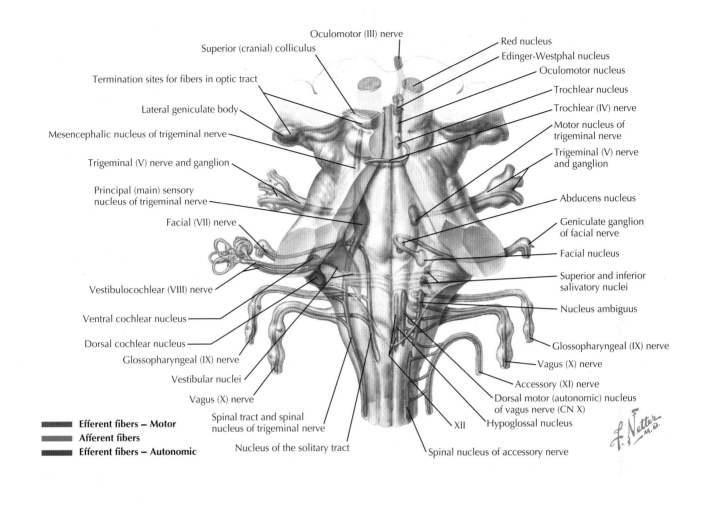

Oculomotor (III) nerve

Superior (cranial) colliculus

Termination sites for fibers in optic tract

Lateral geniculate body

Mesencephalic nucleus of trigeminal nerve

Trigeminal (V) nerve and ganglion

Principal (main) sensory nucleus of trigeminal nerve

Facial (VII) nerve

Vestibulocochlear (VIII) nerve

Ventral cochlear nucleus

Dorsal cochlear nucleus

Glossopharyngeal (IX) nerve

Vestibular nuclei

Vagus (X) nerve

Red nucleus

Edinger-Westphal nucleus

Oculomotor nucleus

Trochlear nucleus

Trochlear (IV) nerve

Motor nucleus of trigeminal nerve

Trigeminal (V) nerve and ganglion

Abducens nucleus

Geniculate ganglion of facial nerve

Facial nucleus

Superior and inferior salivatory nuclei

Nucleus ambiguus

Glossopharyngeal (IX) nerve

Vagus (X) nerve

Accessory (XI) nerve

Dorsal motor (autonomic) nucleus of vagus nerve (CN X)

Hypoglossal nucleus

XII

Efferent fibers – Motor
Afferent fibers
Efferent fibers – Autonomic

Spinal tract and spinal nucleus of trigeminal nerve

Nucleus of the solitary tract

Spinal nucleus of accessory nerve

11.17 CRANIAL NERVES AND THEIR NUCLEI: SCHEMATIC VIEW FROM ABOVE

The LMNs of the brainstem are localized in a medial column (CN motor nuclei for III [oculomotor], IV [trochlear], VI [abducens], and XII [hypoglossal]) and a lateral column (CN motor nuclei for V [trigeminal], VII [facial], IX and X [ambiguus], and XI [spinal accessory]). Preganglionic parasympathetic nuclei are found medially in the Edinger-Westphal nucleus (CN III) and the dorsal (motor) vagal nucleus (CN X) and laterally in the superior (CN VII) and inferior (CN IX) salivatory nuclei. Secondary sensory nuclei include the main sensory and descending nuclei of CN V, the vestibular nuclei and cochlear nuclei (CN VIII), and the nucleus solitarius (CNs VII, IX, and X). The superior colliculus and the lateral geniculate body (nucleus) receive secondary sensory axonal projections from the optic tract; the inferior colliculus receives input from the cochlear nuclei and other accessory auditory nuclei. The nuclei gracilis and cuneatus, located in the medulla, receive input from dorsal root ganglion cells, which convey epicritic somatosensory modalities (fine, discriminative touch; vibratory sensation; joint position sense).

CLINICAL POINT

CNs I, II, V, and VII–X have primary afferent components. CN I, the olfactory nerve, is a CNS tract and terminates directly in limbic forebrain structures, unlike any other CNs. CN II, the optic nerve, also is a CNS tract; its retinal ganglion cells act as a secondary sensory nucleus, projecting to the thalamus (lateral geniculate body), superior colliculus, pretectum, suprachiasmatic nucleus of the hypothalamus, and other brainstem sites. CNs V and VII–X can be affected by peripheral nerve problems, such as demyelinating disease (Guillain-Barré syndrome), neuropathies (diabetic), tumors, vascular infarcts, traumas, and other pathology; these nerve problems generally result in loss of the specific sensory modality carried by that nerve. Secondary sensory CN nuclei associated with the peripheral CNs (III–XII) include the trigeminal nuclei (main sensory, descending [spinal] nucleus), nucleus solitarius, cochlear nuclei (dorsal and ventral), and vestibular nuclei (medial, lateral, inferior, superior). These nuclei can be damaged by vascular infarcts, tumors, and other pathology; such pathology often involves other central nuclei and long tracts and produces syndromes that clearly indicate CNS pathology (e.g., UMN damage). Involvement of some secondary sensory cranial nerve nuclei (e.g., the descending nucleus of CN V damaged by a posterior inferior cerebellar artery infarct) results in a dissociated loss of a specific set of modalities (pain and temperature) in the innervated territory (ipsilateral face); a trigeminal nerve lesion on one side results in total anesthesia in the innervated territory.

Medial dissection

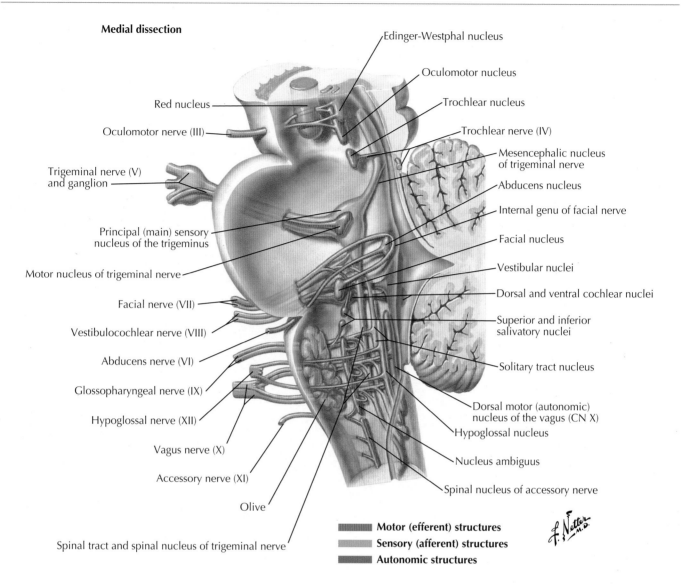

Edinger-Westphal nucleus

Oculomotor nucleus

Trochlear nucleus

Red nucleus

Oculomotor nerve (III)

Trochlear nerve (IV)

Mesencephalic nucleus of trigeminal nerve

Trigeminal nerve (V) and ganglion

Abducens nucleus

Internal genu of facial nerve

Principal (main) sensory nucleus of the trigeminus

Facial nucleus

Vestibular nuclei

Motor nucleus of trigeminal nerve

Dorsal and ventral cochlear nuclei

Facial nerve (VII)

Superior and inferior salivatory nuclei

Vestibulocochlear nerve (VIII)

Abducens nerve (VI)

Solitary tract nucleus

Glossopharyngeal nerve (IX)

Hypoglossal nerve (XII)

Dorsal motor (autonomic) nucleus of the vagus (CN X)

Hypoglossal nucleus

Vagus nerve (X)

Nucleus ambiguus

Accessory nerve (XI)

Spinal nucleus of accessory nerve

Olive

Spinal tract and spinal nucleus of trigeminal nerve

▬ Motor (efferent) structures
▬ Sensory (afferent) structures
▬ Autonomic structures

11.18 CRANIAL NERVES AND THEIR NUCLEI: SCHEMATIC LATERAL VIEW

CN III exits from the ventral and medial surface of the midbrain. CN IV is the only CN to exit from the dorsal surface of the brainstem, in the midbrain near the pons-midbrain junction. CN V exits from the lateral surface of the mid pons. CN VI exits from the pons medially, just rostral to the medullopontine junction. CNs VII and VIII exit from the cerebellopontine angle at the junction of the medulla and pons. CNs IX and X exit from the lateral part of the medulla and are joined by CN XI, which ascends through the foramen magnum. CN XII exits medially from the preolivary sulcus. These CN sites of entry and exit are important localizing features in the brainstem that permit regional localization of lesions resulting from vascular insults, tumors, and degenerative disorders.

CLINICAL POINT

The CN nuclei that contain LMNs are found in two longitudinal columns, including a medial column (CN nuclei III, IV, VI, and XII) and a lateral column (motor CN nuclei V, VII, and nucleus ambiguus). These LMN groups are found in the CNS and send axons into the peripheral nervous system to synapse on their appropriate groups of skeletal muscles using acetylcholine, and they exert important trophic influences on their innervated muscles. An **LMN lesion** (bulbar polio, amyotrophic lateral sclerosis, and other LMN palsies) results in total paralysis of the affected muscle; atrophy is caused by denervation, loss of tone, and loss of reflexes. Denervated muscles commonly demonstrate denervation hypersensitivity, with resultant fibrillation as seen on an electromyogram. As LMNs die (particularly conspicuous in amyotrophic lateral sclerosis), their agonal electrical responses occur as spontaneous discharges of individual motor units (an LMN and its innervated muscle fibers); each discharge produces a visible fasciculation (or twitch). With some LMN disorders such as polio, if enough neighboring LMNs survive, their axons can sprout and reinnervate previously denervated skeletal muscle fibers; this process must occur within approximately 1 year, or the atrophy becomes permanent. In UMN paralysis, in which the LMNs do not die, the affected muscle fibers are not denervated; reflexes are brisk, tone is increased with passive stretch (spasticity), and pathological reflexes (plantar extensor response) are seen.

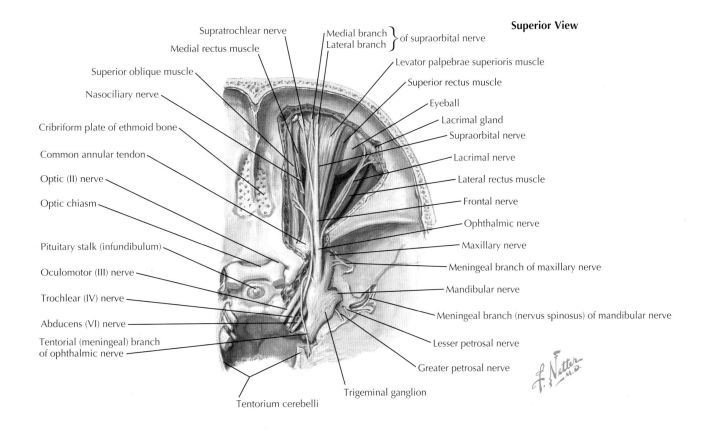

Superior View

Supratrochlear nerve

Medial rectus muscle

Medial branch ⎫
Lateral branch ⎭ of supraorbital nerve

Superior oblique muscle

Levator palpebrae superioris muscle

Nasociliary nerve

Superior rectus muscle

Eyeball

Cribriform plate of ethmoid bone

Lacrimal gland

Supraorbital nerve

Common annular tendon

Lacrimal nerve

Optic (II) nerve

Lateral rectus muscle

Optic chiasm

Frontal nerve

Ophthalmic nerve

Pituitary stalk (infundibulum)

Maxillary nerve

Oculomotor (III) nerve

Meningeal branch of maxillary nerve

Trochlear (IV) nerve

Mandibular nerve

Abducens (VI) nerve

Meningeal branch (nervus spinosus) of mandibular nerve

Tentorial (meningeal) branch
of ophthalmic nerve

Lesser petrosal nerve

Greater petrosal nerve

Tentorium cerebelli

Trigeminal ganglion

11.19 NERVES OF THE ORBIT

CN II carries visual information from the ipsilateral retina. Axons from the temporal hemiretinas remain ipsilateral, whereas axons from the nasal hemiretinas cross the midline in the optic chiasm. All axons then enter the optic tract. CNs III (from oculomotor nuclei), IV, and VI innervate the extrinsic muscles of the eye. Sensory portions of the ophthalmic division of V supply general sensation to the cornea and eyeball and provide the afferent limb of the corneal reflex. Motor fibers of CN VII innervate the orbicularis oculi muscle, closing the eye; these fibers constitute the efferent limb of the corneal reflex.

CLINICAL POINT

CN II (the optic nerve) is a CNS tract myelinated by oligodendroglia. It can be damaged by demyelinating disease (optic neuritis in multiple sclerosis), by optic nerve gliomas, by ischemic injury (central retinal artery), or by trauma (sphenoid fracture). The resultant defect is ipsilateral blindness or a scotoma (blind spot). The ipsilateral nature of the deficit rules out optic chiasm, optic tract, or central visual lesions. The retina also is CNS tissue and can undergo neurodegenerative changes. Macular degeneration involves damage to the cone-intensive regions of the retina (macula) and leads to the inability to read and the loss of acuity. Increased intracranial pressure can result in papilledema, a condition in which pressure pushes the optic nerve head inward (toward the center of the eyeball), producing a swollen appearance on ophthalmoscopy. This process takes 24 hours to occur after onset of intracranial pressure; the presence of papilledema is used diagnostically to identify increased intracranial pressure.

A. Superior view with extraocular muscles partially cut away

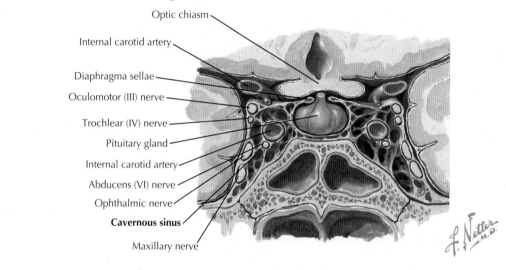

Supratrochlear nerve *(cut)*

Medial and lateral branches of supraorbital nerve *(cut)*

Infratrochlear nerve

Anterior ethmoidal nerve

Long ciliary nerves

Optic (II) nerve

Posterior ethmoidal nerve

Nasociliary nerve

Ophthalmic nerve

Trochlear (IV) nerve *(cut)*

Oculomotor (III) nerve

Abducens (VI) nerve

Levator palpebrae superioris muscle *(cut)*

Superior rectus muscle *(cut)*

Lacrimal nerve *(cut)*

Short ciliary nerves

Branch of oculomotor nerve to inferior oblique muscle

Ciliary ganglion

Motor (parasympathetic) root from oculomotor nerve

Sympathetic root from internal carotid plexus

Sensory root from nasociliary nerve

Branches to medial and inferior rectus muscles

Abducens (VI) nerve (to lateral rectus muscle)

Inferior division of oculomotor nerve

Superior division of oculomotor nerve

B. Coronal section through the cavernous sinus

Optic chiasm

Internal carotid artery

Diaphragma sellae

Oculomotor (III) nerve

Trochlear (IV) nerve

Pituitary gland

Internal carotid artery

Abducens (VI) nerve

Ophthalmic nerve

Cavernous sinus

Maxillary nerve

11.20 NERVES OF THE ORBIT (CONTINUED)

Parasympathetic preganglionic fibers from the nucleus of Edinger-Westphal distribute to the ciliary ganglion, which supplies the pupillary constrictor muscle and the ciliary muscle (accommodation for near vision). Preganglionic parasympathetic axons from the superior salivatory nucleus distribute to the pterygopalatine ganglion, which supplies the lacrimal glands (tear production). Sympathetic postganglionic nerve fibers from the superior cervical ganglion supply the pupillary dilator muscle and the superior tarsal muscle (damage results in mild ptosis). CNs III, IV, VI, and V (ophthalmic and maxillary divisions) traverse the cavernous sinus and are vulnerable to damage by cavernous sinus thrombosis.

CLINICAL POINT

The extraocular nerves can be damaged by trauma, vascular infarcts, tumors, aneurysms, pressure (compression of CN III against the free edge of the tentorium with transtentorial herniation), or other pathology. Oculomotor palsy (CN III) results in paralysis or weakness of the medial rectus, superior and inferior rectus, inferior oblique, and levator palpebrae superioris muscles. The most conspicuous deficit is the inability to adduct the ipsilateral eye, a lateral strabismus (resulting from unopposed action of the lateral rectus), and diplopia. Damage to the levator palpebrae superioris muscle results in profound ptosis of the ipsilateral eye. Lesions in CN III also disrupt the outflow from the Edinger-Westphal nucleus to the ciliary ganglion, producing a fixed (unresponsive) and dilated ipsilateral pupil.

A lesion in CN IV (trochlear) results in paralysis or weakness of the superior oblique muscle. This muscle is a depressor of the eye when it is directed nasally. Thus, a patient has difficulty walking down stairs and stepping off curbs and has trouble reading while lying down. The patient tries to compensate for a lesion in CN IV by turning the head away from the side of the lesion to avoid having to use the paralyzed muscle.

A lesion in CN VI (abducens) results in paralysis or weakness of the ipsilateral lateral rectus muscle, with a resultant medial strabismus and diplopia upon attempted lateral gaze.

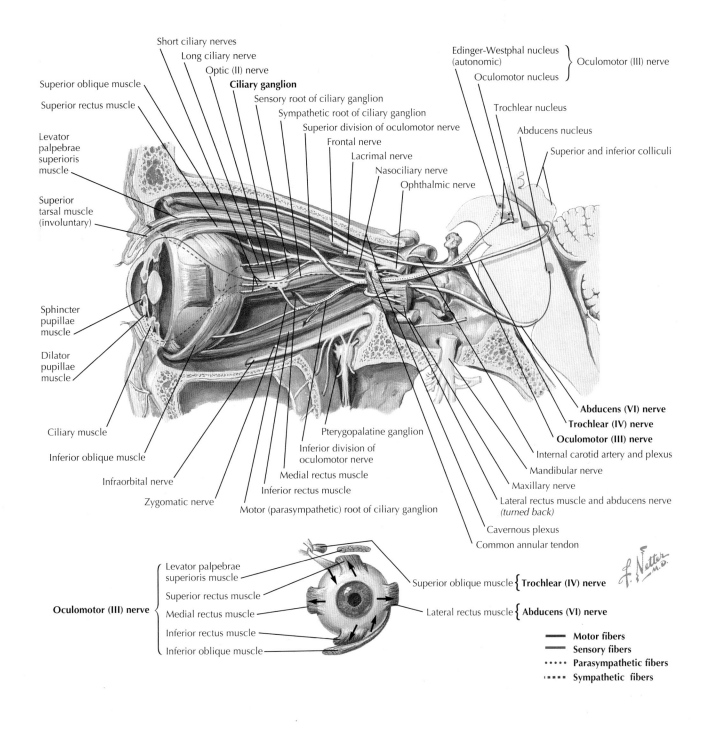

Short ciliary nerves
Long ciliary nerve
Optic (II) nerve
Ciliary ganglion
Sensory root of ciliary ganglion
Sympathetic root of ciliary ganglion
Superior division of oculomotor nerve
Frontal nerve
Lacrimal nerve
Nasociliary nerve
Ophthalmic nerve

Edinger-Westphal nucleus
(autonomic)
Oculomotor nucleus
} Oculomotor (III) nerve

Trochlear nucleus
Abducens nucleus
Superior and inferior colliculi

Superior oblique muscle
Superior rectus muscle
Levator palpebrae superioris muscle
Superior tarsal muscle (involuntary)
Sphincter pupillae muscle
Dilator pupillae muscle
Ciliary muscle
Inferior oblique muscle
Infraorbital nerve
Zygomatic nerve
Motor (parasympathetic) root of ciliary ganglion
Inferior rectus muscle
Medial rectus muscle
Inferior division of oculomotor nerve
Pterygopalatine ganglion

Abducens (VI) nerve
Trochlear (IV) nerve
Oculomotor (III) nerve
Internal carotid artery and plexus
Mandibular nerve
Maxillary nerve
Lateral rectus muscle and abducens nerve *(turned back)*
Cavernous plexus
Common annular tendon

Oculomotor (III) nerve {
Levator palpebrae superioris muscle
Superior rectus muscle
Medial rectus muscle
Inferior rectus muscle
Inferior oblique muscle

Superior oblique muscle { **Trochlear (IV) nerve**
Lateral rectus muscle { **Abducens (VI) nerve**

— Motor fibers
— Sensory fibers
···· Parasympathetic fibers
▪▪▪▪ Sympathetic fibers

11.21 EXTRAOCULAR NERVES (III, IV, AND VI) AND THE CILIARY GANGLION: VIEW IN RELATION TO THE EYE

CN VI innervates the lateral rectus muscle; damage results in ipsilateral paralysis of lateral gaze. CN IV innervates the superior oblique muscle; damage results in inability to look in and down (most conspicuous when climbing stairs, stepping off a curb, reading in bed). CN III (oculomotor nuclei) innervates the medial rectus, superior rectus, inferior rectus, and inferior oblique muscles (damage results in paralysis of the ipsilateral medial gaze) and also innervates the levator palpebrae superioris muscle (damage results in profound ptosis). The ciliary ganglion gives rise to postganglionic parasympathetic axons that supply the pupillary constrictor muscle and the ciliary muscle; damage results in a fixed and dilated pupil that does not constrict for the pupillary light reflex and does not accommodate to near vision.

Motor fibers
Sensory fibers
· · · · Proprioceptive fibers
· · · · Parasympathetic fibers
- - - - Sympathetic fibers

Ophthalmic nerve
Tentorial (meningeal) branch
Nasociliary nerve
Sensory root of ciliary ganglion
Lacrimal nerve
Frontal nerve
Ciliary ganglion
Posterior ethmoidal nerve
Long ciliary nerve
Short ciliary nerves
Supratrochlear nerve
Supraorbital nerve (medial and lateral branches)
Anterior ethmoidal nerve
Infratrochlear nerve
External nasal and internal nasal (medial and lateral rami) branches of anterior ethmoidal nerve

Maxillary nerve
Meningeal branch
Zygomaticotemporal nerve
Zygomaticofacial nerve
Zygomatic nerve
Infraorbital nerve
Ganglionic branches and pterygopalatine ganglion
Superior alveolar branches (anterior, middle, posterior) of infraorbital nerve
Nasal branches (postero-superior lateral, nasopalatine and posterosuperior medial)
Nerve of pterygoid canal
Pharyngeal branch
Palatine nerves; major (anterior), minor (middle and posterior)
Deep temporal nerves (anterior, middle, and posterior) to temporalis muscle
Lateral pterygoid and masseteric nerves
Buccal nerve
Mental nerve
Tensor veli palatini and medial pterygoid nerves

Trigeminal (V) nerve and trigeminal (semilunar) ganglion
Motor nucleus of trigeminal nerve
Mesencephalic nucleus of trigeminal nerve (proprioception)
Principal sensory nucleus of trigeminal nerve (discriminatory sensation)
Spinal tract and spinal nucleus of trigeminal nerve (pain and temperature)

Facial (VII) nerve
Chorda tympani
Superficial temporal branches
Articular and auricular branches
Auriculotemporal nerve
Parotid branches
Meningeal (nervus spinosus) branch
Lesser petrosal nerve (from glossopharyngeal nerve)
Tensor tympani nerve
Otic ganglion
Inferior alveolar nerve
Mylohyoid nerve (to mylohyoid and anterior belly of digastric muscles)

Lingual nerve
Submandibular ganglion
Mandibular nerve

Inferior dental plexus (inferior dental and gingival nerves)

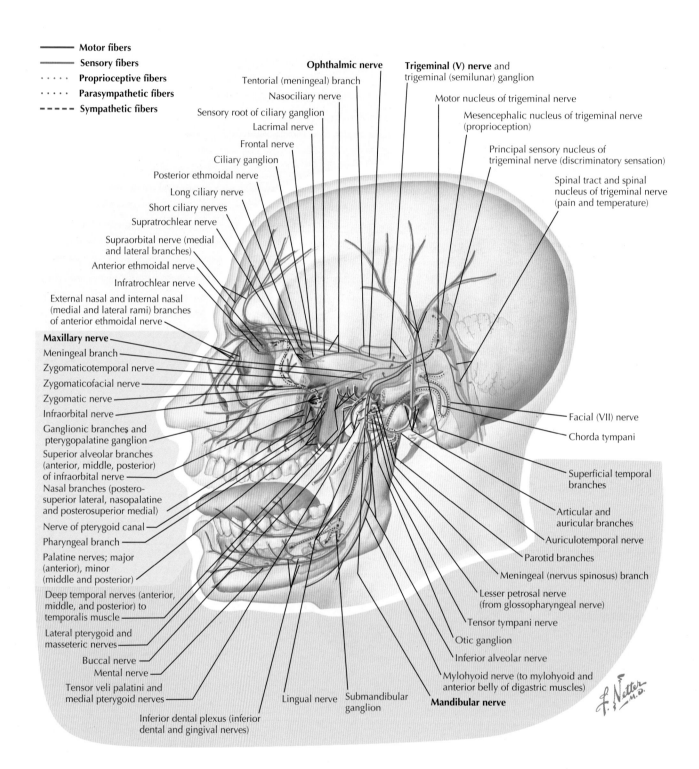

11.22 TRIGEMINAL NERVE (V)

See next page.

11.22 TRIGEMINAL NERVE (V)

The trigeminal nerve (CN V) carries sensory information from the face, sinuses, teeth, and anterior portion of the oral cavity. It has three subdivisions: (1) ophthalmic—sensory innervation, (2) maxillary—sensory innervation, and (3) mandibular—sensory innervation and motor innervation of the masticatory muscles and tensor tympani muscles. Each of the subdivisions has a distinct distribution and sharp boundaries. Unlike the somatosensory dermatomes, which exhibit considerable overlap with nerve fibers of adjacent roots, the trigeminal subdivisions show no overlap at all. Damage to one of the subdivisions results in total anesthesia in the territory of sensory distribution.

Primary sensory axons from trigeminal (semilunar, gasserian) ganglion cells that process fine, discriminative touch (epicritic sensation) terminate in the main sensory nucleus of CN V and the rostral portion of the descending (spinal) nucleus of CN V. Axons that process pain and temperature sensation (protopathic sensation) terminate in the caudal and middle regions of the descending (spinal) nucleus of CN V. The trigeminal nerve also carries proprioceptive information from muscle spindles in muscles of mastication and extraocular muscles. Those primary sensory cell bodies are found in the mesencephalic nucleus of CN V within the CNS, the only example of primary sensory neurons residing in the CNS.

CLINICAL POINT

Trigeminal neuralgia (tic douloureux) involves sudden, brief (lasting less than a minute), excruciating paroxysms of pain, sometimes described as stabbing or lancinating, usually in the territory of one of the divisions of the trigeminal nerve. The maxillary and mandibular divisions are more common targets than the ophthalmic division, and the disorder is more common in older individuals. These episodes of pain may recur several times a day, with paroxysms experienced for weeks on end. Often there is a trigger point, at which mild stimuli such as light touch, chewing, or even talking can provoke an attack. During an attack, no loss of sensation occurs in the distribution of the affected branch. Trigeminal neuralgia can be idiopathic or symptomatic of other disorders. In some cases, compression of the trigeminal nerve root by a small aberrant branch of the superior cerebellar artery or another nearby artery is the suspected cause; in other cases a tumor, an inflammation, or a demyelinating plaque may precipitate such attacks. If trigeminal neuralgia occurs in the accompaniment of other progressive pathology, the neurological examination reveals sensory and motor deficits associated with the involved branch of the trigeminal nerve. Idiopathic trigeminal neuralgia usually can be treated with carbamazepine or other antiseizure and membrane-stabilizing agents, which sometimes permits the condition to regress. Surgical decompression of a compressing blood vessel may help. In other cases, the nerve root is ablated temporarily or permanently; the resultant functional deficit is often better tolerated than the excruciating paroxysms of pain.

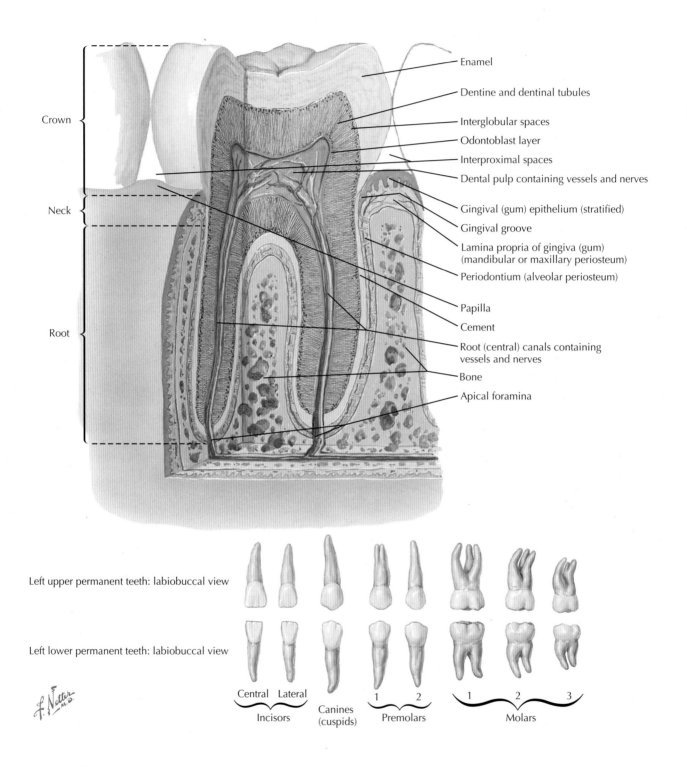

Crown

Neck

Root

Enamel

Dentine and dentinal tubules

Interglobular spaces

Odontoblast layer

Interproximal spaces

Dental pulp containing vessels and nerves

Gingival (gum) epithelium (stratified)

Gingival groove

Lamina propria of gingiva (gum) (mandibular or maxillary periosteum)

Periodontium (alveolar periosteum)

Papilla

Cement

Root (central) canals containing vessels and nerves

Bone

Apical foramina

Left upper permanent teeth: labiobuccal view

Left lower permanent teeth: labiobuccal view

Central   Lateral

Incisors

Canines (cuspids)

1   2

Premolars

1   2   3

Molars

11.23 INNERVATION OF THE TEETH

Sensory nerve fibers of the maxillary (upper teeth) and mandibular (lower teeth) subdivisions of the trigeminal nerve innervate the dental pulp of the teeth. With erosion of a lesion (decay) into the dental pulp or close to the dental pulp, these nerve fibers may become exquisitely sensitive to temperature changes (especially cold) or pressure (by edema or mechanical force), resulting in the sensation of severe pain.

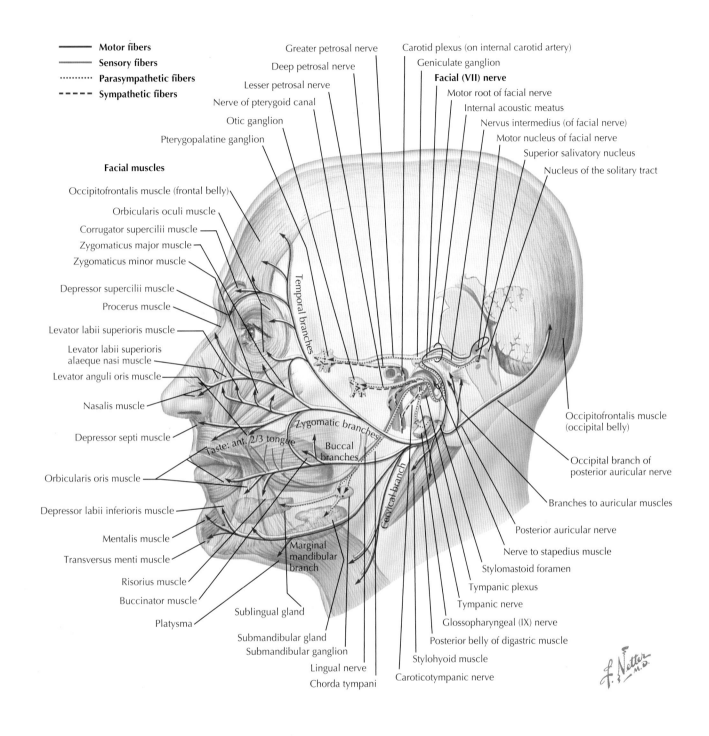

Motor fibers
Sensory fibers
Parasympathetic fibers
Sympathetic fibers

Greater petrosal nerve
Deep petrosal nerve
Lesser petrosal nerve
Nerve of pterygoid canal
Otic ganglion
Pterygopalatine ganglion

Carotid plexus (on internal carotid artery)
Geniculate ganglion
Facial (VII) nerve
Motor root of facial nerve
Internal acoustic meatus
Nervus intermedius (of facial nerve)
Motor nucleus of facial nerve
Superior salivatory nucleus
Nucleus of the solitary tract

Facial muscles
Occipitofrontalis muscle (frontal belly)
Orbicularis oculi muscle
Corrugator supercilii muscle
Zygomaticus major muscle
Zygomaticus minor muscle
Depressor supercilii muscle
Procerus muscle
Levator labii superioris muscle
Levator labii superioris alaeque nasi muscle
Levator anguli oris muscle
Nasalis muscle
Depressor septi muscle
Orbicularis oris muscle
Depressor labii inferioris muscle
Mentalis muscle
Transversus menti muscle
Risorius muscle
Buccinator muscle
Platysma

Temporal branches
Taste: ant. 2/3 tongue
Zygomatic branches
Buccal branches
Cervical branch
Marginal mandibular branch

Sublingual gland
Submandibular gland
Submandibular ganglion
Lingual nerve
Chorda tympani

Occipitofrontalis muscle (occipital belly)
Occipital branch of posterior auricular nerve
Branches to auricular muscles
Posterior auricular nerve
Nerve to stapedius muscle
Stylomastoid foramen
Tympanic plexus
Tympanic nerve
Glossopharyngeal (IX) nerve
Posterior belly of digastric muscle
Stylohyoid muscle
Caroticotympanic nerve

11.24 FACIAL NERVE (VII)

The facial nerve (VII) is a mixed nerve with motor, parasympathetic, and sensory components. The motor fibers distribute to the muscles of facial expression, including the scalp, the auricle, the buccinator, the stapedius, and the stylohyoid muscles, and to the posterior belly of the digastric muscle. Damage results in ipsilateral paralysis of facial expression, including the forehead (Bell's palsy); facial palsy caused by central corticobulbar lesions spare the upper face. Activation of the stapedius muscle dampens the ossicles in the presence of sustained loud noise; damage to CN VII results in hyperacusis. Parasympathetic nerve fibers of CN VII from the superior salivatory nucleus distribute to the pterygopalatine ganglion, which innervates the lacrimal glands, and to the submandibular ganglion, which innervates the submandibular and sublingual salivary glands. Special sensory taste fibers from the anterior two-thirds of the tongue (via the chorda tympani) and the soft palate (via the greater petrosal nerve), whose primary sensory cell bodies are located in the geniculate ganglion, convey that information to the rostral portion of nucleus solitarius in the medulla.

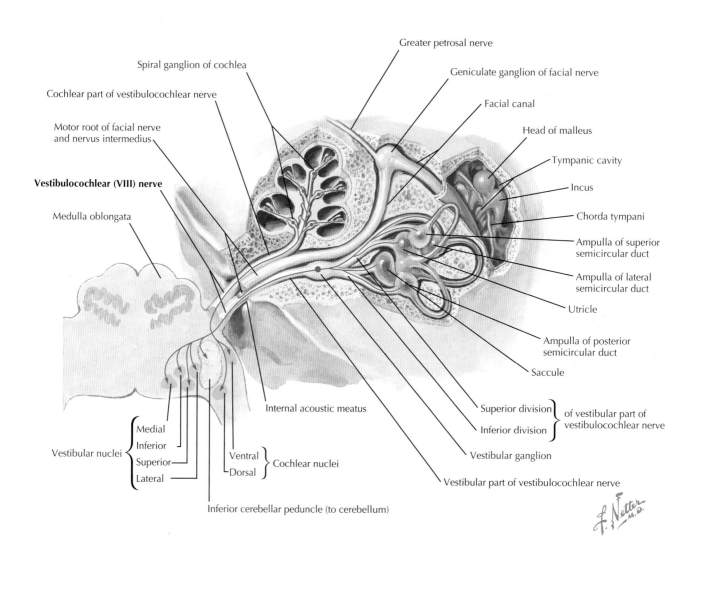

Greater petrosal nerve

Geniculate ganglion of facial nerve

Facial canal

Head of malleus

Spiral ganglion of cochlea

Tympanic cavity

Cochlear part of vestibulocochlear nerve

Incus

Motor root of facial nerve
and nervus intermedius

Chorda tympani

Vestibulocochlear (VIII) nerve

Ampulla of superior
semicircular duct

Medulla oblongata

Ampulla of lateral
semicircular duct

Utricle

Ampulla of posterior
semicircular duct

Saccule

Internal acoustic meatus

Superior division } of vestibular part of
vestibulocochlear nerve

Inferior division }

Medial
Inferior
Superior
Lateral

Vestibular nuclei

Ventral } Cochlear nuclei
Dorsal }

Vestibular ganglion

Vestibular part of vestibulocochlear nerve

Inferior cerebellar peduncle (to cerebellum)

11.27 VESTIBULOCOCHLEAR NERVE (VIII)

The vestibulocochlear nerve (CN VIII) arises from bipolar primary sensory neurons in the vestibular ganglion (Scarpa's ganglion) and the spiral (cochlear) ganglion. The peripheral process of the vestibular ganglion neurons innervates hair cells in the utricle and saccule that respond to linear acceleration (gravity) and in the ampullae of the semicircular ducts that respond to angular acceleration (movement). The utricle, the saccule, and the semicircular ducts provide neural signals for coordination and equilibration of position and for movement of the head and neck. The central processes of the vestibular ganglion cells terminate in vestibular nuclei (medial, lateral, superior, and inferior) in the medulla and pons and in the cerebellum. The peripheral processes of spiral ganglion cells innervate hair cells that lie along the cochlear duct in the organ of Corti. They convey hearing information via central axonal processes into the cochlear nuclei (dorsal and ventral). A lesion in CN VIII results in ipsilateral deafness, vertigo, and loss of equilibrium.

CLINICAL POINT

The vestibulocochlear nerve emerges from the ventrolateral margin of the brainstem near the junction of the medulla, pons, and cerebellum (the cerebellopontine angle). At this site, Schwann cell tumors of CN VIII, **acoustic schwannomas**, can arise, usually from the vestibular portion of CN VIII. Initial irritation of the vestibular division of CN VIII can result in vertigo, dizziness, nausea, and unsteadiness or spatial disorientation. These symptoms persist with nerve destruction. Initial irritation of the auditory division of CN VIII by a schwannoma may first produce tinnitus, followed by slow loss of hearing and the inability to determine the direction from which a sound is coming. As nerve destruction occurs, tinnitus diminishes and ipsilateral deafness ensues. Because of the proximity of CNs VII and VIII, acoustic schwannomas also often produce ipsilateral facial paralysis or palsy. The tumor may extend rostrally to the trigeminal nerve or caudally to the glossopharyngeal and vagus nerves and also may affect the adjacent brainstem and cerebellum. At this point, hydrocephalus and increased intracranial pressure can occur.

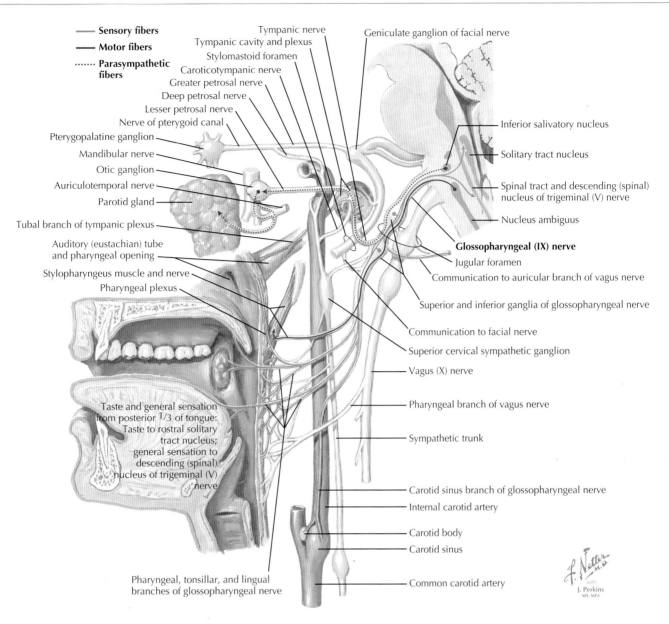

Sensory fibers
Motor fibers
Parasympathetic fibers

Tympanic nerve
Tympanic cavity and plexus
Stylomastoid foramen
Caroticotympanic nerve
Greater petrosal nerve
Deep petrosal nerve
Lesser petrosal nerve
Nerve of pterygoid canal
Pterygopalatine ganglion
Mandibular nerve
Otic ganglion
Auriculotemporal nerve
Parotid gland
Tubal branch of tympanic plexus
Auditory (eustachian) tube and pharyngeal opening
Stylopharyngeus muscle and nerve
Pharyngeal plexus

Geniculate ganglion of facial nerve
Inferior salivatory nucleus
Solitary tract nucleus
Spinal tract and descending (spinal) nucleus of trigeminal (V) nerve
Nucleus ambiguus
Glossopharyngeal (IX) nerve
Jugular foramen
Communication to auricular branch of vagus nerve
Superior and inferior ganglia of glossopharyngeal nerve
Communication to facial nerve
Superior cervical sympathetic ganglion
Vagus (X) nerve
Pharyngeal branch of vagus nerve
Sympathetic trunk
Carotid sinus branch of glossopharyngeal nerve
Internal carotid artery
Carotid body
Carotid sinus
Common carotid artery

Taste and general sensation from posterior 1/3 of tongue: Taste to rostral solitary tract nucleus; general sensation to descending (spinal) nucleus of trigeminal (V) nerve

Pharyngeal, tonsillar, and lingual branches of glossopharyngeal nerve

11.28 GLOSSOPHARYNGEAL NERVE (IX)

CN IX is a mixed nerve with motor, parasympathetic, and sensory components. Motor fibers from the nucleus ambiguus supply the stylopharyngeus muscle and may assist in the innervation of pharyngeal muscles for swallowing. Preganglionic parasympathetic axons from the inferior salivatory nucleus travel with CN IX to the otic ganglion, whose neurons innervate the parotid and mucous glands. Special sensory axons from the petrosal (inferior) ganglion carry information from taste buds on the posterior one-third of the tongue (including numerous taste buds in the vallate papillae) and part of the soft palate. These axons terminate in the rostral portion of nucleus solitarius. Axons from additional primary sensory neurons in the inferior ganglion also carry general sensation from the posterior one-third of the tongue and from the pharynx, the fauces, the tonsils, the tympanic cavity, the eustachian tube, and the mastoid cells. The central axon branches terminate in the descending (spinal) nucleus of CN V. The general sensory fibers from the pharynx provide the afferent limb of the gag reflex. Additional primary sensory neurons innervate the

carotid body (chemoreception of carbon dioxide) and the carotid sinus (baroceptors) and convey their central axons to the caudal nucleus solitarius (solitary tract nucleus). Primary sensory neurons in the superior ganglion innervate a small region behind the ear and convey general sensation into the descending nucleus of CN V.

CLINICAL POINT

The glossopharyngeal nerve can be affected by brief, excruciating paroxysms of pain (glossopharyngeal neuralgia) similar to those experienced in trigeminal neuralgia. The pain originates in the throat (tonsillar fossa) or sometimes the jaw and radiates to the ear. Some patients experience pain in the tongue, face, or jaw. The triggering activity is usually swallowing, coughing, sneezing, or yawning. If the irritative process activates glossopharyngeal afferents associated with brainstem vasomotor responses, the patient may experience bradycardia and syncope. The treatment of glossopharyngeal neuralgia is similar to treatment of trigeminal neuralgia. Successful treatment also has occurred surgically through decompression of a tortuous aberrant vessel.

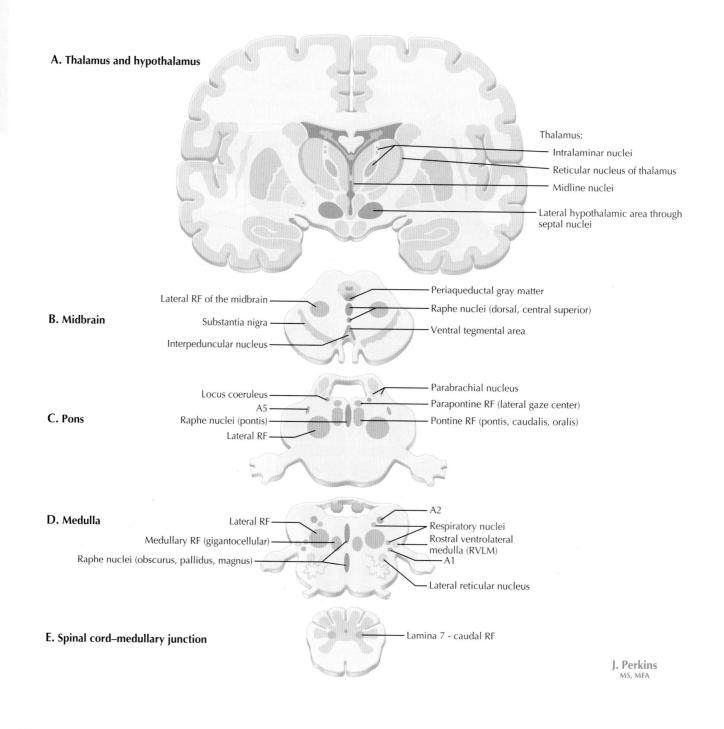

A. Thalamus and hypothalamus

Thalamus:
- Intralaminar nuclei
- Reticular nucleus of thalamus
- Midline nuclei
- Lateral hypothalamic area through septal nuclei

B. Midbrain

Lateral RF of the midbrain
Substantia nigra
Interpeduncular nucleus

Periaqueductal gray matter
Raphe nuclei (dorsal, central superior)
Ventral tegmental area

C. Pons

Locus coeruleus
A5
Raphe nuclei (pontis)
Lateral RF

Parabrachial nucleus
Parapontine RF (lateral gaze center)
Pontine RF (pontis, caudalis, oralis)

D. Medulla

Lateral RF
Medullary RF (gigantocellular)
Raphe nuclei (obscurus, pallidus, magnus)

A2
Respiratory nuclei
Rostral ventrolateral medulla (RVLM)
A1
Lateral reticular nucleus

E. Spinal cord–medullary junction

Lamina 7 - caudal RF

J. Perkins
MS, MFA

11.33 RETICULAR FORMATION: NUCLEI AND AREAS IN THE BRAINSTEM AND DIENCEPHALON

Many of the named nuclei of the RF are present in the medulla, the pons, and the midbrain. Important medial RF groups include the medullary (gigantocellular) and the pontine (caudal and rostral) RF regions, which are involved in reticulospinal regulation of spinal cord LMNs, and the parapontine RF, also known as the horizontal (lateral) gaze center. Lateral RF areas and nuclei (such as the lateral reticular nucleus) are involved in polymodal sensory functions. RF respiratory and cardiovascular neurons are found in the medulla. Catecholaminergic neurons are found in the locus coeruleus (group A6) and tegmental groups denoted here as groups A1, A2, and A5 (norepinephrine-containing neurons). Raphe nuclei are found in the midline and in wings of cells that extend laterally. The core of the RF continues rostrally from the lateral regions of the brainstem into the lateral hypothalamic area and extends through the hypothalamus to the septal nuclei. Several thalamic nuclei (intralaminar, midline, and reticular nucleus of the thalamus) also are classified as part of the RF.

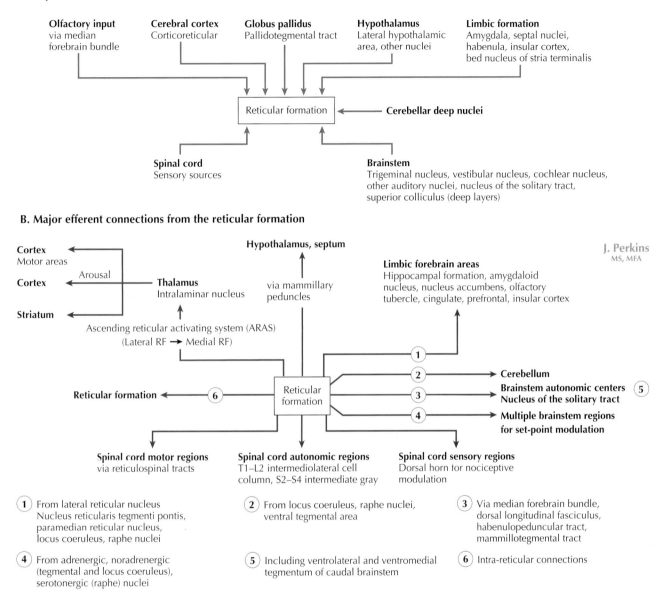

A. Major afferent connections to the reticular formation

Olfactory input
via median
forebrain bundle

Cerebral cortex
Corticoreticular

Globus pallidus
Pallidotegmental tract

Hypothalamus
Lateral hypothalamic
area, other nuclei

Limbic formation
Amygdala, septal nuclei,
habenula, insular cortex,
bed nucleus of stria terminalis

Reticular formation ← **Cerebellar deep nuclei**

Spinal cord
Sensory sources

Brainstem
Trigeminal nucleus, vestibular nucleus, cochlear nucleus,
other auditory nuclei, nucleus of the solitary tract,
superior colliculus (deep layers)

B. Major efferent connections from the reticular formation

Cortex
Motor areas

Arousal

Cortex

Striatum

Thalamus
Intralaminar nucleus

Hypothalamus, septum

via mammillary
peduncles

J. Perkins
MS, MFA

Limbic forebrain areas
Hippocampal formation, amygdaloid
nucleus, nucleus accumbens, olfactory
tubercle, cingulate, prefrontal, insular cortex

Ascending reticular activating system (ARAS)
(Lateral RF → Medial RF)

Reticular formation ← ⑥

Reticular formation

①
② → **Cerebellum**
③ → **Brainstem autonomic centers** ⑤
Nucleus of the solitary tract
④ → **Multiple brainstem regions
for set-point modulation**

Spinal cord motor regions
via reticulospinal tracts

Spinal cord autonomic regions
T1–L2 intermediolateral cell
column, S2–S4 intermediate gray

Spinal cord sensory regions
Dorsal horn for nociceptive
modulation

① From lateral reticular nucleus
Nucleus reticularis tegmenti pontis,
paramedian reticular nucleus,
locus coeruleus, raphe nuclei

② From locus coeruleus, raphe nuclei,
ventral tegmental area

③ Via median forebrain bundle,
dorsal longitudinal fasciculus,
habenulopeduncular tract,
mammillotegmental tract

④ From adrenergic, noradrenergic
(tegmental and locus coeruleus),
serotonergic (raphe) nuclei

⑤ Including ventrolateral and ventromedial
tegmentum of caudal brainstem

⑥ Intra-reticular connections

11.34 MAJOR AFFERENT AND EFFERENT CONNECTIONS TO THE RETICULAR FORMATION

A, Extensive sensory information from spinal cord somatosensory sources (particularly nociceptive information) and from virtually all brainstem sensory modalities is sent to the lateral regions of the RF. Olfactory input arrives through olfactory tract projections into forebrain regions. Many limbic and hypothalamic structures provide input into the RF, particularly for visceral and autonomic regulatory functions. The cerebral cortex, the globus pallidus, and the cerebellum also provide input into the RF medial zones involved in motor regulation. **B,** The ascending reticular activating system (ARAS) of the RF is responsible for consciousness and arousal.

It projects through nonspecific nuclei of the thalamus to the cerebral cortex; lesions in this area lead to coma. The RF sends extensive axonal projections to sensory, motor, and autonomic regions of the spinal cord, modulating nociceptive input, preganglionic autonomic outflow, and LMN outflow, respectively. The RF sends extensive connections to brainstem nuclei (such as nucleus tractus solitarius) and to autonomic regulatory centers and nuclei for modulation of visceral functions. Efferent RF projections to the hypothalamus, septal nuclei, and limbic forebrain areas help to modulate visceral autonomic functions, neuroendocrine outflow, and emotional responsiveness and behavior. Efferent RF projections to the cerebellum and basal ganglia participate in modulating UMN control of LMNs.

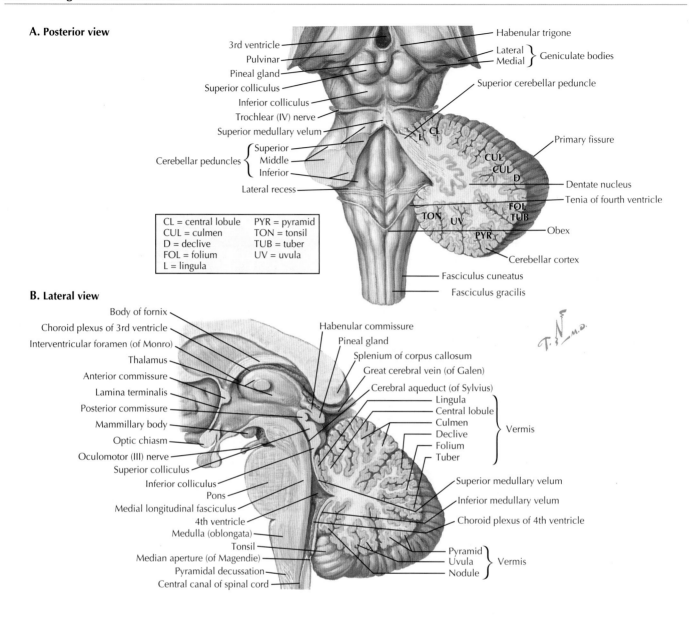

A. Posterior view

Habenular trigone
3rd ventricle
Pulvinar
Pineal gland
Lateral
Medial — Geniculate bodies
Superior colliculus
Superior cerebellar peduncle
Inferior colliculus
Trochlear (IV) nerve
Superior medullary velum
Primary fissure
Superior
Cerebellar peduncles — Middle
Inferior
CUL
CUL
D
Dentate nucleus
Lateral recess
Tenia of fourth ventricle
FOL
TUB
TON
UV
Obex
PYR
Cerebellar cortex
Fasciculus cuneatus
Fasciculus gracilis

CL = central lobule | PYR = pyramid
CUL = culmen | TON = tonsil
D = declive | TUB = tuber
FOL = folium | UV = uvula
L = lingula

B. Lateral view
Body of fornix
Choroid plexus of 3rd ventricle
Interventricular foramen (of Monro)
Thalamus
Anterior commissure
Lamina terminalis
Posterior commissure
Mammillary body
Optic chiasm
Oculomotor (III) nerve
Superior colliculus
Inferior colliculus
Pons
Medial longitudinal fasciculus
4th ventricle
Medulla (oblongata)
Tonsil
Median aperture (of Magendie)
Pyramidal decussation
Central canal of spinal cord

Habenular commissure
Pineal gland
Splenium of corpus callosum
Great cerebral vein (of Galen)
Cerebral aqueduct (of Sylvius)
Lingula
Central lobule
Culmen
Declive — Vermis
Folium
Tuber
Superior medullary velum
Inferior medullary velum
Choroid plexus of 4th ventricle
Pyramid
Uvula — Vermis
Nodule

11.37 CEREBELLAR ANATOMY: LOBULES

A, Posterior view. In this horizontal (axial) section through the right cerebellar hemisphere, the left hemisphere has been removed, the cerebellar peduncles cut, and the fourth ventricle opened to show the dorsal surface of the brainstem below. The cerebellar cortex is organized into 10 lobules. The cerebellar peduncles provide the large white matter regions through which afferents and efferents pass, connecting the cerebellum with the brainstem and diencephalon. **B,** Lateral view. The lobules of the cerebellum are shown in midsagittal section. Inputs into the cerebellar hemispheres show a similar general organization, with variation from lobule to lobule, particularly for noradrenergic inputs from the locus coeruleus. Inputs from a vast majority of nuclei projecting to the cerebellar hemispheres arrive as mossy fibers; the inferior olivary nucleus sends climbing fibers to end on Purkinje cell dendrites in the cerebellar hemispheres, and the locus coeruleus sends diffuse varicose inputs into all three layers of many regions of the cerebellar cortex. The deep nuclei provide the "coarse adjustment" upon which is superimposed the "fine adjustment" by the cerebellar cortex. The cerebellar cortex sends its output via Purkinje cell projections, using GABA as the principal neurotransmitter, to deep nuclei, which in turn project to UMNs.

CLINICAL POINT
Cerebellar tumors commonly start in a specific region of the cerebellum. **Cerebellar medulloblastomas** are childhood malignant tumors that often begin in the flocculonodular lobe and are detected initially because of truncal ataxia and a broad-based uncoordinated gait. However, as the tumor slowly grows, it involves additional areas of the cerebellum by means of pressure or by invading neighboring areas. Then, in addition to the truncal ataxia, additional limb ataxia, dysmetria, dysdiadochokinesia, intention tremor, hypotonia, and other characteristics of lateral cerebellar damage are seen. Because the posterior fossa is involved, and not supratentorial regions, papilledema does not occur and does not provide a clue for diagnosis; rather, the increased posterior fossa pressure results in occipital headaches with nausea, vomiting, and nystagmus. The two most common cerebellar tumors of childhood are medulloblastomas, which can spread to adjacent portions of the CNS, and astrocytomas, which commonly are not highly invasive in the cerebellum but do grow as space-occupying masses.

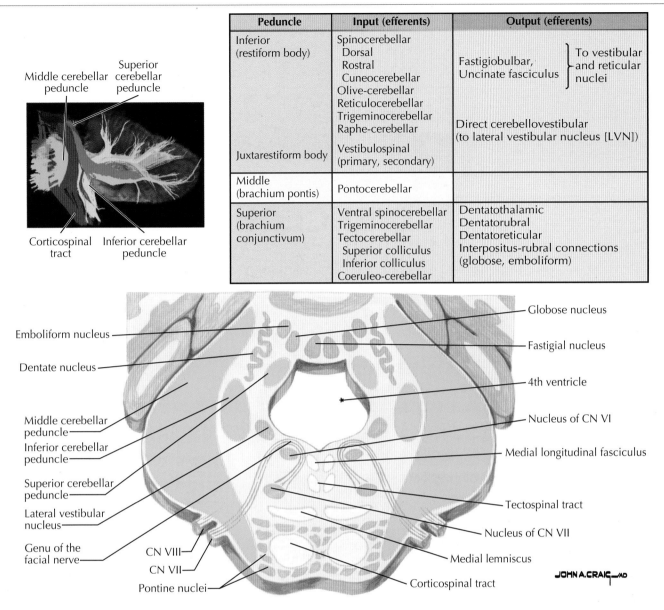

Peduncle	Input (efferents)	Output (efferents)	

Inferior (restiform body)	Spinocerebellar
	  Dorsal
	  Rostral
	  Cuneocerebellar
	Olive-cerebellar
	Reticulocerebellar
	Trigeminocerebellar
	Raphe-cerebellar
		Fastigiobulbar,
		Uncinate fasciculus
			To vestibular and reticular nuclei

Juxtarestiform body	Vestibulospinal (primary, secondary)	Direct cerebellovestibular (to lateral vestibular nucleus [LVN])	
Middle (brachium pontis)	Pontocerebellar		

Superior (brachium conjunctivum)	Ventral spinocerebellar
	Trigeminocerebellar
	Tectocerebellar
	  Superior colliculus
	  Inferior colliculus
	Coeruleo-cerebellar
		Dentatothalamic
		Dentatorubral
		Dentatoreticular
		Interpositus-rubral connections (globose, emboliform)	

11.38 CEREBELLAR ANATOMY: DEEP NUCLEI AND CEREBELLAR PEDUNCLES

The deep cerebellar nuclei are found at the roof of the fourth ventricle in a cross-sectional view of the pons at the level of cranial motor nuclei for CNs VI and VII. The fastigial nucleus receives input from the vermis and sends projections to reticular and vestibular nuclei, the cells of origin of the reticulospinal and vestibulospinal tracts. Some vermal and flocculonodular Purkinje cells project directly to the lateral vestibular nuclei, which some authors consider to be a fifth deep cerebellar nucleus; this nucleus also is the UMN cell group for the vestibulospinal tract. The globose and emboliform nuclei receive input from the paravermis and project to the red nucleus, the cells of origin for the rubrospinal tract. The dentate nucleus receives input from the lateral hemispheres and projects to the ventrolateral and ventral anterior nuclei of the thalamus; these thalamic nuclei project to the cells of origin of the corticospinal and corticobulbar tracts. All three cerebellar peduncles can be seen in this cross-section. The table lists the major afferent and efferent projections through the three cerebellar peduncles and are depicted by color.

CLINICAL POINT

The inferior cerebellar peduncle conveys many afferents to the cerebellum from the spinocerebellar system, reticular formation, vestibular system, and trigeminal system, and it conveys efferents from the fastigial nucleus and flocculonodular lobe to vestibulospinal and reticulospinal UMN systems. The middle cerebellar peduncle mainly conveys afferents to the cerebellum from the cortico-ponto-cerebellar system. The superior cerebellar peduncle conveys selective afferents to the cerebellum and carries extensive efferents from the globose, emboliform, and dentate nuclei to the red nucleus and ventrolateral thalamus for regulation of the rubrospinal and corticospinal UMN systems. An infarct in the superior cerebellar artery can damage the blood supply to the superior and middle peduncles and the deep nuclei on one side. Lesions in these structures commonly have longer lasting and more severe clinical effects than lesions that affect only the cerebellar cortex. A superior cerebellar artery infarct can result in ipsilateral limb ataxia, dysmetria, dysdiadochokinesia, intention tremor, hypotonus, and other characteristics of lateral cerebellar damage. In addition, some midbrain structures are supplied by this artery; an infarct causes added brainstem problems, such as nystagmus and eye movement problems.

12

DIENCEPHALON

Thalamocortical radiations

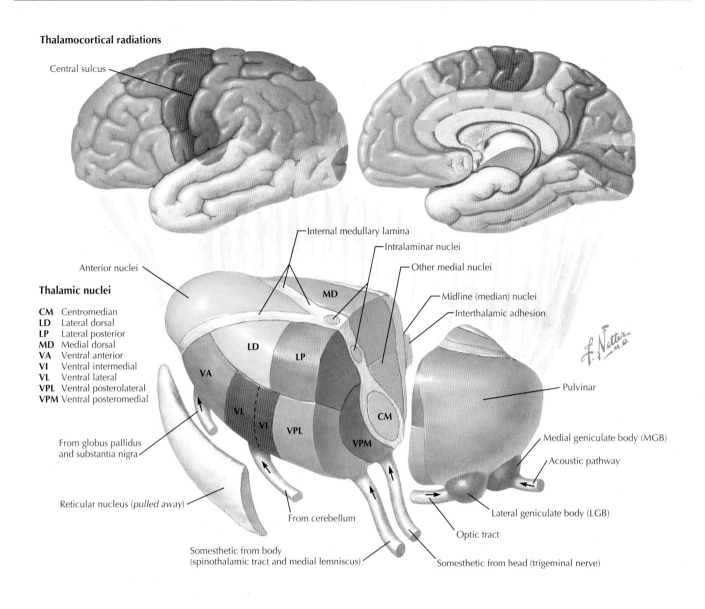

Central sulcus

Internal medullary lamina

Intralaminar nuclei

Anterior nuclei

Other medial nuclei

MD

Midline (median) nuclei

Thalamic nuclei

Interthalamic adhesion

CM	Centromedian
LD	Lateral dorsal
LP	Lateral posterior
MD	Medial dorsal
VA	Ventral anterior
VI	Ventral intermedial
VL	Ventral lateral
VPL	Ventral posterolateral
VPM	Ventral posteromedial

LD

LP

VA

Pulvinar

VL

VI

CM

VPL

Medial geniculate body (MGB)

VPM

Acoustic pathway

From globus pallidus and substantia nigra

Reticular nucleus (*pulled away*)

From cerebellum

Lateral geniculate body (LGB)

Optic tract

Somesthetic from body
(spinothalamic tract and medial lemniscus)

Somesthetic from head (trigeminal nerve)

12.1 THALAMIC ANATOMY AND INTERCONNECTIONS WITH THE CEREBRAL CORTEX

The thalamus, the gateway to the cerebral cortex, conveys extensive sensory, motor, and autonomic information from the brainstem and spinal cord to the cortex. All sensory projections to the cortex except olfaction are processed through thalamic nuclei. Thalamic nuclei are reciprocally interconnected with regions of cortex. Specific thalamic nuclei project to circumscribed regions of cortex. These nuclei include (1) sensory projection nuclei (VPL: somatosensory; VPM: trigeminal; LGB: visual; MGB: auditory; pulvinar: sensory); (2) motor-related nuclei (VL and VI), cerebellum (VA and VL), and basal ganglia (VA, VL, CM); (3) autonomic- and limbic-related nuclei (anterior and LD: cingulate cortex; MD: frontal and cingulate cortex); and (4) nuclei related to association areas (pulvinar and LP: parietal cortex). Nonspecific thalamic nuclei (intralaminar nuclei, such as CM, parafascicular, and medial VA) send diffuse connections to widespread regions of the cerebral cortex and to other thalamic nuclei. The reticular nucleus of the thalamus helps to regulate the excitability

of thalamic projection nuclei. Specific lesions of the thalamus can result in diminished sensory, motor, or autonomic activity related to loss of the specific modalities processed. Some thalamic lesions can lead to excruciating paroxysms of neuropathic pain, which is referred to as thalamic syndrome.

CLINICAL POINT

The thalamus has a complex blood supply that is derived extensively from the penetrating posterior cerebral, posterior communicating, and other nearby arteries. Thalamic nuclei are seldom individually affected by infarcts and lesions but are damaged along with nearby regions. Lesions that affect one side of the thalamus seldom produce permanent deficits unless sensory nuclei are involved. Thalamic lesions can result in changes in consciousness and alertness (intralaminar, reticular nuclei), affective behavior (medial dorsal, ventral anterior, intralaminar nuclei), memory functions (midline, medial, mammillary, and possibly anterior nuclei), motor activity (ventrolateral, ventral anterior, posterior, other nuclei), somatic sensation (ventral posterolateral and posteromedial nuclei), vision (lateral geniculate nuclei), and perceptions and hallucinations (dorsomedial, intralaminar nuclei). Medial dorsal lesions may produce a reciprocal disconnect with the prefrontal cortex and bring about a deficit in frontal functions.

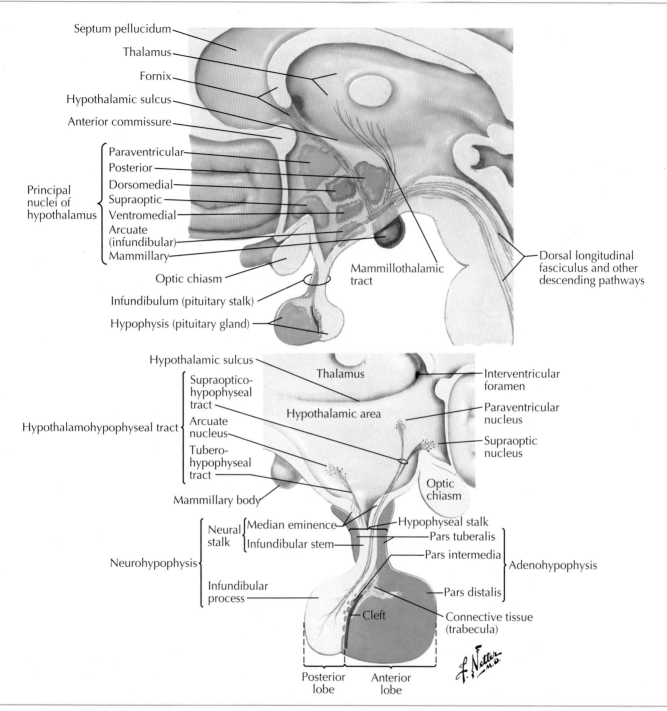

12.2 HYPOTHALAMUS AND PITUITARY GLAND

The hypothalamus is the major region of the central nervous system involved in neuroendocrine regulation and control of visceral functions, such as temperature regulation, food and appetite regulation, thirst and water balance, reproduction and sexual behavior, parturition and control of lactation, respiratory and cardiovascular regulation, gastrointestinal regulation, stress responses, and reparative states. The hypothalamus is located between the rostral midbrain and the lamina terminalis, ventral to the thalamus; it surrounds the third ventricle. The hypothalamus is subdivided in rostral-to-caudal zones (preoptic, anterior or supraoptic, tuberal, and mammillary or posterior) as well as medial-to-lateral zones (periventricular, medial, lateral). These zones contain some discrete nuclei and even discrete chemical-specific subnuclei, such as the paraventricular

nucleus (PVN); and more diffuse centers, regions, or areas (such as anterior, posterior, and lateral regions). The neuroendocrine portion of the hypothalamus consists of (1) magnocellular portions of the PVN and the supraoptic nucleus, which send axons directly to the posterior pituitary and release vasopressin and oxytocin into the general circulation; (2) releasing factor and inhibitory factor neurons, which project axons to the hypophyseal-portal vasculature in the contact zone of the median eminence, through which very high concentrations of these factors (hormones) induce the release of anterior pituitary hormones into the general circulation; and (3) the tuberoinfundibular system and ascending systems (monoamine and other chemically specific neurons) that modulate the release of releasing and inhibitory factors into the hypophyseal-portal vasculature.

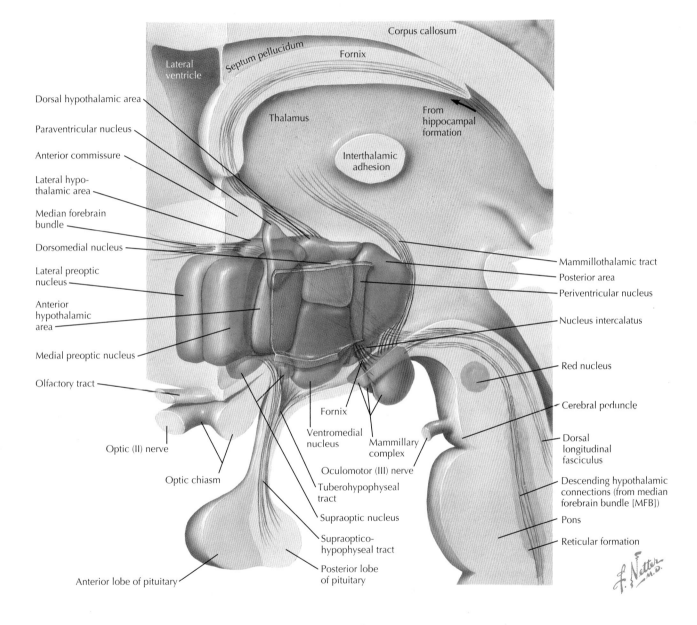

Corpus callosum

Septum pellucidum

Fornix

Lateral ventricle

Thalamus

From hippocampal formation

Interthalamic adhesion

Dorsal hypothalamic area

Paraventricular nucleus

Anterior commissure

Lateral hypo-thalamic area

Median forebrain bundle

Dorsomedial nucleus

Lateral preoptic nucleus

Anterior hypothalamic area

Medial preoptic nucleus

Olfactory tract

Optic (II) nerve

Optic chiasm

Anterior lobe of pituitary

Fornix

Ventromedial nucleus

Mammillary complex

Oculomotor (III) nerve

Tuberohypophyseal tract

Supraoptic nucleus

Supraoptico-hypophyseal tract

Posterior lobe of pituitary

Mammillothalamic tract

Posterior area

Periventricular nucleus

Nucleus intercalatus

Red nucleus

Cerebral peduncle

Dorsal longitudinal fasciculus

Descending hypothalamic connections (from median forebrain bundle [MFB])

Pons

Reticular formation

12.3 **HYPOTHALAMIC NUCLEI**

Hypothalamic nuclei and areas are associated with many visceral and neuroendocrine functions. The magnocellular neurons of the PVN and supraoptic nucleus release oxytocin and vasopressin into the posterior pituitary general circulation. PVN parvocellular neurons containing corticotrophin-releasing hormone project to the hypophyseal portal system in the contact zone of the median eminence and induce the release of adrenocorticotropic hormone (which stimulates the release of cortisol from the adrenal cortex). Descending axons of the PVN also project to the dorsal (motor) nucleus of CN X, the nucleus solitarius, and the intermediolateral cell column preganglionic sympathetic neurons and regulate preganglionic outflow from the autonomic nervous system. The anterior and posterior areas coordinate parasympathetic and sympathetic outflow, respectively. The dorsomedial (DM) and ventromedial (VM) nuclei and the lateral hypothalamic area regulate appetite, drinking, and reproductive behavior. The preoptic area regulates cyclic neuroendocrine behavior, thermoregulation, and the sleep-wake cycle. The suprachiasmatic nucleus receives visual inputs from the optic tract and regulates circadian rhythms. Several hypothalamic regions are involved in the regulation of sleep.

CLINICAL POINT

Hypothalamic nuclei often appear as discrete nuclei and regions that may subserve discrete functions. Early studies of lesions in the hypothalamus led to this impression, resulting in a description of centers, such as the ventromedial nucleus satiety center (lesions led to hyperphagia and obesity) and a lateral appetitive stimulatory center (lesions led to aphagia and cachexia). However, such lesions often damaged passing fiber tracts (e.g., passing axons of the monoaminergic systems) and connections, sometimes even those not associated with the primary functions studied. We now know that many hormones are involved in the **control of appetite and food intake**. When food is ingested, cholecyctokinin and glucagon-like peptide-1 are released by neuroendocrine cells in the intestine, and they act in the brain to suppress appetite and give the sensation of satiety. In the absence of food, these hormone levels are low, permitting appetite and food-seeking behavior. Long-term regulation of food intake also involves the hormone leptin, produced by fat cells. When fat stores are high, leptin is released and acts on the hypothalamus to suppress appetite. When body nutrient stores are depleted, leptin levels are lowered. Other hormones, such as ghrelins, also regulate appetite and eating behavior. Hypothalamic physiology awaits further studies to fully integrate the complex hypothalamic circuitry with the complex hormonal regulation, over which volitional and affective control from higher brain regions is further superimposed. Given the epidemic of obesity in the United States and other "fast-food countries," a better understanding of the physiology of eating and appetite is urgently needed.

CLINICAL POINT

The hypothalamus is a small but complex region of the central nervous system that interconnects the limbic forebrain and the brainstem. The principal functions of the hypothalamus are neuroendocrine regulation, especially through the pituitary gland, and regulation of autonomic function. **Thermoregulation** is one example of the latter. Several hypothalamic sites, including the anterior and posterior hypothalamic areas, regulate the set point for body temperature within relatively tight parameters. Damage to these mechanisms by head trauma, tumor, surgery, increased intracranial pressure, or vascular problems can induce a change in thermoregulation. Posterior hypothalamic damage is often accompanied by hypothermia, whereas anterior hypothalamic damage is often accompanied by hyperthermia. In addition, inflammatory mediators such as interleukin-1β and interleukin-6, whether derived from an infectious process (endotoxin or pyrogen) or from other sources of inflammation, can activate some of the anterior regions of the hypothalamus such as the preoptic area and can induce fever. These inflammatory mediators also can produce classic illness behavior and can powerfully activate both the hypothalamo-pituitary-adrenal axis and the hypothalamo-sympathetic axis, driving a classic stress response. Altered internal body temperature also can be affected by intracranial surgery, susceptibility to some anesthetic agents (malignant hyperthermia), and susceptibility to some neuroleptic drugs.

A major role of the hypothalamus is neuroendocrine regulation of the anterior and posterior pituitary. Neurons in the supraoptic and paraventricular nuclei send axonal connections directly to the posterior pituitary to release oxytocin and vasopressin into the general circulation. Many other collections of neurons, in the hypothalamus and elsewhere, send axonal connections to the hypophyseal-portal vascular system in the contact zone of the median eminence and release releasing factors (hormones) and inhibitory factors (hormones) that regulate the secretion of a variety of hormones from pituicytes in the anterior pituitary. These releasing factor neurons and inhibitory factor neurons receive extensive input from brainstem, hypothalamic, and limbic forebrain sources. Some of these neurons (such as the corticotrophin-releasing factor neurons in the PVN) also receive input from chemical sources, such as interleukin-1β, prostaglandin E2, and nitric oxide. Interleukin-1β, both directly and indirectly, can drive the response of corticotrophin-releasing factor, thereby activating the hypothalamo-pituitary-adrenal system to stimulate cortisol production and drive the hypothalamo-sympathetic system to stimulate the release of catecholamines. Some neurotransmitters in these releasing factor neurons and inhibitory factor neurons can be influenced pharmacologically. Dopamine in the arcuate nucleus acts as a prolactin inhibitory factor. A dopamine agonist can suppress prolactin output by a prolactin-secreting pituitary tumor (chromophobe adenoma).

13

TELENCEPHALON

Level 1: Mid Pons

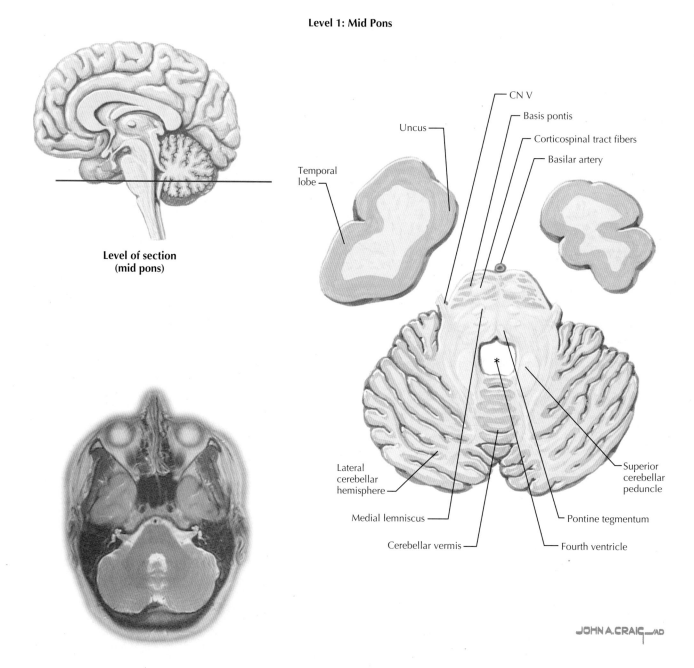

Level of section
(mid pons)

Uncus

Temporal
lobe

CN V

Basis pontis

Corticospinal tract fibers

Basilar artery

*

Lateral
cerebellar
hemisphere

Medial lemniscus

Cerebellar vermis

Superior
cerebellar
peduncle

Pontine tegmentum

Fourth ventricle

JOHN A.CRAIG—AD

13.1A AXIAL (HORIZONTAL) SECTIONS THROUGH THE FOREBRAIN: LEVEL 1—MID PONS

These axial (horizontal) sections compare anatomical sections and high-resolution magnetic resonance (MR) images. They are cut in the true horizontal (axial) plane, not in the older 25-degree tilt. The most important anatomical relationships in these sections center on the internal capsule (IC). The head of the caudate nucleus is medial to the anterior limb of the IC and forms the lateral margin of the frontal pole of the lateral ventricle. The thalamus is medial to the posterior limb of the IC. The globus pallidus and putamen are lateral to the wedge-shaped IC. The

posterior limb of the IC carries the major descending corticospinal, corticorubral, and corticoreticular fibers and the ascending sensory fibers of the somatosensory and trigeminal systems. The most posterior portions of the posterior limb also carry the auditory and visual projections to their respective cortices. The genu of the IC carries the corticobulbar fibers. The anterior limb of the IC carries cortical projections to the striatum and the pontine nuclei (pontocerebellar system). The full-plate MR images are T1-weighted; the ventricles appear dark. The scout MR images that accompany the drawings are T2-weighted MR images, in which the cerebrospinal fluid (CSF) appears white.

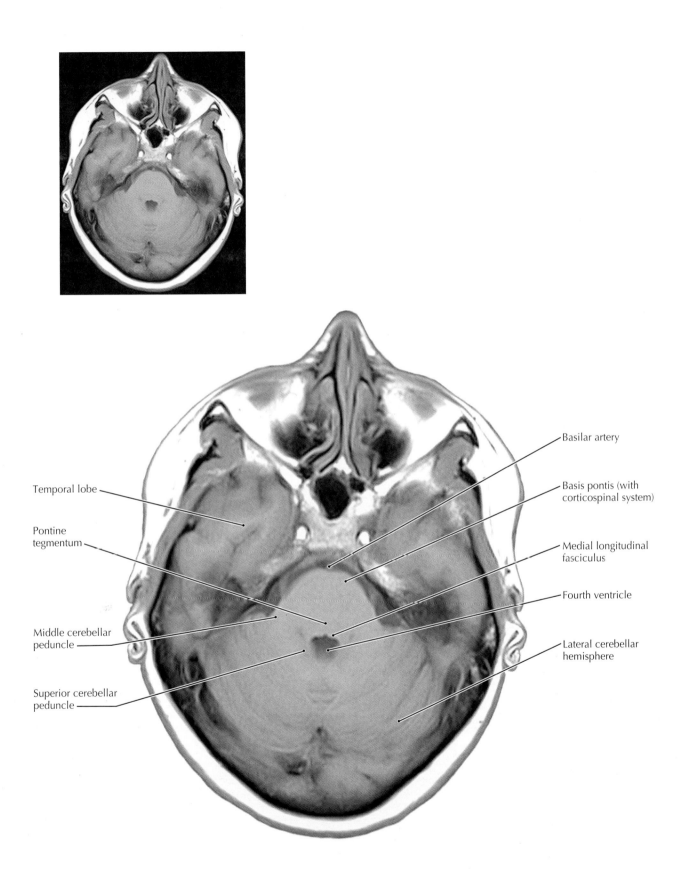

Basilar artery

Basis pontis (with corticospinal system)

Temporal lobe

Medial longitudinal fasciculus

Pontine tegmentum

Fourth ventricle

Middle cerebellar peduncle

Lateral cerebellar hemisphere

Superior cerebellar peduncle

13.1B AXIAL (HORIZONTAL) SECTIONS THROUGH THE FOREBRAIN: LEVEL 1—MID PONS (CONTINUED)

Level 2: Rostral Pons

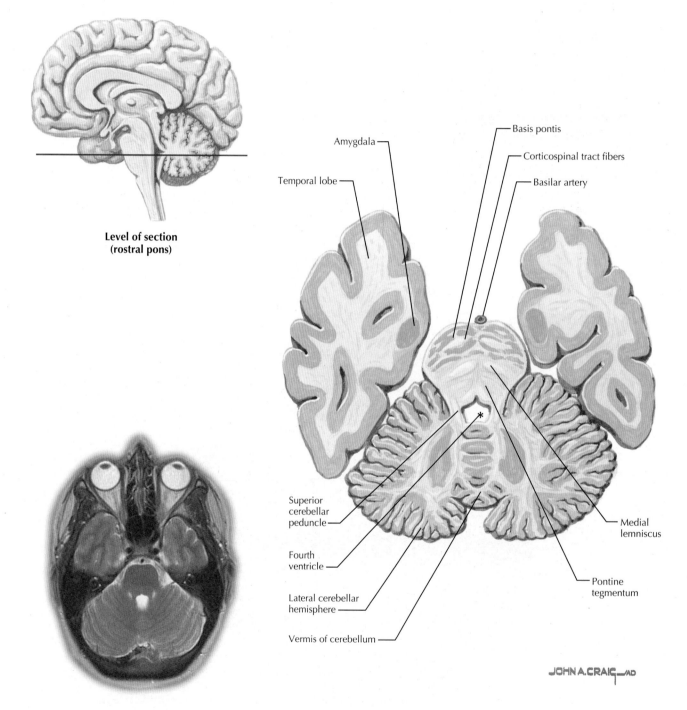

Level of section
(rostral pons)

Amygdala

Temporal lobe

Basis pontis

Corticospinal tract fibers

Basilar artery

Superior
cerebellar
peduncle

Fourth
ventricle

Lateral cerebellar
hemisphere

Vermis of cerebellum

Medial
lemniscus

Pontine
tegmentum

JOHN A. CRAIG—AD

13.2A AXIAL (HORIZONTAL) SECTIONS THROUGH THE FOREBRAIN: LEVEL 2—ROSTRAL PONS

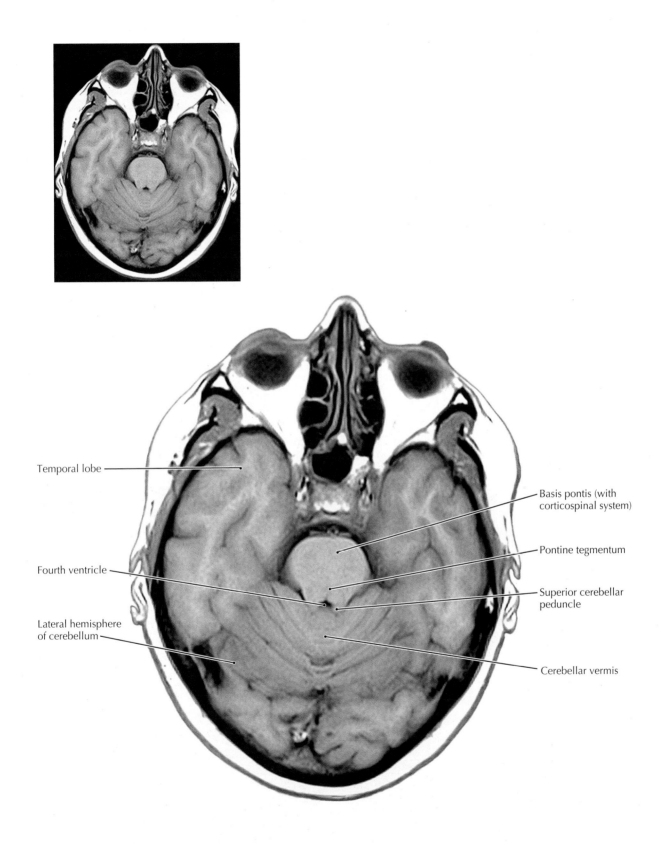

Temporal lobe

Fourth ventricle

Lateral hemisphere
of cerebellum

Basis pontis (with
corticospinal system)

Pontine tegmentum

Superior cerebellar
peduncle

Cerebellar vermis

**13.2B AXIAL (HORIZONTAL) SECTIONS THROUGH THE FOREBRAIN: LEVEL 2—ROSTRAL PONS
(CONTINUED)**

Level 3: Midbrain

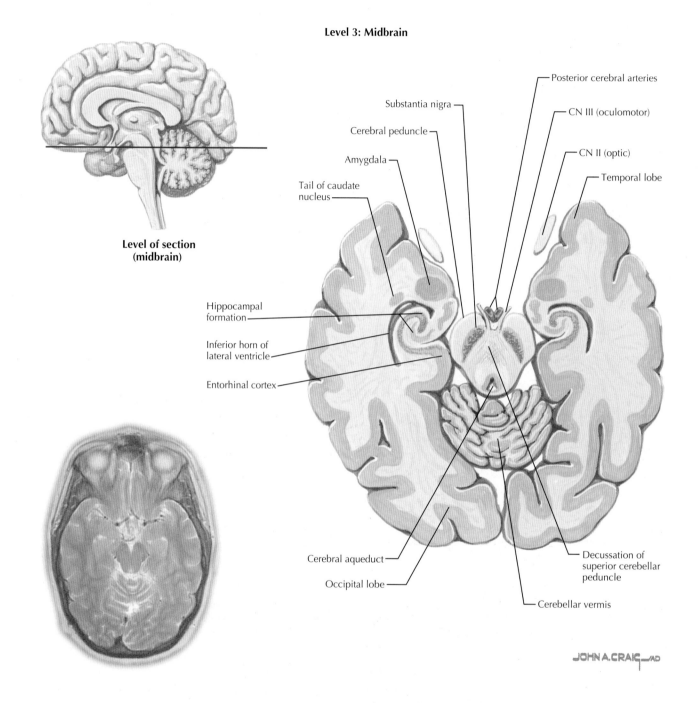

Level of section
(midbrain)

Posterior cerebral arteries

CN III (oculomotor)

Substantia nigra

CN II (optic)

Cerebral peduncle

Temporal lobe

Amygdala

Tail of caudate
nucleus

Hippocampal
formation

Inferior horn of
lateral ventricle

Entorhinal cortex

Cerebral aqueduct

Decussation of
superior cerebellar
peduncle

Occipital lobe

Cerebellar vermis

JOHN A. CRAIG—AD

13.3A AXIAL (HORIZONTAL) SECTIONS THROUGH THE FOREBRAIN: LEVEL 3—MIDBRAIN

CLINICAL POINT

The temporal lobe includes the amygdaloid nuclei, the hippocampal formation and associated cortex, the transverse gyrus of Heschl, some language-associated cortical regions (Wernicke's area in the dominant hemisphere), Meyer's loop of geniculocalcarine axons, the inferior horn of the lateral ventricle, and extensive cortical areas (superior, middle, and inferior temporal gyri). The temporal lobe can be damaged by trauma, infarcts, tumors, abscesses, and other pathological conditions. Such damage can result in auditory hallucinations, delirium and psychotic behavior, sometimes a contralateral upper quadrantanopia (if Meyer's loop is damaged), and receptive aphasia (Wernicke's aphasia) that involves a lack of understanding of verbal information (in a lesion of the dominant hemisphere). Some very specific lesions in the temporal lobe result in an agnosia for recognition of faces (prosopagnosia).

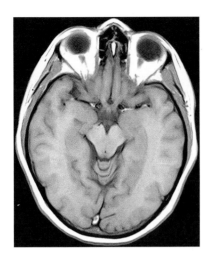

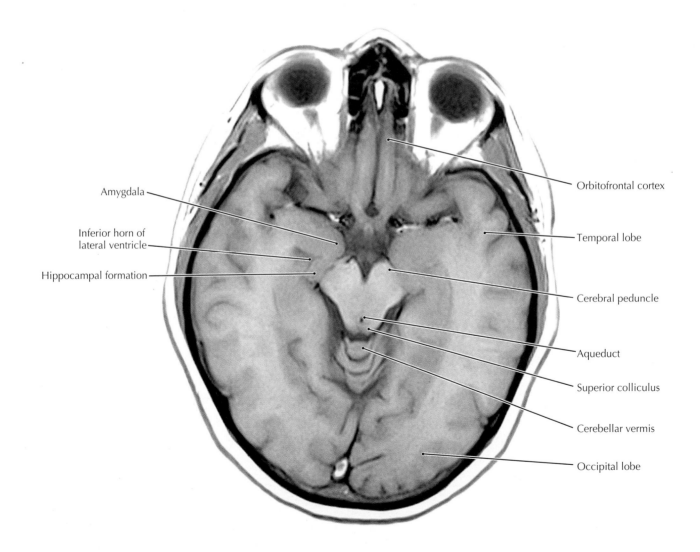

Amygdala

Inferior horn of
lateral ventricle

Hippocampal formation

Orbitofrontal cortex

Temporal lobe

Cerebral peduncle

Aqueduct

Superior colliculus

Cerebellar vermis

Occipital lobe

**13.3B AXIAL (HORIZONTAL) SECTIONS THROUGH THE FOREBRAIN: LEVEL 3—MIDBRAIN
(CONTINUED)**

Level 4: Rostral Midbrain and Hypothalamus

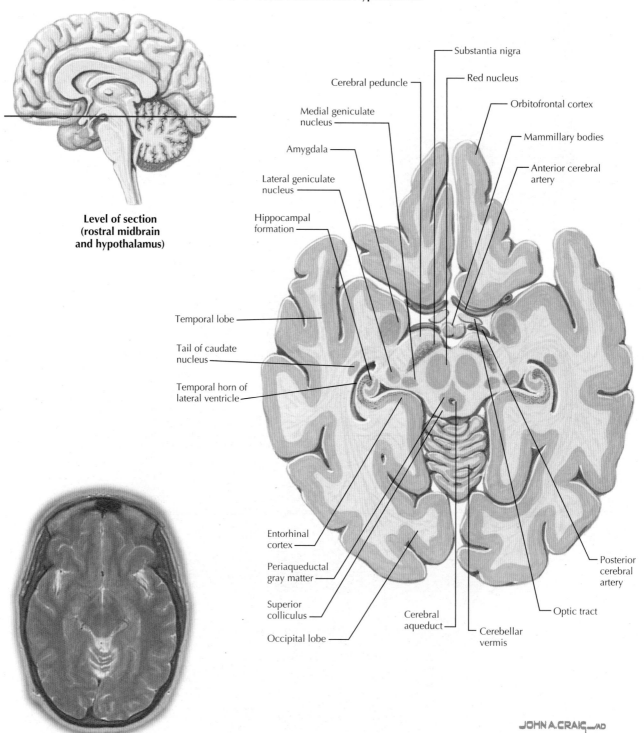

Level of section
(rostral midbrain
and hypothalamus)

Substantia nigra

Red nucleus

Cerebral peduncle

Orbitofrontal cortex

Medial geniculate
nucleus

Mammillary bodies

Amygdala

Anterior cerebral
artery

Lateral geniculate
nucleus

Hippocampal
formation

Temporal lobe

Tail of caudate
nucleus

Temporal horn of
lateral ventricle

Entorhinal
cortex

Periaqueductal
gray matter

Superior
colliculus

Occipital lobe

Cerebral
aqueduct

Cerebellar
vermis

Optic tract

Posterior
cerebral
artery

JOHN A. CRAIG—AD

13.4A AXIAL (HORIZONTAL) SECTIONS THROUGH THE FOREBRAIN: LEVEL 4—ROSTRAL MIDBRAIN AND HYPOTHALAMUS

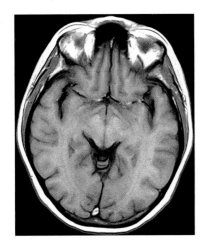

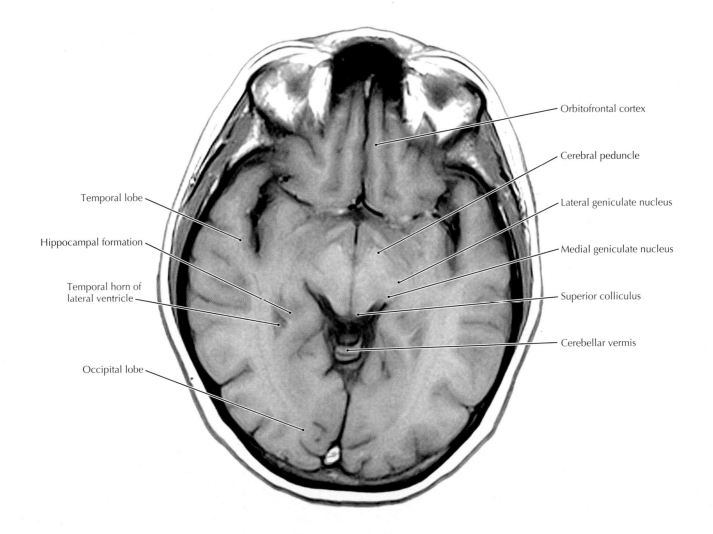

Orbitofrontal cortex

Cerebral peduncle

Temporal lobe

Lateral geniculate nucleus

Hippocampal formation

Medial geniculate nucleus

Temporal horn of
lateral ventricle

Superior colliculus

Cerebellar vermis

Occipital lobe

**13.4B AXIAL (HORIZONTAL) SECTIONS THROUGH THE FOREBRAIN: LEVEL 4—ROSTRAL MIDBRAIN
AND HYPOTHALAMUS (CONTINUED)**

Level 5: Anterior Commissure and Caudal Thalamus

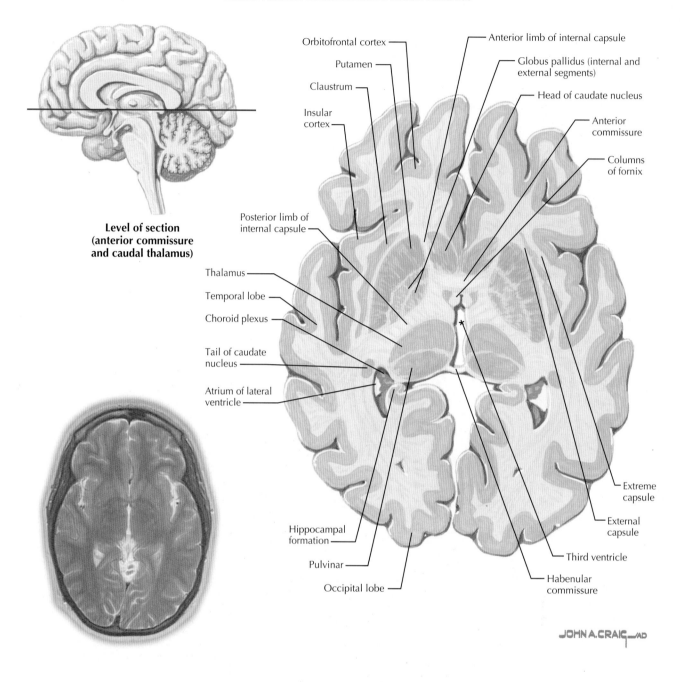

**Level of section
(anterior commissure
and caudal thalamus)**

Orbitofrontal cortex

Putamen

Claustrum

Insular
cortex

Posterior limb of
internal capsule

Thalamus

Temporal lobe

Choroid plexus

Tail of caudate
nucleus

Atrium of lateral
ventricle

Hippocampal
formation

Pulvinar

Occipital lobe

Anterior limb of internal capsule

Globus pallidus (internal and
external segments)

Head of caudate nucleus

Anterior
commissure

Columns
of fornix

Extreme
capsule

External
capsule

Third ventricle

Habenular
commissure

JOHN A. CRAIG—AD

13.5A AXIAL (HORIZONTAL) SECTIONS THROUGH THE FOREBRAIN: LEVEL 5—ANTERIOR COMMISSURE AND CAUDAL THALAMUS

CLINICAL POINT

The basal ganglia assist the cerebral cortex in planning and generating desired programs of activity and suppressing undesired programs of activity. The most conspicuous arena in which these functions are observed is motor activity. **Basal ganglia disorders** produce movement problems that are often involuntary in nature and are commonly accompanied by cognitive and affective symptoms (e.g., Huntington's disease). The principal route of information flow from the basal ganglia is from the thalamus and cerebral cortex to the striatum (caudate nucleus and putamen), then to the globus pallidus, then back to the thalamus and cortex, completing the loop. Disruption of this loop can produce excessive movements (e.g., choreiform and athetoid movements, tremor) or diminished movements (bradykinesia). In some instances, specific nuclei are known to be associated with such changes. A small lacunar infarct in the subthalamic nucleus results in wild, flinging (ballistic) movements in the contralateral limbs. However, a surgical lesion in the subthalamic nucleus may ameliorate some of the movement problems seen in Parkinson's disease. The subthalamus most likely drives activity in the internal segment of the globus pallidus, which in turn can be modified by the external segment. A pathological lesion in the globus pallidus can produce rigidity and akinesia; a surgical pallidal lesion may reduce excessive movements in other basal ganglia disorders.

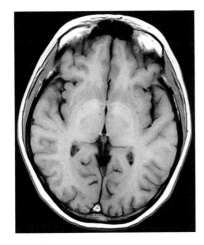

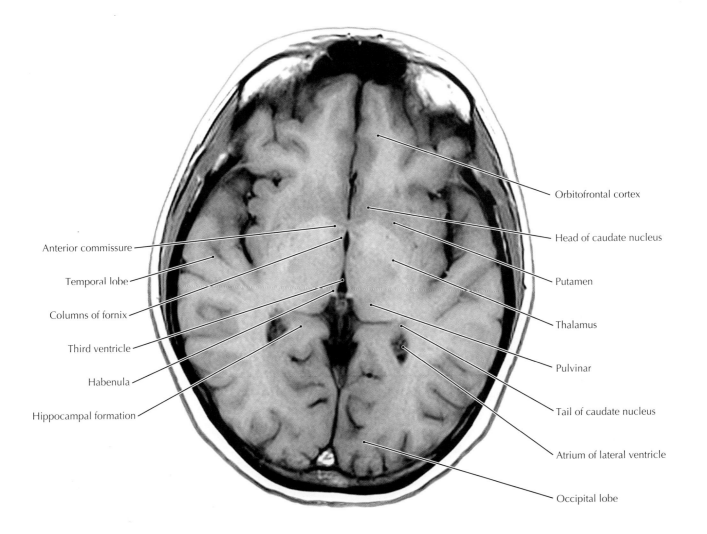

Orbitofrontal cortex

Head of caudate nucleus

Anterior commissure

Putamen

Temporal lobe

Columns of fornix

Thalamus

Third ventricle

Pulvinar

Habenula

Tail of caudate nucleus

Hippocampal formation

Atrium of lateral ventricle

Occipital lobe

13.5B AXIAL (HORIZONTAL) SECTIONS THROUGH THE FOREBRAIN: LEVEL5—ANTERIOR COMMISSURE AND CAUDAL THALAMUS (CONTINUED)

Level 7: Basal Ganglia and Internal Capsule

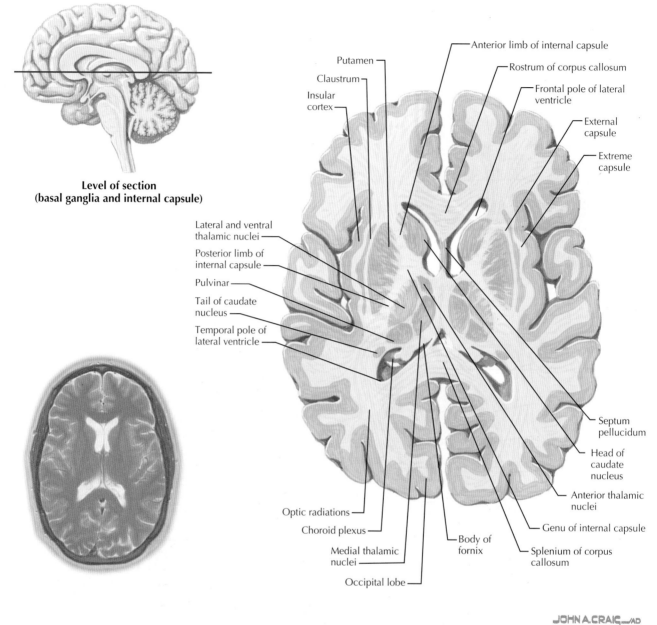

Level of section
(basal ganglia and internal capsule)

Putamen

Claustrum

Insular
cortex

Anterior limb of internal capsule

Rostrum of corpus callosum

Frontal pole of lateral
ventricle

External
capsule

Extreme
capsule

Lateral and ventral
thalamic nuclei

Posterior limb of
internal capsule

Pulvinar

Tail of caudate
nucleus

Temporal pole of
lateral ventricle

Septum
pellucidum

Head of
caudate
nucleus

Anterior thalamic
nuclei

Optic radiations

Choroid plexus

Medial thalamic
nuclei

Occipital lobe

Body of
fornix

Genu of internal capsule

Splenium of corpus
callosum

JOHN A.CRAIG—AD

13.7A AXIAL (HORIZONTAL) SECTIONS THROUGH THE FOREBRAIN: LEVEL 7—BASAL GANGLIA AND INTERNAL CAPSULE

CLINICAL POINT

Huntington's disease is an autosomal dominant disorder caused by a trinucleotide repeat (CAG) on the short arm of chromosome 4. It results in a progressive, untreatable disease that includes a movement disorder (choreiform movements: brisk, jerky, forcible, arrhythmic movements), progressive cognitive impairment, and affective disorders (such as depression, psychotic behavior). This disease progresses from a state of minor impairment (clumsiness) with minor behavioral problems (irritability and depression) to major impairment, dementia, and a decline that leads to incapacitation and ultimately to an early death. The anatomical hallmark of this disease is marked degeneration of the caudate nucleus (also the putamen). The characteristic bulge of the head of the caudate into the frontal pole of the lateral ventricle is lost. Most of the medium spiny caudate neurons that project to the globus pallidus degenerate as the result of damage from excess Ca^{2+} influx caused by glutamate excitotoxic damage via activation of the N-methyl-D-aspartate (NMDA) receptors. The intrinsic cholinergic interneurons of the striatum also degenerate in Huntington's disease.

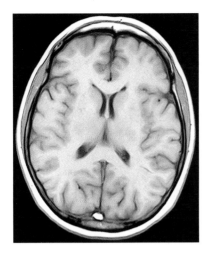

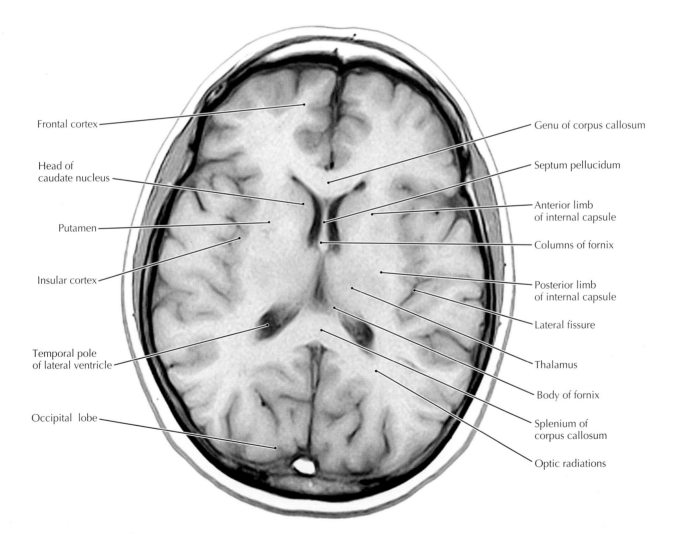

Frontal cortex

Head of
caudate nucleus

Putamen

Insular cortex

Temporal pole
of lateral ventricle

Occipital lobe

Genu of corpus callosum

Septum pellucidum

Anterior limb
of internal capsule

Columns of fornix

Posterior limb
of internal capsule

Lateral fissure

Thalamus

Body of fornix

Splenium of
corpus callosum

Optic radiations

13.7B AXIAL (HORIZONTAL) SECTIONS THROUGH THE FOREBRAIN: LEVEL 7—BASAL GANGLIA AND INTERNAL CAPSULE (CONTINUED)

Level 8: Dorsal Caudate, Splenium, and Genu of Corpus Callosum

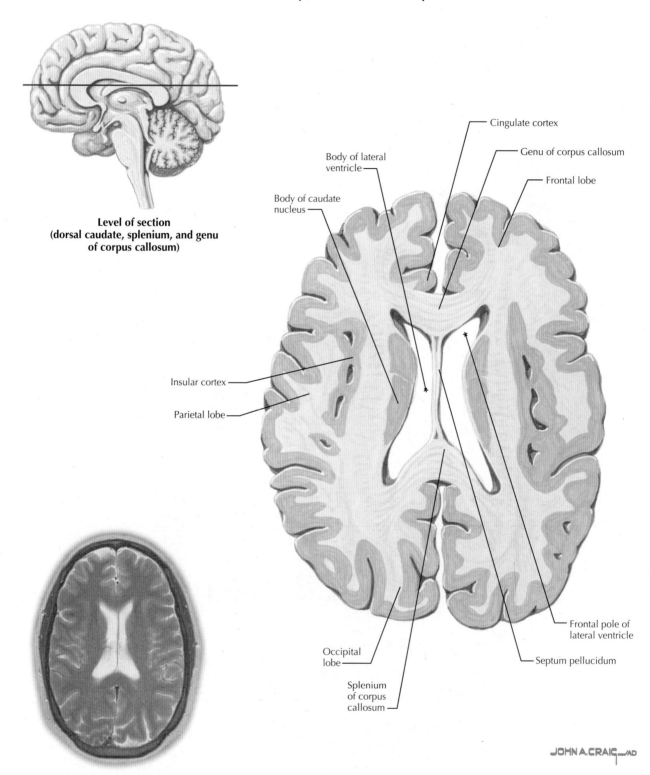

Level of section
(dorsal caudate, splenium, and genu
of corpus callosum)

Body of lateral ventricle

Body of caudate nucleus

Cingulate cortex

Genu of corpus callosum

Frontal lobe

Insular cortex

Parietal lobe

Frontal pole of lateral ventricle

Septum pellucidum

Occipital lobe

Splenium of corpus callosum

JOHN A. CRAIG___AD

13.8A AXIAL (HORIZONTAL) SECTIONS THROUGH THE FOREBRAIN: LEVEL 8—DORSAL CAUDATE, SPLENIUM, AND GENU OF CORPUS CALLOSUM

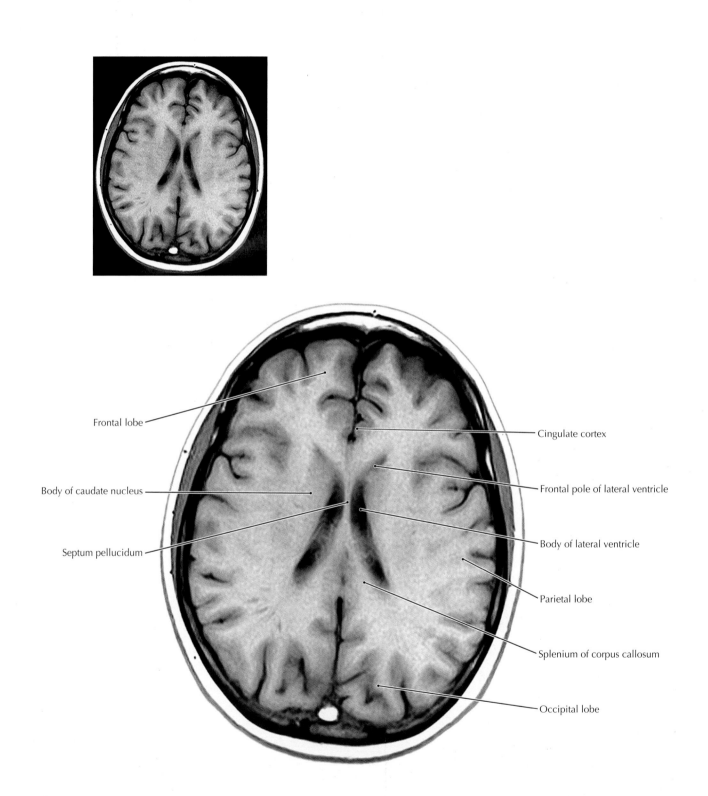

Frontal lobe

Cingulate cortex

Frontal pole of lateral ventricle

Body of caudate nucleus

Body of lateral ventricle

Septum pellucidum

Parietal lobe

Splenium of corpus callosum

Occipital lobe

13.8B AXIAL (HORIZONTAL) SECTIONS THROUGH THE FOREBRAIN: LEVEL 8—DORSAL CAUDATE, SPLENIUM, AND GENU OF CORPUS CALLOSUM (CONTINUED)

Level 9: Body of Corpus Callosum

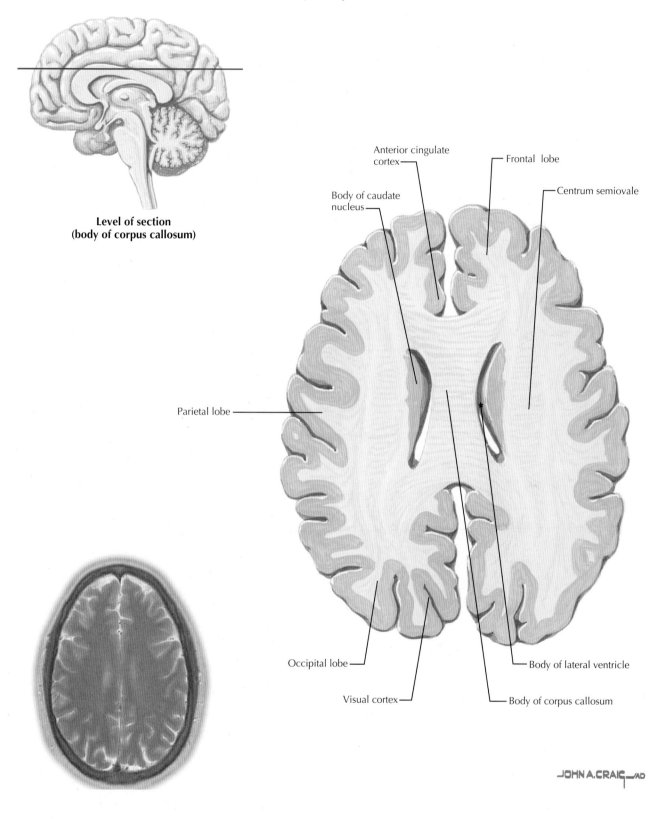

**Level of section
(body of corpus callosum)**

Anterior cingulate
cortex

Frontal lobe

Body of caudate
nucleus

Centrum semiovale

Parietal lobe

Occipital lobe

Body of lateral ventricle

Visual cortex

Body of corpus callosum

JOHN A.CRAIG—AD

13.9A AXIAL (HORIZONTAL) SECTIONS THROUGH THE FOREBRAIN: LEVEL 9—BODY OF CORPUS CALLOSUM

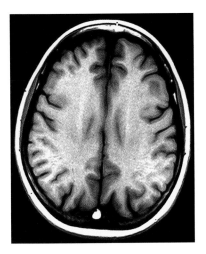

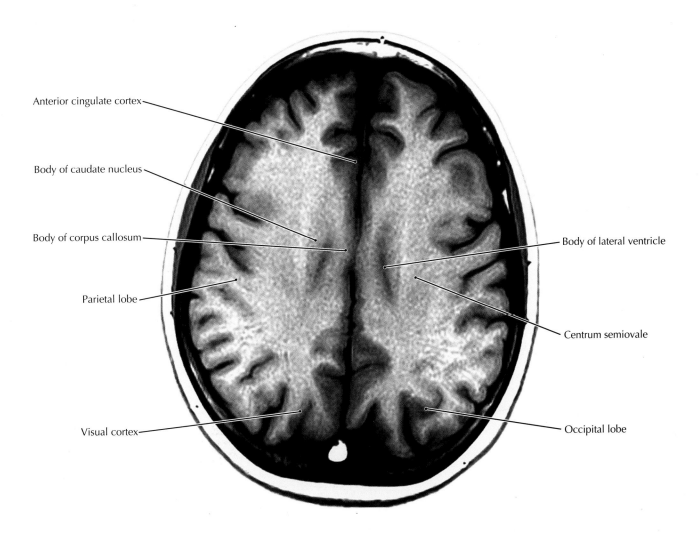

Anterior cingulate cortex

Body of caudate nucleus

Body of corpus callosum

Parietal lobe

Visual cortex

Body of lateral ventricle

Centrum semiovale

Occipital lobe

13.9B AXIAL (HORIZONTAL) SECTIONS THROUGH THE FOREBRAIN: LEVEL 9—BODY OF CORPUS CALLOSUM (CONTINUED)

Level 10: Centrum Semiovale

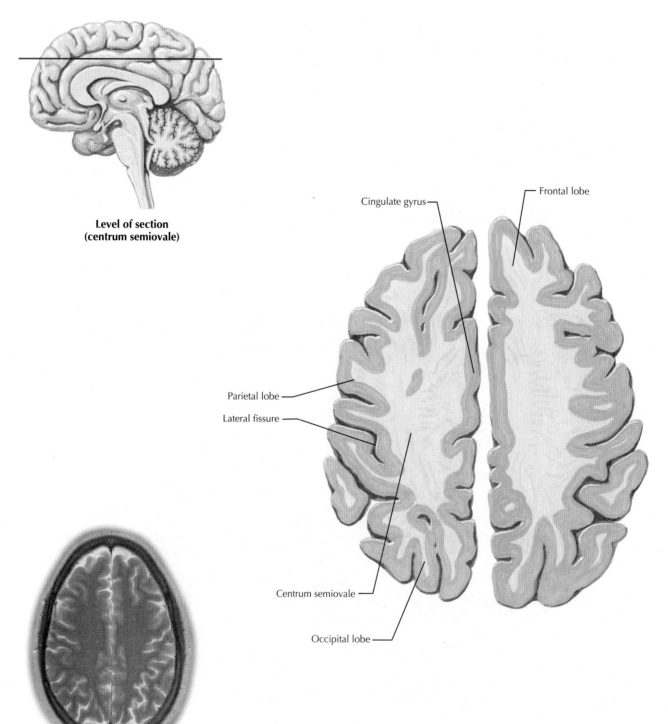

Level of section
(centrum semiovale)

Cingulate gyrus

Frontal lobe

Parietal lobe

Lateral fissure

Centrum semiovale

Occipital lobe

JOHN A.CRAIG—AD

13.10A AXIAL (HORIZONTAL) SECTIONS THROUGH THE FOREBRAIN: LEVEL 10—CENTRUM SEMIOVALE

See Video 13.1.

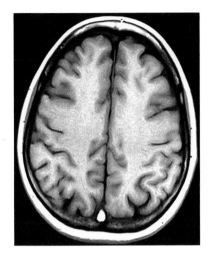

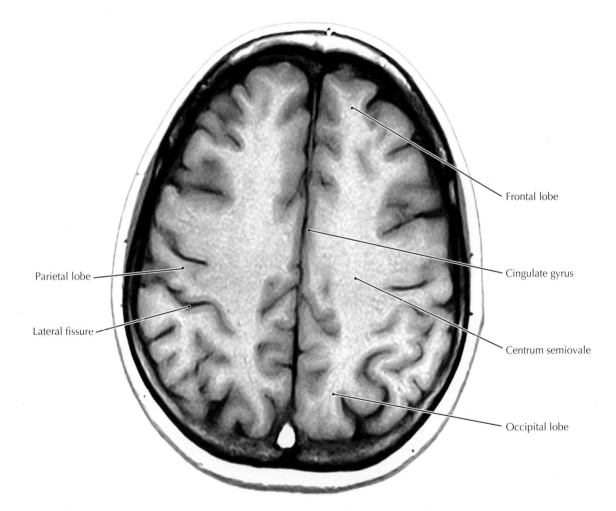

Frontal lobe

Cingulate gyrus

Parietal lobe

Centrum semiovale

Lateral fissure

Occipital lobe

13.10B AXIAL (HORIZONTAL) SECTIONS THROUGH THE FOREBRAIN: LEVEL 10—CENTRUM SEMIOVALE (CONTINUED)

Level 1: Genu of Corpus Callosum

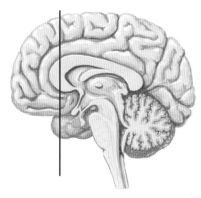

Level of section
(genu of corpus callosum)

Superior frontal gyrus

Cingulate gyrus

Middle frontal gyrus

Genu of corpus callosum

Inferior frontal gyrus

Frontal pole of lateral ventricle

Subcallosal gyrus

Lateral fissure

Temporal pole

JOHN A. CRAIG—AD

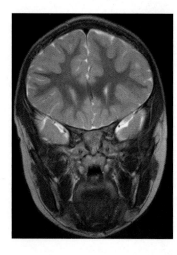

13.11A CORONAL SECTIONS THROUGH THE FOREBRAIN: LEVEL 1—GENU OF CORPUS CALLOSUM

These coronal sections compare anatomical sections and high-resolution MR images. They show important relationships among the internal capsule, basal ganglia, and thalamus. These sections show basal forebrain structures, such as nucleus accumbens, substantia innominata, and nucleus basalis (cholinergic forebrain nucleus), some individual thalamic nuclei, and the important temporal lobe structures (amygdaloid nuclei, hippocampal formation) and pathways (fornix, stria terminalis). The full-page MR images are T1-weighted; the ventricles appear dark. The scout MR images that accompany the drawings are T2-weighted MR images in which the CSF appears white.

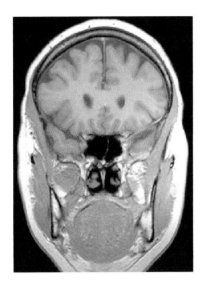

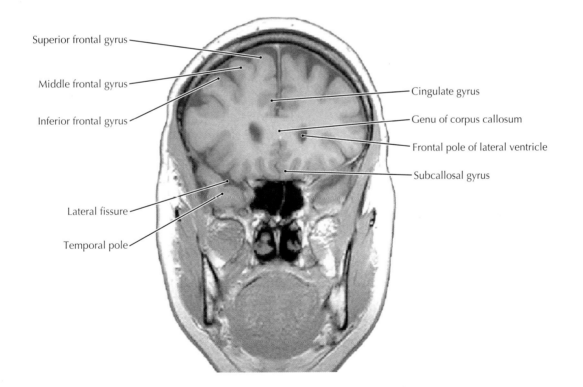

Superior frontal gyrus

Middle frontal gyrus

Inferior frontal gyrus

Cingulate gyrus

Genu of corpus callosum

Frontal pole of lateral ventricle

Subcallosal gyrus

Lateral fissure

Temporal pole

13.11B CORONAL SECTIONS THROUGH THE FOREBRAIN: LEVEL 1—GENU OF CORPUS CALLOSUM (CONTINUED)

Level 3: Anterior Commissure/Columns of Fornix

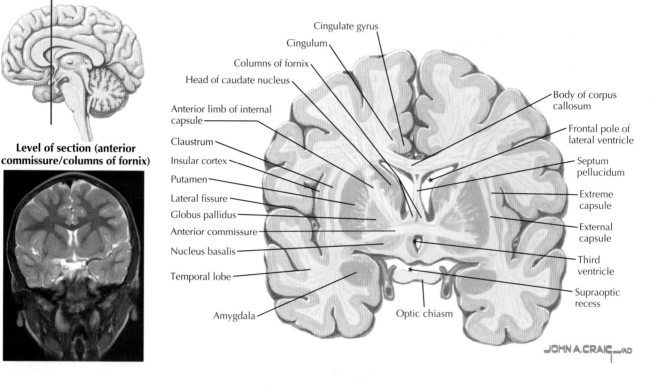

Level of section (anterior commissure/columns of fornix)

Labels on illustration:
- Cingulate gyrus
- Cingulum
- Columns of fornix
- Head of caudate nucleus
- Anterior limb of internal capsule
- Claustrum
- Insular cortex
- Putamen
- Lateral fissure
- Globus pallidus
- Anterior commissure
- Nucleus basalis
- Temporal lobe
- Amygdala
- Body of corpus callosum
- Frontal pole of lateral ventricle
- Septum pellucidum
- Extreme capsule
- External capsule
- Third ventricle
- Supraoptic recess
- Optic chiasm

JOHN A. CRAIG—AD

13.13A CORONAL SECTIONS THROUGH THE FOREBRAIN: LEVEL 3—ANTERIOR COMMISSURE/COLUMNS OF FORNIX

CLINICAL POINT

Most infections in the brain are caused by viruses, bacteria, fungi, and other living organisms. A review of these infections is beyond the scope of this atlas. A prominent but rare exception to the norm is an unusual and unexpected *protein infection* (or *prion*) that is readily transmissible by a nonliving molecule, a protein. A normal neural protein, prion protein (PrP^c, c = cellular) functions as a copper-binding protein and is involved in cellular adhesion and cellular communication in neurons. An aberrant form of this protein (PrP^{Sc}, Sc = scrapie) displays an altered, aberrant folding structure. This aberrant protein form can recruit normal protein PrP^c to transform to the aberrant form, PrP^{Sc}, and form large, insoluble clusters of highly damaging amyloid-like plaques. The end result, after an incubation period, is a rapid, progressive chain reaction leading to vacuolization and degeneration/destruction of virtually all central nervous system (CNS) regions. This is referred to as a spongiform encephalopathy, and the **prion disease** is also known as **Creutzfeldt-Jakob disease (CJD)**.

The clinical symptoms of prion disease are myriad and include cognitive decline, emotional alterations, behavioral and personality changes, speech and language loss, motor and myoclonic changes, severe ataxia, swallowing problems, perceptual changes, seizures, and many others. No brain region is protected, and prominent structural damage can be found in the cerebral cortex, limbic structures, basal ganglia, thalamus, cerebellum, brainstem, and spinal cord.

There are three major forms of prion disease. A genetic form (10% to 15% of cases) arises from an altered *PRNP* gene, which codes for the aberrant protein PrP^{Sc}. A spontaneous form, by far the largest number of cases, arises for unknown reasons (one case per million individuals). A transmissible acquired form (variant CJD) arises from consumption of meat or body tissue from infected sheep and goats (scrapie); from cows (bovine spongiform encephalopathy) who were fed contaminated feed, leading to *bovine spongiform encephalopathy* in cows and *mad cow disease* in humans who eat the contaminated beef; and from wild game (deer, elk, with *chronic wasting disease*) and others. A rare acquired form was found many decades ago in Papua, New Guinea, in an indigenous tribe in which eating the brain tissue from other humans was practiced; this led to the disease *kuru*, which is also a prion disease.

These insoluble aberrant proteins also can be transmitted from individual to individual by medical procedures and the use of contaminated surgical instruments. It was found that even prolonged, vigorous autoclaving of surgical instruments or treatment with standard chemical disinfectants does not inactivate PrP^{Sc}. A special protocol is now required to ensure that prion disease can no longer be transmitted via this route. Ensurance of inactivation of the PrP^{Sc} protein occurs with incineration at 1000°C. There is no evidence for person-to-person transmission through normal human contact. At present, there is no known successful treatment for prion disease.

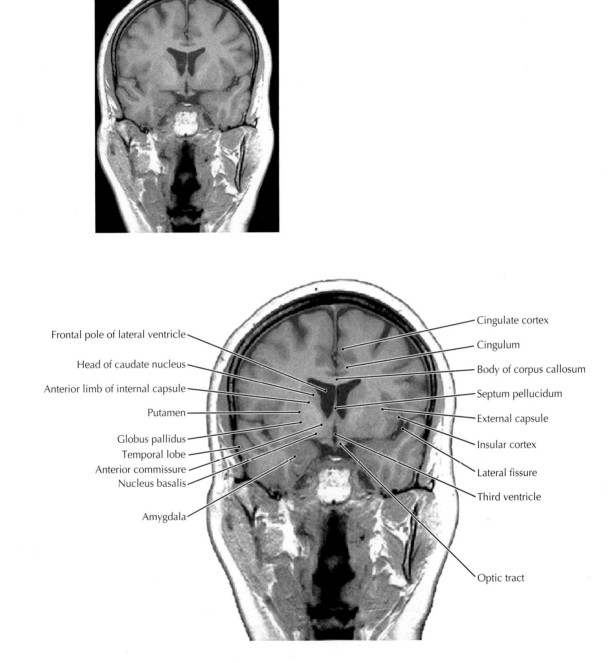

Frontal pole of lateral ventricle

Head of caudate nucleus

Anterior limb of internal capsule

Putamen

Globus pallidus

Temporal lobe

Anterior commissure

Nucleus basalis

Amygdala

Cingulate cortex

Cingulum

Body of corpus callosum

Septum pellucidum

External capsule

Insular cortex

Lateral fissure

Third ventricle

Optic tract

**13.B CORONAL SECTIONS THROUGH THE FOREBRAIN: LEVEL 3—ANTERIOR COMMISSURE/
COLUMNS OF FORNIX (CONTINUED)**

Level 4: Amygdala, Anterior Limb of Internal Capsule

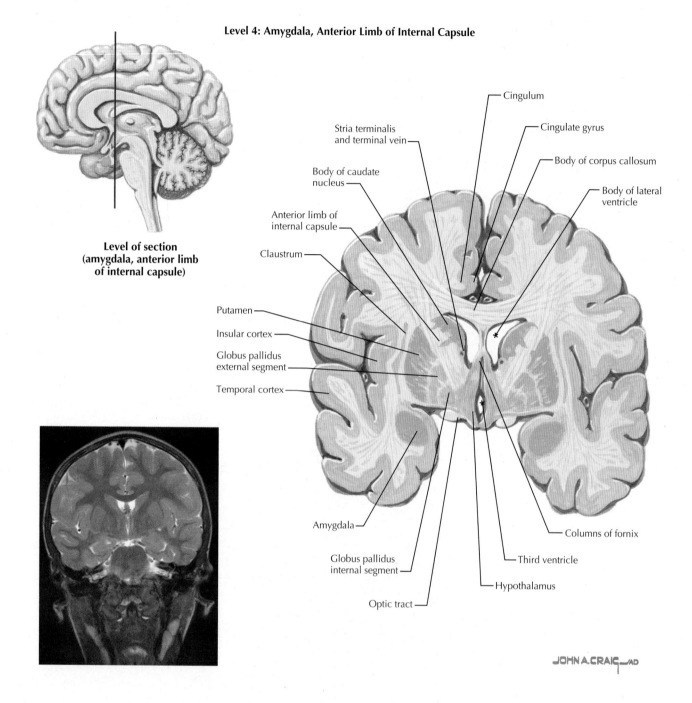

Level of section
(amygdala, anterior limb
of internal capsule)

Stria terminalis and terminal vein

Body of caudate nucleus

Anterior limb of internal capsule

Claustrum

Putamen

Insular cortex

Globus pallidus external segment

Temporal cortex

Cingulum

Cingulate gyrus

Body of corpus callosum

Body of lateral ventricle

Amygdala

Globus pallidus internal segment

Optic tract

Columns of fornix

Third ventricle

Hypothalamus

JOHN A. CRAIG—AD

13.14A CORONAL SECTIONS THROUGH THE FOREBRAIN: LEVEL 4—AMYGDALA, ANTERIOR LIMB OF INTERNAL CAPSULE

CLINICAL POINT

The corpus callosum is the principal interhemispheric or commissural pathway in the brain. It interconnects one hemisphere with its counterpart on the other side, with the exception of part of the temporal lobe that is interconnected by the anterior commissure. Some large lesions resulting from trauma or tumor can damage the corpus callosum, but this is usually accompanied by a large amount of additional forebrain

damage. However, specific **surgical sectioning of the corpus callosum** has been performed in an attempt to alleviate the spread of seizure activity from one side of the brain to the other. This "split brain" surgery causes each hemisphere to be unaware of specific activity occurring in the other hemisphere. Thus, the left brain cannot identify a visual or somatosensory stimulus presented to the right hemisphere and does not know where the left hand and arm are located if they are kept from the left hemisphere's view. Sometimes, the left hand may act independently of the conscious intent of the left hemisphere. Some emotional information appears to transfer through brainstem regions between the two parts of the split brain, providing a limbic context that may be perceived to some extent by both hemispheres.

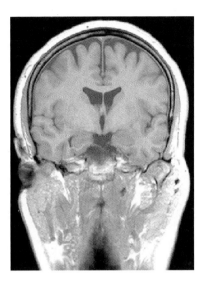

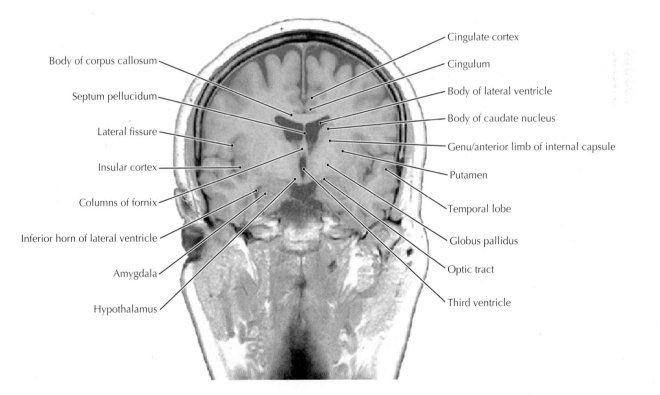

Body of corpus callosum

Septum pellucidum

Lateral fissure

Insular cortex

Columns of fornix

Inferior horn of lateral ventricle

Amygdala

Hypothalamus

Cingulate cortex

Cingulum

Body of lateral ventricle

Body of caudate nucleus

Genu/anterior limb of internal capsule

Putamen

Temporal lobe

Globus pallidus

Optic tract

Third ventricle

13.14B CORONAL SECTIONS THROUGH THE FOREBRAIN: LEVEL 4—AMYGDALA, ANTERIOR LIMB OF INTERNAL CAPSULE (CONTINUED)

Level 5: Mammillary Bodies

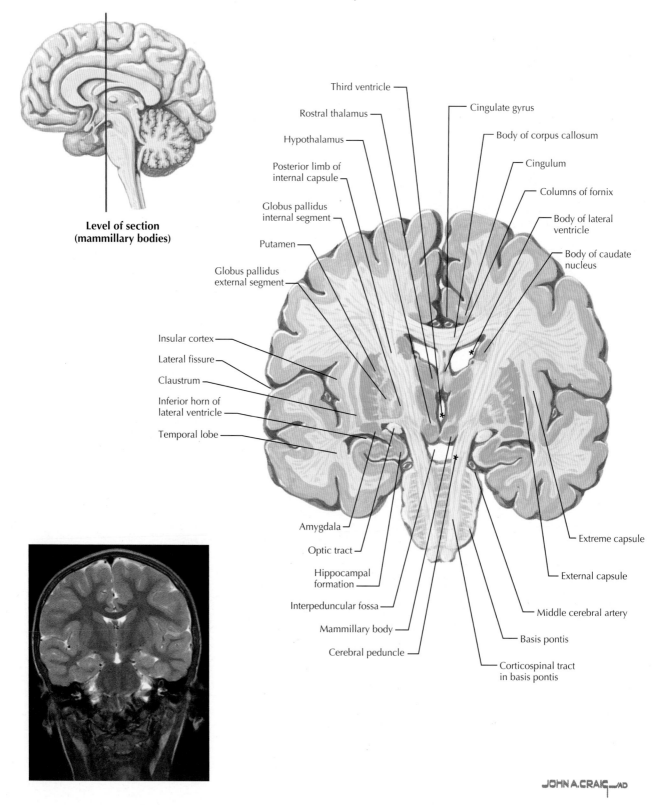

Level of section
(mammillary bodies)

Third ventricle

Rostral thalamus

Hypothalamus

Posterior limb of
internal capsule

Globus pallidus
internal segment

Putamen

Globus pallidus
external segment

Insular cortex

Lateral fissure

Claustrum

Inferior horn of
lateral ventricle

Temporal lobe

Amygdala

Optic tract

Hippocampal
formation

Interpeduncular fossa

Mammillary body

Cerebral peduncle

Cingulate gyrus

Body of corpus callosum

Cingulum

Columns of fornix

Body of lateral
ventricle

Body of caudate
nucleus

Extreme capsule

External capsule

Middle cerebral artery

Basis pontis

Corticospinal tract
in basis pontis

JOHN A. CRAIG—AD

13.15A CORONAL SECTIONS THROUGH THE FOREBRAIN: LEVEL 5—MAMMILLARY BODY

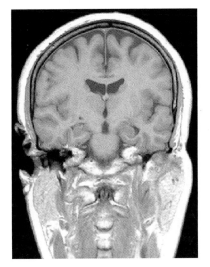

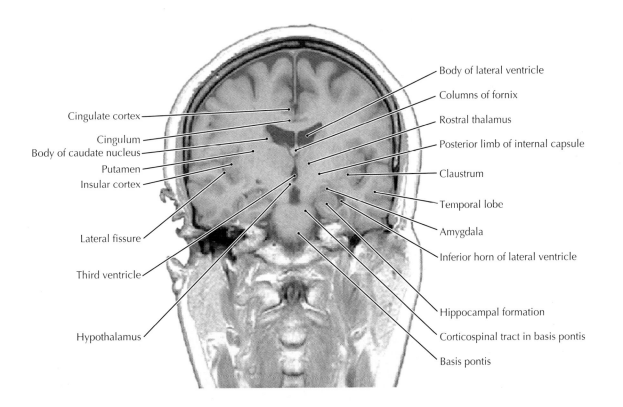

Cingulate cortex

Cingulum

Body of caudate nucleus

Putamen

Insular cortex

Lateral fissure

Third ventricle

Hypothalamus

Body of lateral ventricle

Columns of fornix

Rostral thalamus

Posterior limb of internal capsule

Claustrum

Temporal lobe

Amygdala

Inferior horn of lateral ventricle

Hippocampal formation

Corticospinal tract in basis pontis

Basis pontis

13.15B CORONAL SECTIONS THROUGH THE FOREBRAIN: LEVEL 5—MAMMILLARY BODY (CONTINUED)

Level 6: Mammillothalamic Tract/Substantia Nigra, Rostral Hippocampus

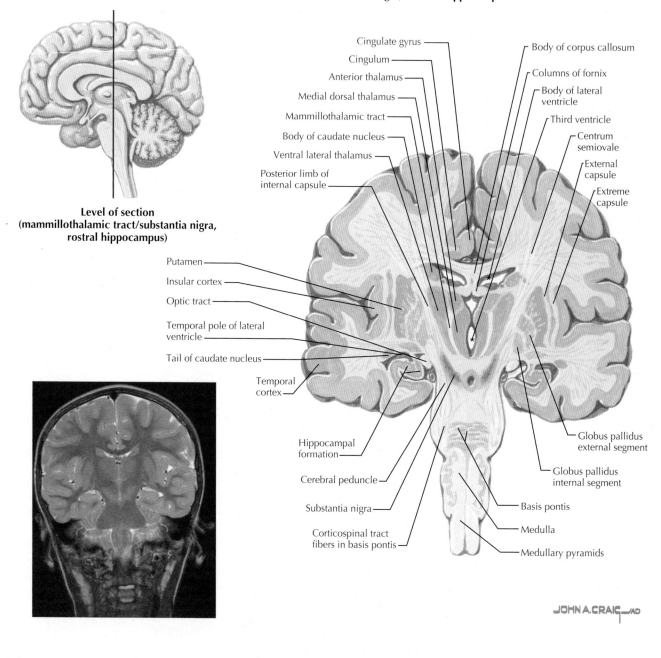

Level of section
(mammillothalamic tract/substantia nigra,
rostral hippocampus)

Cingulate gyrus
Cingulum
Anterior thalamus
Medial dorsal thalamus
Mammillothalamic tract
Body of caudate nucleus
Ventral lateral thalamus
Posterior limb of internal capsule

Body of corpus callosum
Columns of fornix
Body of lateral ventricle
Third ventricle
Centrum semiovale
External capsule
Extreme capsule

Putamen
Insular cortex
Optic tract
Temporal pole of lateral ventricle
Tail of caudate nucleus
Temporal cortex

Hippocampal formation
Cerebral peduncle
Substantia nigra
Corticospinal tract fibers in basis pontis

Globus pallidus external segment
Globus pallidus internal segment
Basis pontis
Medulla
Medullary pyramids

JOHN A. CRAIG—AD

13.16A CORONAL SECTIONS THROUGH THE FOREBRAIN: LEVEL 6— MAMMILLOTHALAMIC TRACT/ SUBSTANTIA NIGRA, ROSTRAL HIPPOCAMPUS

CLINICAL POINT

The **posterior limb of the IC** is the major afferent and efferent route through which the cerebral cortex is connected with the rest of the brain. The cerebral cortex sends descending fibers through the IC that are destined for the spinal cord, brainstem, cerebellum (via pontine nuclei), striatum and related nuclei, thalamus, and limbic structures. Of particular importance for movement are the corticospinal system and cortical connections to other upper motor neuron regions (such as the red nucleus) arising from the motor and premotor/supplemental motor cortices, which help to control skilled movements of the contralateral limbs, and the corticobulbar tract, which supplies motor cranial nerve nuclei with descending control, all bilaterally except for the lower facial nucleus, which receives exclusively contralateral input. The corticospinal tract travels in the posterior limb of the IC, and the corticobulbar tract travels in the genu of the IC. The posterior limb of the IC also conveys the ascending somatosensory and trigeminal sensory axons from the ventral posterolateral and posteromedial thalamus, respectively, which are susceptible to vascular infarcts in the middle cerebral artery and fine penetrating lenticulostriate arteries. Such an infarct acutely produces contralateral hemiplegia and a drooping lower face, with loss of somatic sensation. With time, the hemiplegia becomes spastic, with hyperreflexia, hypertonus, and pathological reflexes (Babinski's reflex, or plantar extensory response).

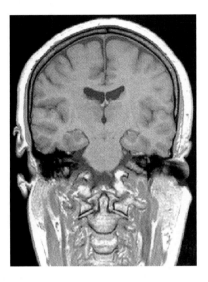

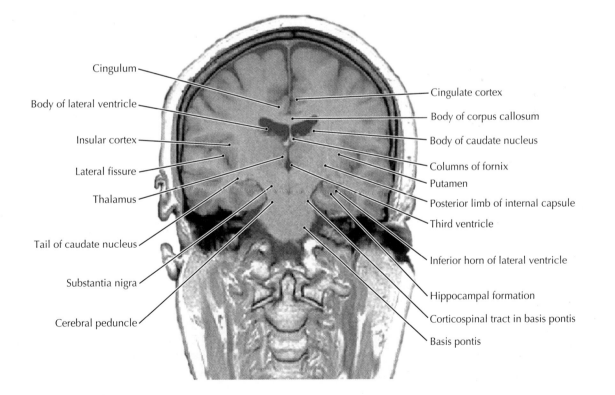

Cingulum

Body of lateral ventricle

Insular cortex

Lateral fissure

Thalamus

Tail of caudate nucleus

Substantia nigra

Cerebral peduncle

Cingulate cortex

Body of corpus callosum

Body of caudate nucleus

Columns of fornix

Putamen

Posterior limb of internal capsule

Third ventricle

Inferior horn of lateral ventricle

Hippocampal formation

Corticospinal tract in basis pontis

Basis pontis

13.16B CORONAL SECTIONS THROUGH THE FOREBRAIN: LEVEL 6—MAMMILLOTHALAMIC TRACT/ SUBSTANTIA NIGRA, ROSTRAL HIPPOCAMPUS (CONTINUED)

Level 7: Midthalamus

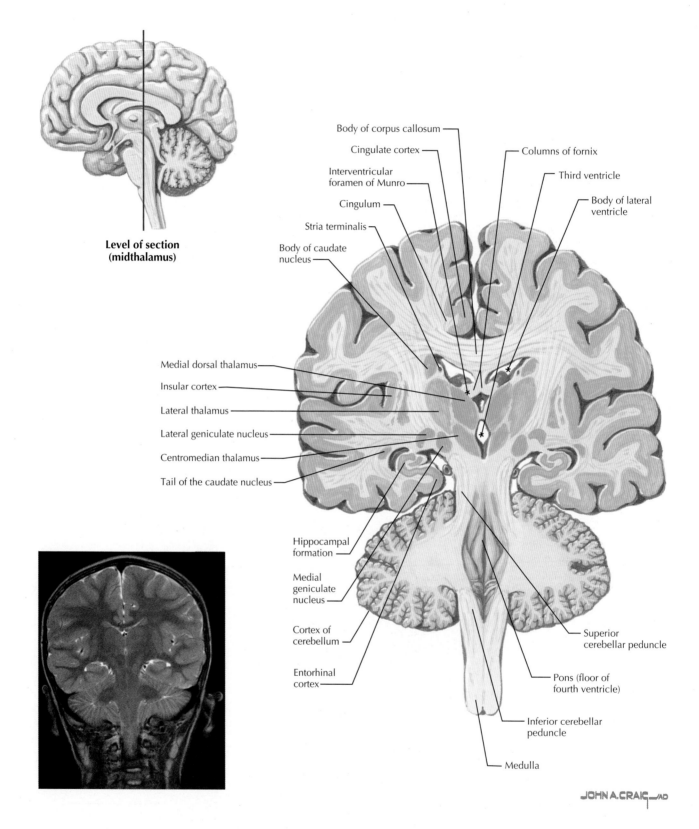

**Level of section
(midthalamus)**

Body of corpus callosum

Cingulate cortex

Interventricular
foramen of Munro

Cingulum

Stria terminalis

Body of caudate
nucleus

Columns of fornix

Third ventricle

Body of lateral
ventricle

Medial dorsal thalamus

Insular cortex

Lateral thalamus

Lateral geniculate nucleus

Centromedian thalamus

Tail of the caudate nucleus

Hippocampal
formation

Medial
geniculate
nucleus

Cortex of
cerebellum

Entorhinal
cortex

Superior
cerebellar peduncle

Pons (floor of
fourth ventricle)

Inferior cerebellar
peduncle

Medulla

JOHN A. CRAIG—AD

13.17A CORONAL SECTIONS THROUGH THE FOREBRAIN: LEVEL 7—MIDTHALAMUS

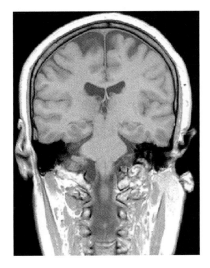

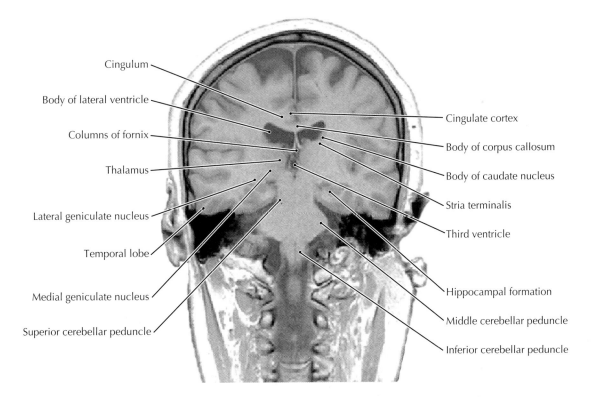

Cingulum

Body of lateral ventricle

Columns of fornix

Thalamus

Lateral geniculate nucleus

Temporal lobe

Medial geniculate nucleus

Superior cerebellar peduncle

Cingulate cortex

Body of corpus callosum

Body of caudate nucleus

Stria terminalis

Third ventricle

Hippocampal formation

Middle cerebellar peduncle

Inferior cerebellar peduncle

13.17B CORONAL SECTIONS THROUGH THE FOREBRAIN: LEVEL 7—MIDTHALAMUS (CONTINUED)

Level 8: Geniculate Nuclei

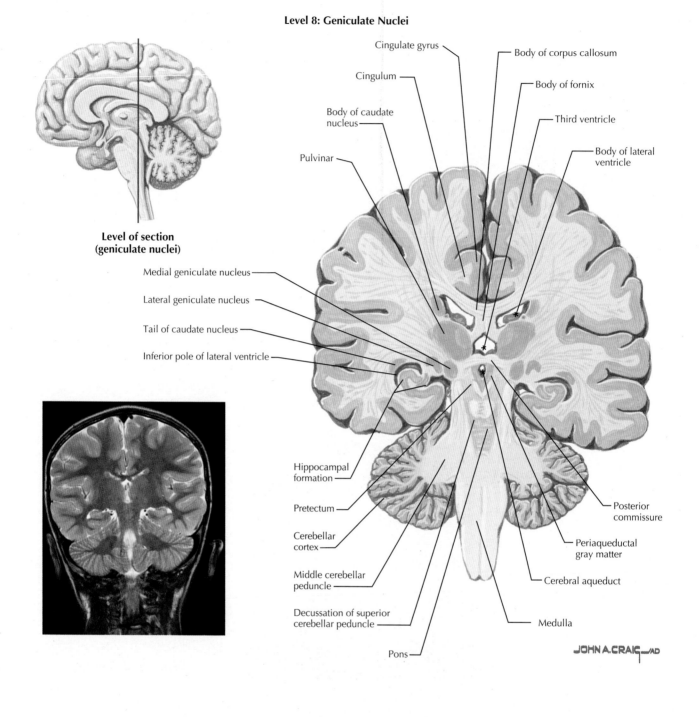

Level of section (geniculate nuclei)

Cingulate gyrus
Body of corpus callosum
Cingulum
Body of fornix
Body of caudate nucleus
Third ventricle
Pulvinar
Body of lateral ventricle
Medial geniculate nucleus
Lateral geniculate nucleus
Tail of caudate nucleus
Inferior pole of lateral ventricle
Hippocampal formation
Pretectum
Posterior commissure
Cerebellar cortex
Periaqueductal gray matter
Middle cerebellar peduncle
Cerebral aqueduct
Decussation of superior cerebellar peduncle
Medulla
Pons

JOHN A. CRAIG _AD

13.18A CORONAL SECTIONS THROUGH THE FOREBRAIN: LEVEL 8—GENICULATE NUCLEI

CLINICAL POINT

Several **thalamic nuclei in the posterior thalamus** are important for conveying visual and auditory information to the cerebral cortex. The lateral geniculate nucleus receives segregated input from the temporal hemiretina of the ipsilateral eye and from the nasal hemiretina of the contralateral eye, and it conveys this topographical information to area 17, the primary visual cortex, located on the banks of the calcarine fissure. A lesion in the lateral geniculate nucleus results in contralateral hemianopia. The pulvinar receives visual input from the superior colliculus and also conveys visual information to the visual cortex, to areas 18 and 19 (associative visual cortex). A lesion in the pulvinar can lead to contralateral visual neglect. The medial geniculate nucleus receives input from the inferior colliculus through the brachium of the inferior colliculus. However, because the auditory system is bilaterally represented at this level, a lesion in the medial geniculate nucleus on one side does not result in contralateral deafness. There may be some diminution of hearing contralateral to the lesion, but it is not a profound deficit. Visual areas 17, 18, and 19 correspond to visual cortices I, II, and III, as illustrated in Fig. 13.26.

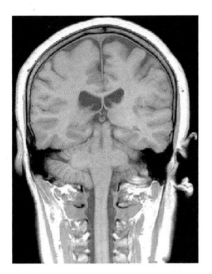

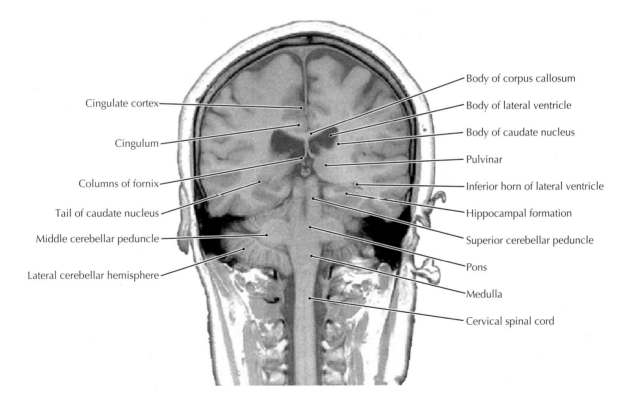

Cingulate cortex

Cingulum

Columns of fornix

Tail of caudate nucleus

Middle cerebellar peduncle

Lateral cerebellar hemisphere

Body of corpus callosum

Body of lateral ventricle

Body of caudate nucleus

Pulvinar

Inferior horn of lateral ventricle

Hippocampal formation

Superior cerebellar peduncle

Pons

Medulla

Cervical spinal cord

13.18B CORONAL SECTIONS THROUGH THE FOREBRAIN: LEVEL 8—GENICULATE NUCLEI (CONTINUED)

Level 9: Caudal Pulvinar and Superior Colliculus

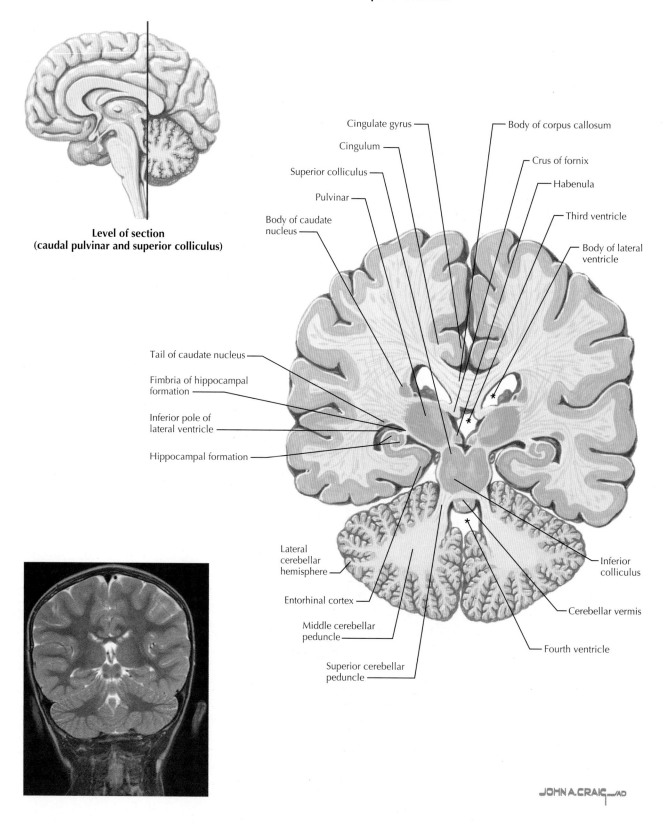

Level of section
(caudal pulvinar and superior colliculus)

Cingulate gyrus

Cingulum

Superior colliculus

Pulvinar

Body of caudate nucleus

Body of corpus callosum

Crus of fornix

Habenula

Third ventricle

Body of lateral ventricle

Tail of caudate nucleus

Fimbria of hippocampal formation

Inferior pole of lateral ventricle

Hippocampal formation

Lateral cerebellar hemisphere

Entorhinal cortex

Middle cerebellar peduncle

Superior cerebellar peduncle

Inferior colliculus

Cerebellar vermis

Fourth ventricle

JOHN A. CRAIG—AD

13.19A CORONAL SECTIONS THROUGH THE FOREBRAIN: LEVEL 9—CAUDAL PULVINAR AND SUPERIOR COLLICULUS

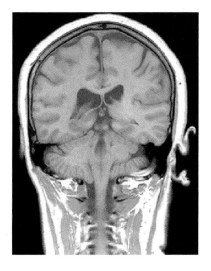

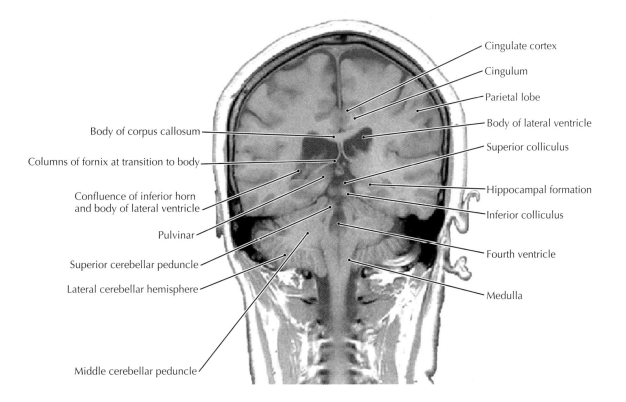

Cingulate cortex

Cingulum

Parietal lobe

Body of lateral ventricle

Body of corpus callosum

Superior colliculus

Columns of fornix at transition to body

Confluence of inferior horn and body of lateral ventricle

Hippocampal formation

Pulvinar

Inferior colliculus

Superior cerebellar peduncle

Fourth ventricle

Lateral cerebellar hemisphere

Medulla

Middle cerebellar peduncle

13.19B CORONAL SECTIONS THROUGH THE FOREBRAIN: LEVEL 9—CAUDAL PULVINAR AND SUPERIOR COLLICULUS (CONTINUED)

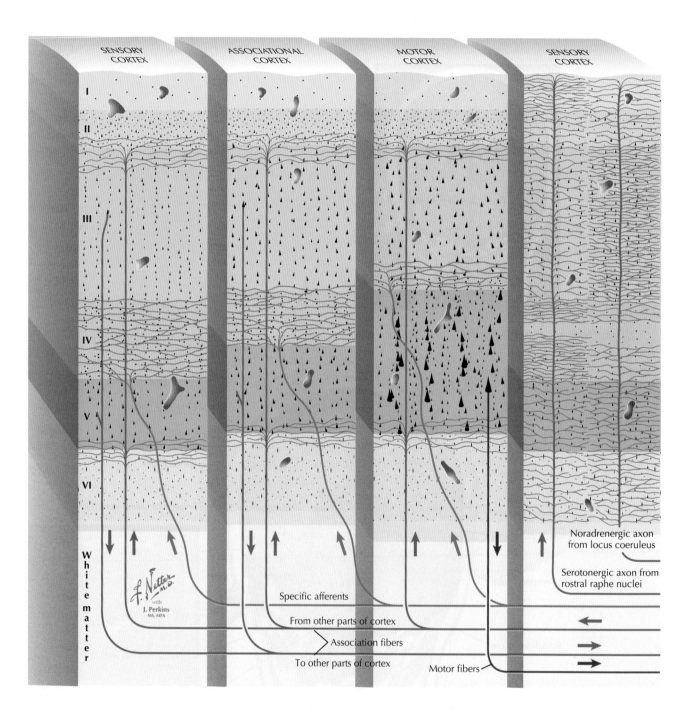

I

II

III

IV

V

VI

White matter

SENSORY CORTEX

ASSOCIATIONAL CORTEX

MOTOR CORTEX

SENSORY CORTEX

Noradrenergic axon from locus coeruleus

Serotonergic axon from rostral raphe nuclei

Specific afferents

From other parts of cortex

Association fibers

To other parts of cortex

Motor fibers

13.21 LAYERS OF THE CEREBRAL CORTEX

Regions of cerebral cortex with specific functional roles, such as the somatosensory cortex and the motor cortex, demonstrate histological characteristics that reflect that function. The sensory cortex has large granule cell layers (granular cortex) for receiving extensive input, whereas the motor cortex has sparse granule cell layers and extensive pyramidal cell layers, reflecting extensive output. Specific and nonspecific afferents terminate differentially in these structurally unique regions of the cortex. Monoamine inputs (noradrenergic and serotonergic) terminate more diffusely than do the specific inputs, reflecting the role of monoamines as modulators and enhancers of the activity of other neuronal systems.

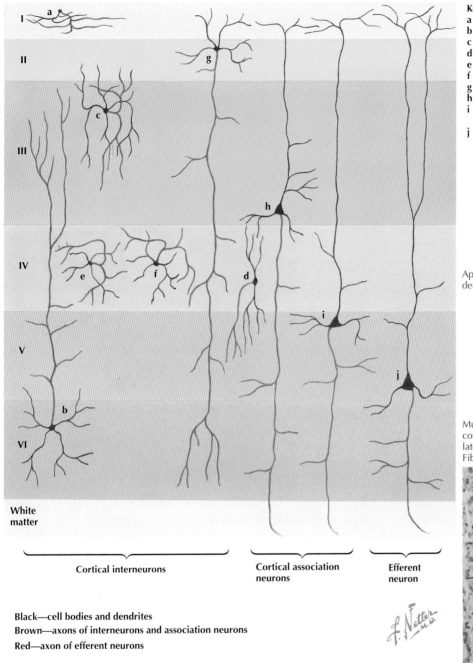

Key for Abbreviations
a Horizontal cell
b Cell of Martinotti
c Chandelier cell
d Aspiny granule cell
e Spiny granule cell
f Stellate (granule) cell
g Small pyramidal cell of layers II, III
h Small pyramidal association cell
i Small pyramidal association
   and projection cells of layer V
j Large pyramidal projection cell
   (Betz cell)

I
II
III
IV
V
VI

White
matter

Cortical interneurons

Cortical association
neurons

Efferent
neuron

Black—cell bodies and dendrites
Brown—axons of interneurons and association neurons
Red—axon of efferent neurons

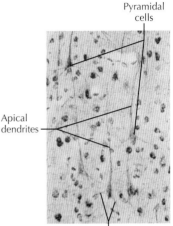

Pyramidal
cells

Apical
dendrites

Basolateral
dendrites

Multiple cortical pyramidal cells with
conspicuous apical dendrites and basolateral dendrites, and other cortical cells.
Fiber stain.

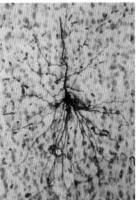

Pyramidal neuron with massive dendritic
branching, particularly the basolateral
dendrites. Golgi stain with background
cell stain.

13.22 CORTICAL NEURONAL CELL TYPES

The cerebral cortex has many anatomically unique cell types
that have characteristic cell bodies, dendritic arborizations, and
axonal distributions. Granule cells are local circuit neurons with
small cell bodies, localized dendritic trees, and axons that distribute locally. Granule cells function as receiving neurons for
thalamic and other inputs, and they modulate the excitability of
other cortical neurons. Pyramidal cells possess more varied cell

bodies (some large, some small) that have large basolateral dendritic branching patterns and apical dendritic arborizations that
run perpendicular to the cortical surface and arborize in upper
layers. The axons of pyramidal cells, which function as projection neurons (e.g., corticospinal tract neurons), leave the cortex
and may extend for as long as a meter before synapsing on target
neurons. These unique anatomical characteristics give rise to the
concept that neuronal structure explains neuronal function.

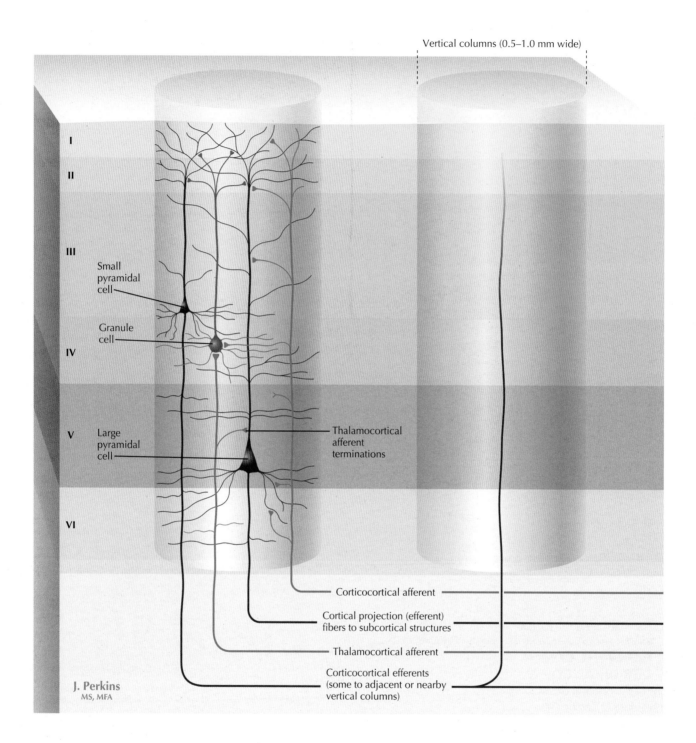

Vertical columns (0.5–1.0 mm wide)

I

II

III

Small pyramidal cell

Granule cell

IV

Large pyramidal cell

Thalamocortical afferent terminations

V

VI

J. Perkins
MS, MFA

Corticocortical afferent

Cortical projection (efferent) fibers to subcortical structures

Thalamocortical afferent

Corticocortical efferents (some to adjacent or nearby vertical columns)

13.23 VERTICAL COLUMNS: FUNCTIONAL UNITS OF THE CEREBRAL CORTEX

Experimental studies of sensory regions of the cerebral cortex provided anatomical and physiological evidence that discrete information that comes from a specific region or that conveys specific functional characteristics is processed in a cylindrical vertical zone of neurons in the cortex that spans all six layers of the neocortex. These vertical units vary from 0.5 to 1.0 mm in diameter. The diameter corresponds to the major horizontal expanse of a larger pyramidal cell in that unit. Both thalamic and cortical afferents arborize in the vertical column and synapse on both stellate (granule) cells and pyramidal neuron dendrites. Information from a vertical column can be sent to an adjacent or nearby column via corticocortical efferents or can be sent to distant structures by commissural fibers (cortex on the other side) or by projection fibers (subcortical structures). The minimal elements of the vertical unit are shown.

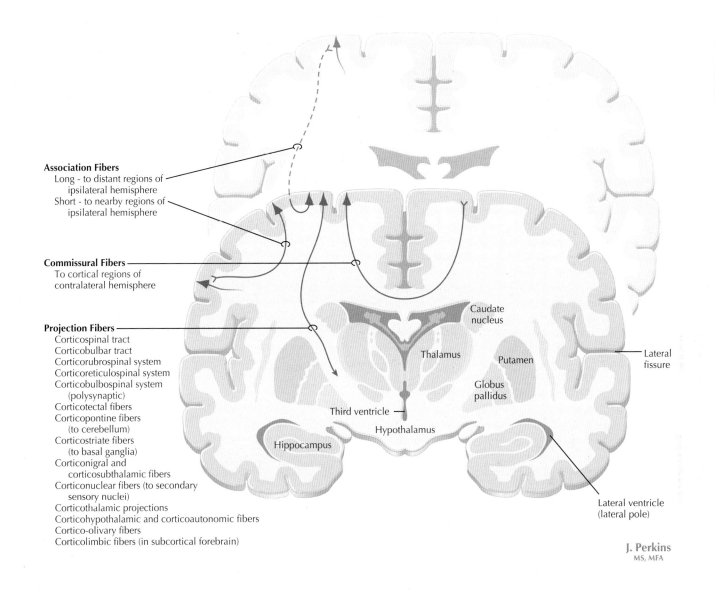

Association Fibers
Long - to distant regions of
ipsilateral hemisphere
Short - to nearby regions of
ipsilateral hemisphere

Commissural Fibers
To cortical regions of
contralateral hemisphere

Projection Fibers
Corticospinal tract
Corticobulbar tract
Corticorubrospinal system
Corticoreticulospinal system
Corticobulbospinal system
   (polysynaptic)
Corticotectal fibers
Corticopontine fibers
   (to cerebellum)
Corticostriate fibers
   (to basal ganglia)
Corticonigral and
   corticosubthalamic fibers
Corticonuclear fibers (to secondary
   sensory nuclei)
Corticothalamic projections
Corticohypothalamic and corticoautonomic fibers
Cortico-olivary fibers
Corticolimbic fibers (in subcortical forebrain)

Caudate
nucleus

Thalamus   Putamen   Lateral
                                   fissure
Globus
pallidus

Third ventricle

Hypothalamus

Hippocampus

Lateral ventricle
(lateral pole)

J. Perkins
MS, MFA

13.24 EFFERENT CONNECTIONS OF THE CEREBRAL CORTEX

Neurons of the cerebral cortex send efferent connections to three major regions: (1) association fibers are sent to other cortical regions of the same hemisphere, either nearby (short association fibers) or at a distance (long association fibers); (2) commissural fibers are sent to cortical regions of the other hemisphere through the corpus callosum or the anterior commissure; and (3) projection fibers are sent to numerous subcortical structures in the telencephalon, diencephalon, brainstem, and spinal cord. The major sites of termination of these connections are listed in the diagram.

The cortex does this through three types of efferent pathways: (1) association fibers; (2) commissural fibers; and (3) projection fibers. Association fibers interconnect with either nearby (short) or distant (long) regions of cortex. Damage to long association fibers can disconnect regions of cortex that normally need to communicate; this can result in altered language function, altered behavior, and other cortex-related problems. Damage to commissural fibers, especially the corpus callosum and anterior commissure, sometimes done deliberately to alleviate the spread of seizure activity, can result in a disconnection between the left and right hemispheres, with each hemisphere not being fully aware of what the other is doing because it does not have separate input. Damage to the projection fibers, which commonly accompanies infarcts or lesions in the internal capsule, can disrupt cortical outflow to the spinal cord, brainstem, cerebellum, thalamus and hypothalamus, basal ganglia, and limbic forebrain structures. As a consequence, major sensory deficits (especially in the opposite side for somatic sensation and vision), contralateral spastic hemiplegia with central facial involvement, hemianopia, and other motor, sensory, and behavioral deficits may occur.

CLINICAL POINT
The cerebral cortex provides the highest level of regulation over motor and sensory systems, behavior, cognition, and the functional capacities of the brain that are most characteristic of human accomplishment.

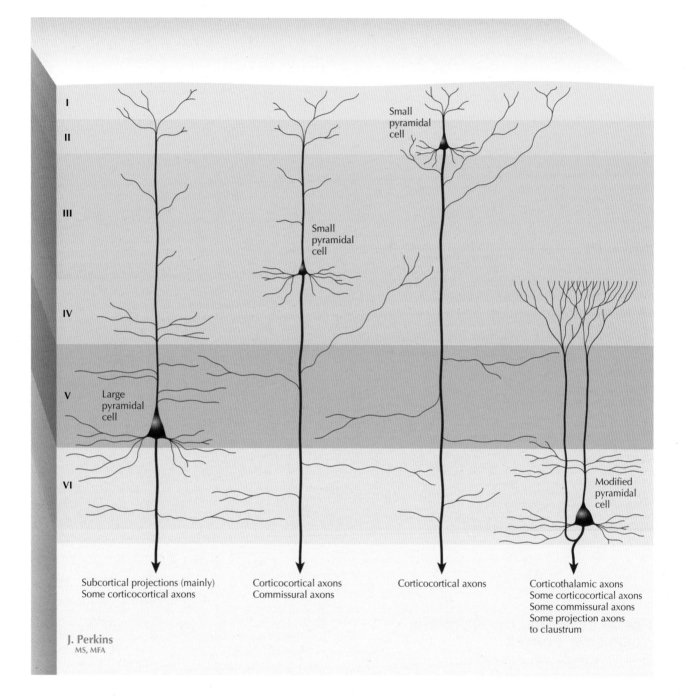

I

II

III

Small
pyramidal
cell

Small
pyramidal
cell

IV

V

Large
pyramidal
cell

VI

Modified
pyramidal
cell

Subcortical projections (mainly)
Some corticocortical axons

Corticocortical axons
Commissural axons

Corticocortical axons

Corticothalamic axons
Some corticocortical axons
Some commissural axons
Some projection axons
to claustrum

J. Perkins
MS, MFA

13.25 NEURONAL ORIGINS OF EFFERENT CONNECTIONS OF THE CEREBRAL CORTEX

Association fibers destined for cortical regions of the same hemisphere arise mainly from smaller pyramidal cells in cortical layers II and III and from modified pyramidal cells in layer VI.

Commissural fibers destined for cortical regions of the opposite hemisphere arise mainly from small pyramidal cells in cortical layer III and from some modified pyramidal cells in layer VI. Projection fibers arise from larger pyramidal cells in layer V and also from smaller pyramidal cells in layers V and VI. Only a small number of projection fibers arise from the giant Betz cells in layer V.

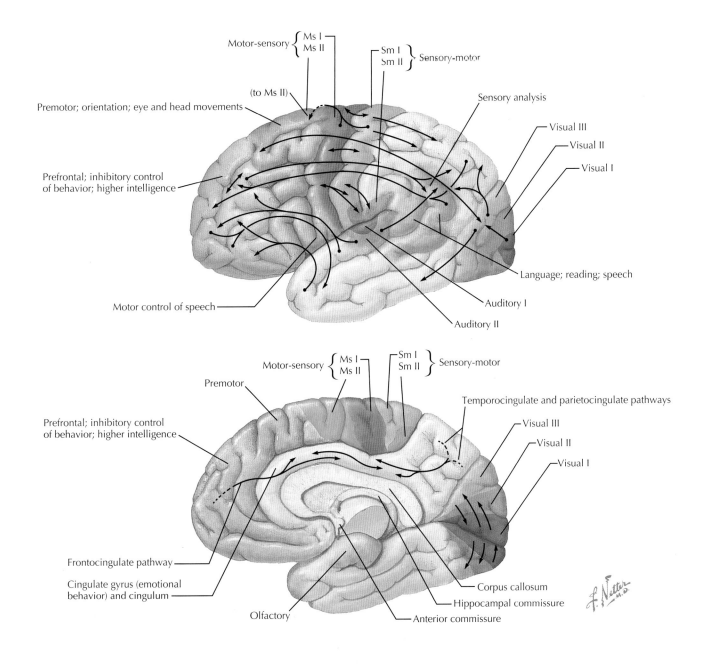

13.26 CORTICAL ASSOCIATION PATHWAYS

Neurons of the cerebral cortex have extensive connections with other regions of the brain (projection neurons), with the opposite hemisphere (commissural neurons), and with other regions of the ipsilateral hemisphere (association fibers). The cortical association fibers may connect a primary sensory cortex with adjacent association areas (e.g., visual cortex, somatosensory cortex) or may link multiple regions of cortex into complex association areas (e.g., polysensory analysis regions) or interlink important areas involved in language function, cognitive function, and emotional behavior and analysis. Damage to these pathways and associated cortical regions can result in loss of specific sensory and motor capabilities, aphasias (language disorders), agnosias (failures of recognition), and apraxias (performance deficits).

Broca's area of the frontal cortex and Wernicke's area in the parieto-temporal region are interconnected by long association fibers of the arcuate fasciculus or superior longitudinal fasciculus. When these association fibers are damaged, Broca's area and Wernicke's area are disconnected. The patient does not demonstrate a classic expressive or receptive aphasia but demonstrates the inability to repeat complex words or sentences. This is called conduction aphasia.

Subcortical white matter plays an important role in human behavior. Many types of pathology can affect subcortical white matter, such as multi-infarct damage or demyelination. These conditions cause a disconnection between regions of cerebral cortex or between subcortical regions and cortex. With multiple regions of **white matter damage**, dementia can occur, including inattention, emotional changes, and memory problems; such changes generally occur in the absence of movement disorders or aphasias. Multi-infarct damage to the ascending catecholamine and serotonin pathways from the brainstem can occur with destruction of the axons in the cingulum, resulting in depression and bipolar disorder, as well as attention deficits, especially with lesions involving ascending noradrenergic and reticular activating circuitry. Bilateral damage to white matter of the frontal lobe may result in euphoria and inappropriate affect, whereas damage to the long association fibers interconnecting the frontal lobes with limbic forebrain structures may result in psychotic behavior.

CLINICAL POINT

Long cortical association pathways link regions of cortex with each other. Some pathways link multiple sensory areas with multimodal cortical association cortex, providing the substrate for integrated interpretation of the outside world. Some association pathways connect language areas in the dominant hemisphere with each other.

A. Sagittal view

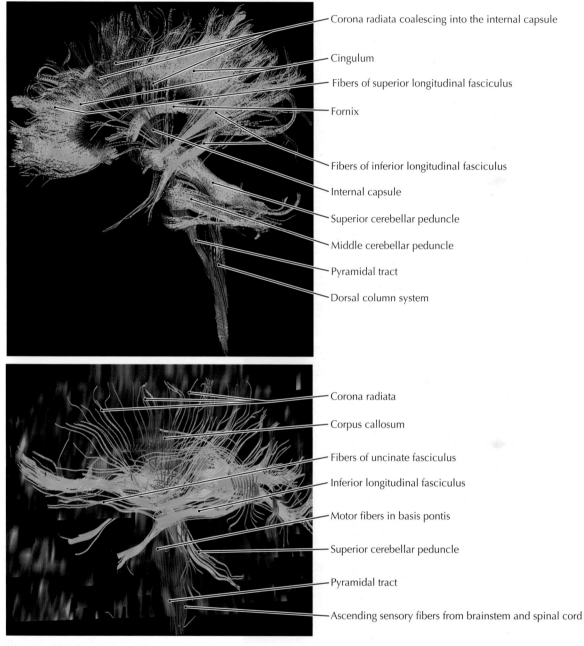

Corona radiata coalescing into the internal capsule

Cingulum

Fibers of superior longitudinal fasciculus

Fornix

Fibers of inferior longitudinal fasciculus

Internal capsule

Superior cerebellar peduncle

Middle cerebellar peduncle

Pyramidal tract

Dorsal column system

Corona radiata

Corpus callosum

Fibers of uncinate fasciculus

Inferior longitudinal fasciculus

Motor fibers in basis pontis

Superior cerebellar peduncle

Pyramidal tract

Ascending sensory fibers from brainstem and spinal cord

B. Sagittal view

13.29 COLOR IMAGING OF PROJECTION PATHWAYS FROM THE CEREBRAL CORTEX

These diffusion tensor images show the projection pathways of the forebrain in blue in two sagittal sections. The widespread cortical projection bundles channel into a narrow zone of the internal capsule and then proceed to their sites of projection in the forebrain, brainstem, or spinal cord. The descending corticospinal/corticobulbar system is particularly prominent. Projection systems associated with the cerebellum also are present. In addition, green association fibers and red commissural fibers can be seen. See Videos 13.3 and 13.4.

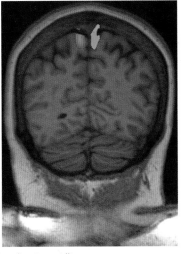

A. Coronal section showing midline motor cortex response to alternating movement of the toes.

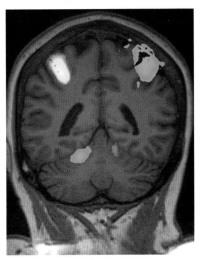

B. Coronal section showing contralateral convexity motor cortex response and ipsilateral cerebellar response to rapid alternating sequential tapping movement of the fingers bilaterally.

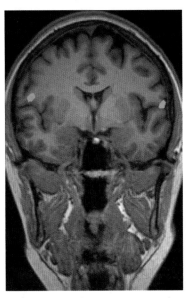

C. Coronal section showing Broca's area response to a language task in which subjects must silently discriminate word characteristics as abstract, concrete, single, double, upper case, or lower case over a 30-second time span.

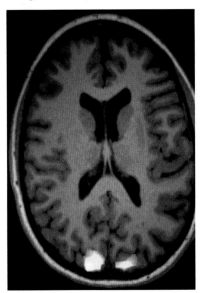

D. Axial section showing occipital cortex response to a visual task of viewing flickering alternating bands on a screen.

13.30 FUNCTIONAL MAGNETIC RESONANCE IMAGING

Functional magnetic resonance imaging (fMRI) is a noninvasive method that uses no radioactive tracers; it takes advantage of the fact that there is a difference in magnetic states of arterial and venous blood, thus providing an intrinsic mechanism of contrast for brain activation studies. The origin of this dual state of blood is due to the fact that the magnetic state of hemoglobin (Hb) depends on its oxygenation; the oxyhemoglobin state (arterial blood) is diamagnetic, and the venous deoxyhemoglobin state (venous blood) is paramagnetic. The change in oxygen saturation of the hemoglobin produces a detectable small signal change; hence, it is called the blood oxygenation level–dependent (BOLD) effect.

During neural activity, the supposition behind BOLD-fMRI is that the involved neurons represent a region of relatively greater oxygenated hemoglobin compared with nonactive regions in T2*-weighted images. However, there is a delay of several seconds between increased neural activity and increased oxygenated arterial blood flow to that region. BOLD-fMRI compares images during specific activity to images of the same region without such activity and can be used for processes that occur rapidly, such as language function, vision, audition, movement, cognitive tasks, and emotional responsiveness. The above images are taken from a sequence of coronal and axial sections showing regions of brain that are activated during (**A**) movement of toes, (**B**) sequential finger tapping, (**C**) language task, and (**D**) visual stimulation.

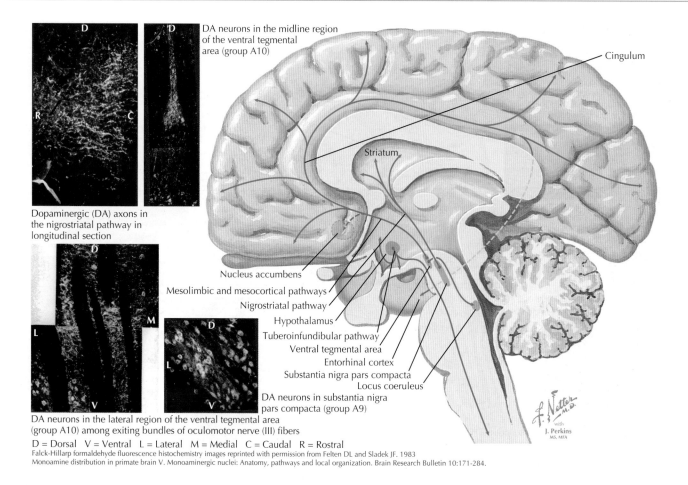

DA neurons in the midline region of the ventral tegmental area (group A10)

Cingulum

Striatum

Dopaminergic (DA) axons in the nigrostriatal pathway in longitudinal section

Nucleus accumbens
Mesolimbic and mesocortical pathways
Nigrostriatal pathway
Hypothalamus
Tuberoinfundibular pathway
Ventral tegmental area
Entorhinal cortex
Substantia nigra pars compacta
Locus coeruleus
DA neurons in substantia nigra pars compacta (group A9)

DA neurons in the lateral region of the ventral tegmental area (group A10) among exiting bundles of oculomotor nerve (III) fibers

D = Dorsal   V = Ventral   L = Lateral   M = Medial   C = Caudal   R = Rostral

Falck-Hillarp formaldehyde fluorescence histochemistry images reprinted with permission from Felten DL and Sladek JF. 1983
Monoamine distribution in primate brain V. Monoaminergic nuclei: Anatomy, pathways and local organization. Brain Research Bulletin 10:171-284.

13.33 DOPAMINERGIC PATHWAYS

DA neurons are found in the midbrain and hypothalamus. In the midbrain, neurons in the substantia nigra pars compacta (A9) project axons (along the nigrostriatal pathway) mainly to the striatum (caudate nucleus and putamen) and to the globus pallidus and subthalamus. This nigrostriatal projection is involved in basal ganglia circuitry that aids in the planning and execution of cortical activities, the most conspicuous of which involve the motor system. Damage to the nigrostriatal system results in Parkinson's disease, a disease characterized by resting tremor, muscular rigidity, bradykinesia (difficulty initiating movements or stopping them once they are initiated), and postural deficits. The antiparkinsonian drugs such as levodopa target this system and its receptors. Dopamine neurons in the ventral tegmental area and mesencephalic RF (A10) send mesolimbic projections to the nucleus accumbens, the amygdala, and the hippocampus, and they send mesocortical projections to the frontal cortex and some cortical association areas. The mesolimbic pathway to the nucleus accumbens is involved in motivation, reward, biological drives, and addictive behaviors, particularly substance abuse. The DA projections to limbic structures can induce stereotyped, repetitive behaviors and activities. The mesocortical projections influence cognitive functions in the planning and carrying out of frontal cortical activities and in attention mechanisms. The mesolimbic and mesocortical DA systems and their receptors are the targets of neuroleptic and antipsychotic agents that influence behaviors in schizophrenia, obsessive-compulsive disorder, attention deficit–hyperactivity disorder, Tourette's syndrome, and other

behavioral states. Dopamine neurons in the hypothalamus form the tuberoinfundibular dopamine pathway, which projects from the arcuate nucleus to the contact zone of the median eminence, where dopamine acts as prolactin inhibitory factor. Intrahypothalamic dopamine neurons also influence other neuroendocrine and visceral/autonomic hypothalamic functions.

CLINICAL POINT

Several discrete DA systems are found in the brain. The midbrain nigrostriatal DA system projects from the substantia nigra pars compacta to the striatum; these neurons degenerate in **Parkinson's disease**. The tuberoinfundibular and intrahypothalamic DA systems are involved in neuroendocrine regulation. A midbrain mesolimbic and mesocortical system sends widespread projections to the forebrain. The mesolimbic pathway to the nucleus accumbens regulates motivation, reward, biological drives, and addictive behaviors, playing an important role in substance abuse. Activation of this circuit can induce stereotyped, repetitive behaviors and activities. The mesolimbic and mesocortical DA systems are involved in many psychiatric disorders, including schizophrenia, obsessive-compulsive disorders, attention deficit–hyperactivity disorder, Tourette's syndrome, and other behavioral states. The use of neuroleptic and antipsychotic medications, which are D2 receptor antagonists, to treat schizophrenia led to the hypothesis that schizophrenia is related to the regulation of dopamine. The current hypothesis is that this disease may involve excessive activity in the mesolimbic DA system and a relative decrease in activity in the mesocortical DA system in the frontal lobes. Use of neuroleptic agents must be monitored carefully because chronic D2 receptor antagonism may lead to tardive dyskinesia, or permanent drug-induced movements.

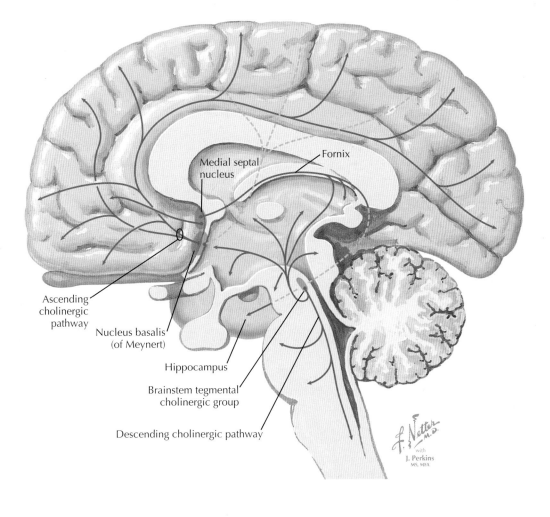

Medial septal nucleus

Fornix

Ascending cholinergic pathway

Nucleus basalis (of Meynert)

Hippocampus

Brainstem tegmental cholinergic group

Descending cholinergic pathway

13.34 CENTRAL CHOLINERGIC PATHWAYS

Central cholinergic neurons are found mainly in the nucleus basalis (of Meynert) and in septal nuclei. Nucleus basalis neurons project cholinergic axons to the cerebral cortex, and the septal cholinergic neurons project to the hippocampal formation. These cholinergic projections are involved in cortical activation and memory function, particularly consolidation of short-term memory. They often appear to be damaged in patients with Alzheimer's disease (AD). Drugs that enhance cholinergic function are used for improvement of memory. Other cholinergic neurons found in the brainstem tegmentum project to structures in the thalamus, brainstem, and cerebellum. The projections to the thalamus modulate arousal and the sleep-wake cycle and appear to be important in the initiation of REM sleep. Cholinergic interneurons are present in the striatum and may participate in basal ganglia control of tone, posture, and initiation of movement or selection of wanted patterns of activity. In some cases, pharmacological agents are targeted at reducing cholinergic activity in the basal ganglia in Parkinson's disease, as a complementary approach to enhancing DA activity. Acetylcholine also is used as the principal neurotransmitter in all preganglionic autonomic neurons and lower motor neurons in the spinal cord and brainstem.

CLINICAL POINT

Central cholinergic neurons are found in the basal forebrain (nucleus basalis of Meynert and nucleus of the diagonal band) and medial septum. The nucleus basalis cholinergic neurons are found in the substantia innominata and also along the ventral extent of the forebrain. The nucleus basalis and the nucleus of the diagonal band cholinergic neurons provide the major cholinergic input to the cerebral cortex. Cholinergic neurons of the medial septum send axons through the fornix to innervate the hippocampal formation. In patients with AD, a loss of cholinergic neurons (positive for choline acetyltransferase, the rate-limiting enzyme for acetylcholine synthesis) is most closely correlated with cognitive impairment. AD patients also show a loss of muscarinic and nicotinic cholinergic receptors and high-affinity choline uptake. Pharmacological agents such as the cholinesterase inhibitor tetrahydroaminoacridine (tacrine) have targeted cholinergic neurons in AD, and some data show a slowing in short-term memory dysfunction. Because choline is recycled for resynthesis of acetylcholine, some studies have used choline or lecithin in an attempt to boost precursor availability for added synthesis of acetylcholine; this approach has not met with great success. It may reflect the fact that AD alters many other neurotransmitter systems in the CNS in addition to the cholinergics, such as substance P, CRF, somatostatin, norepinephrine, and neuropeptide Y.

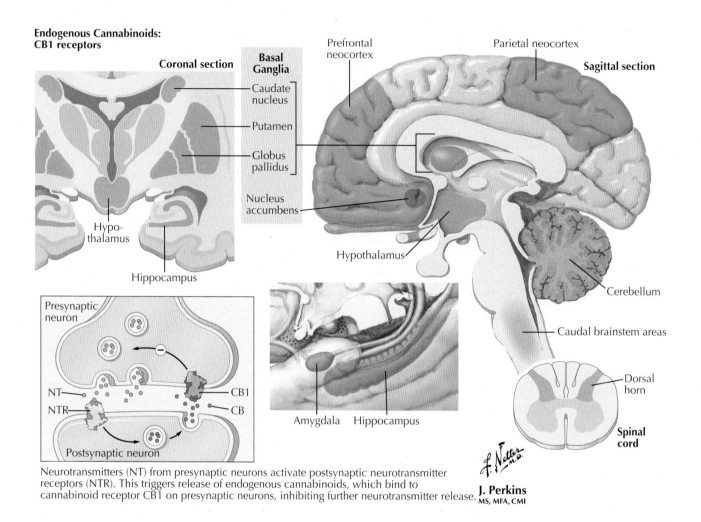

Endogenous Cannabinoids: CB1 receptors

Coronal section

Basal Ganglia

Caudate nucleus

Putamen

Globus pallidus

Nucleus accumbens

Hypothalamus

Hippocampus

Prefrontal neocortex

Parietal neocortex

Sagittal section

Hypothalamus

Cerebellum

Caudal brainstem areas

Dorsal horn

Spinal cord

Presynaptic neuron

NT

NTR

CB1

CB

Postsynaptic neuron

Amygdala Hippocampus

Neurotransmitters (NT) from presynaptic neurons activate postsynaptic neurotransmitter receptors (NTR). This triggers release of endogenous cannabinoids, which bind to cannabinoid receptor CB1 on presynaptic neurons, inhibiting further neurotransmitter release.

J. Perkins
MS, MFA, CMI

13.35 ENDOGENOUS CANNABINOID SYSTEMS

Endogenous cannabinoids (endocannabinoids, ECs) are arachidonic acid derivatives synthesized from membrane-associated lipids. Two principal ECs, anandamine (N-arachidonoylethanolamine) and 2DG (2-arachidonoylglycerol), are released from neurons as "reverse neurotransmitters" and activate cannabinoid receptors. They are taken up into neurons and astrocytes and catabolized by an enzyme (fatty acid hydrolase); an attempt to block this enzyme with an experimental pharmaceutical agent led to toxic consequences, including death. These ECs are the endogenous ligands for cannabinoid receptors (CB1: found mainly on neurons, axons, and nerve terminals; CB2: in periphery on macrophages and lymphocytes, with a role in inflammation). CB receptors are G1/G0 proteins and can initiate signaling events. CB1 receptors in the CNS are found in high concentrations in the neocortex, limbic forebrain structures (amygdala, hippocampus),

basal ganglia, nucleus accumbens, hypothalamic areas, cerebellum, brainstem nuclei, and spinal cord (especially on primary afferents).

At synapses, ECs act as reverse or retrograde signal molecules. Membrane activation postsynaptically produces ECs (from precursors in the neuron), which are released to act on CB1 receptors on the presynaptic terminals, which mainly results in inhibition of other neurotransmitters (both excitatory and inhibitory transmitters). Exogenous cannabinoid administration also can activate CB1 receptors in the brain. ECs are implicated in cognitive activities and judgment, learning and memory of new information, emotional responsiveness (panic, paranoia, euphoria), reaction time, coordination, antinausea effects, increased appetite, pain sensitivity, and many other physiological activities. ECs also may play a neuroprotective role in traumatic brain injury and in neuronal repair in neurodegenerative diseases.

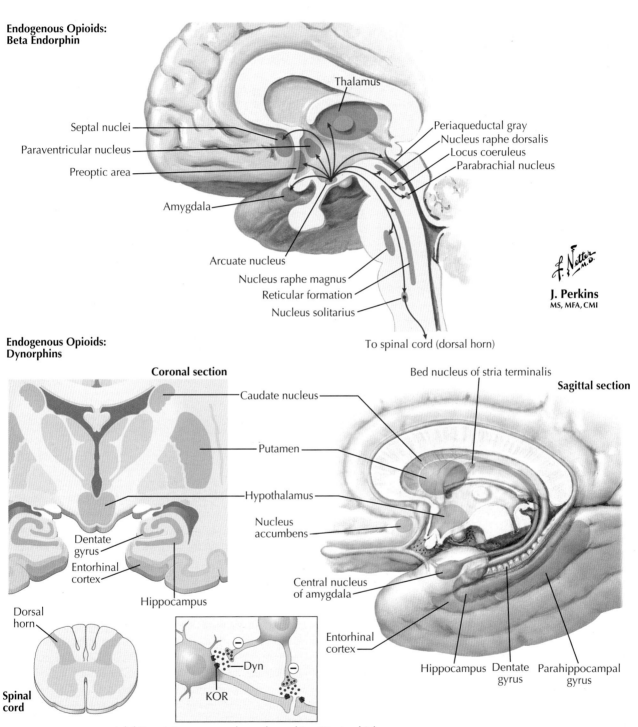

Endogenous Opioids: Beta Endorphin

Thalamus

Septal nuclei

Paraventricular nucleus

Preoptic area

Amygdala

Periaqueductal gray

Nucleus raphe dorsalis

Locus coeruleus

Parabrachial nucleus

Arcuate nucleus

Nucleus raphe magnus

Reticular formation

Nucleus solitarius

To spinal cord (dorsal horn)

J. Perkins
MS, MFA, CMI

Endogenous Opioids: Dynorphins

Coronal section

Bed nucleus of stria terminalis

Sagittal section

Caudate nucleus

Putamen

Hypothalamus

Nucleus accumbens

Dentate gyrus

Entorhinal cortex

Hippocampus

Central nucleus of amygdala

Entorhinal cortex

Dorsal horn

Dyn

KOR

Spinal cord

Hippocampus Dentate gyrus Parahippocampal gyrus

Inhibitory interneurons release dynorphins (Dyn), which bind to kappa opioid receptors (KOR) on target neurons

13.36A ENDOGENOUS OPIOID SYSTEMS: BETA-ENDORPHIN, DYNORPHINS, AND MET-ENKEPHALIN

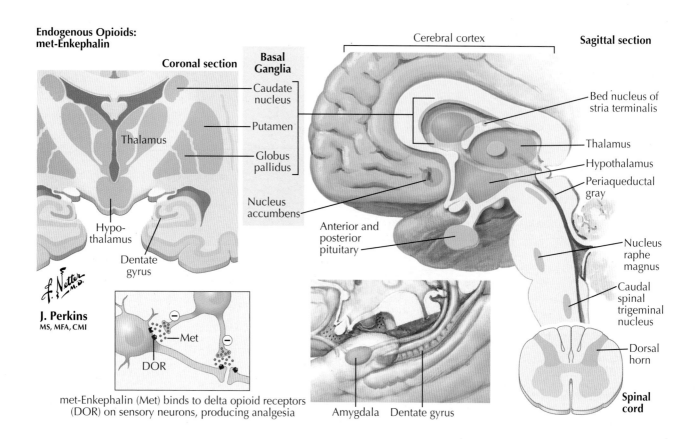

Endogenous Opioids: met-Enkephalin

Coronal section

Basal Ganglia

Cerebral cortex

Sagittal section

Caudate nucleus

Putamen

Thalamus

Globus pallidus

Nucleus accumbens

Hypo-thalamus

Dentate gyrus

J. Perkins
MS, MFA, CMI

Met

DOR

met-Enkephalin (Met) binds to delta opioid receptors (DOR) on sensory neurons, producing analgesia

Anterior and posterior pituitary

Amygdala   Dentate gyrus

Bed nucleus of stria terminalis

Thalamus

Hypothalamus

Periaqueductal gray

Nucleus raphe magnus

Caudal spinal trigeminal nucleus

Dorsal horn

Spinal cord

13.36B ENDOGENOUS OPIOID SYSTEMS: BETA-ENDORPHIN, DYNORPHINS, AND MET-ENKEPHALIN (CONTINUED)

Beta-endorphin neurons. Beta-endorphin neurons are found mainly in the arcuate nucleus in the hypothalamus (sometimes referred to as the peri-arcuate region) and, to a lesser extent, in the nucleus of the solitary tract (nucleus solitarius). Beta-endorphin neurons in the arcuate nucleus project axons to limbic structures, numerous hypothalamic regions, some thalamic sites, and numerous brainstem nuclei. Beta-endorphin neurons in nucleus solitarius project axons to the spinal cord. In the hypothalamus, beta-endorphin neurons innervate corticotropin-releasing hormone (CRH) neurons and inhibit CRH release. Beta-endorphin also inhibits activity of the stress axes. Beta-endorphin plays an important physiological role in analgesia, regulation and release of pituitary hormones, amelioration of anxiety, appetitive behavior, temperature regulation, and other visceral functions. Beta-endorphin binds to mu, kappa, and delta opioid receptors.

Dynorphin neurons. Dynorphins are found in neurons in the hippocampus (dentate gyrus mossy fibers), entorhinal cortex, other limbic structures (central amygdaloid nucleus, bed nucleus of the stria terminalis), basal forebrain (nucleus accumbens), striatum (caudate nucleus, putamen), brainstem nuclei, and

the spinal cord. Dynorphins act mainly on kappa opioid receptors and generally inhibit excitatory neurons. Dynorphins play a functional role in pain responses, stress responses, appetitive behaviors, temperature regulation, learning and memory, and emotional control. Dynorphins also are involved in neurological disorders, including seizure disorders, addictive behaviors, and psychiatric disorders (depression, schizophrenia).

met-Enkephalin neurons. met-Enkephalin is found in small, local circuit neurons in widespread CNS sites, including the cerebral cortex, basal ganglia (medium spiny neurons), limbic sites (amygdala, hippocampal granule cells in the dentate gyrus, bed nucleus of the stria terminalis), basal forebrain (nucleus accumbens), thalamic and hypothalamic regions, many brainstem nuclei, and the spinal cord. met-Enkephalin cells also are found in the adrenal medulla and the anterior and posterior pituitary. met-Enkephalin acts mainly on delta opioid receptors and, to a lesser extent, on mu receptors. met-Enkephalin integrates sensory information related to pain perception and emotional responsiveness. met-Enkephalin also helps to modulate memory responses, some visceral hypothalamic responses (food and water regulation), and dopamine release in the mesolimbic and mesocortical pathways from neurons in the ventral tegmental area.

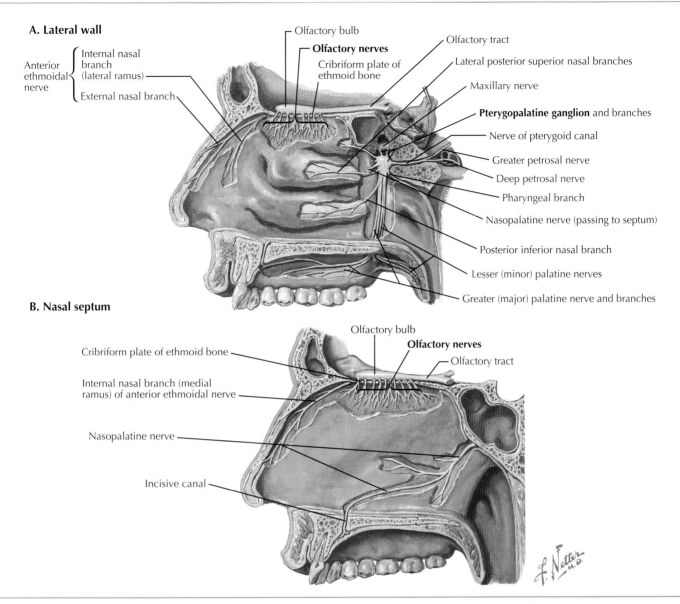

A. Lateral wall

Anterior ethmoidal nerve
- Internal nasal branch (lateral ramus)
- External nasal branch

Olfactory bulb
Olfactory nerves
Cribriform plate of ethmoid bone

Olfactory tract
Lateral posterior superior nasal branches
Maxillary nerve
Pterygopalatine ganglion and branches
Nerve of pterygoid canal
Greater petrosal nerve
Deep petrosal nerve
Pharyngeal branch
Nasopalatine nerve (passing to septum)
Posterior inferior nasal branch
Lesser (minor) palatine nerves
Greater (major) palatine nerve and branches

B. Nasal septum

Cribriform plate of ethmoid bone
Internal nasal branch (medial ramus) of anterior ethmoidal nerve
Nasopalatine nerve
Incisive canal

Olfactory bulb
Olfactory nerves
Olfactory tract

13.37 THE OLFACTORY NERVE AND NERVES OF THE NOSE

The olfactory nerves and their projections into the CNS are important components of forebrain function. Bipolar cells in the olfactory epithelium are the primary sensory neurons. The peripheral axon, a chemosensory transducer, and its branches respond to the unique chemical stimuli of airborne molecules entering the nose. The central axons of the bipolar neurons aggregate into groups of approximately 20 slender olfactory nerves that traverse the cribriform plate and end in glomeruli of the ipsilateral olfactory bulb. These nerves are vulnerable to tearing, which results in anosmia. Unlike neurons in other sensory systems, these bipolar neurons can proliferate and regenerate. After processing information in the olfactory bulb, mitral neurons and tufted neurons project via the olfactory tract directly and indirectly to limbic forebrain structures, including septal nuclei and amygdaloid nuclei. These projections bypass the thalamus, have immediate access to limbic forebrain structures, and directly influence the hypothalamus and its regulation of neuroendocrine and visceral/autonomic function. The olfactory system is essential for survival in many species and is involved in territorial recognition and defense, food and water acquisition, social behavior, reproductive behavior, signaling of danger, stress responses, and other visceral functions.

CLINICAL POINT

The olfactory nerves possess receptors that can detect a wide range of unique odorants. This information is conveyed through the olfactory bulb to central forebrain sites, particularly those in the limbic forebrain, bypassing the thalamus, usually a processing zone for sensory projections to the forebrain. Olfaction is particularly important in recognizing the taste of food. What many people interpret as taste actually has a major olfactory component. Even very strong-tasting substances cannot be readily discerned by most people when the olfactory system is blocked, perhaps explaining the reduced gustatory experience of a good meal when someone has a cold. Clearly, both taste and smell must work together for full appreciation of food. Several regions of the brain have been identified as important sites for the interpretation of smell, including the orbitofrontal cortex and its major interconnected thalamic nucleus (medial dorsal) as well as the anterior temporal lobe. Ablation of the anterior temporal lobe, particularly on the dominant side, leads to olfactory agnosias. The involvement of the temporal lobe in the interpretation and processing of olfaction is further emphasized by olfactory auras of highly aversive or foul smells during temporal lobe seizures. Stimulation of specific olfactory receptors with odorant molecules can influence visceral responses such as appetite, relaxation, alertness, motion sickness, nausea, insomnia, headache pain, and others.

14

SENSORY SYSTEMS

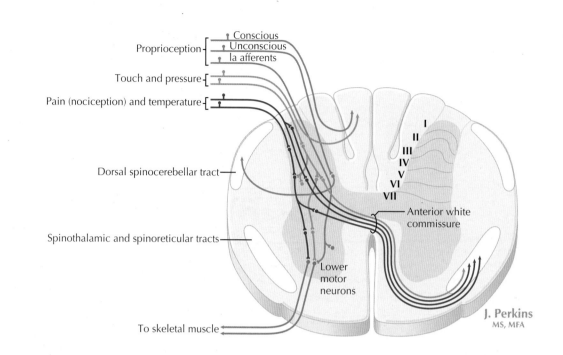

Proprioception — Conscious / Unconscious / Ia afferents

Touch and pressure

Pain (nociception) and temperature

Dorsal spinocerebellar tract

Spinothalamic and spinoreticular tracts

Lower motor neurons

Anterior white commissure

To skeletal muscle

J. Perkins
MS, MFA

SOMATOSENSORY SYSTEMS

14.1 SOMATOSENSORY AFFERENTS TO THE SPINAL CORD

Unmyelinated (UNM) and small myelinated (M) axons that convey nociception and temperature sensation terminate in laminae I and V (origin of the spinothalamic tract). Other UNM axons terminate in the dorsal horn, from which neurons for polysynaptic reflexes and for the spinoreticular system originate. M axons for touch and pressure terminate in the dorsal horn, from which additional reflex connections, spinothalamic projections, and supplementary epicritic projections to the dorsal column (DC) nuclei originate. M axons also project directly into fasciculi gracilis and cuneatus, destined for nuclei gracilis and cuneatus; these lemniscal pathways process epicritic information for conscious interpretation. M proprioceptive axons (Ia afferents) terminate directly on lower motor neurons (LMNs) and on the Ia interneuronal pool. Additional M axons terminate in the dorsal horn on neurons of origin for the spinocerebellar tracts.

CLINICAL POINT

Primary afferents include both epicritic afferents (mainly larger diameter M axons that convey fine, discriminative touch; vibratory sensation; and joint position sense) and protopathic afferents (mainly small M or UNM axons that convey mainly nociceptive information and temperature sensation). These axons can be affected differentially in neuropathies. Some **peripheral neuropathies** can affect all modalities, leading to a total loss of sensation; other peripheral neuropathies affect selected populations of axons and their related modalities. Selective loss of protopathic modalities may occur in leprosy, in amyloid neuropathy, and in some cases of diabetic neuropathy, leading to insensitivity to pain and temperature. Selective loss of epicritic sensation may occur in some distal symmetrical polyneuropathies, neuropathy with vitamin B_{12} deficiency, Guillain-Barré syndrome, and others, accompanied by paresthesias (numbness and tingling,

"pins and needles," abnormal sensations), dysesthesias (disagreeable or abnormal sensations in the absence of stimulation), hyperesthesia (increased sensation with stimulation), or hypesthesia (diminished sensation with stimulation). Some neuropathic conditions also are accompanied by allodynia (pain evoked by normally nonpainful stimuli) and burning, stabbing, radiating pain. Peripheral neuropathies that affect larger diameter M axons often can also affect the motor axons, leading to weakness and hyporeflexia or areflexia. Some small fiber neuropathies, especially diabetic neuropathies, may affect small autonomic axons to bowel, bladder, reproductive organs, and peripheral blood vessels, leading to orthostatic hypotension, bladder dysfunction, chronic gastrointestinal problems, or erectile dysfunction.

CLINICAL POINT

The monosynaptic reflex (the **muscle stretch reflex**) is tested in a clinical neurological examination. Specific muscle tendons are tapped, with the expected result of contraction of the homonymous muscle (e.g., tapping of the patellar tendon resulting in contraction of the ipsilateral quadriceps muscle). The muscle stretch reflexes routinely tested in a neurological examination include the biceps reflex, triceps reflex, brachioradialis reflex, patellar (knee-jerk) reflex, and ankle-jerk reflex on both sides. The reflexes are graded on a numerical scale ranging from hyporeflexic to normoreflexic to hyperreflexic; normal physiological reflexes may vary in responsiveness, so the result of reflex testing must be considered in conjunction with other clinical signs and symptoms. For example, hyperreflexia in a pathological state such as stroke or spinal cord injury may be accompanied by hypertonia of the affected muscle, spasticity, abnormal reflexes (extensor plantar response), and repetitive alternating hyperreflexic responses (clonus). In contrast, hyporeflexia or areflexia accompanying peripheral neuropathy may be accompanied by muscle weakness and flaccidity and diminished sensation of epicritic modalities, protopathic modalities, or both. More formal testing of reflexic responses can be done with electromyography and conduction velocity studies.

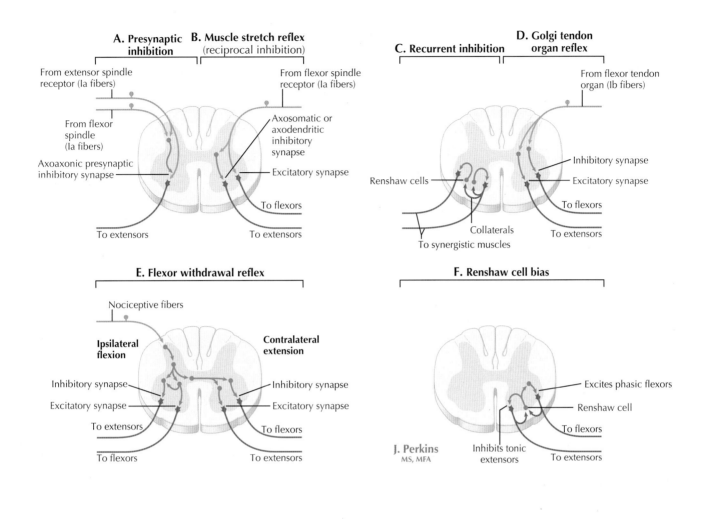

A. Presynaptic inhibition

B. Muscle stretch reflex (reciprocal inhibition)

From extensor spindle receptor (Ia fibers)

From flexor spindle receptor (Ia fibers)

From flexor spindle (Ia fibers)

Axosomatic or axodendritic inhibitory synapse

Axoaxonic presynaptic inhibitory synapse

Excitatory synapse

To flexors

To extensors

To extensors

C. Recurrent inhibition

D. Golgi tendon organ reflex

From flexor tendon organ (Ib fibers)

Renshaw cells

Inhibitory synapse

Excitatory synapse

To flexors

Collaterals

To synergistic muscles

To extensors

E. Flexor withdrawal reflex

Nociceptive fibers

Ipsilateral flexion

Contralateral extension

Inhibitory synapse

Inhibitory synapse

Excitatory synapse

Excitatory synapse

To extensors

To flexors

To flexors

To extensors

F. Renshaw cell bias

Excites phasic flexors

Renshaw cell

To flexors

J. Perkins
MS, MFA

Inhibits tonic extensors

To extensors

14.2 SPINAL SOMATIC REFLEX ACTIONS AND PATHWAYS

A, Presynaptic inhibition. Some interneurons synapse on the terminal arborizations of other axons, as in the case of some afferent pools associated with muscle stretch reflexes. These axoaxonic contacts permit the modulation of neurotransmitter release from the second (target) axon terminal by depolarization of the terminal membrane, altering the influx of Ca^{++}. **B,** Muscle stretch reflex. In the muscle stretch reflex, Ia afferents excite the homonymous LMN pool directly and inhibit the antagonist LMN pool reciprocally via Ia inhibitory interneurons. **C,** Recurrent inhibition. Some interneurons receive recurrent collaterals from axons (e.g., LMN axons) and project back onto the dendrites or cell body of origin of that axon, usually inhibiting that neuron. This process can help to regulate the excitability and timing of excitation of the target neurons. Collaterals of LMN axons excite Renshaw cells (large interneurons), which inhibit the LMN of origin as well as LMNs projecting to synergistic muscles. Renshaw inhibition permits wiping the slate clean, after original excitation, of pools of LMNs, requiring additional incoming stimulation in order to excite these LMNs again. **D,** Golgi tendon organ reflex. Ib axons from Golgi tendon organs in muscle tendons terminate on pools of interneurons that inhibit LMNs to the homonymous muscle disynaptically and excite LMNs to the antagonist muscle

reciprocally. The action of this reflex as a protective mechanism to prevent damage to a muscle during generation of maximal tension on the tendon is seen in attempted passive stretch of a spastic muscle; the resultant inhibition of the homonymous LMN pool is called a clasp-knife reflex. **E,** Flexor withdrawal reflex. A flexor reflex (also called a withdrawal reflex or a nociceptive reflex) occurs when afferents derived from a noxious stimulus terminate on pools of interneurons that excite appropriate pools of LMNs (often flexor LMNs) to bring about a protective withdrawal from the source of the noxious stimulus. These interneurons also inhibit the antagonist LMNs through reciprocal inhibition. Flexor reflexes can extend throughout the spinal cord, as happens when one touches a hot stove with a finger; the result is the removal of the entire arm, or even the entire body, away from the source of heat. These flexor reflexes may involve both sides of spinal cord. **F,** Renshaw cell bias. Some reflex responses such as Renshaw reflexes (see part C) may result in the distribution of influence (bias) in a manner that favors a particular type of action. Renshaw cells receive inputs from axon collaterals of both flexor and extensor LMNs, but their projections are directed mainly toward the inhibition of tonic extensor LMNs (and through reciprocal inhibition with the excitation of phasic flexor LMNs). Thus, the Renshaw cell response favors flexor movements and helps to inhibit extensor movements.

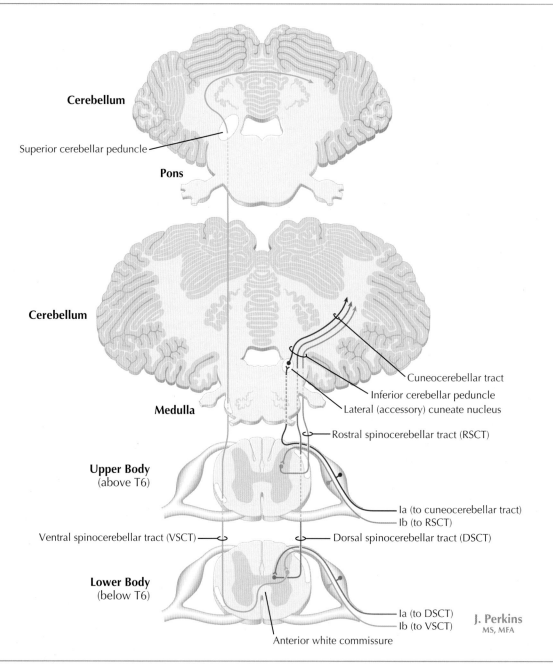

Cerebellum

Superior cerebellar peduncle

Pons

Cerebellum

Medulla

Cuneocerebellar tract

Inferior cerebellar peduncle

Lateral (accessory) cuneate nucleus

Rostral spinocerebellar tract (RSCT)

Upper Body
(above T6)

Ia (to cuneocerebellar tract)

Ib (to RSCT)

Ventral spinocerebellar tract (VSCT)

Dorsal spinocerebellar tract (DSCT)

Lower Body
(below T6)

Ia (to DSCT)

Ib (to VSCT)

J. Perkins
MS, MFA

Anterior white commissure

14.3 SOMATOSENSORY SYSTEM: SPINOCEREBELLAR PATHWAYS

Proprioceptive primary somatosensory axons from joints, tendons, and ligaments (represented in this figure by Ib afferents from Golgi tendon organs) terminate on neurons of origin (border cells, dorsal horn) of the ventral spinocerebellar tract (VSCT) and the rostral spinocerebellar tract (RSCT) from the lower and upper body, respectively (level T6 is the cut-off point). Proprioceptive primary somatosensory axons from muscle spindles (represented in this figure by Ia afferents) terminate on neurons of origin (Clarke's nucleus, lateral [external] cuneate nucleus of the medulla) of the dorsal spinocerebellar tract (DSCT) and the cuneocerebellar tract from the lower and upper body, respectively (level T6 is the cut-off point). The DSCT, RSCT, and cuneocerebellar tracts remain ipsilateral. The VSCT crosses twice, once in the anterior white commissure of the spinal cord and again in the cerebellum.

CLINICAL POINT

The dorsal and ventral spinocerebellar pathways travel in a conspicuous site at the lateral edge of the lateral funiculus throughout most of its length; these pathways are vulnerable to lesions that impinge on this zone of the spinal cord. They include tumors, radiculopathies with accompanying myelopathies, combined-system degeneration, demyelinating diseases, vascular infarcts in the anterior circulation of the cord, Brown-Séquard lesions, and other pathologies. Such a lesion, if superficial in the lateral funiculus, results in ipsilateral ataxia, dysmetria, clumsiness, and mild hypotonia, with impaired ability to perform heel-to-shin testing and tandem walking. However, lesions of the lateral funiculus often also involve the descending upper motor axons of the lateral corticospinal tract and the rubrospinal tract. Lesions that involve these tracts cause ipsilateral spastic hemiparesis or monoparesis below the level of the lesion, depending on the level of the lesion. The resulting spastic weakness, hyperreflexia, and hypertonus predominate in the clinical picture, thus masking the spinocerebellar symptomatology. Thus, an initial picture of **spinocerebellar damage** may give way to a progressive picture of spastic paresis on the same side.

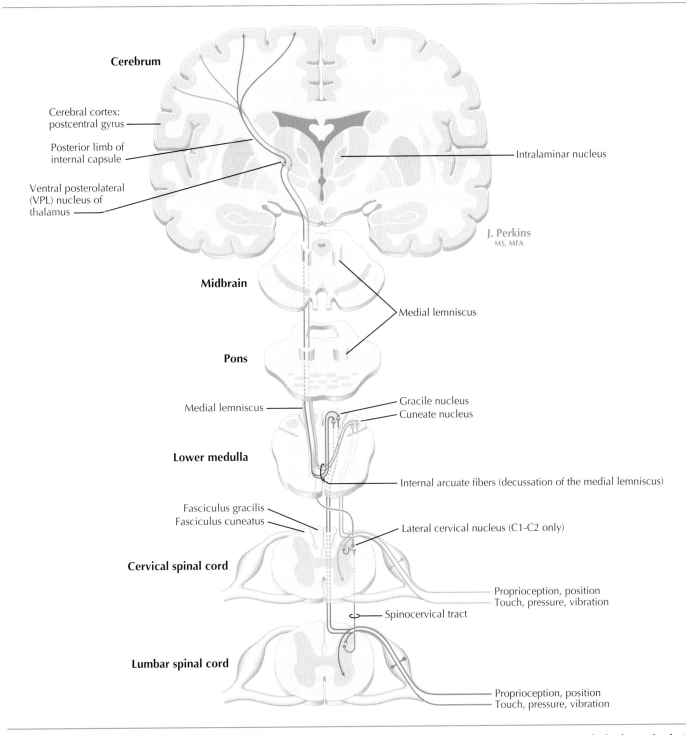

Cerebrum

Cerebral cortex: postcentral gyrus

Posterior limb of internal capsule

Ventral posterolateral (VPL) nucleus of thalamus

J. Perkins
MS, MFA

Intralaminar nucleus

Midbrain

Medial lemniscus

Pons

Medial lemniscus

Gracile nucleus
Cuneate nucleus

Lower medulla

Internal arcuate fibers (decussation of the medial lemniscus)

Fasciculus gracilis
Fasciculus cuneatus

Lateral cervical nucleus (C1-C2 only)

Cervical spinal cord

Proprioception, position
Touch, pressure, vibration

Spinocervical tract

Lumbar spinal cord

Proprioception, position
Touch, pressure, vibration

14.4 SOMATOSENSORY SYSTEM: THE DORSAL COLUMN SYSTEM AND EPICRITIC MODALITIES

Primary somatosensory myelinated axons conveying fine, discriminative touch, pressure, vibratory sensation, and consciousness of joint position project directly into the DC system (fasciculus gracilis for lower body, below T6, and fasciculus cuneatus for upper body, T6 and above), where they are topographically organized. They terminate in nuclei gracilis and cuneatus, respectively, from which the medial lemniscus originates. This tract crosses (decussates) in the medulla, rostral to the decussation of the pyramids, and projects to the ventroposterolateral (VPL) nucleus of the thalamus. Axons of neurons in the VPL nucleus terminate in the primary sensory cortex topographically. The entire DC/medial

lemniscal system is topographically organized; the lower body is represented medially in the primary somatosensory cortex, and the upper body (and face from trigeminal projections) is represented laterally. This representation is sometimes drawn proportionally (the resultant figure is called a homunculus); information from the fingers and hands has far greater representation in the cerebral cortex than information from the back. The spinocervical system is a small supplement to the DC system. Primary afferent projections terminate in the medial part of the dorsal horn; these neurons project to the lateral cervical nucleus (in C1 and C2 only). This nucleus contributes additional crossed axons with polysynaptic mechanoreceptive information. The supplemental epicritic information contributing to the dorsal column/medial lemniscal system ascends in the dorsal portion of the lateral funiculus.

14.6 SOMATOSENSORY SYSTEM: THE SPINOTHALAMIC AND SPINORETICULAR SYSTEMS AND PROTOPATHIC MODALITIES (CONTINUED)

Primary somatosensory unmyelinated (C) fibers and small myelinated (A delta) fibers that convey nociceptive information (fast, localizing pain), temperature sensation, and light, moving touch terminate on neurons in laminae I and V. These dorsal horn neurons send crossed axons into the spinothalamic tract, projecting to neurons in the VPL nucleus of the thalamus (red). This pool of neurons in the VPL nucleus is different from the pool receiving input from nuclei gracilis and cuneatus from the DC system. These thalamic neurons in the VPL nucleus project to the second somatosensory cortex (SII) as well as to the primary sensory cortex. Primary sensory C fibers also terminate in the dorsal horn and contribute to a large, cascading network for bilateral projections into the spinoreticular tract (blue). This system ends mainly in the reticular formation, from which polysynaptic projections lead to nonspecific medial dorsal and anterior thalamic nuclei. Some spinoreticular fibers also terminate in the deeper layers of the superior colliculus (spinotectal pathway), in the parabrachial nuclei of the pons, and in the periaqueductal gray. Cortical regions such as the cingulate, insular, and prefrontal regions then process and interpret nociceptive information related to slow, agonizing, excruciating pain. In addition, axonal projections from neurons in the dorsal horn of the spinal cord, descending nucleus of V, and parabrachial nuclei of the pons terminate directly in the hypothalamus. These nociceptive axons to the hypothalamus help to coordinate visceral responses (e.g., fight-or-flight, autonomic reactions to pain such as blood pressure and cardiovascular responses, stress hormone secretion of cortisol and epinephrine, and emotional responses). Direct somatosensory inputs also help to mediate sexual responses and oxytocin release for milk letdown from suckling.

CLINICAL POINT

The spinothalamic tract conveys lemniscal information from primary afferents for nociception and temperature sensation to secondary sensory neurons in laminae I and V of the dorsal horn of the spinal cord. These dorsal horn neurons then project contralateral spinothalamic tract axons to the VPL nucleus of the thalamus, which in turn sends some information about "fast pain" (not outlasting the duration of the stimulus) to sensory cortices I and II in the parietal lobe. This is the principal **protopathic system** tested in the neurological examination, using light pin prick and touching the body with test tubes containing water of various temperatures. This spinothalamic tract system does not convey chronic, agonizing, deep pain that characterizes many chronic diseases; such **chronic "slow" pain** is conveyed through a vast polysynaptic network through the dorsal horn of the spinal cord and then the lateral reticular formation of the brain. This spinoreticular processed information eventually reaches the nonspecific thalamic nuclei (such as the centromedian) and is conveyed to limbic structures for more subjective, interpretative aspects of pain and to the hypothalamus for appropriate visceral autonomic and hormonal responses to pain. This latter spinoreticular network can be influenced by a host of other inputs, including the cortex, the limbic system, the descending forebrain and diencephalic systems, and collaterals of the DC system. Collaterals of the DC system can gate nociceptive processing through the dorsal horn by activating neurons that dampen transmission of information through the cascading dorsal horn network. This process is evoked in a simple fashion by light rubbing on or adjacent to an injured part of the body. In a more chronic fashion, DC stimulation (by a transcutaneous electrical nerve stimulation [TENS] unit) can electrically activate large-diameter axons that then gate the painful stimuli bombarding the dorsal horn nociceptive axons.

CLINICAL POINT

The DC system consists of fasciculus gracilis (lower half of the body, with T6 cutoff) and fasciculus cuneatus (upper half of the body). These pathways consist of primary sensory axons conveying fine, discriminative touch sensation, vibratory sensation, and joint position sense (the epicritic sensations) toward the first synapse in the secondary sensory nuclei gracilis and cuneatus in the caudal medulla. These **epicritic sensations** are called primary DC modalities, the basic information coded mainly by large-diameter myelinated axons. Additional DC modalities are sometimes tested if the primary modalities are intact, including two-point discrimination, stereognosis (knowing what an object is just by touch), and graphesthesia (interpreting a number drawn into the palm of the hand). These are considered cortical modalities of the DC system; they require that the primary DC modalities be intact and also require the ability of the sensory cortices to interpret the information conveyed and to draw conclusions about that information. If the primary modalities are impaired, there is no reason to attempt to test the cortical modalities that depend on unimpaired primary modalities. Pure lesions of the DC system do not entirely eliminate the primary epicritic modalities; they just remove some interpretive capabilities. Such a patient may realize that a vibratory stimulus is being applied to the upper extremity but may be unable to distinguish vibratory stimuli of different frequencies. The dorsal portion of the lateral funiculus carries additional epicritic information to the DC nuclei from the spinal cord dorsal horn. A lesion of both the DC and the dorsal portion of the lateral funiculus results in total loss of epicritic sensation on the affected side.

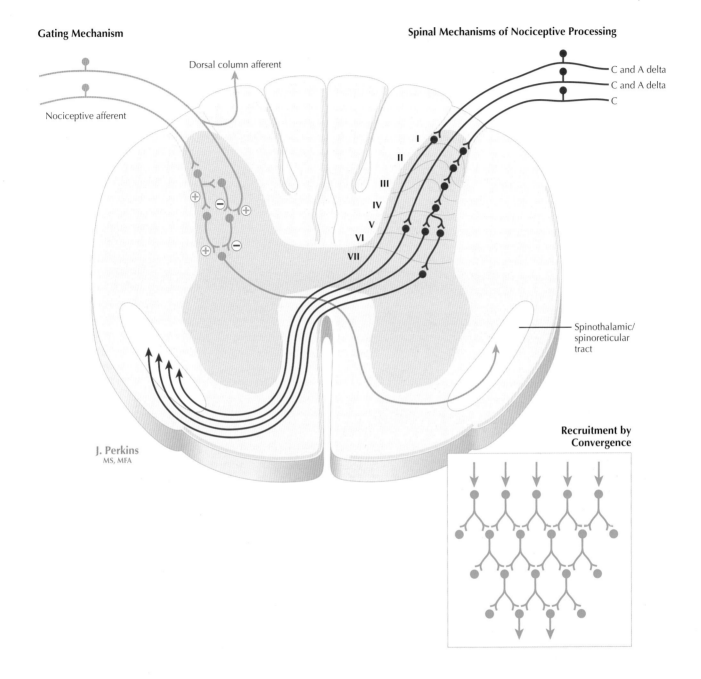

Gating Mechanism

Dorsal column afferent

Nociceptive afferent

Spinal Mechanisms of Nociceptive Processing

C and A delta
C and A delta
C

I
II
III
IV
V
VI
VII

Spinothalamic/
spinoreticular
tract

J. Perkins
MS, MFA

**Recruitment by
Convergence**

14.7 SPINOTHALAMIC AND SPINORETICULAR NOCICEPTIVE PROCESSING IN THE SPINAL CORD

Primary afferents (C and A delta fibers) conveying fast, localized pain and temperature sensation terminate in laminae I and V of the dorsal horn of the spinal cord, from which the crossed spinothalamic axons originate. Unmyelinated primary afferents (C fibers) also terminate on neurons in the dorsal horn, from which a cascading system involving recruitment, convergence, and polysynaptic interconnections originates. This system (shown in red) contributes to the spinoreticular tract (mainly crossed, but some are uncrossed), which projects into the RF and continues polysynaptically to nonspecific medial dorsal and anterior thalamic nuclei. This system contributes to perception of excruciating pain and its emotional connotation via cortical regions such as the cingulate, insular, and prefrontal cortices. The gating mechanism, shown in blue on the left, allows primary DC axon collaterals to dampen pain processing in the dorsal horn via inhibitory interneuronal connections that inhibit the flow of information through the cascading dorsal horn system that contributes to the spinoreticular pathway.

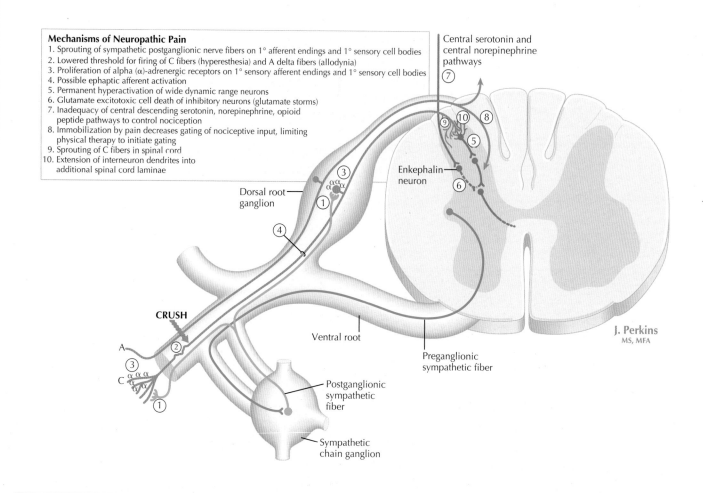

Mechanisms of Neuropathic Pain
1. Sprouting of sympathetic postganglionic nerve fibers on 1° afferent endings and 1° sensory cell bodies
2. Lowered threshold for firing of C fibers (hyperesthesia) and A delta fibers (allodynia)
3. Proliferation of alpha (α)-adrenergic receptors on 1° sensory afferent endings and 1° sensory cell bodies
4. Possible ephaptic afferent activation
5. Permanent hyperactivation of wide dynamic range neurons
6. Glutamate excitotoxic cell death of inhibitory neurons (glutamate storms)
7. Inadequacy of central descending serotonin, norepinephrine, opioid peptide pathways to control nociception
8. Immobilization by pain decreases gating of nociceptive input, limiting physical therapy to initiate gating
9. Sprouting of C fibers in spinal cord
10. Extension of interneuron dendrites into additional spinal cord laminae

Central serotonin and central norepinephrine pathways

Dorsal root ganglion

Enkephalin neuron

CRUSH

Ventral root

Preganglionic sympathetic fiber

J. Perkins
MS, MFA

A

C

Postganglionic sympathetic fiber

Sympathetic chain ganglion

14.8 MECHANISMS OF NEUROPATHIC PAIN AND SYMPATHETICALLY MAINTAINED PAIN

The cascading dorsal horn system receives primary afferent C fibers of nociceptive origin and projects into the spinoreticular system for the conscious interpretation of excruciating pain and neuropathic pain, shown in this illustration. Connections from the sympathetic nervous system can innervate terminals and cell bodies of primary nociceptive neurons directly. In neuropathic pain syndromes such as complex regional pain syndrome (CRPS), formerly called reflex sympathetic dystrophy (RSD), sympathetic postganglionic neurons may activate receptors on greatly sensitized primary afferent nerve terminals and cell bodies, either directly (via synapses) or indirectly (through secretion of norepinephrine into the blood); such activation may exacerbate the perception of the neuropathic pain. Multiple mechanisms are thought to contribute to sensitization of pain-related neurons and presence of chronic, agonizing neuropathic pain in CRPS and related syndromes. These mechanisms are noted in this illustration as numbered sites. Descending central noradrenergic and serotonergic projections are thought to play an important modulatory role in the processing of neuropathic and nonneuropathic pain.

CLINICAL POINT

In some cases of nerve damage or compression, particularly that associated with a sprain, a crush injury, a direct injection into a nerve, or even relatively minor trauma, a pathological reaction of primary afferents can result in a chronic neuropathic pain syndrome called **reflex sympathetic dystrophy**, more recently renamed **CRPS**. It is related to the type of chronic, agonizing central pain experienced in phantom limb syndrome. CRPS affects the hand, arm, and shoulder to a greater extent than the lower extremity. Intense burning or stabbing pain is felt, with allodynia and hyperesthesia (extreme sensitivity to touch and painful stimuli, respectively). When this phenomenon affects one nerve (perhaps following a bullet wound) it is sometimes called causalgia. The primary afferents involved in CRPS appear to proliferate alpha-adrenergic receptors on their sensory receptor endings and on the dorsal root ganglion cell body and often show extraordinary sensitivity to catecholamines, which provoke a lower threshold for response to nociceptive stimuli. In syndromes such as CRPS, permanent destruction of dorsal horn inhibitory interneurons (by glutamate excitotoxicity) and permanently altered thresholds for wide dynamic range spinoreticular neurons also have been observed. Sympathetic-related characteristics may be noted in CRPS, such as changes in skin appearance due to vascular flow changes (vasomotor), atrophic skin and nails (trophic changes), altered sweating and skin temperature (sudomotor), and altered bone density on a triphasic bone scan. Treatment must occur quickly after detection and must employ simultaneous vigorous therapeutic approaches. Treatment choices normally include analgesics, tricyclic or other antidepressants to alter pain threshold in the spinal cord, membrane-stabilizing agents (e.g., Neurontin), physical therapy, and nerve stimulation of large-diameter myelinated "gating" axons.

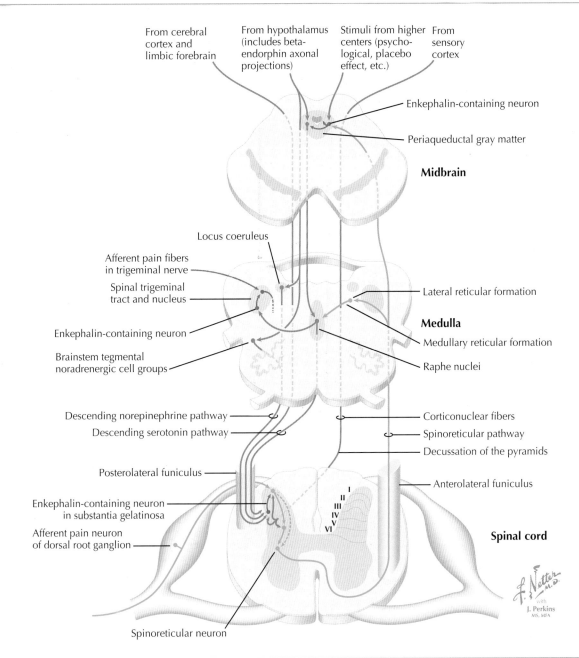

From cerebral cortex and limbic forebrain

From hypothalamus (includes beta-endorphin axonal projections)

Stimuli from higher centers (psychological, placebo effect, etc.)

From sensory cortex

Enkephalin-containing neuron

Periaqueductal gray matter

Midbrain

Locus coeruleus

Afferent pain fibers in trigeminal nerve

Spinal trigeminal tract and nucleus

Enkephalin-containing neuron

Brainstem tegmental noradrenergic cell groups

Lateral reticular formation

Medulla

Medullary reticular formation

Raphe nuclei

Descending norepinephrine pathway

Descending serotonin pathway

Corticonuclear fibers

Spinoreticular pathway

Decussation of the pyramids

Posterolateral funiculus

Anterolateral funiculus

Enkephalin-containing neuron in substantia gelatinosa

Afferent pain neuron of dorsal root ganglion

Spinal cord

Spinoreticular neuron

14.9 DESCENDING CONTROL OF ASCENDING SOMATOSENSORY SYSTEMS

The processing of nociceptive information in the dorsal horn of the spinal cord can be modulated by descending connections from the cerebral cortex, limbic forebrain structures, hypothalamus (paraventricular nucleus), periarcuate beta-endorphin neurons, periaqueductal gray, RF of the brainstem, central noradrenergic neurons (of locus coeruleus and other brainstem tegmental groups), and serotonergic (5HT) neurons (nucleus raphe magnus). The central descending noradrenergic and 5HT pathways, modulated by the periaqueductal gray and other higher centers, are particularly important for endogenous and exogenous (i.e., opioid) modulation of pain.

dorsal horn of the spinal cord for the body and the descending nucleus of V for the face. These areas include regions of cerebral cortex, limbic forebrain areas, hypothalamic regions including endorphin nuclei, and sensory cortical centrifugal connections. Some of these projections use **endogenous opiates**. Enkephalin and dynorphin interneurons are found in pain-processing regions, particularly in the dorsal horn of the spinal cord and the descending nucleus of V, and in many hypothalamic and limbic sites that may be involved in the subjective interpretation of pain. The beta-endorphin neurons of the periarcuate region (sometimes called just the *arcuate nucleus*) of the hypothalamus send connections to the periaqueductal gray, locus coeruleus and brainstem noradrenergic nuclei, raphe nuclei, and many limbic regions. The periaqueductal gray is particularly important for opioid activation of the nucleus raphe magnus and other descending monoamine pathways that activate enkephalins and assist in opiate analgesia. The periaqueductal gray–raphe connection is essential for full functionality of opioid analgesia. Systemic administration of synthetic opiates activates neurons of the periarcuate region of the hypothalamus and periaqueductal gray, resulting in analgesia.

CLINICAL POINT

Several regions of the central nervous system (CNS) send projections, direct and indirect, to regulate nociceptive processing through the

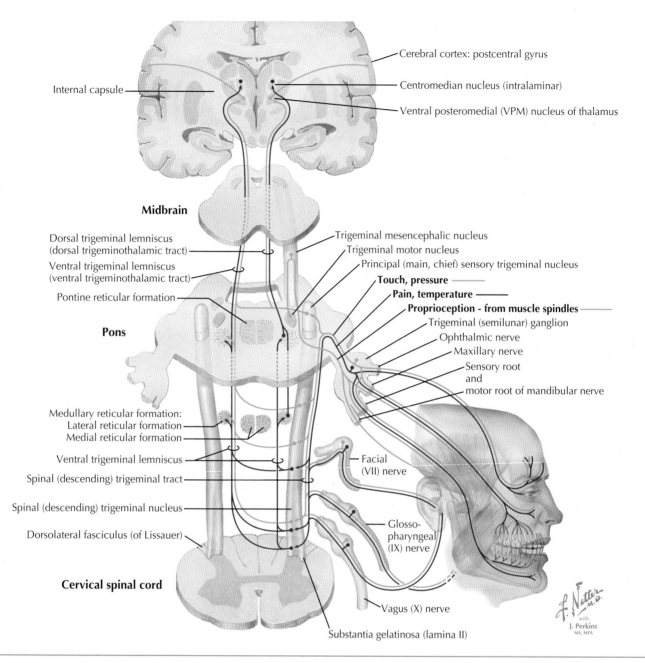

Cerebral cortex: postcentral gyrus

Centromedian nucleus (intralaminar)

Ventral posteromedial (VPM) nucleus of thalamus

Internal capsule

Midbrain

Trigeminal mesencephalic nucleus
Trigeminal motor nucleus
Principal (main, chief) sensory trigeminal nucleus
Touch, pressure
Pain, temperature
Proprioception - from muscle spindles
Trigeminal (semilunar) ganglion
Ophthalmic nerve
Maxillary nerve
Sensory root
and
motor root of mandibular nerve

Dorsal trigeminal lemniscus
(dorsal trigeminothalamic tract)
Ventral trigeminal lemniscus
(ventral trigeminothalamic tract)
Pontine reticular formation

Pons

Medullary reticular formation:
Lateral reticular formation
Medial reticular formation
Ventral trigeminal lemniscus
Spinal (descending) trigeminal tract
Spinal (descending) trigeminal nucleus
Dorsolateral fasciculus (of Lissauer)

Facial
(VII) nerve

Glosso-
pharyngeal
(IX) nerve

Cervical spinal cord

Vagus (X) nerve

Substantia gelatinosa (lamina II)

TRIGEMINAL SENSORY SYSTEM

14.10 TRIGEMINAL SENSORY AND ASSOCIATED SENSORY SYSTEMS

Axons of primary sensory trigeminal neurons enter the brainstem, travel in the descending (spinal) tract of V, and terminate in the descending (spinal) nucleus of V. Axons of the trigeminal ganglion (V) supply the face, anterior oral cavity, and teeth and gums; axons of the geniculate ganglion (VII) and jugular ganglion (X) supply a small zone of the external ear. Axons of the petrosal ganglion (IX) supply general sensation to the posterior oral cavity and pharynx. Axons of the descending nucleus of V project into the ventral trigeminal lemniscus (ventral trigeminothalamic tract; mainly crossed axons) and terminate in the ventral posteromedial (VPM) nucleus of the thalamus. The VPM nucleus projects to the lateral primary sensory cortex and to intralaminar thalamic nuclei, which are associated with nociceptive processing. The caudal descending nucleus also sends contralateral

projections to the RF for processing of excruciating pain (similar to the spinoreticular system). Primary sensory axons carrying fine, discriminative modalities from V (similar to the DC system) terminate in the rostral portion of the descending nucleus of V and in the main (chief) sensory nucleus of V, which contribute to the ventral trigeminothalamic tract. A portion of the main sensory nucleus also projects ipsilaterally to the VPM nucleus via the dorsal trigeminothalamic tract. Although most of the trigeminal system is represented on the lateral portion of the contralateral primary sensory cortex (postcentral gyrus), part of the epicritic trigeminal projections as well as taste are represented in the ipsilateral sensory cortex. The mesencephalic nucleus of V is the only primary sensory nucleus found inside the CNS; these neurons supply muscle spindles for masticatory and extraocular muscles and mediate associated muscle spindle reflexes. See page 433 for a Clinical Point.

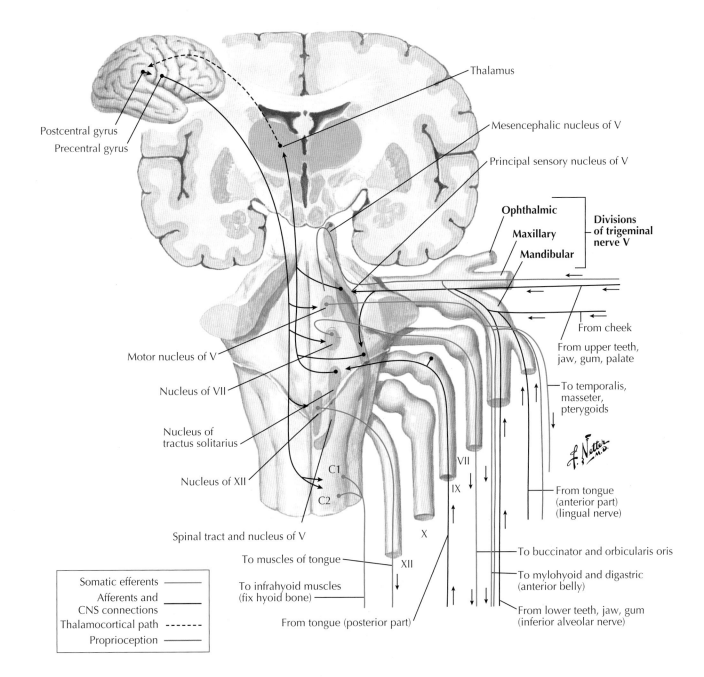

Postcentral gyrus

Precentral gyrus

Thalamus

Mesencephalic nucleus of V

Principal sensory nucleus of V

Ophthalmic

Maxillary

Mandibular

Divisions of trigeminal nerve V

From cheek

From upper teeth, jaw, gum, palate

To temporalis, masseter, pterygoids

Motor nucleus of V

Nucleus of VII

Nucleus of tractus solitarius

Nucleus of XII

Spinal tract and nucleus of V

To muscles of tongue

To infrahyoid muscles (fix hyoid bone)

From tongue (posterior part)

C1

C2

VII

IX

X

XII

From tongue (anterior part) (lingual nerve)

To buccinator and orbicularis oris

To mylohyoid and digastric (anterior belly)

From lower teeth, jaw, gum (inferior alveolar nerve)

Somatic efferents	———
Afferents and CNS connections	———
Thalamocortical path	- - - -
Proprioception	———

14.11 TRIGEMINAL SYSTEM PERIPHERAL AND CENTRAL CONNECTIONS

This illustration is a summary of trigeminal-related pathways and connections, including cortical and reflex connections.

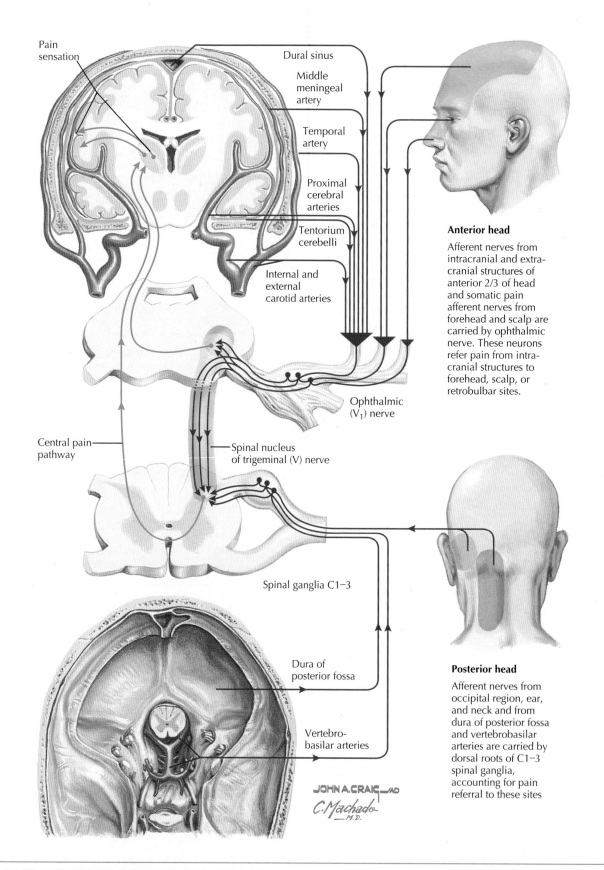

Pain sensation

Dural sinus

Middle meningeal artery

Temporal artery

Proximal cerebral arteries

Tentorium cerebelli

Internal and external carotid arteries

Anterior head

Afferent nerves from intracranial and extra-cranial structures of anterior 2/3 of head and somatic pain afferent nerves from forehead and scalp are carried by ophthalmic nerve. These neurons refer pain from intra-cranial structures to forehead, scalp, or retrobulbar sites.

Ophthalmic (V₁) nerve

Central pain pathway

Spinal nucleus of trigeminal (V) nerve

Spinal ganglia C1–3

Dura of posterior fossa

Vertebro-basilar arteries

JOHN A. CRAIG—MD
C. Machado—M.D.

Posterior head

Afferent nerves from occipital region, ear, and neck and from dura of posterior fossa and vertebrobasilar arteries are carried by dorsal roots of C1–3 spinal ganglia, accounting for pain referral to these sites

14.12 PAIN-SENSITIVE STRUCTURES OF THE HEAD AND PAIN REFERRAL

Pain-sensitive structures of the head include dural structures (e.g., sinuses, tentorium cerebelli), arteries, and muscles. Primary headaches can arise as migraine headaches, tension headaches, and neuralgias. Secondary headaches can arise from tumors, abscesses, hematomas, bleeding (e.g., ruptured berry aneurysm), and meningitis or meningeal irritation.

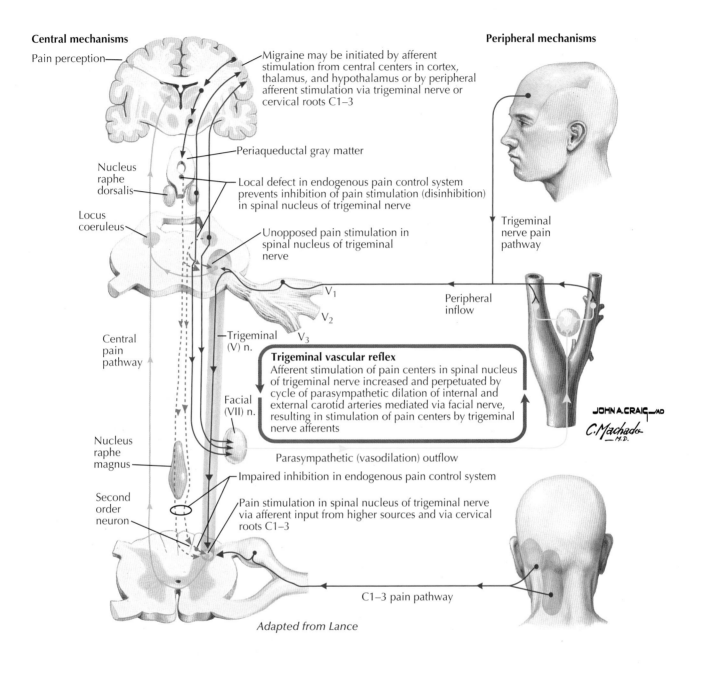

Central mechanisms

Pain perception

Nucleus raphe dorsalis

Locus coeruleus

Central pain pathway

Nucleus raphe magnus

Second order neuron

Migraine may be initiated by afferent stimulation from central centers in cortex, thalamus, and hypothalamus or by peripheral afferent stimulation via trigeminal nerve or cervical roots C1–3

Periaqueductal gray matter

Local defect in endogenous pain control system prevents inhibition of pain stimulation (disinhibition) in spinal nucleus of trigeminal nerve

Unopposed pain stimulation in spinal nucleus of trigeminal nerve

V_1

V_2

V_3

Trigeminal (V) n.

Trigeminal vascular reflex
Afferent stimulation of pain centers in spinal nucleus of trigeminal nerve increased and perpetuated by cycle of parasympathetic dilation of internal and external carotid arteries mediated via facial nerve, resulting in stimulation of pain centers by trigeminal nerve afferents

Facial (VII) n.

Parasympathetic (vasodilation) outflow

Impaired inhibition in endogenous pain control system

Pain stimulation in spinal nucleus of trigeminal nerve via afferent input from higher sources and via cervical roots C1–3

C1–3 pain pathway

Peripheral mechanisms

Trigeminal nerve pain pathway

Peripheral inflow

JOHN A. CRAIG—MD
C. Machado —M.D.

Adapted from Lance

14.13 **MECHANISMS OF MIGRAINE HEADACHES**

A common migraine headache is a headache lasting from 4 to 72 hours, accompanied by nausea, vomiting, and aversion to light (photophobia) and/or sound (phonophobia). The headache is usually unilateral, severe, throbbing or pulsatile, and intensified by physical activity. A classical migraine headache, occurring in 15% of migraine patients, is foreshadowed by an aura, consisting of neurological symptoms such as visual field deficits, scotomas, light flashes, or sensory/motor symptoms. The aura generally lasts less than 1 hour, usually followed by the

headache. Prodromes such as emotional or mood disturbances, fatigue, drowsiness, and other general symptoms often occur. Migraine headaches are three times more common in women than in men.

The mechanisms of migraine headache include dilation of meningeal blood vessels, release of vasoactive neuropeptides, neurogenic inflammation, activation of trigeminal pain pathways, and inhibition of endogenous pain-dampening central mechanisms. Chronic migraines are migraine headaches that persist for at least 15 days a month.

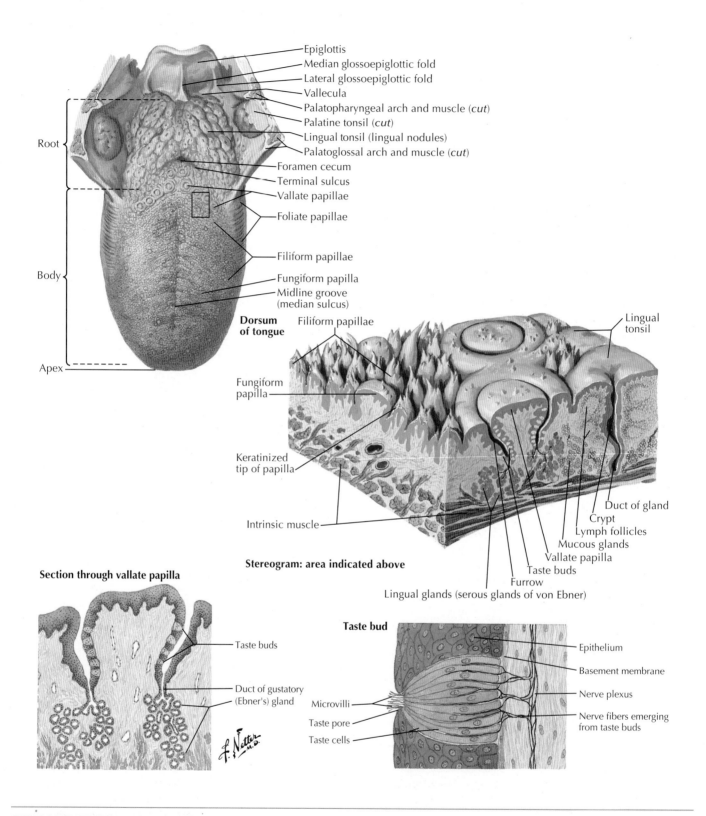

Epiglottis
Median glossoepiglottic fold
Lateral glossoepiglottic fold
Vallecula
Palatopharyngeal arch and muscle (*cut*)
Palatine tonsil (*cut*)
Lingual tonsil (lingual nodules)
Palatoglossal arch and muscle (*cut*)
Foramen cecum
Terminal sulcus
Vallate papillae
Foliate papillae
Filiform papillae
Fungiform papilla
Midline groove (median sulcus)

Root

Body

Apex

Dorsum of tongue

Filiform papillae
Fungiform papilla
Keratinized tip of papilla
Intrinsic muscle

Lingual tonsil
Duct of gland
Crypt
Lymph follicles
Mucous glands
Vallate papilla
Taste buds
Furrow
Lingual glands (serous glands of von Ebner)

Stereogram: area indicated above

Section through vallate papilla

Taste buds
Duct of gustatory (Ebner's) gland

Taste bud

Epithelium
Basement membrane
Nerve plexus
Nerve fibers emerging from taste buds

Microvilli
Taste pore
Taste cells

SENSORY SYSTEM FOR TASTE

14.14 ANATOMY OF TASTE BUDS AND THEIR RECEPTORS

Taste buds are chemosensory transducers that consist of bundles of columnar cells that lie within the epithelium. They translate individual molecular configurations or combinations of molecules for salty, sweet, sour, bitter, and umami (glutamate) sensations into action potentials of both large and small primary sensory axons. The taste buds are found on the anterior and posterior regions of the tongue and, less frequently, on the palate and epiglottis, mainly in children. Nerve fibers for taste show complex responses of electrical activity across populations of many nerve fibers. The integrative interpretation of taste takes place in the CNS.

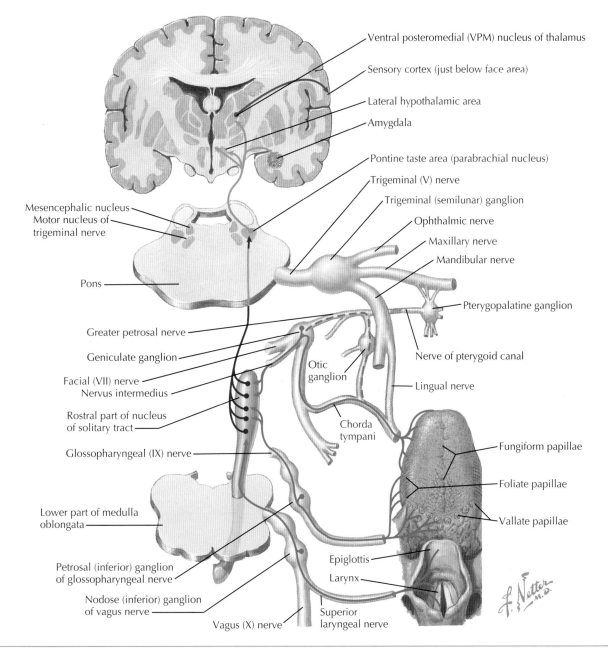

14.15 TASTE PATHWAYS

Primary sensory axons of neurons of the geniculate ganglion (VII), petrosal ganglion (IX), and nodose (inferior) ganglion (X), supply taste buds on the anterior two thirds of the tongue, the posterior one third of the tongue, and the epiglottis and palate, respectively. These axons terminate in the rostral part of nucleus solitarius (nucleus of the solitary tract), which sends ipsilateral projections mainly to the parabrachial nucleus in the pons (and a few projections to nucleus VPM of the thalamus). The parabrachial nucleus projects fibers to nucleus VPM of the thalamus, to the hypothalamus (lateral hypothalamic area, paraventricular nucleus), and to amygdaloid nuclei. These nonthalamic projections are associated with the emotional, motivational, and behavioral aspects of taste and food intake.

one third), and X (epiglottis). The taste buds detect sweet, salty, bitter, sour, and umami (glutamate); each taste bud appears to be associated mainly with one such modality. Combined taste receptor activation can code for a tremendous array of subtle tastes and flavors. Olfaction plays a major role in the discrimination of what an individual perceives to be taste. The primary taste afferents terminate in the rostral nucleus solitarius, which projects mainly to a pontine parabrachial nucleus and then to the parvicellular part of the VPM nucleus of the thalamus, several hypothalamic sites, and the amygdaloid complex. Some cortical areas, such as the anterior portion of the insular cortex and a lateral zone of the posterior orbitofrontal cortex, are involved in subjective aspects of taste and the gustatory experience. These pathways are mainly ipsilateral. Chemical influences can also have a profound effect on taste. Smoking may blunt taste. Many illnesses, including severe nasal congestion, liver dysfunction, autonomic problems, postradiation responses, some vitamin deficiencies, and some medications, may distort or alter the tastes of foods or may leave a lingering, unpleasant, distinctive taste. Many chemotherapeutic agents also profoundly alter taste sensation, perhaps accounting in part for loss of appetite in such individuals. The sequelae of COVID-19 viral infection may include temporary or long-term loss of taste and smell.

CLINICAL POINT

Taste pathways arise from primary receptors, the taste buds, which are associated with cranial nerves VII (anterior two thirds), IX (posterior

Frontal section

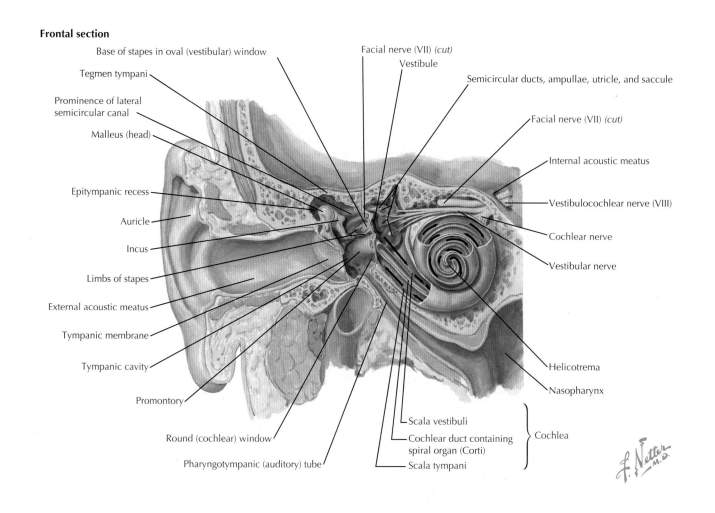

Base of stapes in oval (vestibular) window

Tegmen tympani

Prominence of lateral semicircular canal

Malleus (head)

Epitympanic recess

Auricle

Incus

Limbs of stapes

External acoustic meatus

Tympanic membrane

Tympanic cavity

Promontory

Round (cochlear) window

Pharyngotympanic (auditory) tube

Facial nerve (VII) *(cut)*

Vestibule

Semicircular ducts, ampullae, utricle, and saccule

Facial nerve (VII) *(cut)*

Internal acoustic meatus

Vestibulocochlear nerve (VIII)

Cochlear nerve

Vestibular nerve

Helicotrema

Nasopharynx

Scala vestibuli

Cochlear duct containing spiral organ (Corti)

Cochlea

Scala tympani

AUDITORY SYSTEM

14.16 PERIPHERAL PATHWAYS FOR SOUND RECEPTION

The sound transduction process involves complex mechanical transduction of sound waves through the external ear and the external acoustic meatus and across the tympanic membrane; there it is leveraged as a mechanical force by the bones of the middle ear (ossicles) via the oval window to produce a fluid wave in the cochlear duct. This fluid wave causes differential movement of the basilar membrane, stimulating hairs on the apical portion of hair cells to release neurotransmitters that stimulate primary sensory axons of neurons of the cochlear (spiral) ganglion. The basilar membrane in the cochlea shows maximal displacement spatially according to the frequency of impinging tones, with low frequencies maximally stimulating the apex (helicotrema) and high frequencies maximally stimulating the base. The eustachian (pharyngotympanic) tube permits pressure equilibrium between the middle ear and the outside world.

CLINICAL POINT

Hearing loss may be partial or total and can involve virtually any range of detectable frequencies. The most devastating for human communication is a loss in the frequencies of speech (300 to 3000 Hz) of 40 or more decibels. In general, hearing loss can be subdivided into two categories: sensorineural and conductive. **Sensorineural hearing** loss involves damage to the hair cells, the auditory nerve, or central auditory pathways. Because of the neural damage, both air conduction and bone conduction are diminished. **Conductive hearing** loss involves damage to the outer or middle ear. Air conduction is impaired because the sound is not properly transduced into the inner ear, but bone conduction is normal. These two types of hearing loss can be tested for at the bedside by using a tuning fork of 512 Hz. The Weber test involves placing the vibrating tuning fork on the center of the forehead. Normally, the patient hears the fork equally in both ears. With sensorineural loss, the sound is heard best in the unaffected ear; with conductive loss, the sound is heard best in the affected ear. The Rinne test involves holding the vibrating tuning fork against the mastoid bone. When the fork is no longer heard, it is immediately placed just outside the external auditory meatus. Normally, air conduction is more effective than bone conduction, and the fork will again be heard when moved adjacent to the external auditory meatus (air conducting sound better than bone). If conductive hearing loss is present, once bone conduction is no longer heard, air conduction also will not be heard (bone conducting sound better than air). If sensorineural hearing loss is present, air conduction may be greater than bone conduction, although both may be diminished.

Bony and membranous labyrinths

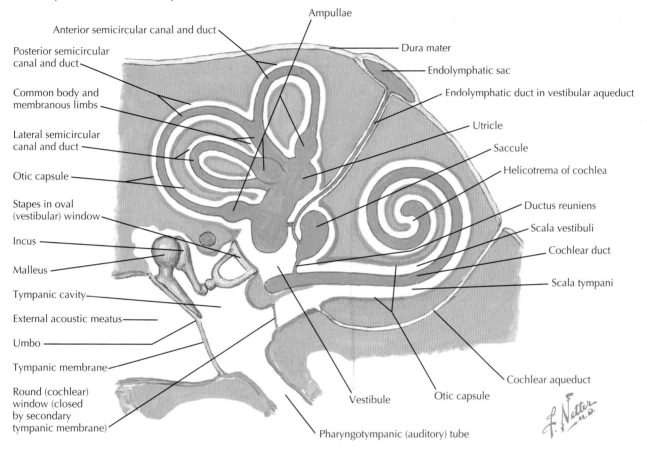

Ampullae

Anterior semicircular canal and duct

Posterior semicircular canal and duct

Common body and membranous limbs

Lateral semicircular canal and duct

Otic capsule

Stapes in oval (vestibular) window

Incus

Malleus

Tympanic cavity

External acoustic meatus

Umbo

Tympanic membrane

Round (cochlear) window (closed by secondary tympanic membrane)

Dura mater

Endolymphatic sac

Endolymphatic duct in vestibular aqueduct

Utricle

Saccule

Helicotrema of cochlea

Ductus reuniens

Scala vestibuli

Cochlear duct

Scala tympani

Cochlear aqueduct

Vestibule

Otic capsule

Pharyngotympanic (auditory) tube

14.17 BONY AND MEMBRANOUS LABYRINTHS

The relationship between the cochlea and the vestibular apparatus (utricle, saccule, semicircular canals, and ducts) and the bony labyrinth that surrounds them is illustrated. The ossicles (malleus, incus, stapes) leverage the movement of the tympanic membrane to produce movement of the oval window. Movement of the oval window causes a fluid wave to move through the scala vestibuli and the scala tympani of the cochlea and ricochet onto the round window, causing differential movement of the basilar membrane and stimulation of selected responsive hair cells. The three semicircular canals are located at 90-degree angles to each other, representing tilted *x, y,* and *z* axes.

A mismatch of vestibular inputs from the two sides is interpreted as turning, resulting in vertigo, an internal or external sensation of spinning, usually accompanied by nausea and dizziness. Vertigo can arise from CN VIII (neuritis, acoustic Schwannoma), cerebellum (tumor, hemorrhage, infarct), brainstem (infarct, demyelination), or temporal lobe (tumor, abscess).

CLINICAL POINT

The semicircular canals (ducts) contain the ampullae that have hair cells that respond to angular acceleration. The utricle contains the otolith organ in the macula that responds to linear acceleration and detects gravitation. The saccule responds best to low-frequency vibratory stimuli. The cochlea contains the hair cells that respond to fluid movements in the scalae vestibuli and tympani, brought about by the leveraging of the ossicles against the oval window; this movement affects hair cells in the cochlear duct.

The activity of the utricle can sometimes become distorted when debris moves away from the hairs and induces activation of the hair cells in the ampulla of the posterior semicircular canal. This produces vertigo and nystagmus that are associated with a specific position of the head (**benign postural or positional vertigo**). This disorder is the most common cause of vertigo seen in neurological practice. These attacks commonly occur when the patient is lying down, moving to a particular position, or tilting the head back; they may recur either briefly or for a longer period of days or weeks. Attacks can be induced by an examiner through the Hallpike maneuver (tilting the patient's head back and then 30 degrees to the side), resulting in a brief attack of vertigo and nystagmus. No pharmacological treatment is available. Attempts to reposition the debris by deliberate Hallpike-like head movements have met with some success.

Section through turn of cochlea

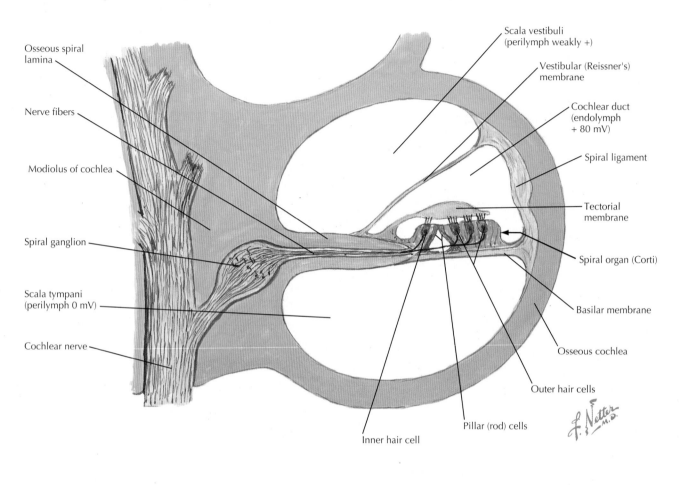

Osseous spiral lamina

Nerve fibers

Modiolus of cochlea

Spiral ganglion

Scala tympani (perilymph 0 mV)

Cochlear nerve

Scala vestibuli (perilymph weakly +)

Vestibular (Reissner's) membrane

Cochlear duct (endolymph + 80 mV)

Spiral ligament

Tectorial membrane

Spiral organ (Corti)

Basilar membrane

Osseous cochlea

Outer hair cells

Pillar (rod) cells

Inner hair cell

14.18 VIII NERVE INNERVATION OF HAIR CELLS OF THE ORGAN OF CORTI

Primary sensory axons of the spiral (cochlear) ganglion innervate inner and outer hair cells of the organ of Corti, located on the basilar membrane. The axons are activated by release of neurotransmitters from the hair cells, which occurs when the hairs on the apical surface are moved by shearing forces resulting from movement of the basilar membrane (fluid wave through the scalae vestibuli and tympani) in relation to the more rigidly fixed tectorial membrane. This represents the complex transduction process of the conversion of external sound waves to action potentials in spiral ganglion axons. The ionic potentials (in millivolts) are indicated for the scala tympani and vestibuli (perilymph) and the cochlear duct (endolymph). These potential differences contribute to the excitability of the hair cells.

CLINICAL POINT

Hair cells in the organ of Corti respond to fluid movements in the scalae vestibuli and tympani that induce shearing motion of the tectorial membrane relative to the basilar membrane. Each region of the spiraled cochlea contains hair cells that respond optimally to movement of the basilar membrane; low frequencies stimulate hair cell movement in the apex (helicotrema) and high frequencies stimulate hair cell movement in the basilar coils of the cochlea. The **hair cells** can be damaged by many pathological processes, such as viral infections (e.g., mumps), drugs (e.g., quinine), antibiotics, exposure to sustained loud noise, and age-related deterioration caused by free radical damage. Exposure to loud noises above 85 decibels can selectively damage hair cells, especially those in the basilar coils of the cochlea that transduce high-frequency sounds. High-pitched machinery noise (jet engines), gunfire without ear protection, exposure to loud music at concerts or by earphones, and loud ambient noise in construction or industrial sites can induce temporary damage that can become permanent with repeated exposure. Environmental protection regulations now require ear protection in personnel working at such sites.

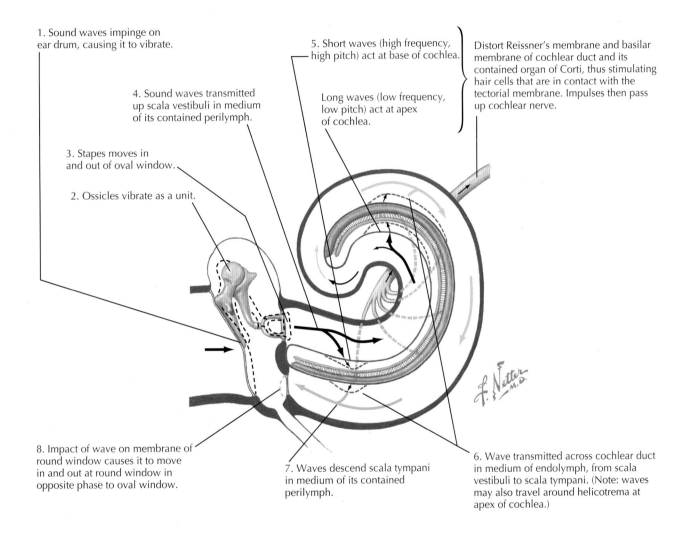

1. Sound waves impinge on ear drum, causing it to vibrate.

4. Sound waves transmitted up scala vestibuli in medium of its contained perilymph.

3. Stapes moves in and out of oval window.

2. Ossicles vibrate as a unit.

5. Short waves (high frequency, high pitch) act at base of cochlea.

Long waves (low frequency, low pitch) act at apex of cochlea.

Distort Reissner's membrane and basilar membrane of cochlear duct and its contained organ of Corti, thus stimulating hair cells that are in contact with the tectorial membrane. Impulses then pass up cochlear nerve.

8. Impact of wave on membrane of round window causes it to move in and out at round window in opposite phase to oval window.

7. Waves descend scala tympani in medium of its contained perilymph.

6. Wave transmitted across cochlear duct in medium of endolymph, from scala vestibuli to scala tympani. (Note: waves may also travel around helicotrema at apex of cochlea.)

14.19 COCHLEAR RECEPTORS

Fluid movement through scala vestibuli, around the helicotrema, and back through the scala tympani differentially moves the basilar membrane on which the organ of Corti and its hair cells reside. Movement of hairs on the apical portion of the hair cells by shearing forces of the tectorial membrane results in their depolarization and the release of neurotransmitters. This release stimulates action potentials in the primary afferent axons of spiral ganglion cells. Efferent axons from the olivocochlear bundle, controlled by descending central auditory pathways, can modulate the excitability of hair cells and the sensory transduction process.

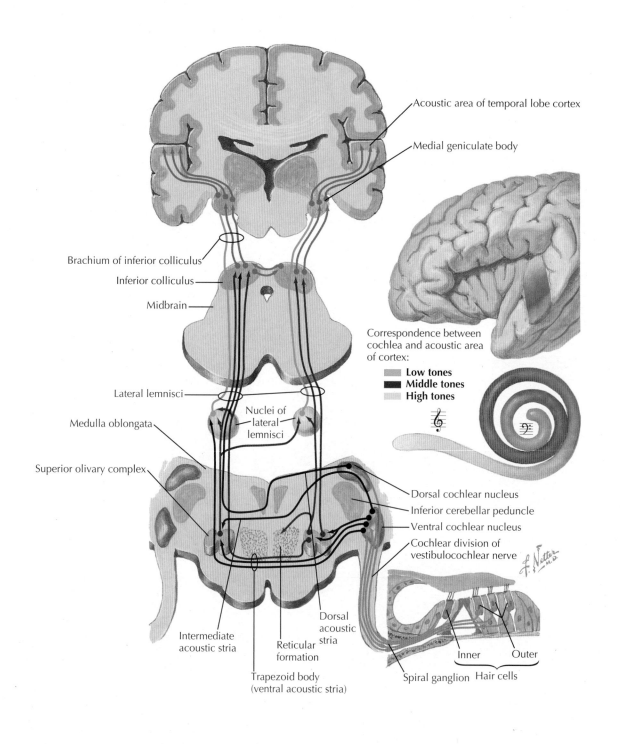

Acoustic area of temporal lobe cortex

Medial geniculate body

Correspondence between cochlea and acoustic area of cortex:

- Low tones
- Middle tones
- High tones

Brachium of inferior colliculus

Inferior colliculus

Midbrain

Lateral lemnisci

Nuclei of lateral lemnisci

Medulla oblongata

Superior olivary complex

Dorsal cochlear nucleus

Inferior cerebellar peduncle

Ventral cochlear nucleus

Cochlear division of vestibulocochlear nerve

Intermediate acoustic stria

Reticular formation

Dorsal acoustic stria

Trapezoid body (ventral acoustic stria)

Spiral ganglion

Inner   Outer

Hair cells

14.20 AFFERENT AUDITORY PATHWAYS

Central axon projections of the spiral ganglion neurons terminate in dorsal and ventral cochlear nuclei in several tonotopic maps (receptor origination shown in the cochlea in colors). These cochlear nuclei project into the lateral lemniscus via acoustic striae; many of these projections remain ipsilateral. The lateral lemniscus terminates in the nucleus of the inferior colliculus, which in turn projects via the brachium of the inferior colliculus to the medial geniculate body (nucleus) of the thalamus. The thalamus sends tonotopical projections to the primary auditory cortex on the transverse gyrus of Heschl. Several accessory auditory brainstem nuclei (the superior olivary nucleus for lateral sound localization, the nuclei of the trapezoid body [not shown], and the lateral lemniscus) send both crossed and uncrossed projections through the lateral lemniscus. Sound is represented throughout the afferent auditory pathways bilaterally; thus a unilateral lesion in the lateral lemniscus, auditory thalamus, auditory radiations, or auditory cortex does not produce contralateral deafness. With such a lesion, there is a diminution in hearing and auditory neglect contralateral to the lesion with bilateral simultaneous stimulation.

Large acoustic Schwannoma intruding in the cerebellopontine angle, causing damage to both the vestibular and cochlear portions of CN VIII, CN VII, other cranial nerves (V, IX, X), and brainstem structures

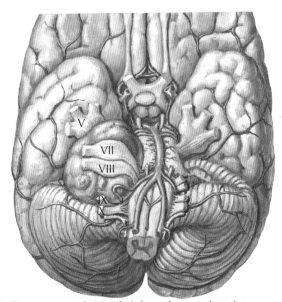

MRI of vestibular schwannoma at the cerebellopontine angle; axial *(left)* and coronal *(right)*

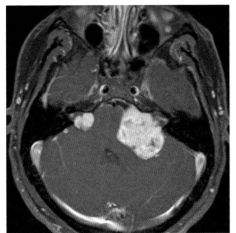

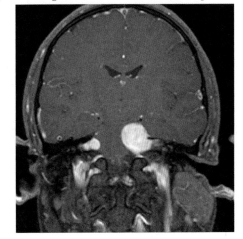

14.21 AFFERENT AUDITORY PATHWAYS (CONTINUED)

CLINICAL POINT

The cochlear nerve contains axons that innervate the hair cells of the organ of Corti in the spirals of the cochlea. Primary cochlear axons enter the lateral portion of the caudal pons, terminating in the dorsal and ventral cochlear nuclei with several tonotopically representative maps of the auditory frequency world. The auditory nerve can be damaged by infections, tumors (e.g., acoustic Schwannoma), and traumas, particularly those associated with the petrous portion of the temporal bone; both the auditory portion and vestibular portion of CN VII are affected clinically. Irritation of auditory nerve fibers can produce tinnitus, a sense of ringing in the ears (or buzzing, humming, clicking, or other sounds). When the nerve is actually destroyed, the tinnitus stops and hearing loss ensues. Auditory nerve damage has symptoms that are present on the ipsilateral side with respect to the damage. In the brainstem, the acoustic striae project axons to a host of nuclei in bilateral fashion, including the superior olivary nuclei, the nuclei of the trapezoid body, the nuclei of the lateral lemnisci, and the inferior colliculi. The inferior colliculi, a mandatory synaptic processing site for central auditory processing, receive information from both ears. These projections proceed to the medial geniculate nucleus and then via the auditory radiations to the auditory cortex (transverse gyrus of Heschl). Damage in the interior of the brainstem or, more likely, in the temporal lobe, generally caused by a vascular infarct, tumor or abscess, or trauma, may result in diminished hearing and auditory neglect from contralateral stimuli but not unilateral deafness. Schwannomas frequently arise from the vestibular division of CN VIII and involve both the vestibular and auditory divisions of this cranial nerve.

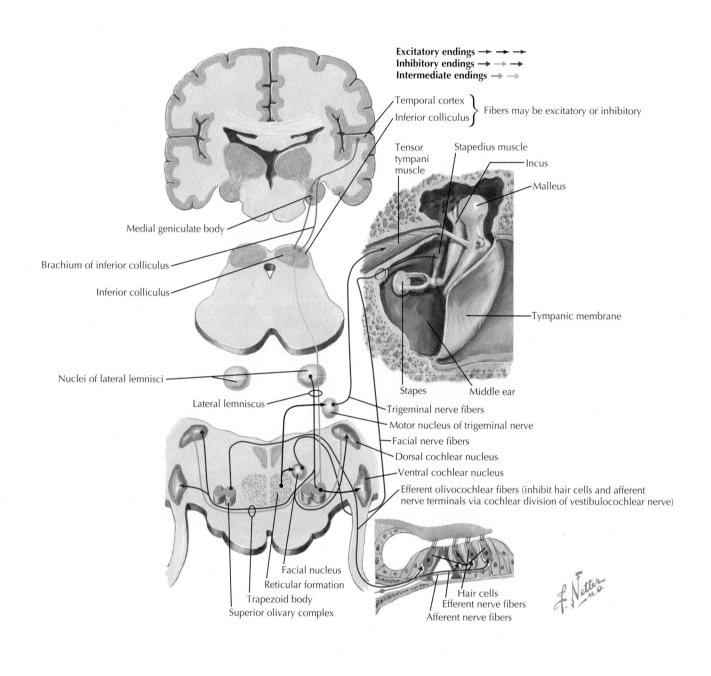

Excitatory endings → → →
Inhibitory endings → → →
Intermediate endings ⇒ ⇒

Temporal cortex
Inferior colliculus } Fibers may be excitatory or inhibitory

Tensor tympani muscle
Stapedius muscle
Incus
Malleus

Medial geniculate body

Brachium of inferior colliculus

Inferior colliculus

Tympanic membrane

Nuclei of lateral lemnisci

Lateral lemniscus

Stapes
Middle ear

Trigeminal nerve fibers
Motor nucleus of trigeminal nerve
Facial nerve fibers
Dorsal cochlear nucleus
Ventral cochlear nucleus
Efferent olivocochlear fibers (inhibit hair cells and afferent nerve terminals via cochlear division of vestibulocochlear nerve)

Facial nucleus
Reticular formation
Trapezoid body
Superior olivary complex

Hair cells
Efferent nerve fibers
Afferent nerve fibers

14.22 CENTRIFUGAL (EFFERENT) AUDITORY PATHWAYS

Descending pathways travel from the auditory cortex, the medial geniculate body of the thalamus, the inferior colliculus, and accessory auditory nuclei of the brainstem to terminate in caudal structures in the pathway, such as the cochlear nuclei and the superior olivary nucleus. These centrifugal connections permit descending control of incoming auditory information. The olivocochlear bundle, from the superior olivary nuclei, projects back to the hair cells in the organ of Corti and modulates the transduction process between the hair cells and the primary afferent axons. The motor nuclei of V and VII send LMN axonal projections to the tensor tympani and stapedius muscles, respectively, for reflex dampening of the ossicles in the presence of sustained loud noise.

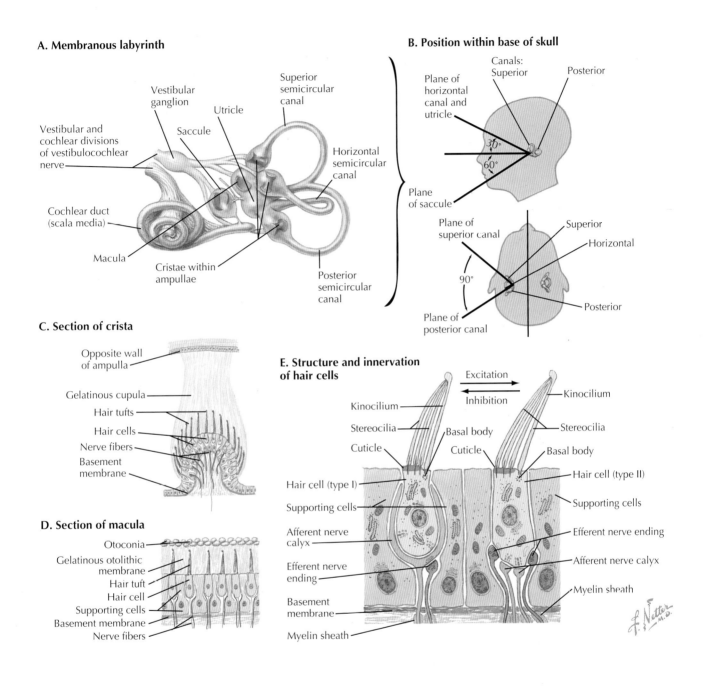

A. Membranous labyrinth

Vestibular and cochlear divisions of vestibulocochlear nerve

Vestibular ganglion

Saccule

Utricle

Superior semicircular canal

Horizontal semicircular canal

Cochlear duct (scala media)

Macula

Cristae within ampullae

Posterior semicircular canal

B. Position within base of skull

Canals: Superior   Posterior

Plane of horizontal canal and utricle

30°

60°

Plane of saccule

Plane of superior canal

Superior

Horizontal

90°

Posterior

Plane of posterior canal

C. Section of crista

Opposite wall of ampulla

Gelatinous cupula

Hair tufts

Hair cells

Nerve fibers

Basement membrane

D. Section of macula

Otoconia

Gelatinous otolithic membrane

Hair tuft

Hair cell

Supporting cells

Basement membrane

Nerve fibers

E. Structure and innervation of hair cells

Excitation

Inhibition

Kinocilium

Stereocilia

Cuticle

Kinocilium

Stereocilia

Basal body

Cuticle

Basal body

Hair cell (type I)

Supporting cells

Afferent nerve calyx

Efferent nerve ending

Basement membrane

Myelin sheath

Hair cell (type II)

Supporting cells

Efferent nerve ending

Afferent nerve calyx

Myelin sheath

VESTIBULAR SYSTEM

14.23 VESTIBULAR RECEPTORS

The vestibular receptors include hair cells in the maculae of the utricle (linear acceleration or gravity) and saccule (low frequency vibration) and in the cristae ampullaris of the orthogonally oriented semicircular canals (angular acceleration or movement of the head). Hair tufts from the cristae ampullaris and the maculae are embedded in a gelatinous substance, which is moved when gravity (utricle) exerts force on the calcium carbonate crystals (otoliths) resting on top of the hairs or when fluid movement occurs in a semicircular canal (head movement). Bending of the kinocilium in the hair tufts depolarizes the hair cell, causing the release of neurotransmitters that stimulate action potentials in primary sensory axons of the vestibular (Scarpa's) ganglion. Additional efferent projections from the CNS modulate this transduction process, similar to centrifugal regulation of auditory transduction.

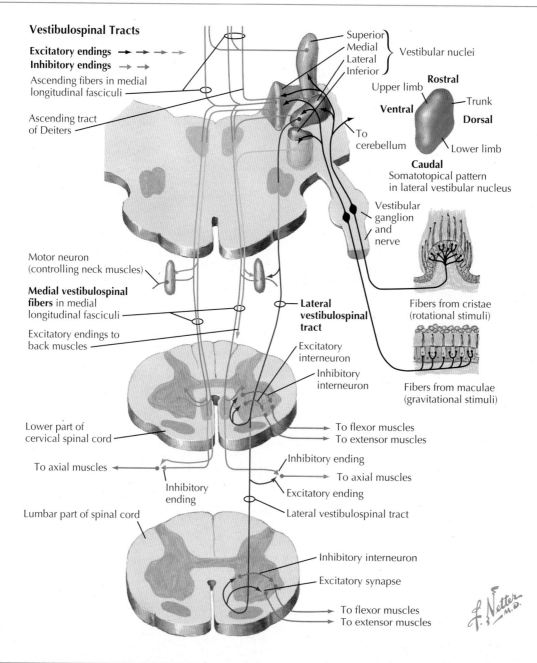

Vestibulospinal Tracts

Excitatory endings → → → →
Inhibitory endings → →

Ascending fibers in medial longitudinal fasciculi

Ascending tract of Deiters

Superior
Medial
Lateral
Inferior } Vestibular nuclei

Rostral
Upper limb
Ventral　**Dorsal**
Trunk
Lower limb
Caudal
Somatotopical pattern in lateral vestibular nucleus

To cerebellum

Vestibular ganglion and nerve

Fibers from cristae (rotational stimuli)

Motor neuron (controlling neck muscles)

Medial vestibulospinal fibers in medial longitudinal fasciculi

Excitatory endings to back muscles

Lateral vestibulospinal tract

Excitatory interneuron

Inhibitory interneuron

Fibers from maculae (gravitational stimuli)

Lower part of cervical spinal cord

To flexor muscles
To extensor muscles

To axial muscles ←

Inhibitory ending

Inhibitory ending
To axial muscles
Excitatory ending
Lateral vestibulospinal tract

Lumbar part of spinal cord

Inhibitory interneuron

Excitatory synapse

To flexor muscles
To extensor muscles

14.24 VESTIBULAR PATHWAYS

Primary afferent vestibular axons from the vestibular ganglion terminate in the four vestibular nuclei (superior, inferior, medial, and lateral) and directly in the cerebellum (deep nuclei and cortex). Descending axons are sent via the medial vestibulospinal tract (from the medial nucleus) to spinal cord LMNs that regulate head and neck movements. Descending axons are sent via the lateral vestibulospinal tract (from the lateral nucleus) to all levels of spinal cord LMNs to activate extensor movements. Multiple vestibular nuclei project to the cerebellum to modulate and coordinate muscle activity for basic tone and posture and to extraocular LMNs via the medial longitudinal fasciculus to coordinate eye movements with head and neck movements. Some ascending axons from the vestibular nuclei may reach the thalamus (near the VPM and posterior nuclei), with thalamic projections to the lateral postcentral gyrus (area 2, motion perception and spatial orientation) and to the insular cortex and temporoparietal cortex.

CLINICAL POINT

The vestibular nerve consists of axons that supply the hair cells of the cristae in the ampullae of the semicircular canals, as well as the maculae of the utricle and saccule. These primary afferent axons terminate in the four vestibular nuclei and directly in the vestibular cerebellum (part of the vermis and flocculonodular lobe). The vestibular nuclei send axonal projections to the LMNs of the spinal cord (via vestibulospinal tracts), the cerebellum, the extraocular nuclei (via the medial longitudinal fasciculus), and the RF. The peripheral vestibular and auditory apparatus can be damaged by increased endolymphatic pressure that gradually destroys hair cells in both the vestibular and auditory peripheral systems. This condition, called **Meniere's disease**, is characterized by abrupt attacks of severe vertigo that can last for as long as several hours. The attacks are incapacitating and immobilizing and produce nausea and vomiting. The vestibular symptoms are accompanied by auditory symptoms, including tinnitus and progressive sensorineural deafness. Most cases are unilateral, but bilateral disease does occur. After many episodes, some remission is occasionally seen, but the disease can progress to the point where the hearing loss and vestibular damage are almost total.

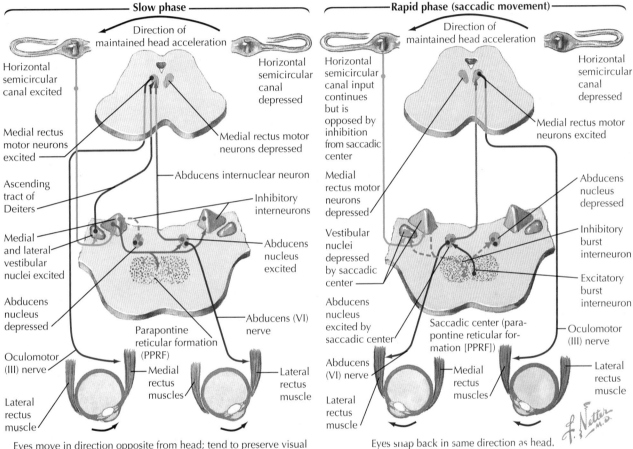

Slow phase

Direction of
maintained head acceleration

Horizontal
semicircular
canal excited

Horizontal
semicircular
canal
depressed

Medial rectus
motor neurons
excited

Medial rectus motor
neurons depressed

Abducens internuclear neuron

Ascending
tract of
Deiters

Inhibitory
interneurons

Medial
and lateral
vestibular
nuclei excited

Abducens
nucleus
excited

Abducens
nucleus
depressed

Abducens (VI)
nerve

Parapontine
reticular formation
(PPRF)

Oculomotor
(III) nerve

Medial
rectus
muscles

Lateral
rectus
muscle

Lateral
rectus
muscle

Eyes move in direction opposite from head; tend to preserve visual
fixation; rate determined by degree of horizontal canal excitation.

Rapid phase (saccadic movement)

Direction of
maintained head acceleration

Horizontal
semicircular
canal input
continues
but is
opposed by
inhibition
from saccadic
center

Horizontal
semicircular
canal
depressed

Medial rectus motor
neurons excited

Medial
rectus motor
neurons
depressed

Abducens
nucleus
depressed

Vestibular
nuclei
depressed
by saccadic
center

Inhibitory
burst
interneuron

Excitatory
burst
interneuron

Abducens
nucleus
excited by
saccadic center

Saccadic center (para-
pontine reticular for-
mation [PPRF])

Oculomotor
(III) nerve

Abducens
(VI) nerve

Medial
rectus
muscles

Lateral
rectus
muscle

Lateral
rectus
muscle

Eyes snap back in same direction as head.

14.25 NYSTAGMUS

Nystagmus is repetitive, alternating back-and-forth movements of
the eye, requiring central coordination of extraocular LMNs and eye
movements. Optokinetic nystagmus is a normal process of visually
activated movement of the eyes via tracking mechanisms, with the
eyes returning to a forward position by means of visual association
cortex projections through the superior colliculus to extraocular
LMNs. Vestibular nystagmus results from asymmetrical input from
receptors in the semicircular canals or from damage to vestibular
nuclei or the vestibular cerebellum and is mediated by vestibular
projections via the medial longitudinal fasciculus to extraocular
nuclei (LMNs); the asymmetrical input provokes the slow phase
(or drift) of vestibular nystagmus, eliciting eye movements as if
the head were turning. The fast phase (saccadic movement) is the
return of the eyes to a forward position, which is provoked when
the slow phase moves the eyes to a maximal position.

Horizontal section

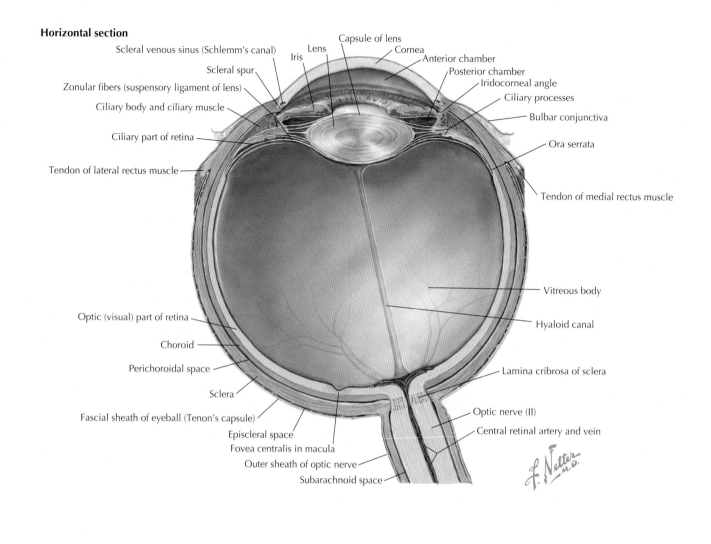

VISUAL SYSTEM

14.26 ANATOMY OF THE EYE

The eye consists of three major layers, or tunics. The outer fibrous layer, the fibrous tunic, consists of the protective cornea (transparent) and the sclera (opaque). The middle layer, the vascular tunic (uveal tract), consists of the choroid, the ciliary body, and the iris. The transparent biconvex lens, with its surrounding capsule of zonular fibers, is suspended from the ciliary process of the ciliary body. The inner layer, or tunic, consists of the neuroretina, the nonpigment epithelium of the ciliary body, and the pigment epithelium of the posterior iris. The retina contains the photoreceptors for transduction of photon energy from light into neuronal activity. Aqueous humor is secreted from blood vessels of the iris into the posterior chamber and flows through the aperture of the pupil into the anterior chamber, where it is absorbed into the trabecular meshwork into Schlemm's canal at the iridocorneal angle. Blockage of this absorption of aqueous humor results in glaucoma. The vitreous humor fills the interior of the eyeball.

CLINICAL POINT

When light impinges on the eye, it is refracted to focus on the photoreceptors of the retina to permit interpretation of the outside visual world. A vast proportion (close to 90%) of the refraction of light is accomplished by the cornea. A smaller percentage (approximately 10%) of the refraction is accomplished by the lens; however, this smaller percentage can be regulated neurologically, via CN III and its influence on accommodation to near vision. If the cornea is opacified (e.g., following abrasion that results in vascularization) it may impede the light pathway and cause a distortion of vision. Accommodation to near vision occurs when one tries to look at an object that is close rather than distant and usually involves simultaneous convergence, constriction (pupil), and accommodation. Accommodation involves a portion of the nucleus of Edinger-Westphal, which acts through CN III axonal projections to the ciliary ganglion. This portion provides postganglionic parasympathetic cholinergic innervation to the ciliary muscle. When this parasympathetic system is activated, the ciliary muscle lifts up and in, releasing tension on the zonular fibers that suspend the lens, permitting the lens to bunch up (fatten) and refract light. Accommodation commonly diminishes with age (presbyopia). A **CN III palsy** damages both pupillary constriction (resulting in a fixed, dilated pupil) and accommodation to near vision. Accommodation also can be damaged by trauma, diabetes, viral infections, and other pathology. If accommodation is impaired, corrective lenses are needed to allow proper focusing of light on the retina.

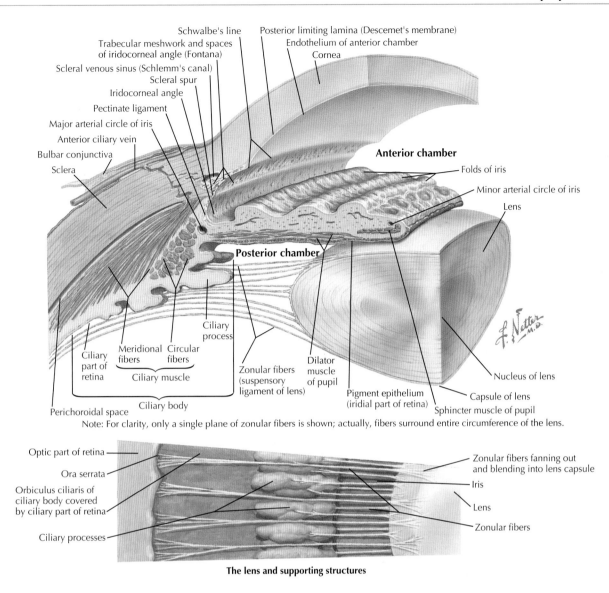

Schwalbe's line
Trabecular meshwork and spaces of iridocorneal angle (Fontana)
Scleral venous sinus (Schlemm's canal)
Scleral spur
Iridocorneal angle
Pectinate ligament
Major arterial circle of iris
Anterior ciliary vein
Bulbar conjunctiva
Sclera

Posterior limiting lamina (Descemet's membrane)
Endothelium of anterior chamber
Cornea

Anterior chamber

Folds of iris
Minor arterial circle of iris
Lens

Posterior chamber

Ciliary part of retina
Meridional fibers
Circular fibers
Ciliary muscle
Ciliary process
Zonular fibers (suspensory ligament of lens)
Dilator muscle of pupil
Pigment epithelium (iridial part of retina)
Sphincter muscle of pupil
Capsule of lens
Nucleus of lens

Perichoroidal space
Ciliary body

Note: For clarity, only a single plane of zonular fibers is shown; actually, fibers surround entire circumference of the lens.

Optic part of retina
Ora serrata
Orbiculus ciliaris of ciliary body covered by ciliary part of retina
Ciliary processes

Zonular fibers fanning out and blending into lens capsule
Iris
Lens
Zonular fibers

The lens and supporting structures

14.27 ANTERIOR AND POSTERIOR CHAMBERS OF THE EYE

The ciliary muscle and the pupillary constrictor muscle are supplied by parasympathetic postganglionic myelinated nerve fibers from the ciliary ganglion (innervated by preganglionics in the nucleus of Edinger-Westphal in CN III). Contraction of the ciliary muscle reduces the tension on zonular fibers and causes the lens to curve or bunch, which induces accommodation for near vision. The pupillary constrictor muscle also is supplied by parasympathetic postganglionic fibers from the ciliary ganglion. In the pupillary light reflex, light shone into one eye stimulates photoreceptors and related neurons in the retina; retinal ganglion cells send neural projections via the optic (II) nerve (afferent limb), which terminate in the pretectum. Neurons of the pretectum project bilaterally (crossed axons through the posterior commissure) to the Edinger-Westphal nucleus. This nucleus projects to the ciliary ganglion via CN III (efferent limb), which causes both direct (ipsilateral) and consensual (contralateral) pupillary constriction. The pupillary dilator muscle is supplied by noradrenergic sympathetic postganglionic unmyelinated nerve fibers from the superior cervical ganglion (innervated by preganglionics in T1 and T2). Schlemm's canals are conspicuous at the iridocorneal angle.

The lens is surrounded by a capsule anchored and suspended by an array of zonular fibers fanning out in circular fashion to attach to the ciliary processes of the ciliary body. Some interior zonular fibers extend along the ciliary body to the junction at the ora serrata.

CLINICAL POINT

Aqueous humor is secreted from the vasculature of the ciliary apparatus into the posterior chamber. It circulates through the pupillary aperture into the anterior chamber. From the anterior chamber, the aqueous humor is resorbed into the scleral venous sinuses, called the canals of Schlemm. If the canals of Schlemm are blocked, preventing absorption of aqueous humor, increased ocular pressure occurs; this results in pressure on the optic nerve head, cupped discs, atrophy, and defective vision of increasing severity, including total blindness. **Glaucoma**, the most common cause of optic nerve damage, occurs in more than 1% of the population over 40 years of age. This condition can be detected through ophthalmoscopy and tonometry. The principal type of glaucoma is called wide-angle glaucoma, which involves gradual sclerosis of the canals of Schlemm. A far less common type of glaucoma is narrow-angle (acute or closed-angle) glaucoma, a medical emergency in which bunching of the dilator muscle or narrowing of the iridocorneal angle blocks resorption of aqueous humor. The eye is red, swollen, and painful, sometimes causing a headache. It can be precipitated by pupillary dilation during an ophthalmological examination and must be reversed by means of pharmacological pupillary constriction.

Section through retina

Retinal Layers

Cells

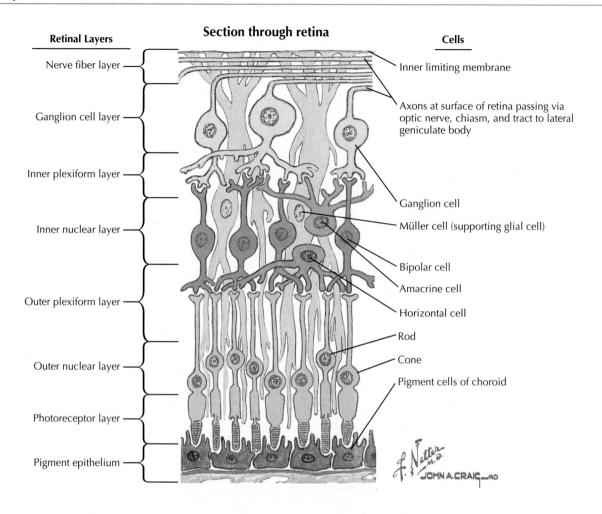

Nerve fiber layer

Ganglion cell layer

Inner plexiform layer

Inner nuclear layer

Outer plexiform layer

Outer nuclear layer

Photoreceptor layer

Pigment epithelium

Inner limiting membrane

Axons at surface of retina passing via optic nerve, chiasm, and tract to lateral geniculate body

Ganglion cell

Müller cell (supporting glial cell)

Bipolar cell

Amacrine cell

Horizontal cell

Rod

Cone

Pigment cells of choroid

14.28 THE RETINA: RETINAL LAYERS

The retina is a tissue paper–thin piece of CNS tissue that contains the photoreceptors; it is attached to the vascular tunic at the ora serrata. The layers of the retina in the interior of the eyeball are oriented from outer to inner. The pigment epithelium is at the outer margin, followed by the outer nuclear layer (photoreceptors), the inner nuclear layer (bipolar neurons, amacrine and horizontal cells), and the ganglion cell layer. The outer and inner plexiform layers are the zones of synaptic connectivity. The ganglion cell axons form an inner nerve fiber layer projecting centrally toward the optic nerve head, into which they collect as the optic nerve, CN II. The outer segments of the photoreceptors, the rods and cones, are embedded in a pigment epithelium in the outer part of the interior eyeball to prevent backscatter of light. The rods and cones connect synaptically with bipolar cells in the outer plexiform layer; these bipolar neurons connect with the ganglion cells of the retina in the inner plexiform layer. The retinal ganglion cells are the equivalent of secondary sensory nuclei for other sensory modalities. Horizontal and amacrine cells provide horizontal interconnections in the retina, mainly at the outer plexiform layer and the inner plexiform layer, respectively. These cells modulate the central flow of information from the photoreceptors to the bipolar neurons to the retinal ganglion cells. The central point for visual focusing is the fovea centralis (0.4 mm in diameter) in the macula (3 mm in diameter), which is found temporally and slightly below the geometric midpoint. The fovea consists purely of cones for color vision (photopic); these cone projections to ganglion cells involve very little convergence. In the fovea, there is close to a one-to-one-to-one relationship among the cones, bipolar neurons, and ganglion cells. The peripheral retinal photoreceptors are mainly rods, for night vision (scotopic); there is huge convergence of rods onto bipolar neurons, which in turn converge onto single ganglion cells. Thus, acuity is best achieved in the fovea, the region for color vision.

CLINICAL POINT

Cones permit color vision and are concentrated in the macula of the retina, the point of focus for high-acuity vision. The center of the macula, the fovea centralis, consists entirely of cones. These cones are connected with bipolar retinal cells, which in turn contact retinal ganglion cells, resulting in conveyance of visual information via the optic nerve into other CNS structures (superior colliculus, pretectum, hypothalamus, lateral geniculate nucleus). The macular pathway is essential for photopic (color, high-acuity) vision. The peripheral retina contains rods as the main photoreceptors; rods massively converge onto bipolar neurons. This peripheral retinal pathway is active in scotopic (night) vision. The macula can undergo a gradual process of depigmentation and degeneration in elderly individuals, leading to the loss of central vision and reading capability. Although there is no immediate cure for **macular degeneration**, carotenoid supplements of lutein and zeaxanthin appear to replenish the macula with these important depleted carotenoids, slowing the degenerative process. Although macular degeneration is mainly a disease of the elderly, some young individuals with inherited storage diseases (Tay-Sachs) or infectious processes may experience macular degeneration.

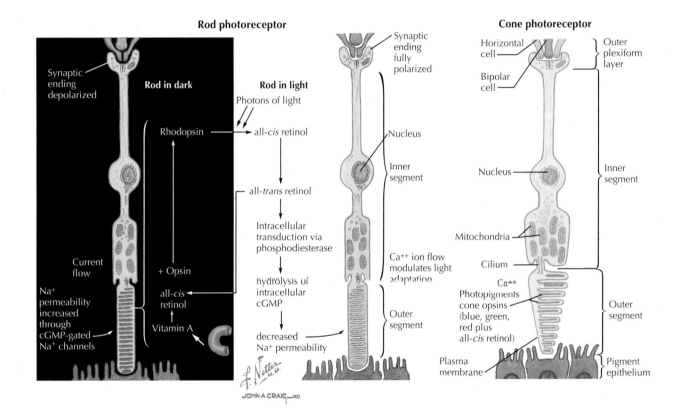

Rod photoreceptor

Synaptic ending depolarized

Rod in dark

Rod in light

Photons of light

Rhodopsin → all-*cis* retinol

all-*trans* retinol

Intracellular transduction via phosphodiesterase

hydrolysis of intracellular cGMP

+ Opsin

all-*cis* retinol

Vitamin A

decreased Na+ permeability

Current flow

Na+ permeability increased through cGMP-gated Na+ channels

Synaptic ending fully polarized

Nucleus

Inner segment

Ca++ ion flow modulates light adaptation

Outer segment

Cone photoreceptor

Horizontal cell

Bipolar cell

Outer plexiform layer

Nucleus

Inner segment

Mitochondria

Cilium

Ca++

Photopigments cone opsins (blue, green, red plus all-*cis* retinol)

Outer segment

Plasma membrane

Pigment epithelium

14.29 THE RETINA: PHOTORECEPTORS

Rods use the photopigment rhodopsin to achieve transduction of photons of energy from light into neurotransmitter release that can activate electrical activity in bipolar neurons. Rod light transduction involves conversion of all-*cis*-retinol (from rhodopsin) to an all-*trans* form, provoking calcium influx and a decrease in sodium conductance with hyperpolarization. This process is outlined in detail in the first two parts of the figure, a rod in the dark and a rod in light. When a rod is activated by light, it hyperpolarizes rather than depolarizes. A cone uses opsin photopigments for blue, green, and red, as well as all-*cis* retinal; these cone pigments permit color vision.

A. Topography of retinal nerve fibers

Arcuate nerve fibers from temporal periphery of retina must arc around macular bundle.

Temporal retina
Median horizontal raphe. Inferior and superior arcuate fibers meet but do not cross.

Macular nerve fibers course directly to optic disc.

Optic disc (blind spot)

Nasal retina

Nerve fibers of nasal retina course directly to optic disc.

Macula (fixation point)

B. Anatomy of optic nerve

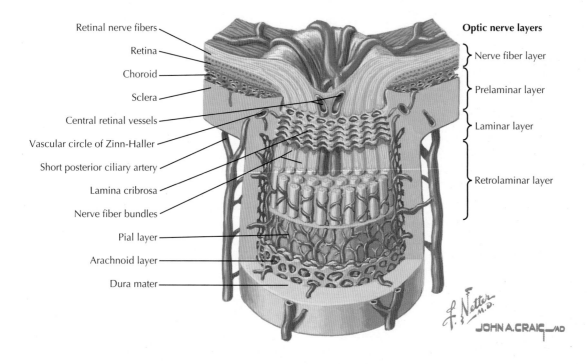

Retinal nerve fibers

Retina

Choroid

Sclera

Central retinal vessels

Vascular circle of Zinn-Haller

Short posterior ciliary artery

Lamina cribrosa

Nerve fiber bundles

Pial layer

Arachnoid layer

Dura mater

Optic nerve layers

Nerve fiber layer

Prelaminar layer

Laminar layer

Retrolaminar layer

JOHN A. CRAIG—AD

14.30 THE RETINA: OPTIC NERVE

A, The retina is topographically organized; a representation of the visual world (referred to as a visual field) is mapped onto the retina of each eye. Because the eye acts like a camera, the visual world is inverted as it projects onto the retina. The temporal (lateral) visual field falls on the nasal hemiretina, and the nasal (medial) visual field falls on the temporal hemiretina. The upper visual field falls on the lower hemiretina, and the lower visual field falls on the upper hemiretina. When viewing the retina directly using ophthalmoscopy, the macula is located temporally and slightly inferior to the geometric midpoint of the retina. The optic disc (zone of optic nerve fibers, sometimes called the blind spot) is located nasally and slightly above (superior to) the geometric midpoint. The precise retinotopic organization is maintained throughout the projections of the main visual pathway (the

retino-geniculo-calcarine pathway). **B,** The optic nerve (CN II) is a CNS tract that consists of myelinated axons of the ganglion cells of the retina. These axons collect across the innermost layer of the neuroretina and form the optic nerve, which exits from the eyeball nasally, slightly above the horizontal midline. These optic nerve fibers are myelinated by oligodendroglia. The optic nerve is surrounded by meninges, as part of the CNS. A subarachnoid space containing cerebrospinal fluid is present between the arachnoid and pial layers of the meninges. Elevated intracranial pressure can exert pressure on the optic nerve head (where the ganglion cell axons first form the optic nerve), forcing it inward; this phenomenon is called papilledema and is evidence of increased intracranial pressure; approximately 24 hours are required for increased intracranial pressure to cause papilledema. Major retinal vessels from the central retinal artery and vein travel in the optic nerve.

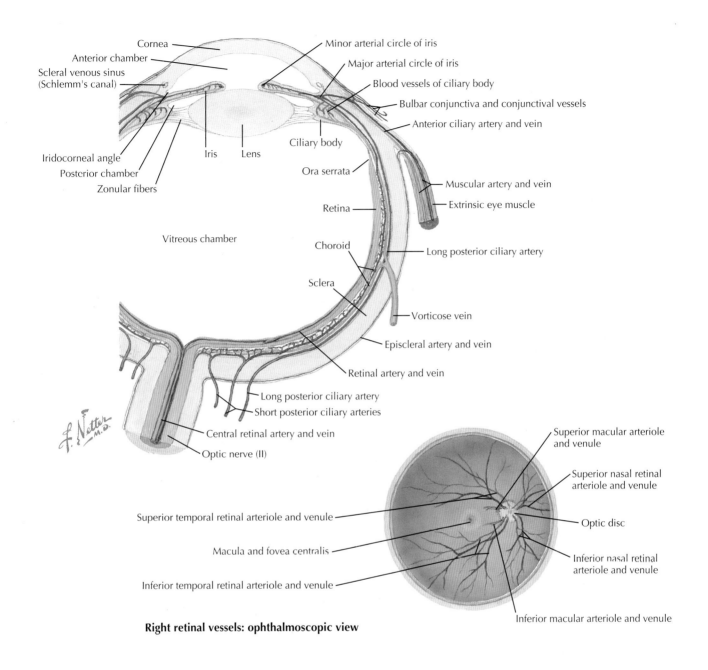

Cornea

Anterior chamber

Scleral venous sinus
(Schlemm's canal)

Iridocorneal angle

Posterior chamber

Zonular fibers

Iris   Lens

Vitreous chamber

Minor arterial circle of iris

Major arterial circle of iris

Blood vessels of ciliary body

Bulbar conjunctiva and conjunctival vessels

Anterior ciliary artery and vein

Ciliary body

Ora serrata

Retina

Choroid

Sclera

Muscular artery and vein

Extrinsic eye muscle

Long posterior ciliary artery

Vorticose vein

Episcleral artery and vein

Retinal artery and vein

Long posterior ciliary artery

Short posterior ciliary arteries

Central retinal artery and vein

Optic nerve (II)

Superior temporal retinal arteriole and venule

Macula and fovea centralis

Inferior temporal retinal arteriole and venule

Superior macular arteriole
and venule

Superior nasal retinal
arteriole and venule

Optic disc

Inferior nasal retinal
arteriole and venule

Inferior macular arteriole and venule

Right retinal vessels: ophthalmoscopic view

14.31 ARTERIES AND VEINS OF THE EYE

The central retinal artery and its branches supply blood to the retina. This arterial system, derived from the ophthalmic artery (the first branch off the internal carotid artery), is commonly the first site where ischemic or embolic events (transient ischemic attacks) herald the presence of serious vascular disease and high risk for a future stroke. Ciliary arteries supply the middle vascular tunic, which also contributes partial blood supply to the retina; this component of blood supply can be disrupted by a detached retina. Blood vessels enter and exit the retina at the optic disc (nerve head), located nasally and slightly superiorly from the geometric midpoint of the eyeball. The macula is located temporally and slightly inferiorly from this midpoint.

CLINICAL POINT
The central retinal artery is a common site of emboli in impending cerebrovascular disease; such emboli are forerunners of stroke and indications of carotid atherosclerosis or occlusion. An embolus in the central retinal artery may produce temporary (fleeting) blindness in the affected eye, called amaurosis fugax, which lasts for several minutes but less than an hour; such an episode is called a **transient ischemic attack**. An infarct in the central retinal artery produces characteristic ophthalmologic findings, such as loss of opalescence in the fovea (a so-called cherry-red spot). If the central retinal vein is occluded, a hemorrhage is seen, and the resultant visual loss may be significant. In addition to hemorrhages, edema and exudates may be present, indicative of hypertension or diabetic problems. If the retina becomes detached, it may be separated from part of its blood supply from the ciliary arteries in the middle vascular tunic, which also results in loss of vision.

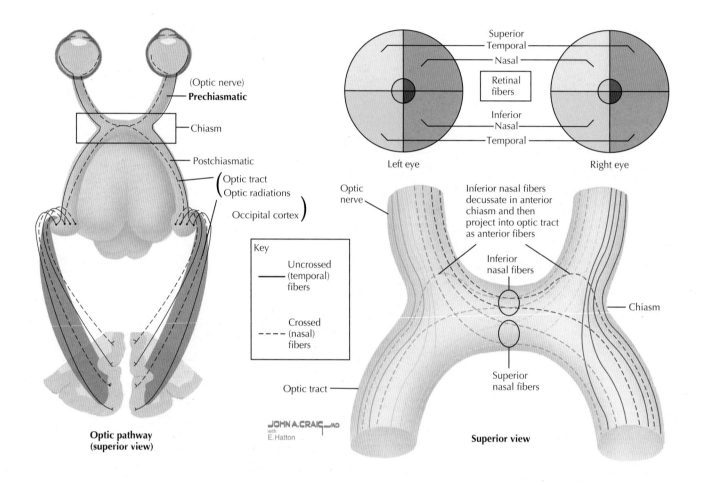

**Optic pathway
(superior view)**

Superior view

JOHN A. CRAIG
with
E. Hatton

14.32 ANATOMY AND RELATIONSHIPS OF THE OPTIC CHIASM

Axons from ganglion cells in the temporal hemiretinas (carrying information from the nasal visual fields) travel into the optic nerve and remain ipsilateral in the optic chiasm; they synapse in the ipsilateral lateral geniculate body or nucleus. Axons from ganglion cells in the nasal hemiretinas (carrying information from the temporal visual fields) travel into the optic nerve and cross the midline in the optic chiasm; they synapse in the contralateral lateral geniculate body. Therefore, crossing axons in the optic chiasm carry information from the temporal visual fields, which are derived from retinal ganglion cells in the nasal hemiretinas. These crossing axons are susceptible to disruption by a pituitary adenoma; such a lesion can produce a bitemporal hemianopia, starting first as an upper visual quadrant defect and progressing to full hemianopia. The optic tract contains axons from the ipsilateral temporal hemiretina and the contralateral nasal hemiretina, representing the contralateral visual field; disruption of the optic tract results in contralateral hemianopia.

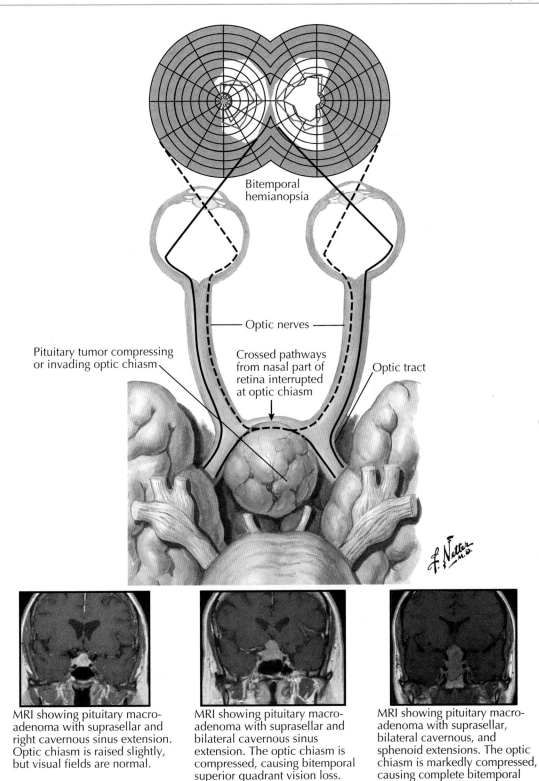

Bitemporal
hemianopsia

Pituitary tumor compressing
or invading optic chiasm

— Optic nerves —

Crossed pathways
from nasal part of
retina interrupted
at optic chiasm

Optic tract

f. Netter
M.D.

MRI showing pituitary macro-
adenoma with suprasellar and
right cavernous sinus extension.
Optic chiasm is raised slightly,
but visual fields are normal.

MRI showing pituitary macro-
adenoma with suprasellar and
bilateral cavernous sinus
extension. The optic chiasm is
compressed, causing bitemporal
superior quadrant vision loss.

MRI showing pituitary macro-
adenoma with suprasellar,
bilateral cavernous, and
sphenoid extensions. The optic
chiasm is markedly compressed,
causing complete bitemporal
hemianopsia.

Reprinted with permission from Young WF. The Netter Collection of Medical Illustrations, Volume 2 – Endocrine System. Elsevier, Philadelphia, 2011.

14.33 **DAMAGE AFFECTING THE OPTIC CHIASM**

Tumors, aneurysms, and infarcts can produce damage to the
optic chiasm. This illustration demonstrates increasing severity
(as noted by MRIs) of pituitary adenomas impinging on the optic
chiasm.

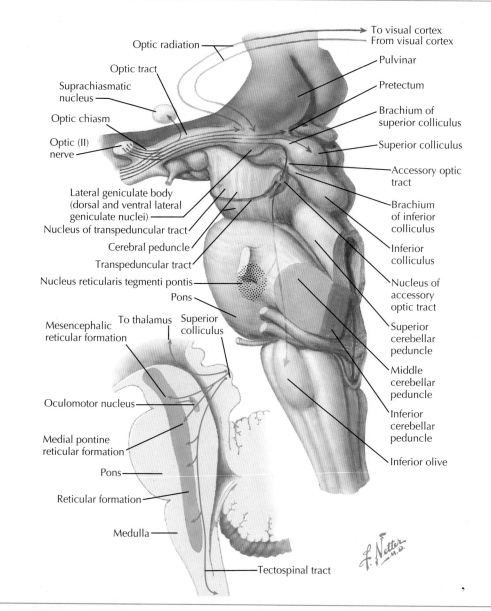

Optic radiation

To visual cortex
From visual cortex

Optic tract

Pulvinar

Suprachiasmatic nucleus

Pretectum

Optic chiasm

Brachium of superior colliculus

Optic (II) nerve

Superior colliculus

Accessory optic tract

Lateral geniculate body (dorsal and ventral lateral geniculate nuclei)

Brachium of inferior colliculus

Nucleus of transpeduncular tract

Inferior colliculus

Cerebral peduncle

Nucleus of accessory optic tract

Transpeduncular tract

Nucleus reticularis tegmenti pontis

Superior cerebellar peduncle

Pons

Mesencephalic reticular formation

To thalamus

Superior colliculus

Middle cerebellar peduncle

Oculomotor nucleus

Inferior cerebellar peduncle

Medial pontine reticular formation

Inferior olive

Pons

Reticular formation

Medulla

Tectospinal tract

14.34 VISUAL PATHWAYS: RETINAL PROJECTIONS TO THE THALAMUS, HYPOTHALAMUS, AND BRAINSTEM

Retinal projections travel through the optic nerve, chiasm, and tract and terminate in several regions, including the lateral geniculate body or nucleus, the upper layers of the superior colliculus, the pretectum, the hypothalamus (suprachiasmatic nucleus), and the nucleus of the accessory optic tract. The lateral geniculate body mediates conscious visual interpretation of visual input via the retino-geniculo-calcarine (area 17) pathway. The superior colliculus provides a second visual pathway through projections to the pulvinar, which in turn projects to the associative visual cortex (areas 18 and 19), providing localizing information for coordinating movement of the eyes to novel or moving visual stimuli. Neurons in deeper layers of the superior colliculus also provide descending contralateral connections (tectospinal tract) to cervical LMNs to mediate reflex visual effects on head and neck movements; collaterals of this descending system terminate in the brainstem reticular formation. The superior colliculus receives input from the visual cortex. The pretectum mediates the pupillary light reflex. The suprachiasmatic nucleus of the hypothalamus integrates light flux and regulates circadian rhythms and diurnal cycles. The nucleus of the inferior accessory optic tract may help to mediate brainstem responses for visual tracking and may interconnect with sympathetic preganglionic neurons in T1 and T2 (regulating the superior cervical ganglion).

CLINICAL POINT

Ganglion cells of the retina (the neural equivalents of the secondary sensory nuclei in other sensory systems, such as the nuclei gracilis and cuneatus) send projections through the optic nerve, chiasm, and tract to terminate in the superior colliculus, the lateral geniculate nucleus of the thalamus, the pretectum, the suprachiasmatic nucleus of the hypothalamus, and some brainstem sites. However, they all require the projection of axons through the optic nerve, chiasm, and tract. If the **optic nerve** is damaged (by multiple sclerosis, glaucoma, inflammatory disorder, trauma, vascular pathology), there is visual loss in a selected area (scotoma) or in the entire ipsilateral eye (monocular blindness). If the **optic chiasm** is damaged, usually by a pituitary tumor, the growth of the tumor impinges on the crossing fibers in a manner that disrupts the outer visual fields (bitemporal hemianopia), usually from the upper to the lower fields (much like pulling down the shades). If the **optic tract** is damaged, axons from the ipsilateral temporal hemiretina and the contralateral nasal hemiretina are disrupted, producing a contralateral visual field deficit (homonymous contralateral hemianopia).

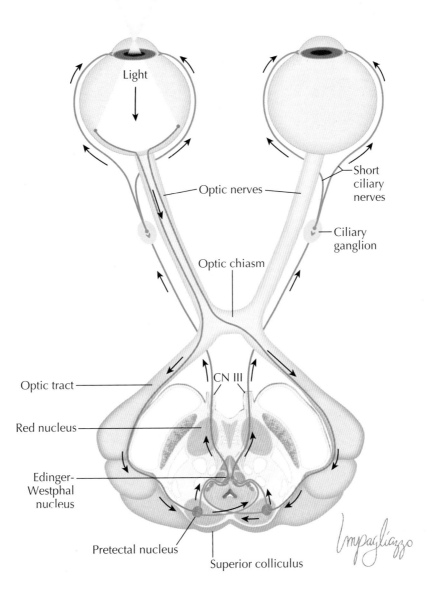

Light

Optic nerves

Short ciliary nerves

Ciliary ganglion

Optic chiasm

Optic tract

CN III

Red nucleus

Edinger-Westphal nucleus

Pretectal nucleus

Superior colliculus

Impagliazzo

14.35 PUPILLARY LIGHT REFLEX

The pupillary light reflex requires CN II, CN III, and central brainstem connections. Light shined in one eye stimulates retinal photoreceptors, and subsequently retinal ganglion cells, whose axons travel through the optic nerve, chiasm, and tract to terminate in the pretectum (pretectal nucleus). The pretectal neurons project to a portion of the nucleus of Edinger-Westphal on both sides. This preganglionic parasympathetic nucleus projects to ciliary ganglion neurons, which in turn send postganglionic cholinergic axons to innervate the pupillary constrictor muscle.

Thus, light shined in one eye normally results in the constriction of both pupils (ipsilateral pupillary constriction—direct response; contralateral pupillary constriction—consensual response).

Lesions of CN II produce an unresponsive pupillary light reflex on both sides (afferent pupillary defect) from light shined in the eye on the side of the CN II lesion. With light shined in the unaffected eye, both pupils constrict.

Lesions of CN III result in unresponsive ipsilateral pupillary constriction on the affected side (the pupil is "fixed and dilated") when light is shined in either eye (efferent pupillary defect).

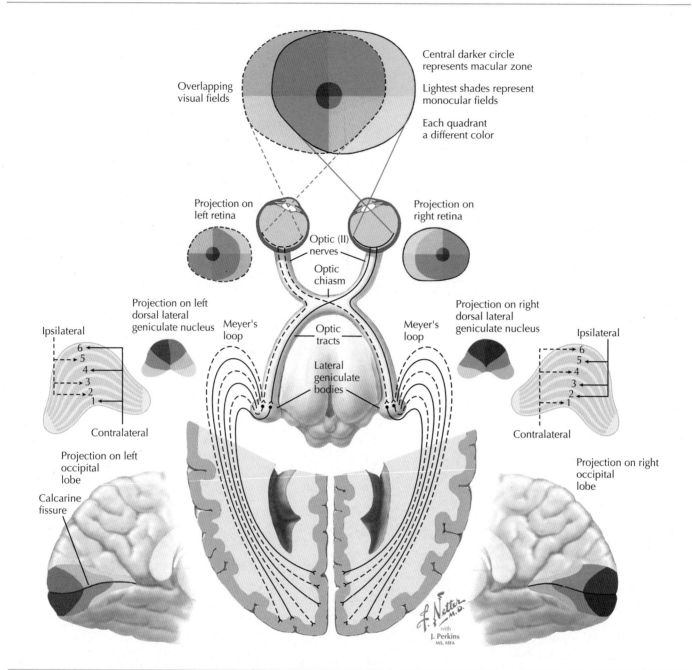

Overlapping visual fields

Central darker circle represents macular zone

Lightest shades represent monocular fields

Each quadrant a different color

Projection on left retina

Projection on right retina

Optic (II) nerves

Optic chiasm

Projection on left dorsal lateral geniculate nucleus

Projection on right dorsal lateral geniculate nucleus

Ipsilateral

Meyer's loop

Optic tracts

Meyer's loop

Ipsilateral

Lateral geniculate bodies

Contralateral

Contralateral

Projection on left occipital lobe

Projection on right occipital lobe

Calcarine fissure

14.36 VISUAL PATHWAY: THE RETINO-GENICULO-CALCARINE PATHWAY

The retino-geniculo-calcarine pathway conveys information about fine-grained conscious visual analysis of the outside world. It is organized topographically (retinotopic) throughout its course to the calcarine (visual) cortex in the occipital lobe. The nasal hemiretinal ganglion cell axons cross the midline in the optic chiasm, whereas the temporal hemiretinal ganglion cell axons remain ipsilateral. Thus, each optic tract conveys information from the contralateral visual world (or visual field); damage to the optic tract produces contralateral hemianopia. The optic tract terminates in the lateral geniculate body or nucleus and is organized in six layers, as shown. However, binocular convergence does not take place here; ganglion cell axons from the ipsilateral temporal hemiretina terminate in layers 2, 3, and 5, and ganglion cell axons from the contralateral nasal hemiretina terminate in layers 1, 4, and 6. The optic radiations project to the calcarine (striate) cortex (area 17,

the primary visual cortex). A portion of the optic radiations loops through the temporal lobe (Meyer's loop) and can be damaged by a tumor or mass, resulting in contralateral upper quadrantanopia. Bilateral convergence from right and left retinas first takes place in the primary visual cortex, area 17. The retinotopic organization of this pathway is shown in color in this illustration.

CLINICAL POINT

Meyer's loop consists of axons of the lateral geniculate nucleus that loop downward through the temporal lobe before extending posteriorly to synapse on cortical neurons in layer 4 of the lower bank of the ipsilateral calcarine fissure (area 17, primary visual cortex). The temporal lobe is a site at which tumor or abscess formation is far more likely than it is in the parietal or occipital lobes. If such a mass lesion damages fibers of Meyer's loop, the individual loses vision in the upper quadrant of the contralateral visual field (**upper contralateral quadrantanopia**), reflecting the persistent "retinotopic" organization of the entire retino-geniculo-calcarine pathway that is depicted in this illustration. This visual deficit is sometimes referred to as a "pie in the sky" deficit.

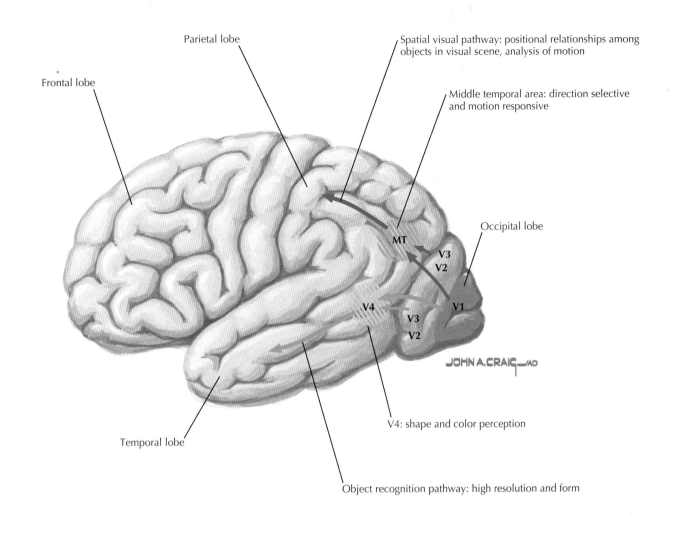

Frontal lobe

Parietal lobe

Spatial visual pathway: positional relationships among objects in visual scene, analysis of motion

Middle temporal area: direction selective and motion responsive

Occipital lobe

MT

V3
V2

V1

V4

V3
V2

JOHN A.CRAIG—AD

V4: shape and color perception

Temporal lobe

Object recognition pathway: high resolution and form

14.37 VISUAL PATHWAYS IN THE PARIETAL AND TEMPORAL LOBES

Neurons in the primary visual cortex (V1, area 17) send axons to association visual cortices (V2 and V3, areas 18 and 19). V2 and V3 also receive input from the superior colliculus via the pulvinar. V1, V2, and V3 project to the middle temporal (MT) area and V4. Middle temporal neurons are direction selective and motion responsive and further project into the parietal lobe for spatial visual processing. The parietal neurons provide analysis of motion and positional relationships among objects in the visual field. V4 neurons are involved in shape and color perception. Neurons in V4 project into the temporal lobe, in which further neuronal processing provides high-resolution object recognition, including faces, animate and inanimate objects, and the classification and orientation of objects. Small infarcts in the temporal lobe may produce specific agnosias, or the inability to recognize specific types of objects, such as faces or animate objects.

CLINICAL POINT

The retino-geniculo-calcarine pathway projects to area 17, the primary visual cortex; subsequent axonal projections are sent to areas 18 and 19. In these visual association cortices, feature extraction from simple to complex to hypercomplex cells occurs, giving form to new visual information. A parietal cortical pathway further processes information related to the direction and motion of objects—a spatial visual pathway. A temporal cortical pathway conveys further information about the shape, color, and form of objects. Some discrete lesions in these parietal and temporal cortical pathways can produce distinctive visual deficits. Visual agnosias occur when an individual cannot recognize objects that are viewed but has full visual acuity. This can happen with lesions in the occipito-temporal visual pathway. **Visual agnosias** are particularly common with lesions in the dominant mesial portion of the occipital cortex; they accompany a right homonymous hemianopia. Cortical color agnosias (cortical color blindness) also can occur with lesions in the occipito-temporal visual pathway, through V4. Some specific lesions of the occipito-temporal pathway, especially when bilateral, can result in prosopagnosia, or the inability to recognize faces. Some lacunar infarcts in this pathway also may result in the inability to distinguish between animate and inanimate objects. Lesions in the occipito-parietal visual pathway, particularly in the nondominant hemisphere, can cause visual-spatial disorientation, appearing clinically as impaired ability to see.

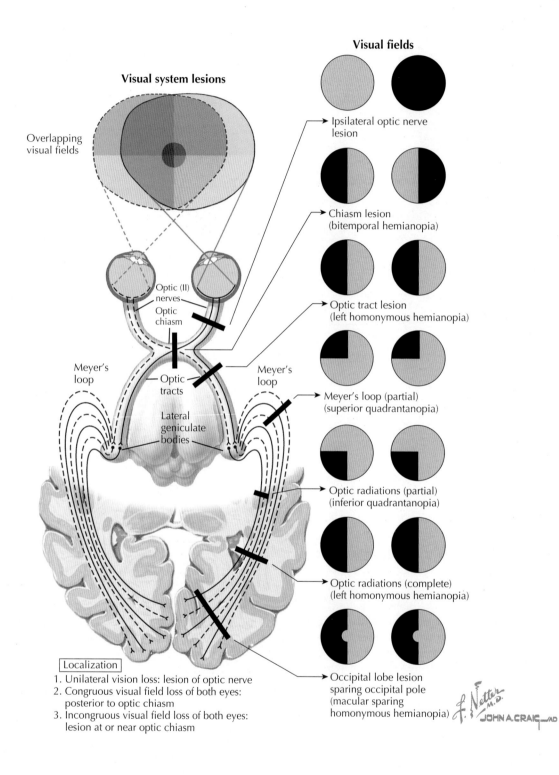

Visual system lesions

Overlapping
visual fields

Optic (II)
nerves
Optic
chiasm

Meyer's
loop

Optic
tracts

Meyer's
loop

Lateral
geniculate
bodies

Visual fields

Ipsilateral optic nerve
lesion

Chiasm lesion
(bitemporal hemianopia)

Optic tract lesion
(left homonymous hemianopia)

Meyer's loop (partial)
(superior quadrantanopia)

Optic radiations (partial)
(inferior quadrantanopia)

Optic radiations (complete)
(left homonymous hemianopia)

Occipital lobe lesion
sparing occipital pole
(macular sparing
homonymous hemianopia)

Localization
1. Unilateral vision loss: lesion of optic nerve
2. Congruous visual field loss of both eyes:
   posterior to optic chiasm
3. Incongruous visual field loss of both eyes:
   lesion at or near optic chiasm

14.38 VISUAL SYSTEM LESIONS

Lesions of the optic nerve, optic chiasm, optic tract, Meyer's loop
in the temporal lobe, optic radiations, and visual cortex produce
specific visual field deficits, as shown in this figure.

15

MOTOR SYSTEMS

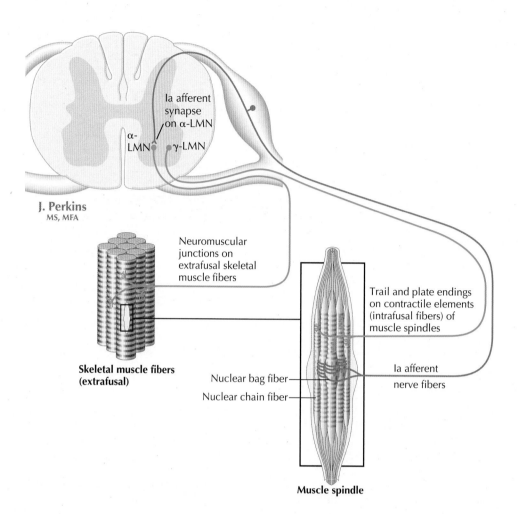

Ia afferent
synapse
on α-LMN

α-
LMN   γ-LMN

J. Perkins
MS, MFA

Neuromuscular
junctions on
extrafusal skeletal
muscle fibers

Trail and plate endings
on contractile elements
(intrafusal fibers) of
muscle spindles

Skeletal muscle fibers
(extrafusal)

Ia afferent
nerve fibers

Nuclear bag fiber
Nuclear chain fiber

Muscle spindle

LOWER MOTOR NEURONS

15.1 ALPHA AND GAMMA LOWER MOTOR NEURONS

All lower motor neuron (LMN) groups except the facial nerve nucleus that supplies the muscles of facial expression consist of both alpha LMNs that supply the skeletal muscle fibers (extrafusal fibers) and gamma LMNs that supply the small contractile elements in the muscle spindles (intrafusal fibers). The muscles of facial expression do not have muscle spindles and are not supplied by gamma LMNs. The alpha LMNs regulate contraction of the skeletal muscles to produce movement. The gamma LMNs regulate the sensitivity of the muscle spindles for group Ia and group II afferent modulation of alpha LMN excitability.

CLINICAL POINT

An alpha LMN supplies a motor axon to a variable number of skeletal muscle fibers (extrafusal fibers), ranging from just a few (e.g., extraocular muscles) to several thousand (large muscles such as the quadriceps). The LMN and its innervated skeletal muscle fibers are called a **motor unit**. Supporting cells (such as Schwann cells) and myocytes produce trophic factors to maintain the nerve-muscle association; when nerve injury occurs, growth factors help to attract motor axonal regrowth to reestablish the prior nerve-muscle association. When motor axons degenerate, the neuromuscular junctions (NMJs) disappear, and the nicotinic cholinergic receptors spread across the membrane of the denervated skeletal muscle fibers. This results in denervation hypersensitivity to nicotinic cholinergic stimulation, noted as random individual muscle fiber twitches (fibrillation), best observed by electromyography. If motor nerves are attracted back to the muscle fibers and NMJs are restored, the nicotinic cholinergic receptors are again restricted to the secondary folds of the NMJ. If the motor axon that was lost cannot regrow, neighboring motor axons of other motor units that supply adjacent skeletal muscle fibers may send sprouts to the denervated muscle fibers and incorporate them into the motor unit; the consequence is a larger motor unit and a greater demand on the LMN cell body that now supplies a greater than normal number of skeletal muscle fibers. This mechanism may account for recovery of physiological function in some LMN diseases such as polio. If the alpha-LMN cell body itself is damaged or is in the process of dying (e.g., in amyotrophic lateral sclerosis), the axon may produce aberrant action potentials (agonal bursts of electrical activity) that result in muscle fiber contraction throughout the motor unit, called a fasciculation, which is visually observable. A denervated muscle fiber must be reinnervated within 1 year or so if it is to restore relatively normal function; a longer period leads to permanent changes that preclude proper reinnervation. Many experimental approaches are seeking to restore innervation or attract a more robust nerve supply to denervated muscle fibers by applying or inducing gene expression of growth factors and trophic factors. Denervated skeletal muscle fibers are flaccidly paralyzed, lack muscle tone, cannot be induced to contract with muscle stretch reflexes, and undergo atrophy; these are classic characteristics of **LMN syndrome**.

A. Cytoarchitecture of the spinal cord gray matter

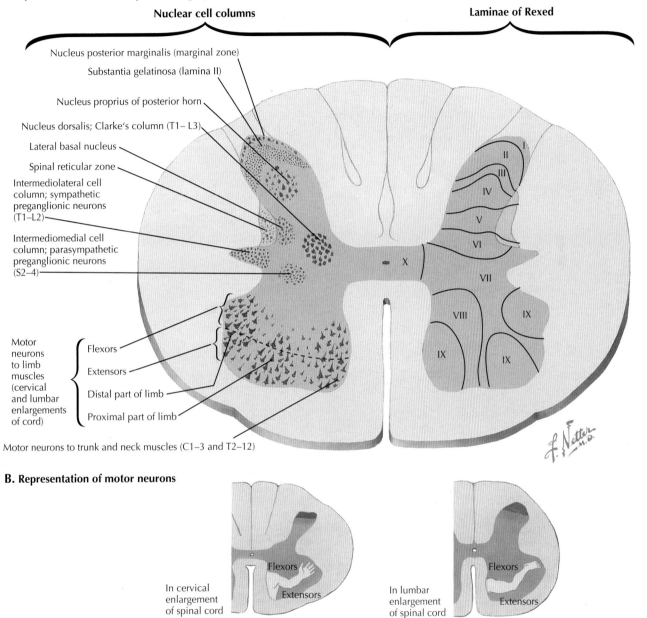

Nuclear cell columns

Laminae of Rexed

Nucleus posterior marginalis (marginal zone)

Substantia gelatinosa (lamina II)

Nucleus proprius of posterior horn

Nucleus dorsalis; Clarke's column (T1– L3)

Lateral basal nucleus

Spinal reticular zone

Intermediolateral cell column; sympathetic preganglionic neurons (T1–L2)

Intermediomedial cell column; parasympathetic preganglionic neurons (S2–4)

Motor neurons to limb muscles (cervical and lumbar enlargements of cord)
- Flexors
- Extensors
- Distal part of limb
- Proximal part of limb

Motor neurons to trunk and neck muscles (C1–3 and T2–12)

I
II
III
IV
V
VI
VII
VIII
IX
IX
IX
X

B. Representation of motor neurons

Flexors
Extensors

In cervical enlargement of spinal cord

Flexors
Extensors

In lumbar enlargement of spinal cord

15.2 DISTRIBUTION OF LOWER MOTOR NEURONS IN THE SPINAL CORD

LMNs are found as clusters of neurons in the anterior (ventral) horn of the spinal cord, represented as lamina IX of Rexed. Distinct clusters of LMNs supply distinct skeletal muscles with motor innervation. These LMN groups are organized topographically; LMNs distributing to trunk and neck muscles are found medially, and LMNs distributing to muscles of distal extremities are found laterally. Within spinal cord segments, LMNs distributing to flexor muscle groups are found dorsally, and LMNs distributing to extensor muscle groups are found ventrally.

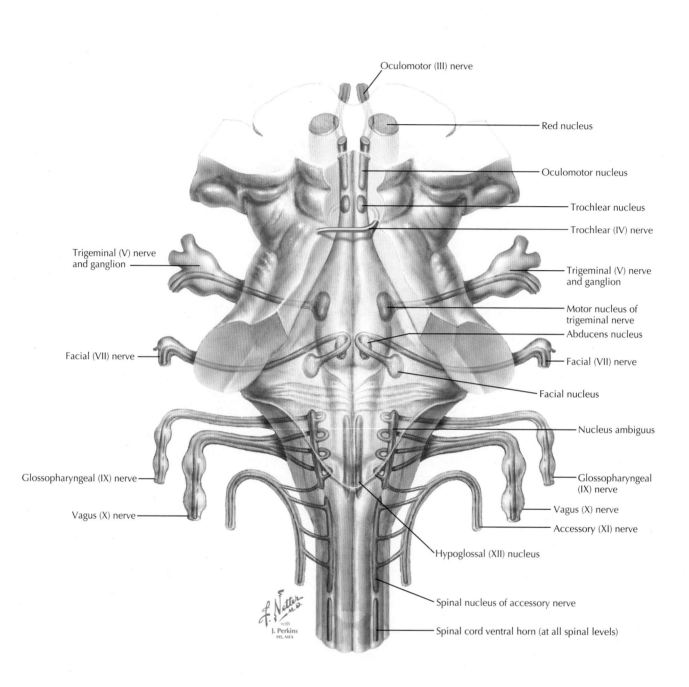

Oculomotor (III) nerve

Red nucleus

Oculomotor nucleus

Trochlear nucleus

Trochlear (IV) nerve

Trigeminal (V) nerve and ganglion

Trigeminal (V) nerve and ganglion

Motor nucleus of trigeminal nerve

Abducens nucleus

Facial (VII) nerve

Facial (VII) nerve

Facial nucleus

Nucleus ambiguus

Glossopharyngeal (IX) nerve

Glossopharyngeal (IX) nerve

Vagus (X) nerve

Vagus (X) nerve

Accessory (XI) nerve

Hypoglossal (XII) nucleus

Spinal nucleus of accessory nerve

Spinal cord ventral horn (at all spinal levels)

15.3 DISTRIBUTION OF LOWER MOTOR NEURONS IN THE BRAINSTEM

LMNs are found in medial and lateral columns in a longitudinal view of the brainstem. The medial column (LMNs of the oculomotor nucleus, trochlear nucleus, abducens nucleus, and hypoglossal nucleus) derives from the general somatic efferent system, and the lateral column (LMNs of motor nucleus V, facial nucleus, nucleus ambiguus, and spinal accessory nucleus) derives from the special visceral efferent system. LMNs in the spinal cord are found in a longitudinal column coursing through the anterior horn at all levels.

Cerebral Cortex: Efferent Pathways

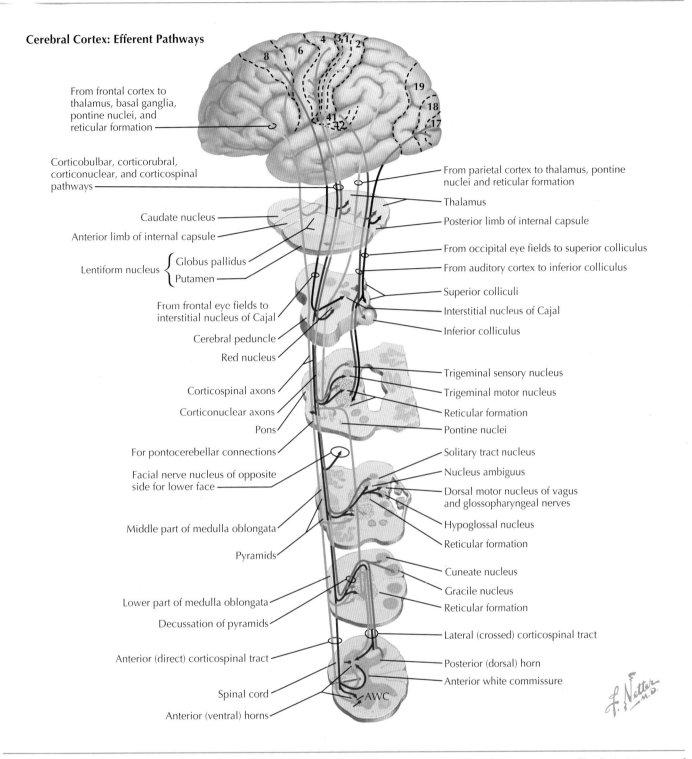

From frontal cortex to thalamus, basal ganglia, pontine nuclei, and reticular formation

Corticobulbar, corticorubral, corticonuclear, and corticospinal pathways

Caudate nucleus

Anterior limb of internal capsule

Lentiform nucleus { Globus pallidus / Putamen

From frontal eye fields to interstitial nucleus of Cajal

Cerebral peduncle

Red nucleus

Corticospinal axons

Corticonuclear axons

Pons

For pontocerebellar connections

Facial nerve nucleus of opposite side for lower face

Middle part of medulla oblongata

Pyramids

Lower part of medulla oblongata

Decussation of pyramids

Anterior (direct) corticospinal tract

Spinal cord

Anterior (ventral) horns

From parietal cortex to thalamus, pontine nuclei and reticular formation

Thalamus

Posterior limb of internal capsule

From occipital eye fields to superior colliculus

From auditory cortex to inferior colliculus

Superior colliculi

Interstitial nucleus of Cajal

Inferior colliculus

Trigeminal sensory nucleus

Trigeminal motor nucleus

Reticular formation

Pontine nuclei

Solitary tract nucleus

Nucleus ambiguus

Dorsal motor nucleus of vagus and glossopharyngeal nerves

Hypoglossal nucleus

Reticular formation

Cuneate nucleus

Gracile nucleus

Reticular formation

Lateral (crossed) corticospinal tract

Posterior (dorsal) horn

Anterior white commissure

AWC

UPPER MOTOR NEURONS

15.4 CORTICAL EFFERENT PATHWAYS

Cortical neurons in the motor cortex (area 4) and the supplemental and premotor cortices (area 6) send axons to the basal ganglia (caudate nucleus and putamen), the thalamus (ventral anterior [VA] and ventral lateral [VL] nuclei), the red nucleus, the pontine nuclei, the cranial nerve (CN) motor nuclei on both sides, and the spinal cord ventral horn, mainly on the contralateral side. These axons form the corticospinal tract, corticobulbar tract, corticostriatal projections, corticopontine projections, corticothalamic projections, and cortical connections to the upper motor neurons (UMNs) of the brainstem (reticular formation

[RF] motor areas, red nucleus, superior colliculus). Neurons of the sensory cortex (areas 3, 1, 2) send axons mainly to secondary sensory nuclei (corticonuclear fibers) to regulate incoming lemniscal sensory projections destined for conscious interpretation. Neurons in the frontal eye fields (area 8) project to the superior colliculus, the horizontal and vertical gaze centers of the brainstem, and the interstitial nucleus of Cajal to coordinate voluntary eye movements and associated head movements. Other regions of sensory cortex project axons to thalamic and brainstem structures that regulate incoming lemniscal sensory information. Some cortical efferent fibers project to limbic forebrain regions, such as the amygdaloid nuclei, hippocampal formation, and septal nuclei.

Lateral/oblique view

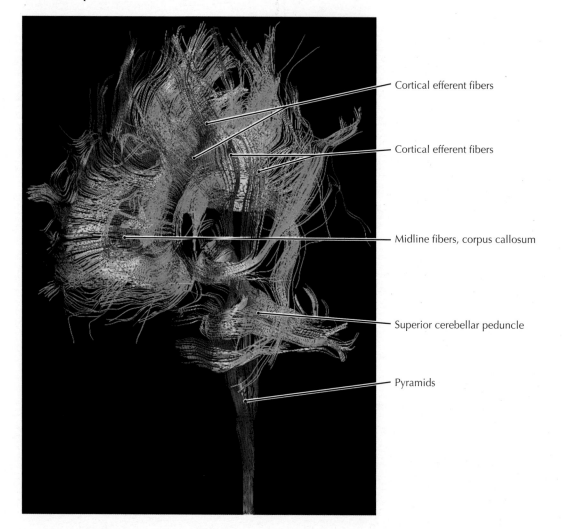

Cortical efferent fibers

Cortical efferent fibers

Midline fibers, corpus callosum

Superior cerebellar peduncle

Pyramids

15.5 **COLOR IMAGING OF CORTICAL EFFERENT PATHWAYS**

This diffusion tensor image shows the cortical efferent pathways in a lateral oblique section. These pathways, shown in blue, channel from widespread areas of the cerebral cortex to structures in the forebrain, the thalamus, the brainstem, the cerebellum (indirectly, through the pontine nuclei), and the spinal cord. Additional cortical association pathways are depicted in green (running in anterior-posterior direction) and commissural pathways are shown in red (running in left-right direction).

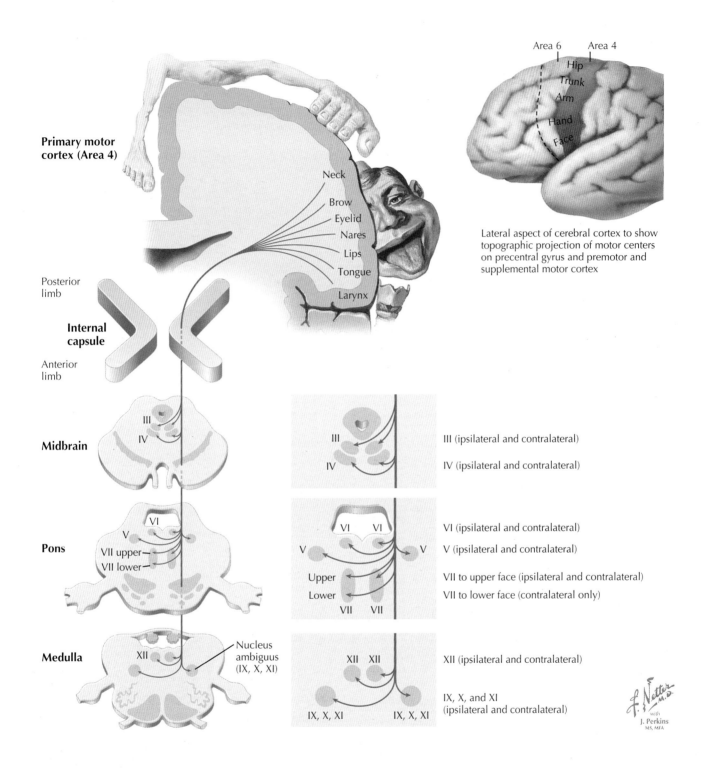

Primary motor cortex (Area 4)

Neck
Brow
Eyelid
Nares
Lips
Tongue
Larynx

Posterior limb

Internal capsule

Anterior limb

Area 6　Area 4
Hip
Trunk
Arm
Hand
Face

Lateral aspect of cerebral cortex to show topographic projection of motor centers on precentral gyrus and premotor and supplemental motor cortex

Midbrain

III
IV

III (ipsilateral and contralateral)

IV (ipsilateral and contralateral)

Pons

VI
V
VII upper
VII lower

VI　VI
V　　V
Upper
Lower
VII　VII

VI (ipsilateral and contralateral)

V (ipsilateral and contralateral)

VII to upper face (ipsilateral and contralateral)

VII to lower face (contralateral only)

Medulla

XII
Nucleus ambiguus (IX, X, XI)

XII　XII

IX, X, XI　　IX, X, XI

XII (ipsilateral and contralateral)

IX, X, and XI (ipsilateral and contralateral)

15.6 CORTICOBULBAR TRACT

The corticobulbar tract (CBT) arises mainly from the lateral portion of the primary motor cortex (area 4). CBT axons project through the genu of the internal capsule into the cerebral peduncle, the basis pontis, and the medullary pyramids on the ipsilateral side. The axons distribute to CN motor nuclei on the ipsilateral and contralateral sides except for the portion of the facial nerve nucleus (CN VII) that supplies the muscles of facial expression for the lower face, which receives exclusively contralateral projections. The CBT projections to the hypoglossal nucleus are mainly contralateral; CBT projections to the spinal accessory nucleus are mainly ipsilateral. CBT lesions result mainly in contralateral drooping of the lower face that is paretic to attempted movements from voluntary commands (central facial palsy), in contrast to Bell's palsy (CN VII palsy), in which the entire ipsilateral face is paralyzed.

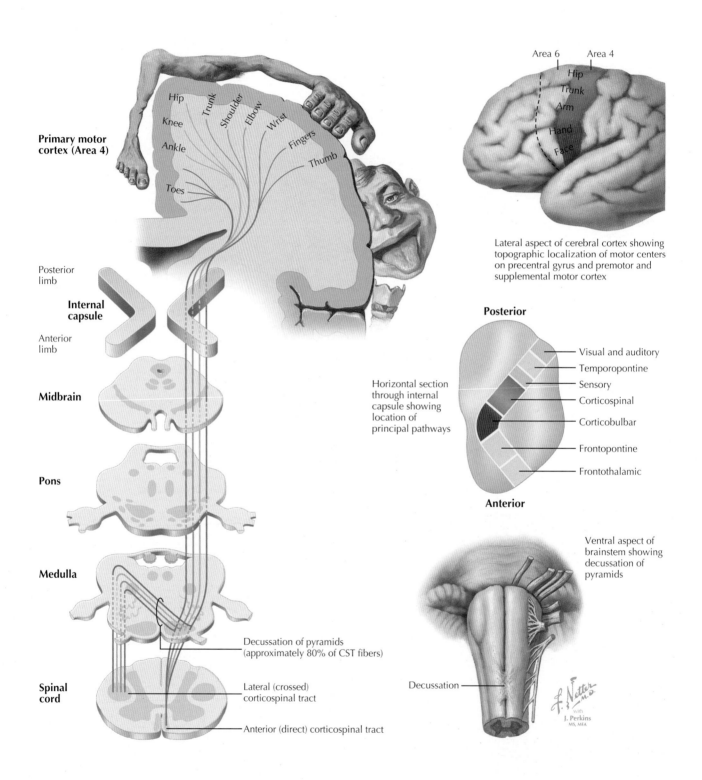

Primary motor cortex (Area 4)

Hip
Trunk
Shoulder
Knee
Elbow
Wrist
Ankle
Fingers
Thumb
Toes

Posterior limb

Internal capsule

Anterior limb

Midbrain

Pons

Medulla

Spinal cord

Decussation of pyramids (approximately 80% of CST fibers)

Lateral (crossed) corticospinal tract

Anterior (direct) corticospinal tract

Area 6   Area 4
Hip
Trunk
Arm
Hand
Face

Lateral aspect of cerebral cortex showing topographic localization of motor centers on precentral gyrus and premotor and supplemental motor cortex

Posterior

Visual and auditory
Temporopontine
Sensory
Corticospinal
Corticobulbar
Frontopontine
Frontothalamic

Horizontal section through internal capsule showing location of principal pathways

Anterior

Ventral aspect of brainstem showing decussation of pyramids

Decussation

J. Netter M.D.
with
J. Perkins
MS, MFA

15.7 CORTICOSPINAL TRACT

See next page.

15.7 **CORTICOSPINAL TRACT (CONTINUED)**

The motor portion of the corticospinal tract (CST) originates from neurons of many sizes, mainly from the primary motor cortex (area 4) and the supplemental and premotor cortices (area 6). The primary sensory cortex (areas 3, 1, 2) contributes axons into the CST, but these axons terminate mainly in secondary sensory nuclei to regulate the processing of incoming lemniscal sensory information. The CST travels through the posterior limb of the internal capsule, the middle region of the cerebral peduncle, numerous fascicles of axons in the basis pontis, and the medullary pyramid on the ipsilateral side. Most of the CST axons (approximately 80% but variable from individual to individual) cross the midline in the decussation of the pyramids at the medullary–spinal cord junction. These crossed fibers descend in the lateral CST in the lateral funiculus of the spinal cord and synapse on alpha and gamma LMNs, both directly and indirectly through interneurons. CST axons that do not decussate continue as the anterior CST in the anterior funiculus of the spinal cord and then decussate at the appropriate level through the anterior white commissure to terminate directly and indirectly on alpha and gamma LMNs contralateral to the cortical cells of origin. Only a very small portion of the motor connections of the corticospinal tract terminate on LMNs on the ipsilateral side of the spinal cord.

CLINICAL POINT

The motor portion of the CST arises mainly from neurons in the primary motor cortex (area 4) and the supplemental and premotor cortices (area 6). The primary sensory cortex and superior parietal lobule contribute corticospinal axons (corticonuclear fibers) to secondary sensory nuclei in the lower brainstem and spinal cord. Approximately 80% of the CST axons cross in the decussation of the pyramids and terminate directly and indirectly with alpha and gamma LMNs that control movements of the distal extremities, especially the hands and fingers. At least 10% of the CST terminates monosynaptically on alpha LMNs, especially those associated with hand and finger musculature. A **lesion in the internal capsule** damages the CST, corticorubral fibers, and corticoreticular fibers, resulting in contralateral hemiplegia. Initially, the hemiplegia is flaccid, with loss of tone and reflexes. Within days to a week or so, the hemiplegia becomes spastic, with hyperreflexia and hypertonus. The affected musculature shows initial resistance to attempted passive movement, followed by a dissipation or "melting" of tone (the clasp-knife reflex), perhaps because of high threshold Ib Golgi tendon organ inhibitory influences on the

homonymous LMNs. The initial suspected mechanism of classical **UMN syndrome** was disinhibition of dynamic gamma LMNs, which drives initial resistance to passive stretch, mediated via subsequent Ia afferent influences over alpha LMNs; this mechanism was reinforced by observations that dorsal root sectioning diminished spasticity in UMN syndromes. Further studies have revealed additional potential mechanisms, including diminished reciprocal inhibition, recurrent Renshaw inhibition, and presynaptic inhibition on Ia afferents, all suggestive of major changes in interneurons of the spinal cord following a classic UMN lesion. In UMN syndrome, the plantar reflexes are extensor (reverting to a developmentally early stage in the absence of the CST), and abdominal reflexes are absent on the affected side. Clonus (repetitive alternating flexor and extensor muscle stretch reflexes) also may occur and is possibly attributable to interneuronal changes such as diminished Renshaw inhibition.

CLINICAL POINT

The CBT arises mainly from the lateral portion of the primary motor cortex; it descends through the genu of the internal capsule and the cerebral peduncle (medial to the corticospinal tract fibers) ipsilaterally, and it distributes bilaterally to the motor CN nuclei (CNN) of the brainstem, except to the facial nucleus for the lower face, which receives almost exclusively contralateral projections. The corticobulbar axons terminate mainly on interneurons that regulate LMN output. Originally, *corticobulbar* was a term reserved for cortical projections to LMNs of the medulla (bulb), but it now has been expanded to include CNN for V, VII, nucleus ambiguus, XII, and the spinal accessory (XI) nucleus. A lesion in the genu of the internal capsule (embolic or thrombotic stroke or hemorrhage of the middle cerebral artery or its branches) or the cerebral peduncle (Weber's syndrome, compression of the peduncle against the free edge of the tentorium cerebelli with transtentorial herniation) results mainly in a drooping lower face (central facial palsy) on the contralateral side. The intact hemisphere can control voluntary movement of the LMNs in the CNN for all other brainstem motor nuclei on both sides. In some individuals, a predominance of contralateral fibers to LMNs for the soft palate or the tongue is noted, resulting in a temporary contralateral palsy, or a predominance of ipsilateral fibers to LMNs of XI may be noted, resulting in an ipsilateral palsy of the sternocleidomastoid and upper trapezius muscles. This central paresis occurs without atrophy. Bilateral corticobulbar lesions result in profound paralysis of voluntary movement in all muscles supplied by CNN, with preservation of muscle bulk, reflex responses, and some emotional responses using those LMNs. The LMNs in CNN III, IV, and VI receive cortical input from the frontal eye fields (area 8) and parietal eye fields of both sides.

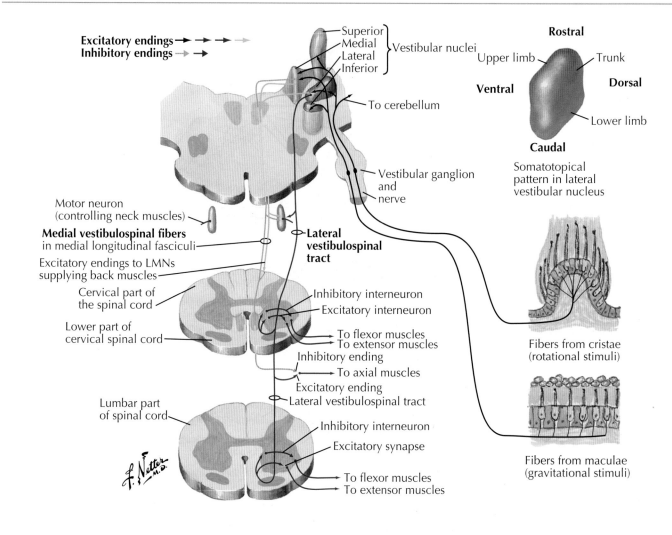

Excitatory endings → → → →
Inhibitory endings → →

Superior
Medial
Lateral
Inferior
} Vestibular nuclei

To cerebellum

Vestibular ganglion and nerve

Motor neuron (controlling neck muscles)

Medial vestibulospinal fibers in medial longitudinal fasciculi

Excitatory endings to LMNs supplying back muscles

Cervical part of the spinal cord

Lower part of cervical spinal cord

Lateral vestibulospinal tract

Inhibitory interneuron
Excitatory interneuron

To flexor muscles
To extensor muscles
Inhibitory ending
To axial muscles
Excitatory ending
Lateral vestibulospinal tract

Lumbar part of spinal cord

Inhibitory interneuron
Excitatory synapse

To flexor muscles
To extensor muscles

Rostral

Upper limb — Trunk

Ventral — **Dorsal**

Lower limb

Caudal

Somatotopical pattern in lateral vestibular nucleus

Fibers from cristae (rotational stimuli)

Fibers from maculae (gravitational stimuli)

15.10 VESTIBULOSPINAL TRACTS

The lateral vestibulospinal tract arises from the lateral vestibular nucleus and terminates directly and mainly indirectly on ipsilateral alpha and gamma LMNs associated with extensor musculature, especially proximal musculature. If this powerful antigravity extensor system were not kept in check by descending connections from the red nucleus and by connections from the cerebellum, it would produce a constant state of extensor hypertonus. Removal of these influences can occur with lesions caudal to the red nucleus, producing decerebration with powerful extensor posturing. The medial vestibulospinal tract arises from the medial vestibular nucleus and provides inhibition of alpha and gamma LMNs controlling neck and axial musculature. The medial vestibulospinal tract terminates mainly on interneurons in the cervical spinal cord ventral horn. These two vestibulospinal tracts stabilize and coordinate the position of the head, neck, and body and provide important reflex and brainstem control over tone and posture. The vestibulospinal tracts work with the reticulospinal tract to control tone and posture.

CLINICAL POINT

Primary vestibular input from both the maculae of the utricle and the cristae of the ampullae of the semicircular canals terminates in the vestibular nuclei of the medulla and pons, including the cells of origin of the vestibular UMN tracts, the lateral and medial vestibular nuclei. This allows influences from the direction of the gravitational field (linear acceleration) and head movement (angular acceleration) to affect the firing of neurons in the vestibular nuclei. The lateral vestibular nuclei give rise to a powerful vestibulospinal antigravity system that terminates mainly indirectly on alpha and gamma LMNs in the medial part of the ventral horn, which is associated with proximal extensor musculature. This system, if left unchecked and uninhibited, would drive the neck and body into marked extensor posturing, called **decerebration** (or decerebrate rigidity). The lateral vestibulospinal system is inhibited mainly by the red nucleus and the anterior cerebellum. In decerebrate posturing, sectioning of the dorsal roots (dorsal rhizotomy) abolishes the extraordinary "rigidity" (it is actually spasticity, not true rigidity), suggesting that decerebration results from the unregulated activity of the reticulospinal and lateral vestibulospinal tract driving the gamma LMNs. This is consistent with the earlier hypothesis of the mechanism of spasticity, although additional spinal interneuronal inhibition is also most likely involved in decerebrate posturing. The medial vestibulospinal tract exerts inhibitory influences on LMNs that innervate neck muscles, permitting unconscious adjustments to move the head in response to vestibular stimuli. Thus, the vestibulospinal tracts help to promote body and head movements to maintain appropriate posture with vestibular activation, particularly during movement; these systems also coordinate with projections via the medial longitudinal fasciculus that synchronize eye movements.

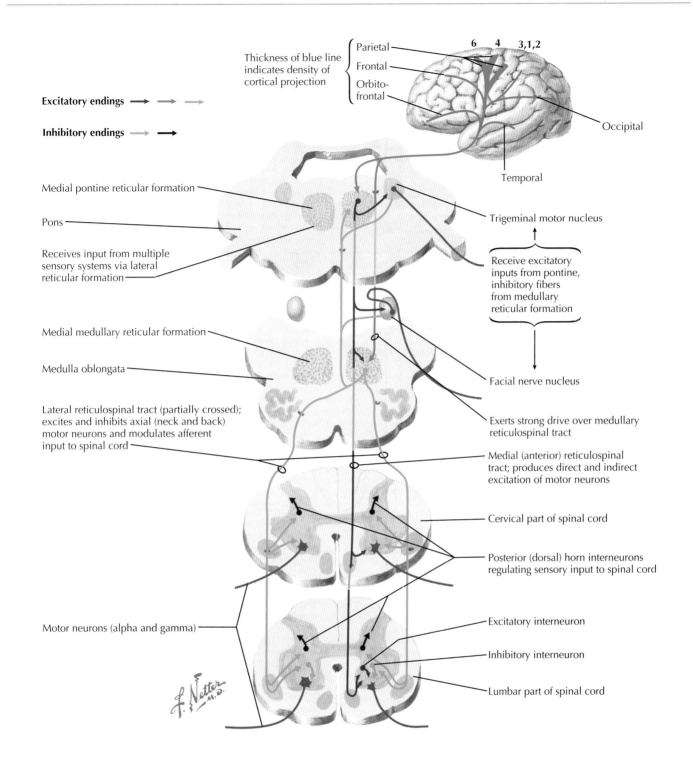

Thickness of blue line indicates density of cortical projection

Excitatory endings

Inhibitory endings

Parietal
Frontal
Orbito-frontal

6 4 3,1,2

Occipital

Temporal

Medial pontine reticular formation

Pons

Receives input from multiple sensory systems via lateral reticular formation

Trigeminal motor nucleus

Receive excitatory inputs from pontine, inhibitory fibers from medullary reticular formation

Medial medullary reticular formation

Medulla oblongata

Facial nerve nucleus

Lateral reticulospinal tract (partially crossed); excites and inhibits axial (neck and back) motor neurons and modulates afferent input to spinal cord

Exerts strong drive over medullary reticulospinal tract

Medial (anterior) reticulospinal tract; produces direct and indirect excitation of motor neurons

Cervical part of spinal cord

Posterior (dorsal) horn interneurons regulating sensory input to spinal cord

Excitatory interneuron

Motor neurons (alpha and gamma)

Inhibitory interneuron

Lumbar part of spinal cord

15.11 RETICULOSPINAL AND CORTICORETICULAR PATHWAYS

The pontine reticulospinal tract (RetST) arises from neurons of the medial pontine RF (nuclei pontis caudalis and oralis). Axons descend as the pontine (medial) RetST, mainly ipsilaterally, and terminate directly and indirectly on alpha and gamma LMNs at all levels. This tract has a distinct extensor bias for axial musculature and reinforces the action of the lateral vestibulospinal tract. Although some cortical axons terminate in the nuclei of origin of the pontine RetST, the cortex provides minimal influence on the activity of this tract; the pontine RetST is driven primarily by polysensory input from trigeminal and somatosensory sources. The medullary RetST originates from the medial RF (nucleus gigantocellularis) and is heavily driven by cortical input, especially from the motor cortex and supplemental and premotor cortices. Axons of the medullary (lateral) RetST terminate bilaterally, directly and indirectly, on alpha and gamma LMNs at all levels. The medullary RetST exerts a flexor bias, reinforcing the CST and RST. The reticulospinal tracts are important regulators of basic tone and posture. They are not organized somatotopically. See page 433 for a Clinical Point.

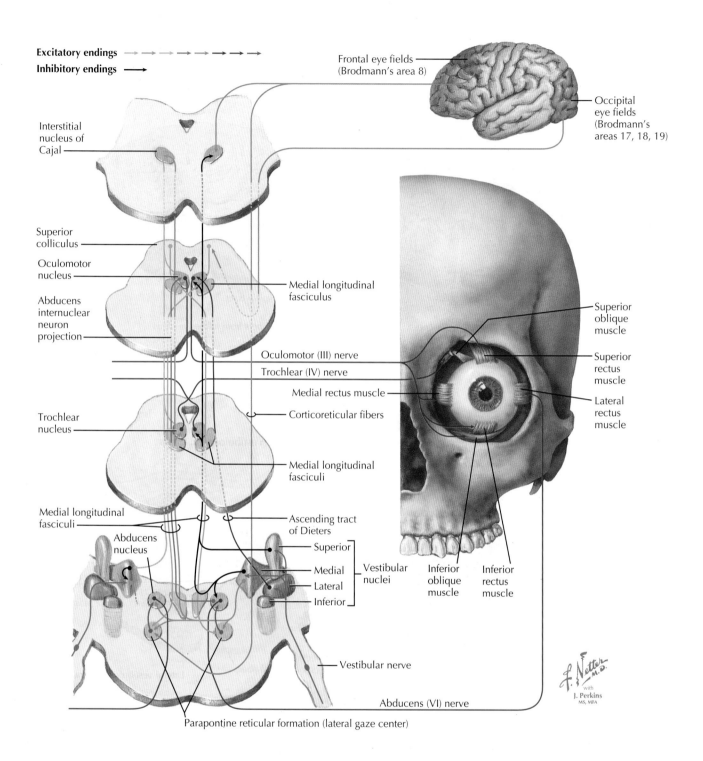

Excitatory endings →→→→→→
Inhibitory endings ⟶

Frontal eye fields
(Brodmann's area 8)

Occipital
eye fields
(Brodmann's
areas 17, 18, 19)

Interstitial
nucleus of
Cajal

Superior
colliculus

Oculomotor
nucleus

Medial longitudinal
fasciculus

Abducens
internuclear
neuron
projection

Oculomotor (III) nerve

Trochlear (IV) nerve

Medial rectus muscle

Corticoreticular fibers

Superior
oblique
muscle

Superior
rectus
muscle

Lateral
rectus
muscle

Trochlear
nucleus

Medial longitudinal
fasciculi

Medial longitudinal
fasciculi

Ascending tract
of Dieters

Superior

Medial
Lateral
Inferior

Vestibular
nuclei

Inferior
oblique
muscle

Inferior
rectus
muscle

Abducens
nucleus

Vestibular nerve

Abducens (VI) nerve

Parapontine reticular formation (lateral gaze center)

15.14 CENTRAL CONTROL OF EYE MOVEMENTS

Central control of eye movements is achieved through the coordination of extraocular motor nuclei for CNs III (oculomotor), IV (trochlear), and VI (abducens). This is achieved by the parapontine reticular formation (horizontal gaze center); it receives input from the vestibular nuclei, the deep layers of the superior colliculus (input from V1, V2, and V3), the cerebral cortex (frontal eye fields), and the interstitial nucleus of Cajal (which receives input from the vestibular nuclei and the frontal eye fields). The parapontine reticular formation supplies the ipsilateral VI nucleus for movement of the lateral rectus muscle and the contralateral III nucleus (via interneurons in VI nucleus) for movement of the medial rectus muscle, thus coordinating horizontal eye movements. The interstitial nucleus of Cajal helps to coordinate vertical and oblique eye movements. Secondary sensory vestibular projections also terminate in the extraocular motor CNN. Axons interconnecting the extraocular motor CNN travel through the medial longitudinal fasciculus. See page 433 for a Clinical Point.

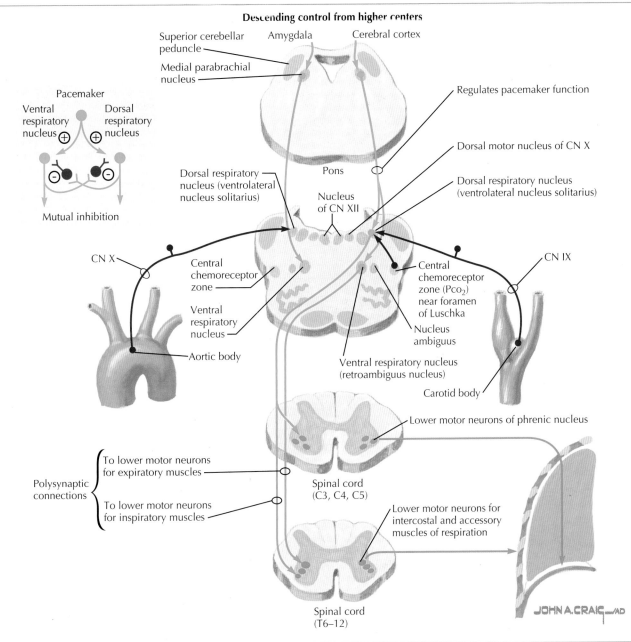

Descending control from higher centers

Superior cerebellar peduncle

Medial parabrachial nucleus

Amygdala

Cerebral cortex

Regulates pacemaker function

Dorsal motor nucleus of CN X

Pacemaker

Ventral respiratory nucleus

Dorsal respiratory nucleus

Mutual inhibition

Dorsal respiratory nucleus (ventrolateral nucleus solitarius)

Pons

Nucleus of CN XII

Dorsal respiratory nucleus (ventrolateral nucleus solitarius)

CN X

Central chemoreceptor zone

Ventral respiratory nucleus

Aortic body

Central chemoreceptor zone (Pco_2) near foramen of Luschka

Nucleus ambiguus

CN IX

Ventral respiratory nucleus (retroambiguus nucleus)

Carotid body

Lower motor neurons of phrenic nucleus

Polysynaptic connections

To lower motor neurons for expiratory muscles

To lower motor neurons for inspiratory muscles

Spinal cord (C3, C4, C5)

Lower motor neurons for intercostal and accessory muscles of respiration

Spinal cord (T6–12)

JOHN A. CRAIG—AD

15.15 CENTRAL CONTROL OF RESPIRATION

Inspiration and expiration are regulated by nuclei of the RF. The dorsal respiratory nucleus (lateral nucleus solitarius) sends crossed axons to terminate on cervical spinal cord LMNs of the phrenic nucleus and on thoracic spinal cord LMNs that supply intercostal muscles and accessory musculature associated with inspiration. The ventral respiratory nucleus (nucleus retroambiguus) sends crossed axons to terminate on thoracic spinal cord LMNs that supply accessory musculature associated with expiration. The dorsal respiratory nucleus receives input from the carotid body (via CN IX), from the aortic body chemosensors (via CN X), and from central chemoreceptive zones of the lateral medulla. The dorsal respiratory nucleus and ventral respiratory nucleus mutually inhibit each other. The medial parabrachial nucleus acts as a respiratory pacemaker to regulate the dorsal respiratory nucleus and the ventral respiratory nucleus. The medial parabrachial nucleus receives input from higher centers, such as the amygdala and the cerebral cortex.

CLINICAL POINT

The dorsal respiratory nucleus (lateral nucleus solitarius) sends axonal projections to the contralateral cervical LMNs of the phrenic nucleus and thoracic LMNs of accessory respiratory muscles, regulating inspiration. The ventral respiratory nucleus (nucleus retroambiguus) sends axonal projections to contralateral thoracic LMNs that supply accessory musculature associated with expiration. The medial parabrachial nucleus functions as a pacemaker and receives input from higher levels of the central nervous system. **Progressive damage to the forebrain and brainstem** elicits relatively predictable **changes in respiration**. Progressive damage through the telencephalon and diencephalon elicits Cheyne-Stokes respiration (crescendo-decrescendo breathing; periods of hyperpnea alternating with brief periods of apnea). The hyperpnea phase is provoked by Pco_2 from the apneic phase and results in the lowering of Pco_2, again provoking apnea. If damage extends through the mesencephalon and upper pons, respiration becomes shallow, with hyperventilation, but the patient still is relatively hypoxic. If damage extends through the lower pons, respiration involves long inspiratory pauses prior to expiration, called apneustic breathing. Damage extending further into the medulla produces ataxic breathing with irregular patterns, including inspiratory gasps and periods of apnea. This pattern of breathing foreshadows total respiratory failure and death as the basic brainstem centers fail.

Peripheral Mechanisms

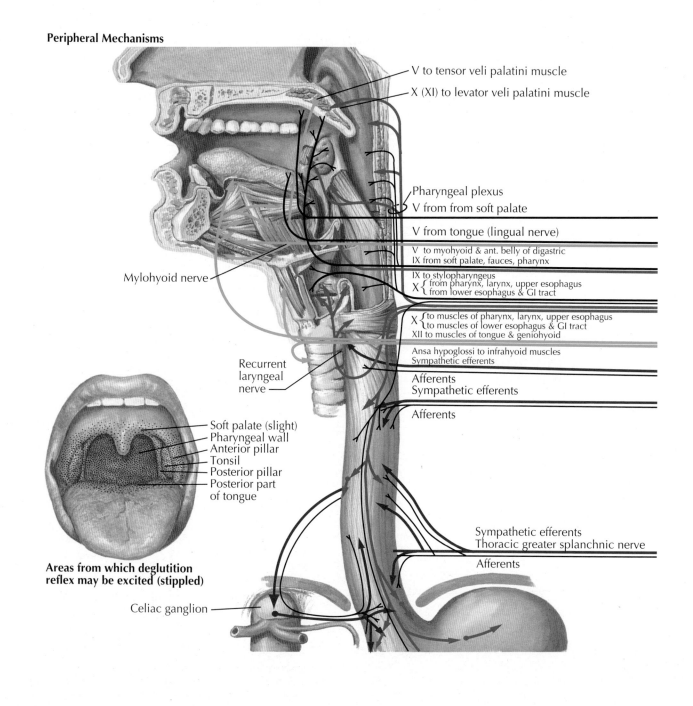

V to tensor veli palatini muscle

X (XI) to levator veli palatini muscle

Pharyngeal plexus
V from from soft palate

V from tongue (lingual nerve)

V to myohyoid & ant. belly of digastric
IX from soft palate, fauces, pharynx

IX to stylopharyngeus
X { from pharynx, larynx, upper esophagus
    { from lower esophagus & GI tract

X { to muscles of pharynx, larynx, upper esophagus
   { to muscles of lower esophagus & GI tract
XII to muscles of tongue & geniohyoid

Ansa hypoglossi to infrahyoid muscles
Sympathetic efferents

Afferents
Sympathetic efferents

Afferents

Mylohyoid nerve

Recurrent
laryngeal
nerve

Sympathetic efferents
Thoracic greater splanchnic nerve

Afferents

Soft palate (slight)
Pharyngeal wall
Anterior pillar
Tonsil
Posterior pillar
Posterior part
of tongue

**Areas from which deglutition
reflex may be excited (stippled)**

Celiac ganglion

15.16 NEURAL CIRCUITRY OF SWALLOWING

Consumption of food and water requires the complex process of swallowing, which involves the coordinated activity of CNs V, VII, IX, X, and XII. Swallowing involves motor and sensory activities of the oral cavity, pharynx, larynx, and esophagus. Protection of the airway from aspiration is a vital component of this process.

Initial processing in the oral cavity requires chewing and mandible movement (CN V), closure of the oral cavity (CN VII), tongue movement (CN XII), soft palate movement (CN IX), and salivation (CNs VII and IX). Taste is perceived by CNs VII (anterior two-thirds of the tongue) and IX (posterior one-third of the tongue), coordinated with CN I (olfaction) for perception of the food. Propulsion of the food into the oropharynx requires timing and movement, as well as prevention of nasal regurgitation, from coordinated activities of CNs V, VII, IX, and X. A swallowing reflex allows the food to move into the pharynx.

Food passes through the pharynx into the esophagus through coordinated action of CNs X (pharyngeal contraction) and XII (tongue movement) at the same time that the larynx is closed off by laryngeal muscles (CN X). If this protective process is not fully functional, a cough or choking reaction occurs (afferent

Central Mechanisms

Thalamus

Hypothalamus

V

VII

IX

X

XI

XII

Stellate ganglion

T4

Thoracic sympathetic ganglionic chain

Dorsal root ganglion

T5

T6

T7

T8

aa

Principal sensory nucleus of V

Motor nucleus of V

Deglutition center

Nucleus of XII

Dorsal nucleus of X (motor and sensory)

Nucleus of solitary tract

Nucleus ambiguus

Key

Sympathetic efferents ──────

Parasympathetic efferents ──────

Somatic efferents ──────

Afferents (and CNS connections) ──────

Indefinite paths ▪ ▪ ▪ ▪ ▪

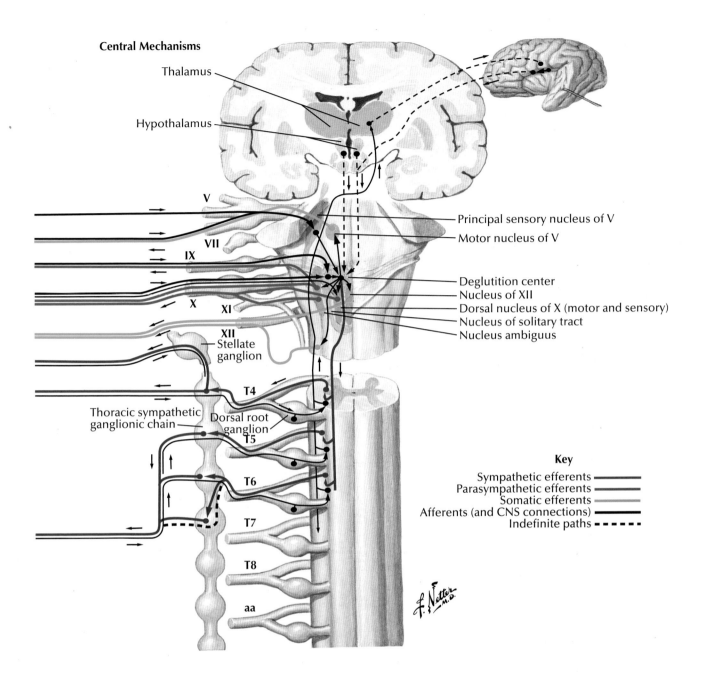

component of CNs IX and X). CNs IX and X are the sensory components of swallowing, projecting to a medullary swallowing center in nucleus solitarius. Nucleus solitarius then connects with nucleus ambiguous to initiate the major motor activation needed for swallowing.

As the food passes by the closed pharynx, the cricopharyngeal muscle (CN X) controls passage through the cricopharyngeal sphincter at the proximal end of the esophagus, into the esophagus. The dorsal motor (visceral) nucleus of the vagus innervates the involuntary muscles of the esophagus and more distal portions of the gastrointestinal tract through part of the colon.

CLINICAL POINT

A swallowing disorder, dysphagia, may occur with a wide range of clinical disorders. Peripheral (cranial) nerve damage may occur with Guillain-Barré syndrome, mass lesions impinging on cranial nerves of the medulla, pharyngeal or myotonic dystrophies, myasthenia gravis, or other pathological processes impinging on the many cranial nerves involved in swallowing.

Central lesions also may be accompanied by dysphagia, including forebrain or brainstem infarcts, movement disorders (Parkinson's disease), demyelinating disorders (multiple sclerosis), motor neuron disorders (amyotrophic lateral sclerosis, motor involvement in syringobulbia), or tumors.

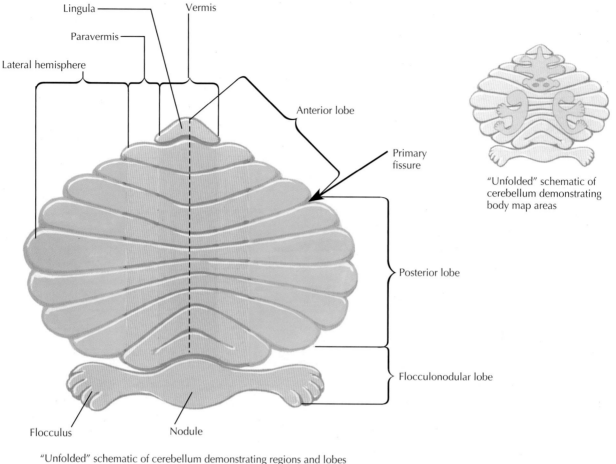

Lingula

Vermis

Paravermis

Lateral hemisphere

Anterior lobe

Primary fissure

Posterior lobe

Flocculonodular lobe

Flocculus

Nodule

"Unfolded" schematic of cerebellum demonstrating regions and lobes

"Unfolded" schematic of cerebellum demonstrating body map areas

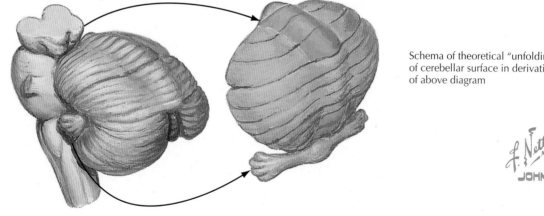

Schema of theoretical "unfolding" of cerebellar surface in derivation of above diagram

CEREBELLUM

15.17 FUNCTIONAL SUBDIVISIONS OF THE CEREBELLUM

The cerebellum is classically subdivided into anterior, middle (posterior), and flocculonodular (FN) lobes, each associated with ipsilateral syndromes, such as stiff-legged gait (anterior lobe) and loss of coordination with dysmetria, action tremor, hypotonus, ataxia, and decomposition of movement (middle lobe) and truncal ataxia (FN lobe). The cerebellum also is classified according to a longitudinal scheme that is based on cerebellar cortical regions that project to deep cerebellar nuclei, which in turn project to and coordinate the activity of specific UMN cell groups. This scheme includes the vermis and FN lobe (projecting to the fastigial nucleus and the lateral vestibular nucleus), the paravermis (projecting to the globose and emboliform nuclei), and the lateral hemispheres (projecting to the dentate nucleus). Each cerebellar subdivision is interlinked with circuitry related to specific UMN systems.

Cerebellar Cortex

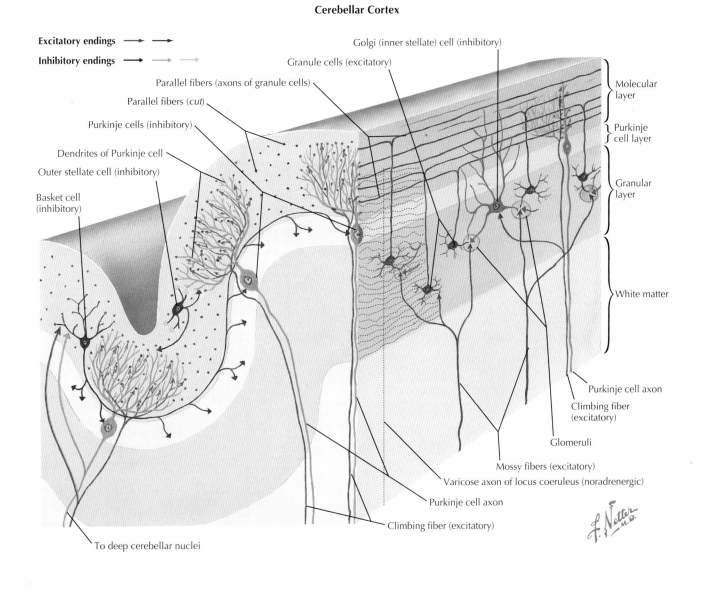

Excitatory endings ⟶ ⟶

Inhibitory endings ⟶ ⟶ ⟶

Golgi (inner stellate) cell (inhibitory)

Granule cells (excitatory)

Parallel fibers (axons of granule cells)

Parallel fibers (*cut*)

Purkinje cells (inhibitory)

Dendrites of Purkinje cell

Outer stellate cell (inhibitory)

Basket cell (inhibitory)

Molecular layer

Purkinje cell layer

Granular layer

White matter

Purkinje cell axon

Climbing fiber (excitatory)

Glomeruli

Mossy fibers (excitatory)

Varicose axon of locus coeruleus (noradrenergic)

Purkinje cell axon

Climbing fiber (excitatory)

To deep cerebellar nuclei

15.18 CEREBELLAR NEURONAL CIRCUITRY

The cerebellum is organized into four parts: an outer three-layer cortex, white matter, deep cerebellar nuclei, and cerebellar peduncles that connect with the spinal cord, brainstem, and thalamus. In the cortex, the Purkinje cells (the major output neurons) have their dendritic trees in the molecular layer (arranged in parallel "plates" adjacent to each other), their cell bodies in the Purkinje cell layer, and their axons in the granular layer and deeper white matter. Inputs into the cerebellar cortex arrive as climbing fibers (from inferior olivary nuclei), mossy fibers (all other inputs except monoaminergic), or fine, highly branched, varicose arborizations (noradrenergic and other monoaminergic inputs). The mossy fibers synapse on granule cells, whose axons form an array of parallel fibers that extend through the dendritic trees of several hundred Purkinje cells. Additional interneurons modulate interconnections in the molecular layer (outer stellate cells), at the Purkinje cell body (basket cells), and at granule cell–molecular layer associations (Golgi cells). Noradrenergic axons of locus coeruleus neurons terminate in all three layers and modulate the excitability of other cerebellar connectivities.

CLINICAL POINT

The cerebellum is a target for significant adverse effects of several types of drugs, sometimes in therapeutic dose ranges and sometimes in toxic dose ranges. Many pharmacologic agents can exert both direct effects on the cerebellum and more global neurological effects, including ischemia or hypoxia. **Cerebellar damage** is usually manifested first as impairment of gait, followed later by limb ataxia. These cerebellar side effects often resolve after discontinuation of the medication, but some deficits may remain. Some antiseizure agents, including phenytoin, carbamazepine, and barbiturates, can lead to cerebellar symptoms; after prolonged treatment, particularly with phenytoin, some permanent deficits such as degeneration of Purkinje cells may occur. Valproate may provoke an intention tremor. Some cancer chemotherapeutic agents also can cause adverse cerebellar effects, occasionally permanently. Treatment of psychiatric disorders by multiple pharmacologic agents, particularly neuroleptics, also can produce adverse cerebellar effects. Toxic damage resulting from exposure to dangerous environmental agents also may damage the cerebellum. Exposure to organophosphate agents and organic solvents may induce cerebellar symptomatology. Exposure to heavy metals, including methylmercury, lead, and thallium, can induce gait disturbance and ataxia.

A. General Scheme

B. Deep Nuclei Relationship with Afferents

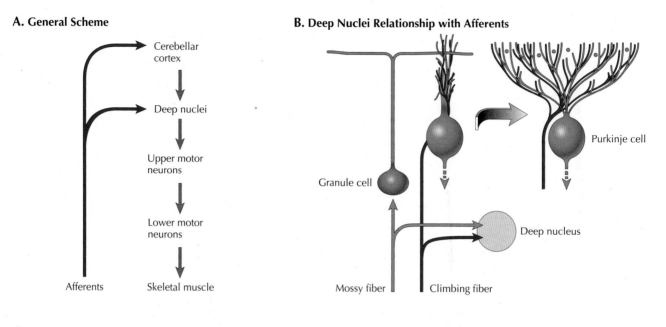

C. Circuitry of Cerebellar Neurons - Mossy Fibers

D. Circuitry of Cerebellar Neurons - Climbing Fibers

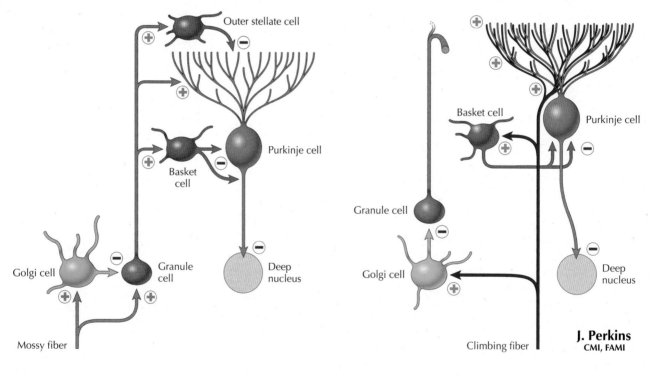

J. Perkins
CMI, FAMI

15.19 CIRCUIT DIAGRAMS OF AFFERENT CONNECTIONS IN THE CEREBELLUM

Afferents to the cerebellum include mossy fibers, climbing fibers, and locus coeruleus noradrenergic fibers. The mossy fibers synapse in deep nuclei and on granule cells. The climbing fibers intertwine around a Purkinje cell dendritic tree. The noradrenergic locus coeruleus axons terminate on all cell types in the cerebellar cortex. The loops and circuits in parts **C** and **D** of the figure show interneuronal modulation of afferent connections and Purkinje cell outflow. The entire circuitry of the cerebellar cortex provides fine-tuning of the original processing in the deep cerebellar nuclei. The entire Purkinje cell output to the deep nuclei is mediated by inhibition, using gamma-aminobutyric acid (GABA) as the neurotransmitter.

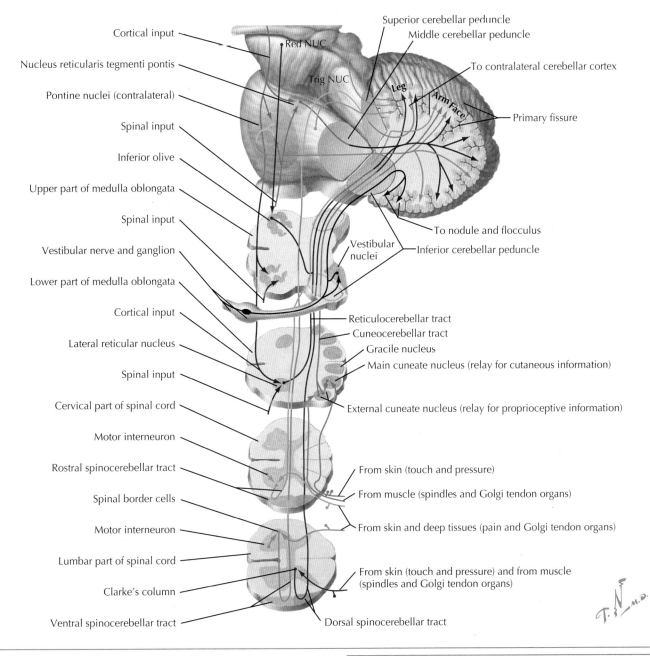

Cortical input

Nucleus reticularis tegmenti pontis

Pontine nuclei (contralateral)

Spinal input

Inferior olive

Upper part of medulla oblongata

Spinal input

Vestibular nerve and ganglion

Lower part of medulla oblongata

Cortical input

Lateral reticular nucleus

Spinal input

Cervical part of spinal cord

Motor interneuron

Rostral spinocerebellar tract

Spinal border cells

Motor interneuron

Lumbar part of spinal cord

Clarke's column

Ventral spinocerebellar tract

Red NUC

Trig NUC

Superior cerebellar peduncle

Middle cerebellar peduncle

To contralateral cerebellar cortex

Leg

Arm Face

Primary fissure

To nodule and flocculus

Vestibular nuclei

Inferior cerebellar peduncle

Reticulocerebellar tract

Cuneocerebellar tract

Gracile nucleus

Main cuneate nucleus (relay for cutaneous information)

External cuneate nucleus (relay for proprioceptive information)

From skin (touch and pressure)

From muscle (spindles and Golgi tendon organs)

From skin and deep tissues (pain and Golgi tendon organs)

From skin (touch and pressure) and from muscle (spindles and Golgi tendon organs)

Dorsal spinocerebellar tract

15.20 AFFERENT PATHWAYS TO THE CEREBELLUM

Afferents to the cerebellum terminate in both the deep nuclei and the cerebellar cortex in topographically organized zones. The body is represented in the cerebellar cortex in at least three separate regions. Afferents traveling through the inferior cerebellar peduncle include spinocerebellar pathways (dorsal and rostral spinocerebellar tracts, cuneocerebellar tract), the inferior olivary input, RF input from the lateral reticular nucleus and other regions, vestibular input from the vestibular ganglion and vestibular nuclei, and some trigeminal input. The middle cerebellar peduncle conveys mainly pontocerebellar axons carrying crossed corticopontocerebellar inputs. Afferents traveling through the superior cerebellar peduncle include the ventral spinocerebellar tract, visual and auditory tectocerebellar input, some trigeminal input, and noradrenergic locus coeruleus input. The dorsal spinocerebellar tract and cuneocerebellar tract derive mainly from muscle spindle afferent information, whereas the ventral and rostral spinocerebellar tracts derive mainly from Golgi tendon and other receptor organ afferent information.

CLINICAL POINT

Several forms of **progressive neuronal degeneration** involve cerebellar neurons and connections, including Friedreich's ataxia and olivopontocerebellar atrophy. **Friedreich's ataxia** is an autosomal recessive disorder that begins in late childhood and progresses over several decades. The disorder commonly starts with ataxia and gait dysfunction, dysmetria and decomposition of movement, and dysarthria. Spastic motor involvement and sensory losses also may occur. Neuropathological examination reveals degeneration of primary afferents and of axons in the spinal cord white matter, especially the dorsal and lateral funiculi, including the spinocerebellar tracts. Some axonal damage also may occur in both the peripheral nervous system and the central nervous system, but the cerebellum itself is usually not a focus of direct neuronal degeneration.

Olivopontocerebellar atrophy is a progressive, mainly autosomal dominant, neurodegenerative disorder that affects adults in midlife. This disorder commonly begins with gait abnormalities and progresses to full-blown cerebellar dysfunction with limb ataxia and dysarthria. Additional symptoms, such as chorea, dystonia, and rigidity, suggest some degenerative involvement of the basal ganglia as well. Neuropathological examination usually reveals neurodegeneration of the cerebellar cortex, the inferior olivary nuclei, and the pontine nuclei. As a consequence, the inferior and middle cerebellar peduncles are diminished. Additional degenerative changes in the cerebral cortex and descending UMN pathways and in the basal ganglia also are commonly present.

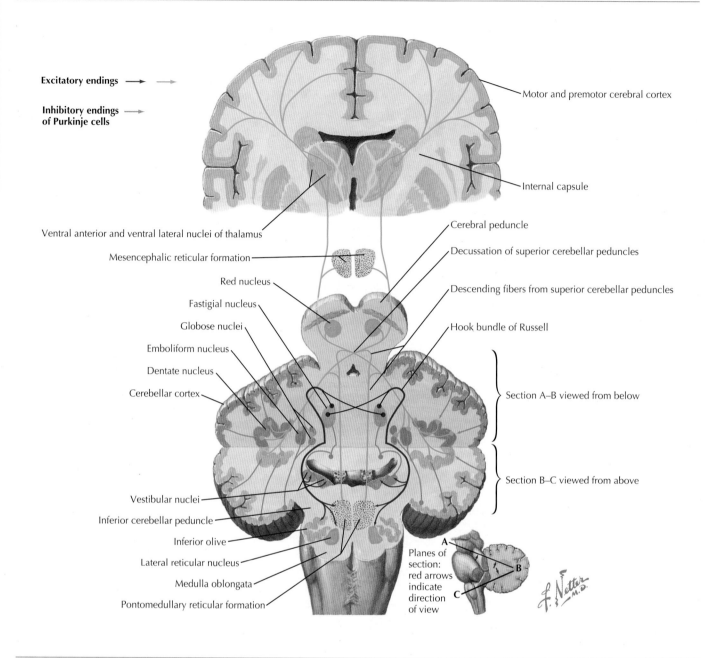

Excitatory endings ⟶ ⟶

Inhibitory endings ⟶
of Purkinje cells

Motor and premotor cerebral cortex

Internal capsule

Ventral anterior and ventral lateral nuclei of thalamus

Mesencephalic reticular formation

Red nucleus

Fastigial nucleus

Globose nuclei

Emboliform nucleus

Dentate nucleus

Cerebellar cortex

Cerebral peduncle

Decussation of superior cerebellar peduncles

Descending fibers from superior cerebellar peduncles

Hook bundle of Russell

Section A–B viewed from below

Section B–C viewed from above

Vestibular nuclei

Inferior cerebellar peduncle

Inferior olive

Lateral reticular nucleus

Medulla oblongata

Pontomedullary reticular formation

Planes of section: red arrows indicate direction of view

A
B
C

f. Netter M.D.

15.21 CEREBELLAR EFFERENT PATHWAYS

Efferents from the cerebellum derive from the deep nuclei. Projections from the fastigial nucleus exit mainly through the inferior cerebellar peduncle and terminate mainly ipsilaterally in the lateral vestibular nucleus and in other vestibular nuclei as well as in pontine and medullary reticular nuclei that give rise to the reticulospinal tracts; there, they primarily modulate the activity of the vestibulospinal and reticulospinal UMN pathways. Axons from neurons of the globose and emboliform nuclei project mainly contralaterally through the decussation of the superior cerebellar peduncle to the red nucleus, with a smaller contribution to the VL nucleus of the thalamus; primarily, they modulate activity of the RST. Axons from neurons in the dentate nucleus project mainly contralaterally through the decussation of the superior cerebellar peduncle to the VL and to a lesser extent to the VA nuclei of the thalamus; mainly, they modulate the activity of the corticospinal tract. A small projection from the dentate nucleus also distributes to the contralateral red nucleus and to brainstem reticular motor nuclei.

CLINICAL POINT

Paraneoplastic syndrome is a relatively uncommon progressive disorder that causes damage to the cerebellum and other neural structures as a secondary effect of cancer. Sometimes the onset of cerebellar symptomatology may precede the detection of the cancer. One major hypothesis about the cause of this disorder is the presence of an autoimmune reaction in which antibodies generated by the immune system against some epitope associated with the cancer cross-react with neural targets. The Purkinje cells appear to be a major target of these immunoglobulin G antibodies. The syndrome often is triggered or exacerbated by chemotherapy or radiation therapy. The entire cerebellum may be targeted, and symptoms may include gait disturbance, ataxia of the limbs with accompanying cerebellar symptoms, dysarthria, and oculomotor coordination problems. Other possible targets of paraneoplastic syndrome include the cerebral cortex and its UMN projections as well as peripheral nerves.

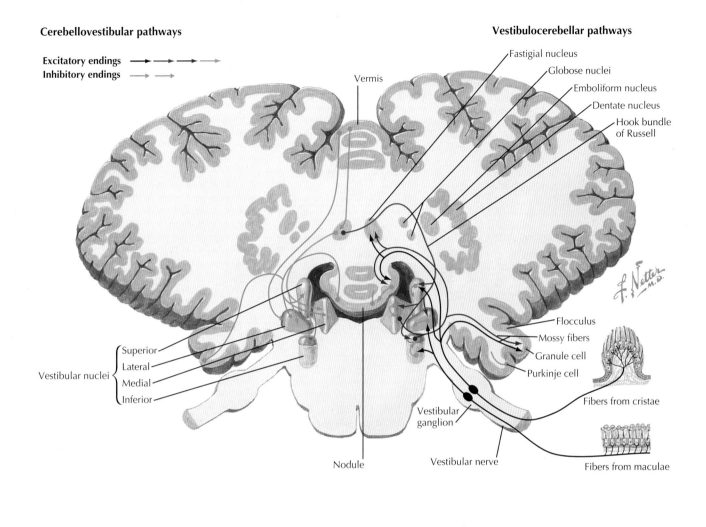

Cerebellovestibular pathways

Excitatory endings ⟶ ⟶ ⟶ ⟶
Inhibitory endings ⟶ ⟶

Vestibulocerebellar pathways

Fastigial nucleus
Globose nuclei
Emboliform nucleus
Dentate nucleus
Hook bundle of Russell

Vermis

Flocculus
Mossy fibers
Granule cell
Purkinje cell

Fibers from cristae

Vestibular nuclei
- Superior
- Lateral
- Medial
- Inferior

Vestibular ganglion

Nodule

Vestibular nerve

Fibers from maculae

15.22 CEREBELLOVESTIBULAR AND VESTIBULOCEREBELLAR PATHWAYS

Primary sensory vestibular inputs terminate in the four vestibular nuclei and in the fastigial nucleus and the cerebellar cortex of the vermis and FN lobe. The vestibular nuclei also project to the cerebellar cortex of the vermis and FN lobe. Purkinje cells in the vermis and FN lobe, in turn, project back to the vestibular nuclei and the fastigial nucleus. The fastigial nucleus projects to the vestibular nuclei and to the pontine and medullary medial reticular formation. Thus, primary and secondary vestibular neurons project to the fastigial nucleus and cerebellar cortex, and both the cerebellar cortex and deep nuclei project back to the vestibular nuclei. This extensive reciprocal vestibulocerebellar circuitry regulates basic spatial position and body tone and posture.

CLINICAL POINT

Alcohol consumption may result in acute **or chronic dysfunction of the cerebellum and its pathways**. Acutely, alcohol intoxication can cause global cerebellar dysfunction, including staggering gait, limb ataxia, dysmetria, dysdiadochokinesia, dysarthria, and oculomotor dysfunction. Cerebellar testing for alcohol intoxication in the field involves tandem walking, finger-to-nose testing, speech patterns and coordination, and gait testing. These more global effects of alcohol on the cerebellum generally subside with catabolism of the alcohol. Chronic alcoholism results in more permanent damage to the cerebellum, with a particular initial predilection for the anterior lobe of the cerebellum and the vermis (paleocerebellum). The patient may show a staggering, broad-based gait with a stiff-legged movement. The mechanism of this unusual appearance of cerebellar damage (in contrast to the hypotonic, ataxic gait that occurs with global cerebellar damage, particularly in the lateral hemispheres) appears to be removal of the anterior cerebellar influence, via cerebellovestibular connections, on the lateral vestibular nucleus, disinhibiting this extensor-dominant system. This anterior cerebellar syndrome may diminish if the patient stops drinking. With further alcohol exposure, the entire cerebellum may become damaged, leading to the classic appearance of global cerebellar dysfunction, including gait disturbance, hypotonia, limb ataxia, dysarthria, and uncoordinated extraocular involvement. In addition to direct toxicity from alcohol, neural damage may occur because of vitamin deficiencies, liver dysfunction, and other metabolic aspects of alcoholism. Other parts of the brain, including the cerebral cortex, also can be significantly damaged in chronic alcoholism.

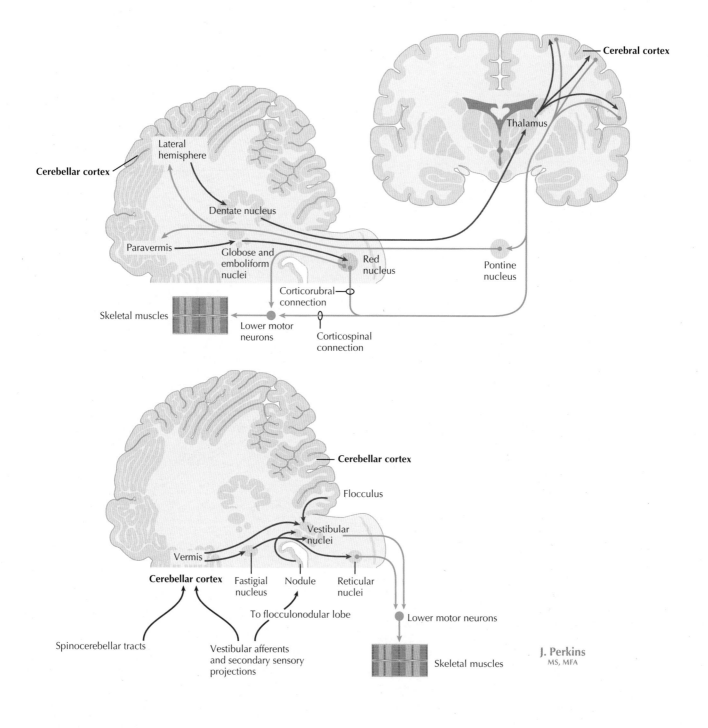

15.23 SCHEMATIC DIAGRAMS OF EFFERENT PATHWAYS FROM THE CEREBELLUM TO UPPER MOTOR NEURON SYSTEMS

The lateral cerebellar hemisphere connects through the dentate nucleus with nuclei VA and VL of the thalamus; the major thalamic inputs to the cells of origin of the CST in the motor cortex and with the supplemental and premotor cortices. The paravermal cerebellar cortex connects through the globose and emboliform nuclei with the red nucleus, cells of origin for the RST. The cerebellar connections to the cells of origin for the CST and RST are mainly crossed, and these UMN systems cross again before terminating on LMNs. Thus, the cerebellum is associated with the ipsilateral LMNs through two crossings. The vermis and FN lobe connect with the fastigial nucleus and lateral vestibular nuclei. The fastigial nucleus projects mainly ipsilaterally to cells of origin of the vestibulospinal and reticulospinal tracts, exerting mainly an ipsilateral influence on spinal cord LMNs through these UMN systems. The lateral vestibular nucleus is the source of the lateral vestibular tract, which exerts a marked extensor influence on ipsilateral LMNs of the spinal cord.

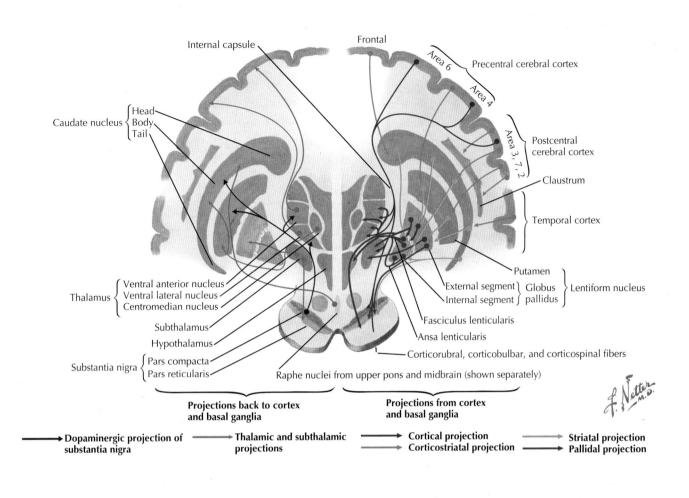

Internal capsule

Frontal

Area 6

Area 4

Precentral cerebral cortex

Caudate nucleus { Head / Body / Tail }

Area 3, 7, 2

Postcentral cerebral cortex

Claustrum

Temporal cortex

Thalamus { Ventral anterior nucleus / Ventral lateral nucleus / Centromedian nucleus }

Putamen

External segment } Globus
Internal segment } pallidus } Lentiform nucleus

Subthalamus

Hypothalamus

Fasciculus lenticularis

Ansa lenticularis

Substantia nigra { Pars compacta / Pars reticularis }

Corticorubral, corticobulbar, and corticospinal fibers

Raphe nuclei from upper pons and midbrain (shown separately)

**Projections back to cortex
and basal ganglia**

**Projections from cortex
and basal ganglia**

→ **Dopaminergic projection of
substantia nigra**

→ **Thalamic and subthalamic
projections**

→ **Cortical projection**
→ **Corticostriatal projection**

→ **Striatal projection**
→ **Pallidal projection**

BASAL GANGLIA

15.24 CONNECTIONS OF THE BASAL GANGLIA

The basal ganglia consist of the striatum (caudate nucleus and putamen) and the globus pallidus. The substantia nigra (SN) and the subthalamic nucleus (STN), which are reciprocally connected with the basal ganglia, are often included as part of the basal ganglia. Inputs into the basal ganglia from the cerebral cortex, the thalamus (intralaminar nuclei), the SN pars compacta (dopaminergic input), and rostral raphe nuclei (serotonergic input) are directed mainly toward the striatum. Inputs from the STN are directed mainly toward the globus pallidus. The striatum projects to the globus pallidus. The internal segment of the globus pallidus projects to the thalamus (VA, VL, and centromedian nuclei), and the external segment projects to the STN. The VA and VL thalamic nuclei provide input into the cells of origin of the corticospinal tract. Damage to basal ganglia components often results in movement disorders. Damage to the dopamine neurons in SN pars compacta results in Parkinson's disease (characterized by resting tremor, muscular rigidity, bradykinesia, and postural instability).

CLINICAL POINT

Disorders of the basal ganglia are frequently referred to as movement disorders and were previously called **involuntary movement disorders**. Despite the conspicuous presence of motor-related symptoms, the basal ganglia also are involved in cognitive and affective processing, particularly in assisting the cerebral cortex to select wanted subroutines of activity and to suppress unwanted patterns. The basal ganglia assist in providing a connection between motivation and emotional context on one hand and movement on the other. Observations of discrete infarcts of parts of the basal ganglia have revealed such abnormalities as abnormal positioning of parts of the body with the presence of increased tone (dystonia) and other movements such as athetosis (slow, writhing movements) or chorea (brisk, dance-like movements). With caudate nucleus damage, more cognitive and affective symptoms may occur, such as apathy and loss of initiative, slowed thinking, and blunted emotional reactivity (abulia), possibly related to the interconnections between the caudate nucleus and the prefrontal cortex. In the classic movement disorders, as in **progressive neurodegenerative diseases**, there is a mixture of symptoms showing loss of action, such as bradykinesia (difficulty in initiating movements or diminished movements such as blinking), and symptoms showing an excess of action, such as rigidity, athetosis, chorea, or dystonia. As an example of excess movement, Tourette's syndrome involves tics and involuntary vocalizations, sometimes accompanied by echolalia, grunts and vocal spasms, explosive cursing, and hyperactive behavior, often starting in childhood. Treatment strategies have included use of D2 dopamine antagonists such as haloperidol.

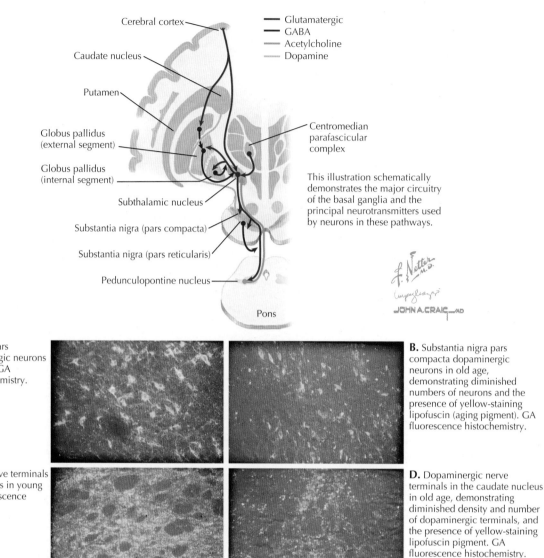

Cerebral cortex

Caudate nucleus

Putamen

Globus pallidus (external segment)

Globus pallidus (internal segment)

Subthalamic nucleus

Substantia nigra (pars compacta)

Substantia nigra (pars reticularis)

Pedunculopontine nucleus

—— Glutamatergic
—— GABA
—— Acetylcholine
----- Dopamine

Centromedian parafascicular complex

This illustration schematically demonstrates the major circuitry of the basal ganglia and the principal neurotransmitters used by neurons in these pathways.

Pons

A. Substantia nigra pars compacta dopaminergic neurons in young adulthood. GA fluorescence histochemistry.

B. Substantia nigra pars compacta dopaminergic neurons in old age, demonstrating diminished numbers of neurons and the presence of yellow-staining lipofuscin (aging pigment). GA fluorescence histochemistry.

C. Dopaminergic nerve terminals in the caudate nucleus in young adulthood. GA fluorescence histochemistry.

D. Dopaminergic nerve terminals in the caudate nucleus in old age, demonstrating diminished density and number of dopaminergic terminals, and the presence of yellow-staining lipofuscin pigment. GA fluorescence histochemistry.

15.25 SIMPLIFIED SCHEMATIC OF BASAL GANGLIA CIRCUITRY AND NEUROCHEMISTRY

CLINICAL POINT

In **Parkinson's disease**, the pars compacta of the substantia nigra shows loss of pigmented (melanin-containing) neurons that use dopamine as their major neurotransmitter. Both the substantia nigra and the target of the axonal projections, the caudate nucleus and putamen, are severely depleted of their dopamine content. By the time symptoms of Parkinson's disease are clinically evident, at least 50% (and sometimes as much as 80%) of the dopamine neurons in the pars compacta of the substantia nigra have degenerated. Neurons in the substantia nigra sometimes demonstrate Lewy inclusion bodies or neurofibrillary tangles, further evidence of the degenerative process in Parkinson's disease. The neuropathology of Parkinson's disease sometimes also includes the degeneration of

dopamine neurons in the ventral tegmental area of the midbrain, of serotonergic neurons in the raphe nuclei, of cholinergic neurons in nucleus basalis, and of other pigmented neurons in regions such as the dorsal (motor) nucleus of CN X. Although the dopamine deficit in the substantia nigra is the most conspicuous pathological hallmark of Parkinson's disease, these other degenerative processes may contribute to some of the symptoms. The major manifestations of Parkinson disease include both negative and positive (excessive) symptomatology, including (1) resting tremor (approximately 2 cps), which dissipates with movement (i.e., not a movement tremor); (2) muscle rigidity *(lead pipe rigidity),* in which limb musculature shows resistance to passive movement through all ranges of movement, both flexion and extension (NOT similar to spasticity); (3) bradykinesia (difficulty initiating movement or halting movement once it is initiated); and (4) postural instability. Also, sometimes present are head tremor (titubation), rigid facies (fixed, austere-appearing facial expression), and depression.

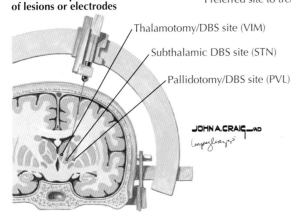

Stereotactic needle guide
Stereotactic frame attached to patient's head creates space with X, Y, and Z coordinates. Any location within that space can be targeted by probes using these coordinates. Specific localization is selected by stereotactic targeting software using common neuroanatomic sites as reference points.

Sites within globus pallidus, thalamus and STN used in control of movement disorders

Stereotactic frame

Patient usually awake

Stereotactic placement of lesions or electrodes

Thalamotomy/DBS site (VIM)

Subthalamic DBS site (STN)

Pallidotomy/DBS site (PVL)

JOHN A. CRAIG—AD

Thalamotomy/DBS site
Ventralis intermedius nucleus (VIM) preferred site for tremor-controlling lesions

Pallidotomy/DBS site
Posteroventrolateral region (PVL) of pars interna of globus pallidus (GPi) preferred site to treat rigidity, tremor, bradykinesia, and dyskinesias.

Subthalamic nucleus—DBS site
Preferred site to treat Parkinson's disease

Deep brain stimulation (DBS)
High-frequency stimulation (DBS) of VIM region of thalamus is predominant treatment of medically refractory tremor. Globus pallidus and STN sites provide relief for Parkinson's disease and dystonia. DBS electrodes are implanted and connected to subclavicular battery pack.

Caudate nucleus

Thalamus

Globus pallidus

Care must be taken to avoid damage to optic tract and internal capsule

DBS electrodes in position in VIM nucleus of each thalamus

Subclavicular battery pack

15.26 SURGICAL APPROACHES TO MOVEMENT DISORDERS

Surgical approaches to ameliorating Parkinson's disease and other movement disorders are based on deliberate disruption or stimulation of specific anatomical components of the complex basal ganglia circuitry involved in the disorder. Initially, stereotaxic lesions were performed in the thalamus (nucleus ventralis intermedius) for tremors; in the internal segment of the globus pallidus (posterior ventrolateral portion) for rigidity, tremors, bradykinesia, and dyskinesias; and in the subthalamus for treating Parkinson's disease. Lesion approaches have been replaced with deep brain stimulation (DBS) with implantable electrodes. Targets for DBS include the internal segment of the globus pallidus, the subthalamic nucleus, and the ventral intermedius nucleus of the thalamus. DBS appears to be more effective in patients with a good response to levodopa-carbidopa. DBS is utilized for patients with PD who show motor fluctuations and drug-involved dyskinesias. Symptom relief is seen contralateral to the side of DBS.

CLINICAL POINT

The mainstay of pharmacological treatment of Parkinson's disease is levodopa-carbidopa (Sinemet). Levodopa does not readily cross the blood-brain barrier but is assisted by blocking aromatic L-amino acid decarboxylase (ALAAD) with carbidopa. This approach constitutes replacement therapy with L-dopa to enhance dopamine presence in the nigrostriatal neurons and nerve terminals. Dopamine agonists also have been used, but the side effects have limited their effective use.

Brain cell transplantation with fetal dopaminergic neurons into the striatum, initially described as dopaminergic neuronal replacement, also has been attempted, but problems with rejection of the transplant, marginal efficacy, and lack of understanding of the mechanism of the treatment have not led to widespread use. The transplants may have temporarily stimulated growth factor production or release in the striatum or contributed to sprouting of remaining dopamine axons in the striatum. Other pharmacologic approaches have attempted to alter the activity of neurotransmitters other than dopamine, such as acetylcholine, to compensate for the loss of dopamine. These many attempted treatments do not appear to halt the pathological process of the disease, but some may provide partial relief of symptoms.

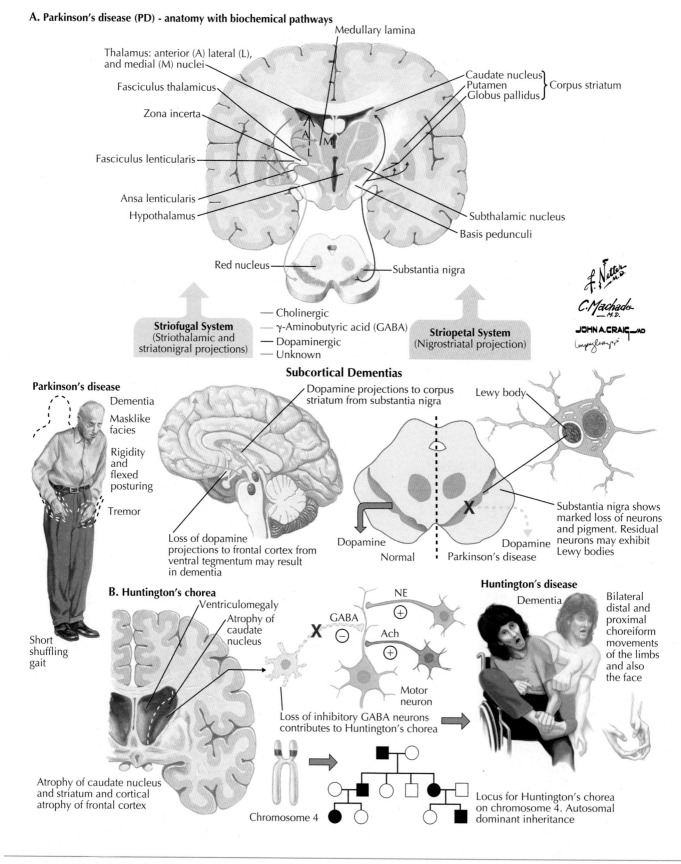

A. Parkinson's disease (PD) - anatomy with biochemical pathways

Medullary lamina

Thalamus: anterior (A) lateral (L), and medial (M) nuclei

Fasciculus thalamicus

Zona incerta

Fasciculus lenticularis

Ansa lenticularis

Hypothalamus

Caudate nucleus
Putamen   } Corpus striatum
Globus pallidus

Subthalamic nucleus

Basis pedunculi

Red nucleus

Substantia nigra

— Cholinergic
— γ-Aminobutyric acid (GABA)
— Dopaminergic
— Unknown

Striofugal System
(Striothalamic and striatonigral projections)

Striopetal System
(Nigrostriatal projection)

Subcortical Dementias

Parkinson's disease

Dementia

Masklike facies

Rigidity and flexed posturing

Tremor

Short shuffling gait

Dopamine projections to corpus striatum from substantia nigra

Loss of dopamine projections to frontal cortex from ventral tegmentum may result in dementia

Lewy body

Dopamine

Normal

Dopamine

Parkinson's disease

Substantia nigra shows marked loss of neurons and pigment. Residual neurons may exhibit Lewy bodies

B. Huntington's chorea

Ventriculomegaly

Atrophy of caudate nucleus

NE

GABA

Ach

Motor neuron

Loss of inhibitory GABA neurons contributes to Huntington's chorea

Atrophy of caudate nucleus and striatum and cortical atrophy of frontal cortex

Chromosome 4

Huntington's disease

Dementia

Bilateral distal and proximal choreiform movements of the limbs and also the face

Locus for Huntington's chorea on chromosome 4. Autosomal dominant inheritance

15.27 NEUROTRANSMITTER INVOLVEMENT IN PARKINSON'S DISEASE AND HUNTINGTON'S DISEASE

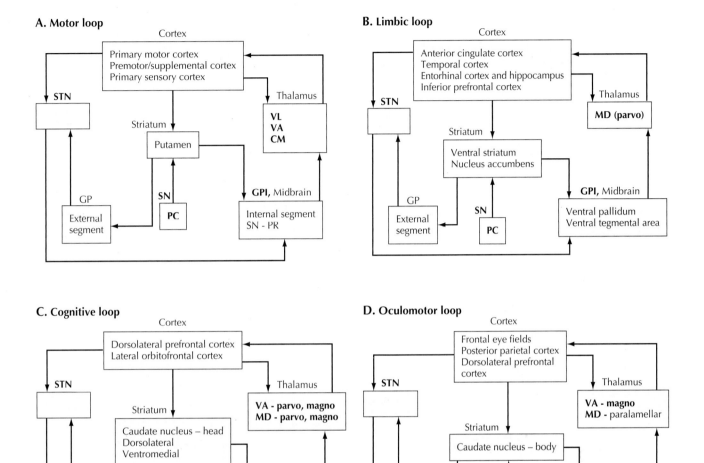

A. Motor loop

Cortex

Primary motor cortex
Premotor/supplemental cortex
Primary sensory cortex

STN

Thalamus

VL
VA
CM

Striatum

Putamen

GP

SN

GPI, Midbrain

External segment

PC

Internal segment
SN - PR

B. Limbic loop

Cortex

Anterior cingulate cortex
Temporal cortex
Entorhinal cortex and hippocampus
Inferior prefrontal cortex

STN

Thalamus

MD (parvo)

Striatum

Ventral striatum
Nucleus accumbens

GP

SN

GPI, Midbrain

External segment

PC

Ventral pallidum
Ventral tegmental area

C. Cognitive loop

Cortex

Dorsolateral prefrontal cortex
Lateral orbitofrontal cortex

STN

Thalamus

VA - parvo, magno
MD - parvo, magno

Striatum

Caudate nucleus – head
Dorsolateral
Ventromedial

GP

SN

GPI, Midbrain

External segment

PC

Internal segment
(lateral and medial)
SN - PR

D. Oculomotor loop

Cortex

Frontal eye fields
Posterior parietal cortex
Dorsolateral prefrontal cortex

STN

Thalamus

VA - magno
MD - paralamellar

Striatum

Caudate nucleus – body

GP

SN

GPI, Midbrain

External segment

PC

Internal segment
(central zone)
SN - PR (ventrolateral)

Midbrain

Horizontal and vertical gaze centers

Superior colliculus

CM = Centromedian nucleus
GPI = Globus pallidus internal segment
magno = Magnocellular
MD = Medial dorsal nucleus

parvo = Parvocellular
PC = Pars compacta
PR = Pars reticulata
SN = Substantia nigra

STN = Subthalamic nucleus
VA = Ventral anterior nucleus
VL = Ventrolateral nucleus

15.28 PARALLEL LOOPS OF CIRCUITRY THROUGH THE BASAL GANGLIA

The corticostriatal, striatopallidal, and pallidothalamic connections form parallel loops for motor, limbic, cognitive, and oculomotor circuitry. The motor circuitry is processed through the putamen, the limbic circuitry through the ventral pallidum and nucleus accumbens, the cognitive circuitry through the head of the caudate nucleus, and the oculomotor circuitry through the body of the caudate nucleus. Connections through the globus pallidus and the pars reticulata of the substantia nigra or ventral tegmental area then project to appropriate regions of the thalamus to link back to the cortical neurons of origin for the initial corticostriatal projections. These parallel loops through the basal ganglia and the cortex serve to modulate specific subroutines of cortical activity distinct to the appropriate function. The pars compacta of the substantia nigra may act as the principal interconnections among these parallel loops.

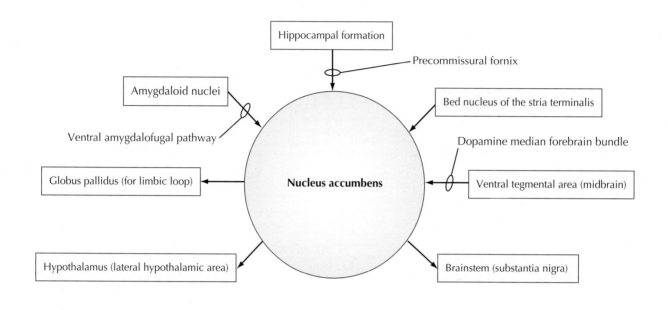

15.29 CONNECTIONS OF NUCLEUS ACCUMBENS

Nucleus accumbens is located at the anterior end of the striatum in the interior of the ventral and rostral forebrain (see Fig. 13.12). Inputs are derived from limbic structures (amygdala, hippocampal formation, bed nucleus of the stria terminalis) and from the ventral tegmental area of the midbrain via a rich dopaminergic projection. Nucleus accumbens is central to motivational states and addictive behaviors. It also appears to be a principal region in brain reward circuits associated with joy, pleasure, and gratification. The involvement of nucleus accumbens with a specific limbic basal ganglia loop (via globus pallidus) helps to provide motor expression of emotional responses and accompanying gestures and behaviors.

CLINICAL POINT

The **extended amygdala** refers to forebrain circuitry involved in processing risk-or-reward perception. This circuitry includes the bed nucleus of the stria terminalis and nucleus accumbens. These forebrain structures have interconnections with the corticomedial and central nuclei of the amygdala (see Plate 16.36 for a summary of amygdaloid circuitry). The bed nucleus of the stria terminalis is involved in processing uncertainty and uncertain threats or risks, in contrast to amygdaloid processing of more specific threats or risks. Nucleus accumbens is involved in processing control of behavioral actions in the face of uncertain threats or risks and, in concert with the amygdala and frontal cortex, is involved with active avoidance behavior (see the work of Joseph LeDoux and colleagues).

When the amygdala and the extended amygdala are activated by potential threats, a quick unconscious response from thalamic input (not the fine-grain analytical lemniscal thalamic components) prepares the brainstem circuitry for needed action. If the amygdaloid-related processing is sent to the prefrontal cortex (medial and lateral) and the parietal cortex, then conscious awareness of the threat and appropriate decision making regarding that threat are activated. More specific threats are processed through the amygdala and specific thalamic projections through sensory cortices to the prefrontal cortex.

CLINICAL POINT

The ventromedial prefrontal cortex (vmPFC) regulates dopamine release in the nucleus accumbens and mediates the response of the amygdala to perceived challenges. The vmPFC inhibits the release of mesolimbic dopamine in the nucleus accumbens, but not of meso-cortical dopamine in the prefrontal cortex, during amygdaloid activation. Thus, medial prefrontal cortex mediates the behavioral impact of amygdaloid reactivity through mesolimbic dopamine in the nucleus accumbens. In turn, the mesolimbic dopamine projections modulate amygdaloid emotional responsiveness, and the mesocortical dopamine projections modulate prefrontal cortical decision making and executive functions.

CLINICAL POINT

See Fig. 14.10. The varicella-zoster virus of childhood chickenpox can reside as a latent virus in dorsal root ganglia, the trigeminal sensory ganglia, and other sensory ganglia. During immunosuppression (medication, cancers, chronic stressors), the reactivation of this virus can cause painful eruptions in the distribution of a sensory nerve root or a division of the trigeminal nerve; this condition is commonly known as **shingles or herpes zoster (postherpetic) neuralgia**. The most common sites are the thoracic nerve roots or the ophthalmic division (Vj) of the trigeminal nerve. The skin erupts with vesicles and a sharp, radiating or burning pain is felt in the region of the eruptions. Sometimes the painful sensations (dysesthesias) occur several days before the eruptions appear. A particular risk related to the ophthalmic division of CN V is corneal ulcerations and subsequent opacities. The nerve, the ganglion, and sometimes the surrounding tissues show inflammatory reactivity. Usually, with combined antiviral therapy and analgesics, the eruptions can subside within a week or so. However, the postherpetic neuralgia, with burning pain, can last for weeks to months and may require the same type of treatment that other neuropathic pain syndromes (reflex sympathetic dystrophy or complex regional pain syndrome) require, including analgesics, tricyclic antidepressants to alter the pain threshold, membrane-stabilizing agents, anti-inflammatory medication, and other approaches.

CLINICAL POINT

See Fig. 15.9. The rubrospinal tract, arising from magnocellular neurons of the red nucleus, is part of a cortico-rubro-spinal system that may represent an indirect corticospinal pathway. Rubrospinal tract connections are contralateral and have mainly indirect effects (through interneurons) on both alpha and gamma LMNs. Some authors believe that the rubrospinal tract has a minor role in humans, although observations of **decorticate and decerebrate posturing** suggest otherwise. In conditions of UMN pathology, the cortico-rubro-spinal system is usually damaged in conjunction with the corticospinal tract (posterior limb of the internal capsule, lateral funiculus of the spinal cord), resulting in a clinical picture of UMN syndrome. Bilateral damage to the forebrain and diencephalon, leaving only the rubrospinal tract, reticulospinal tracts, and vestibulospinal tracts intact, results in a classic UMN appearance bilaterally, with upper limbs in a flexed position and lower limbs in an extended posture (called decorticate posturing). If the lesion extends caudally just below the red nucleus, further removing rubrospinal tract influences, the lateral vestibulospinal tracts are markedly disinhibited, resulting in decerebrate posturing with all four limbs extended. These observations suggest that the rubrospinal system particularly drives flexor activity in the upper extremities and has a lesser role in the lower extremities.

CLINICAL POINT

See Fig. 15.11. The reticulospinal tracts originate from isodendritic neurons in the medial portion of the pontine and medullary RF. The pontine RF gives rise to the pontine (medial) reticulospinal tract, which influences mainly proximal musculature. The medullary RF gives rise to the medullary (lateral) reticulospinal tract, which lies more laterally in the spinal cord and influences muscles of the extremities. The reticulospinal tracts help to **regulate basic tone and postural responses**, sometimes coordinating musculature supplied by LMNs at multiple spinal cord levels. These tracts also may help to direct stereotyped movements such as those involved in extending a limb toward an object. The reticulospinal tracts can selectively influence both alpha and gamma LMNs, thus providing a mechanism for activation of static or dynamic gamma LMNs in conditions of damage to other descending systems, such as the corticospinal and cortico-rubro-spinal systems.

CLINICAL POINT

See Fig 15.14. Vestibular nuclei receive input from the hair cells in the ampullae of the semicircular canals and are connected with extraocular CN motor nuclei, thereby permitting vestibular reflex control of eye movements. This circuitry establishes the connections of the **vestibulo-ocular reflex**. When the head is rotated in one direction, the lateral semicircular canal initiates a vestibulo-ocular reflex that moves the eyes in the opposite direction, thereby maintaining the position of the eyes. Stimulation of the hair cells on one side of the vestibular apparatus with cold water in the external auditory meatus (the caloric response) provides the brainstem on that side with the neural signaling of apparent movement and elicits eye movements that would be appropriate to an actual movement, were one occurring. This elicited movement is called **caloric nystagmus**; it evokes a sense of apparent movement, a tendency to fall to one side, and past-pointing. With caloric nystagmus, there is a slow phase and a compensatory fast phase. Cold water results in the fast phase directed to the opposite side, and warm water results in the fast phase directed to the same side. A lesion or irritative stimulation of the vestibular nerve on one side also gives the neural perception of movement, eliciting **pathological nystagmus**. If a person rotates in one direction to a greater extent than a simple vestibulo-ocular reflex can easily correct through compensatory eye movements, the eyes will be directed sufficiently far to one side that a quick movement (saccade) will be necessary to refocus them straight ahead. This is called **rotational nystagmus**, with the slow phase opposite from the direction of movement and the saccade (fast phase) in the direction of the movement; the saccade is neurally directed from the occipital lobe visual cortices. After the rotation stops, the individual will feel as if she or he is still rotating but in the opposite direction (postrotational nystagmus), with the saccade in the direction opposite from the original movement and past-pointing in the direction of apparent movement. If an individual is stationary and stimuli move past the visual field (telephone poles and a person in a moving car), tracking reflexes move the eyes and a cortically evoked saccade corrects the eye position with a quick movement of the eyes. This normal physiologic process is called **optokinetic nystagmus**.

16

AUTONOMIC-HYPOTHALAMIC-LIMBIC SYSTEMS

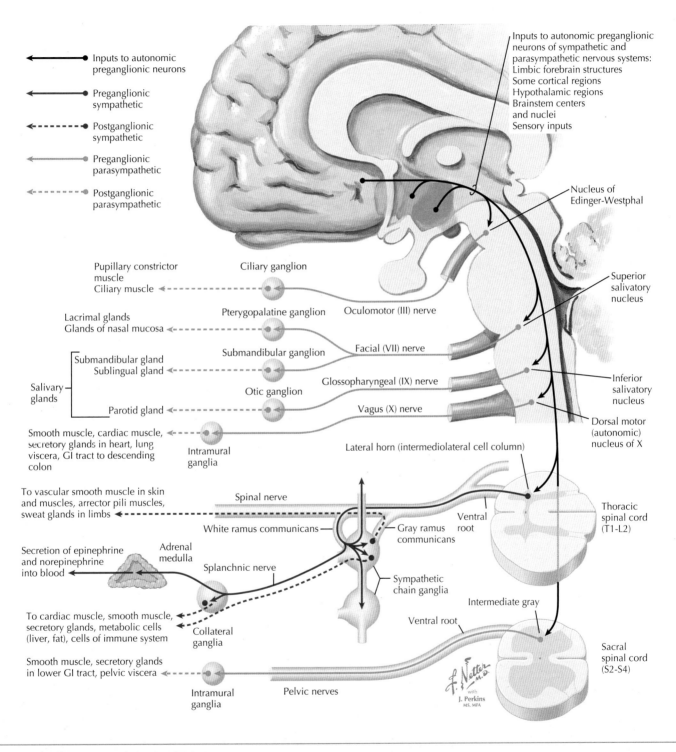

Inputs to autonomic preganglionic neurons

Preganglionic sympathetic

Postganglionic sympathetic

Preganglionic parasympathetic

Postganglionic parasympathetic

Inputs to autonomic preganglionic neurons of sympathetic and parasympathetic nervous systems:
Limbic forebrain structures
Some cortical regions
Hypothalamic regions
Brainstem centers and nuclei
Sensory inputs

Nucleus of Edinger-Westphal

Superior salivary nucleus

Inferior salivary nucleus

Dorsal motor (autonomic) nucleus of X

Pupillary constrictor muscle
Ciliary muscle

Ciliary ganglion

Oculomotor (III) nerve

Lacrimal glands
Glands of nasal mucosa

Pterygopalatine ganglion

Submandibular ganglion

Facial (VII) nerve

Submandibular gland
Sublingual gland

Glossopharyngeal (IX) nerve

Salivary glands

Otic ganglion

Vagus (X) nerve

Parotid gland

Smooth muscle, cardiac muscle, secretory glands in heart, lung viscera, GI tract to descending colon

Intramural ganglia

Lateral horn (intermediolateral cell column)

To vascular smooth muscle in skin and muscles, arrector pili muscles, sweat glands in limbs

Spinal nerve

White ramus communicans

Gray ramus communicans

Ventral root

Thoracic spinal cord (T1-L2)

Secretion of epinephrine and norepinephrine into blood

Adrenal medulla

Splanchnic nerve

Sympathetic chain ganglia

Intermediate gray

To cardiac muscle, smooth muscle, secretory glands, metabolic cells (liver, fat), cells of immune system

Collateral ganglia

Ventral root

Sacral spinal cord (S2-S4)

Smooth muscle, secretory glands in lower GI tract, pelvic viscera

Intramural ganglia

Pelvic nerves

AUTONOMIC NERVOUS SYSTEM

16.1 GENERAL ORGANIZATION OF THE AUTONOMIC NERVOUS SYSTEM

See next page.

16.1 GENERAL ORGANIZATION OF THE AUTONOMIC NERVOUS SYSTEM (CONTINUED)

The autonomic nervous system is a two-neuron chain connecting preganglionic neurons through ganglia to visceral target tissues (cardiac muscle, smooth muscle, secretory glands, metabolic cells, cells of the immune system). The sympathetic division (sympathetic nervous system; SNS) is a thoracolumbar (T1-L2) system arising from the intermediolateral cell column of the lateral horn of the spinal cord, acting through chain ganglia and collateral ganglia; it is a system designed for enhancing activities and for fight-or-flight reactions in an emergency. The parasympathetic division (parasympathetic nervous system) is a craniosacral system arising from brainstem nuclei associated with cranial nerves (CNs) III, VII, IX, and X and from the intermediate gray in the S2–S4 spinal cord. Connections from CNs III, VII, and IX act through cranial nerve ganglia; connections from the vagal system and sacral system act through intramural ganglia in or near the target tissue. The parasympathetic nervous system is a homeostatic reparative system. Central connections from the limbic forebrain, hypothalamus, and brainstem regulating the sympathetic and parasympathetic nervous systems' outflow to the body act mainly through connections to vagal and sympathetic preganglionic neurons.

CLINICAL POINT

Preganglionic parasympathetic neurons in the brainstem and sacral spinal cord, as well as preganglionic sympathetic neurons in the thoracolumbar spinal cord, send projections to ganglion cells and use acetylcholine as the principal neurotransmitter. The ganglion cells possess mainly nicotinic cholinergic receptors for transducing fast neurotransmission responses. Postganglionic sympathetic neurons use mainly norepinephrine as their neurotransmitter, whereas postganglionic parasympathetic neurons use acetylcholine. Target tissue possesses **alpha and beta adrenoceptor subclasses and cholinergic muscarinic receptor subclasses** (M1–M3). In the heart, beta1 receptors increase the force and rate of contraction, increase cardiac output, and dilate coronary arteries, whereas M2 receptors decrease the force and rate of contraction and cardiac output. In vascular smooth muscle and smooth muscles of the pupil, ureters, and bladder, alpha1 receptors cause contraction. In blood vessels, alpha2 receptors also cause constriction. In smooth muscle of the tracheobronchial system, uterus, and gastrointestinal tract vasculature, beta2 receptors cause relaxation. Alpha1 receptors cause relaxation of gastrointestinal smooth muscles, and M1 receptors cause slow contraction. M3 receptors cause contraction of most parasympathetic smooth muscle target structures. In salivary glands, alpha1 receptors cause secretion and beta2 receptors cause mucus secretion. In adipose tissue, alpha1 receptors cause glycogenolysis, beta1 receptors cause lipolysis, and alpha2 receptors inhibit lipolysis. In sweat glands, alpha1 receptors cause secretion. In the kidney, alpha1 receptors enhance reabsorption of Na^+, and beta1 receptors provoke renin release. In liver and skeletal muscles, beta2 receptors cause glycogenolysis. In the pancreas, beta2 receptors stimulate insulin release, and alpha2 receptors inhibit insulin release. On immunocytes, beta-adrenergic receptors decrease natural killer (NK) cell activity and decrease the secretion of Th1 cytokines (interferon-gamma, interleukin 2) by Th1 lymphocytes. The balance of adrenergic and cholinergic neurotransmission determines the relative degree of activation of target tissues, and differential affinity of ligands for the various receptor subclasses helps to determine the final integrative physiological response.

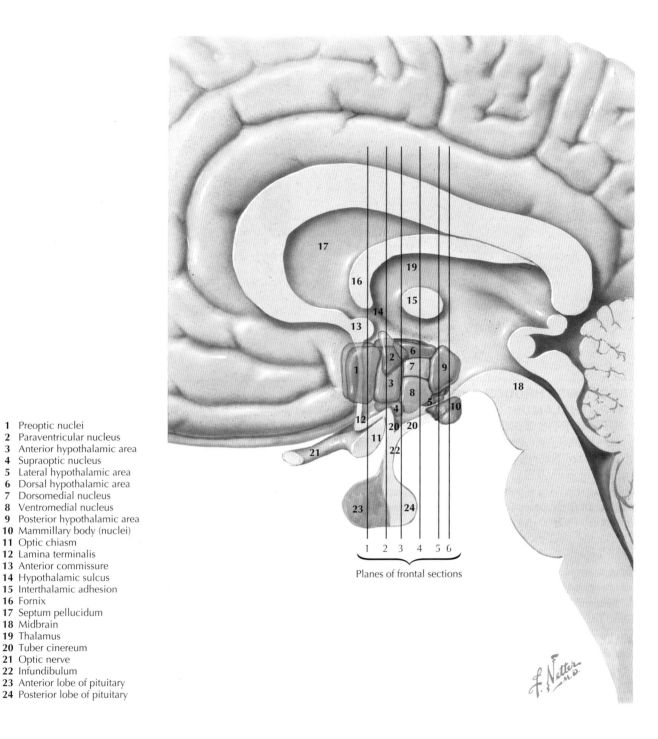

1 Preoptic nuclei
2 Paraventricular nucleus
3 Anterior hypothalamic area
4 Supraoptic nucleus
5 Lateral hypothalamic area
6 Dorsal hypothalamic area
7 Dorsomedial nucleus
8 Ventromedial nucleus
9 Posterior hypothalamic area
10 Mammillary body (nuclei)
11 Optic chiasm
12 Lamina terminalis
13 Anterior commissure
14 Hypothalamic sulcus
15 Interthalamic adhesion
16 Fornix
17 Septum pellucidum
18 Midbrain
19 Thalamus
20 Tuber cinereum
21 Optic nerve
22 Infundibulum
23 Anterior lobe of pituitary
24 Posterior lobe of pituitary

Planes of frontal sections

HYPOTHALAMUS AND PITUITARY

16.2 GENERAL ANATOMY OF THE HYPOTHALAMUS

The hypothalamus is a collection of nuclei and fiber tracts in the ventral diencephalon that regulates visceral autonomic functions and neuroendocrine functions, particularly from the anterior and posterior pituitary. Many nuclei are found between the posterior boundary (mammillary bodies) and the anterior boundary (lamina terminalis, anterior commissure) of the hypothalamus; these nuclei are subdivided into four general hypothalamic zones, from rostral to caudal: (1) preoptic, (2) anterior or supraoptic, (3) tuberal, and (4) mammillary or posterior. From the medial boundary at the III ventricle to the lateral boundary, the nuclei are subdivided into three general zones or areas: (1) periventricular, (2) medial, and (3) lateral. The pituitary gland is attached at the base of the hypothalamus by the infundibulum (pituitary stalk), which possesses an important zone of neuroendocrine transduction, the median eminence.

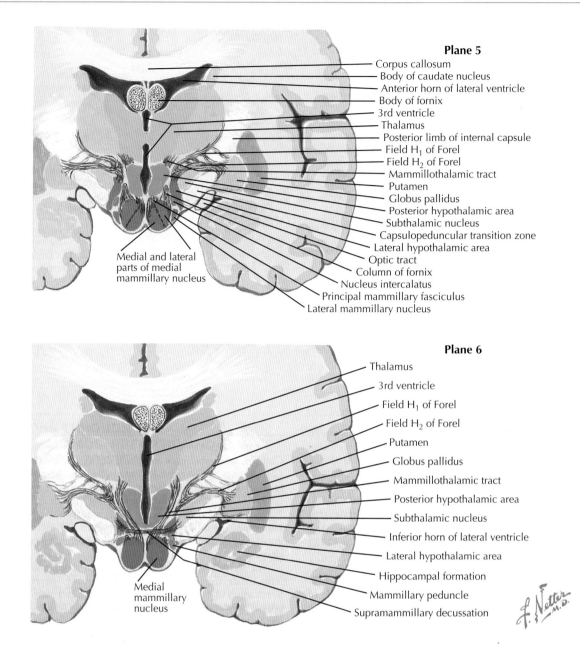

Plane 5
- Corpus callosum
- Body of caudate nucleus
- Anterior horn of lateral ventricle
- Body of fornix
- 3rd ventricle
- Thalamus
- Posterior limb of internal capsule
- Field H$_1$ of Forel
- Field H$_2$ of Forel
- Mammillothalamic tract
- Putamen
- Globus pallidus
- Posterior hypothalamic area
- Subthalamic nucleus
- Capsulopeduncular transition zone
- Lateral hypothalamic area
- Optic tract
- Column of fornix
- Nucleus intercalatus
- Principal mammillary fasciculus
- Lateral mammillary nucleus

Medial and lateral parts of medial mammillary nucleus

Plane 6
- Thalamus
- 3rd ventricle
- Field H$_1$ of Forel
- Field H$_2$ of Forel
- Putamen
- Globus pallidus
- Mammillothalamic tract
- Posterior hypothalamic area
- Subthalamic nucleus
- Inferior horn of lateral ventricle
- Lateral hypothalamic area
- Hippocampal formation
- Mammillary peduncle
- Supramammillary decussation

Medial mammillary nucleus

16.5 SECTIONS THROUGH THE HYPOTHALAMUS: MAMMILLARY ZONE

The major nuclei in the mammillary zone (Planes 5 and 6) include the medial and lateral mammillary nuclei, the posterior hypothalamic area, and the LHA. The LHA extends throughout most of the length of the hypothalamus and shows neuronal characteristics seen in the brainstem reticular formation.

CLINICAL POINT

In the 1930s, James Papez proposed a brain circuit that was viewed as a substrate for control of emotional behavior and later as a substrate for memory, especially for consolidation of immediate and short-term memory into long-term memory. This **Papez circuit** includes hippocampal formation (especially the subiculum) via the fornix to the mammillary nuclei (especially medial nuclei); via the mammillothalamic tract to the anterior thalamic nuclei; via the internal capsule to the anterior cingulate cortex; and via polysynaptic connections in the cingulum to the entorhinal cortex, subiculum, and hippocampus. This

circuit is proposed as a site of major damage in **Wernicke-Korsakoff syndrome**, a disorder that is commonly seen in chronic alcoholic patients with a vitamin B$_1$ (thiamine) deficiency. This syndrome includes Wernicke's encephalopathy and the memory dysfunction of Korsakoff's syndrome. Wernicke's encephalopathy involves a confused and psychotic state involving confabulation (made-up stories derived from a host of confused past memories or experiences), cerebellar ataxia, extraocular and gaze palsies, and nystagmus. Korsakoff amnestic syndrome involves the inability to consolidate immediate and short-term memory into long-term traces (anterograde amnesia) as well as long-term memory loss concerning events that have occurred since the onset of the disease. Degeneration has been described in the mammillary bodies, fornix, hippocampal formation, and anterior and medial dorsal thalamus. However, the extent to which the mammillary nuclei themselves play a role in consolidation of memory traces remains to be shown. Thiamine administration may help to reverse some of the symptoms, but the amnesias may persist. Administration of glucose (carbohydrate loading) without thiamine may cause death as the result of nutritional cardiomyopathy.

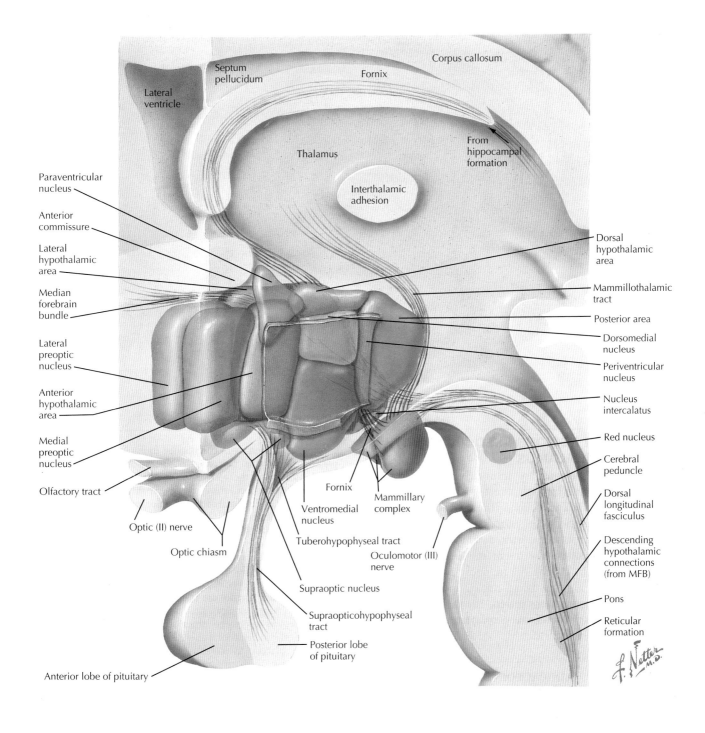

16.6 SCHEMATIC RECONSTRUCTION OF THE HYPOTHALAMUS

A schematic three-dimensional reconstruction of the hypothalamus in sagittal section shows the nuclei, areas, and zones that occupy this small, compact region of the diencephalon. Many pathways are represented in this schematic reconstruction, including the fornix, the mammillothalamic tract, the median forebrain bundle (MFB), the supraopticohypophyseal tract, the tuberohypophyseal (tuberoinfundibular) tract, and brainstem connections with the hypothalamus via the dorsal longitudinal fasciculus, the descending median forebrain bundle, the mammillotegmental tract, and descending connections from the PVN to preganglionic autonomic nuclei.

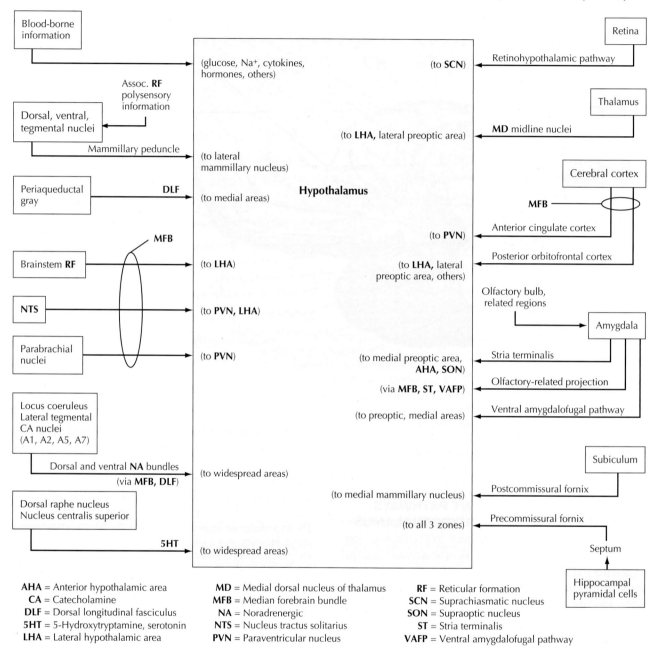

Brainstem and Blood-Borne Inputs

Diencephalon and Telencephalon Inputs

Blood-borne information → (glucose, Na⁺, cytokines, hormones, others) (to **SCN**)

Assoc. **RF** polysensory information

Dorsal, ventral, tegmental nuclei

Mammillary peduncle → (to lateral mammillary nucleus)

Periaqueductal gray — DLF → (to medial areas)

Hypothalamus

MFB

Brainstem **RF** → (to LHA)

NTS → (to PVN, LHA)

Parabrachial nuclei → (to PVN)

Locus coeruleus Lateral tegmental CA nuclei (A1, A2, A5, A7)

Dorsal and ventral **NA** bundles (via **MFB, DLF**) → (to widespread areas)

Dorsal raphe nucleus Nucleus centralis superior

5HT → (to widespread areas)

(to **LHA**, lateral preoptic area)

(to **PVN**)

(to **LHA**, lateral preoptic area, others)

(to medial preoptic area, **AHA, SON**)

(via **MFB, ST, VAFP**)

(to preoptic, medial areas)

(to medial mammillary nucleus)

(to all 3 zones)

Retina — Retinohypothalamic pathway

Thalamus — **MD** midline nuclei

Cerebral cortex — **MFB**

Anterior cingulate cortex

Posterior orbitofrontal cortex

Olfactory bulb, related regions → Amygdala

Stria terminalis

Olfactory-related projection

Ventral amygdalofugal pathway

Subiculum — Postcommissural fornix

Precommissural fornix — Septum

Hippocampal pyramidal cells

AHA = Anterior hypothalamic area
CA = Catecholamine
DLF = Dorsal longitudinal fasciculus
5HT = 5-Hydroxytryptamine, serotonin
LHA = Lateral hypothalamic area

MD = Medial dorsal nucleus of thalamus
MFB = Median forebrain bundle
NA = Noradrenergic
NTS = Nucleus tractus solitarius
PVN = Paraventricular nucleus

RF = Reticular formation
SCN = Suprachiasmatic nucleus
SON = Supraoptic nucleus
ST = Stria terminalis
VAFP = Ventral amygdalofugal pathway

16.9 SCHEMATIC DIAGRAM OF MAJOR HYPOTHALAMIC AFFERENT PATHWAYS

The hypothalamus receives extensive input from many regions of the CNS. Descending inputs arrive from limbic forebrain structures (hippocampal formation, subiculum, amygdaloid nuclei), the cerebral cortex (anterior cingulate, orbitofrontal, prefrontal), and the thalamus (medial dorsal). Ascending inputs arrive from extensive areas of the autonomic brainstem (tegmental nuclei, periaqueductal gray, parabrachial nuclei, nucleus tractus solitarius, locus coeruleus and tegmental catecholamine nuclei, raphe serotonergic nuclei) and from the brainstem reticular formation. The retina sends input directly to the suprachiasmatic nucleus, a nucleus of the hypothalamus that modulates diurnal rhythms. Blood-borne substances (cytokines, hormones, glucose, Na⁺, others) influence the hypothalamus via numerous routes and mechanisms.

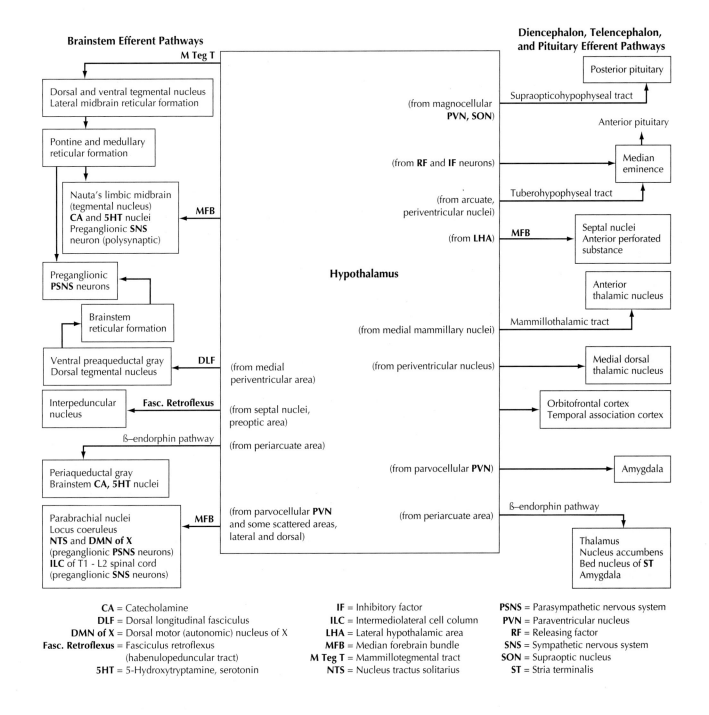

Brainstem Efferent Pathways

M Teg T

Dorsal and ventral tegmental nucleus
Lateral midbrain reticular formation

Pontine and medullary
reticular formation

Nauta's limbic midbrain
(tegmental nucleus)
CA and **5HT** nuclei
Preganglionic **SNS**
neuron (polysynaptic)

MFB

Preganglionic
PSNS neurons

Brainstem
reticular formation

Ventral preaqueductal gray
Dorsal tegmental nucleus

DLF

Interpeduncular
nucleus

Fasc. Retroflexus

ß–endorphin pathway

Periaqueductal gray
Brainstem **CA, 5HT** nuclei

Parabrachial nuclei
Locus coeruleus
NTS and **DMN of X**
(preganglionic **PSNS** neurons)
ILC of T1 - L2 spinal cord
(preganglionic **SNS** neurons)

MFB

(from medial
periventricular area)

(from septal nuclei,
preoptic area)

(from periarcuate area)

(from parvocellular **PVN**
and some scattered areas,
lateral and dorsal)

Hypothalamus

**Diencephalon, Telencephalon,
and Pituitary Efferent Pathways**

Posterior pituitary

(from magnocellular
PVN, SON)

Supraopticohypophyseal tract

Anterior pituitary

(from **RF** and **IF** neurons)

Median
eminence

(from arcuate,
periventricular nuclei)

Tuberohypophyseal tract

(from **LHA**)

MFB

Septal nuclei
Anterior perforated
substance

Anterior
thalamic nucleus

(from medial mammillary nuclei)

Mammillothalamic tract

(from periventricular nucleus)

Medial dorsal
thalamic nucleus

Orbitofrontal cortex
Temporal association cortex

(from parvocellular **PVN**)

Amygdala

(from periarcuate area)

ß–endorphin pathway

Thalamus
Nucleus accumbens
Bed nucleus of **ST**
Amygdala

CA = Catecholamine
DLF = Dorsal longitudinal fasciculus
DMN of X = Dorsal motor (autonomic) nucleus of X
Fasc. Retroflexus = Fasciculus retroflexus
(habenulopeduncular tract)
5HT = 5-Hydroxytryptamine, serotonin

IF = Inhibitory factor
ILC = Intermediolateral cell column
LHA = Lateral hypothalamic area
MFB = Median forebrain bundle
M Teg T = Mammillotegmental tract
NTS = Nucleus tractus solitarius

PSNS = Parasympathetic nervous system
PVN = Paraventricular nucleus
RF = Releasing factor
SNS = Sympathetic nervous system
SON = Supraoptic nucleus
ST = Stria terminalis

16.10 SCHEMATIC DIAGRAM OF MAJOR HYPOTHALAMIC EFFERENT PATHWAYS

The hypothalamus gives rise to extensive efferent projections to many regions of the CNS. Ascending efferents are sent to limbic forebrain structures (amygdaloid nuclei, septal nuclei, the anterior perforated substance), the cerebral cortex (orbito frontal cortex and temporal association cortex), and the thalamus (medial dorsal, anterior). Extensive projections are sent to the median eminence (releasing and inhibitory factors for control of anterior pituitary hormones, dopamine projections from the arcuate nucleus and periventricular nucleus) and to the posterior pituitary. Additional efferent projections are sent directly and indirectly to the preganglionic neurons of the sympathetic and the parasympathetic nervous systems (median forebrain bundle, dorsal longitudinal fasciculus, mammillotegmental tract, and direct projections from the paraventricular nucleus), to widespread autonomic and visceral nuclei (noradrenergic neurons, serotonergic neurons, parabrachial nuclei, nucleus tractus solitarius, periaqueductal gray, tegmental nuclei, interpeduncular nucleus), and to the brainstem reticular formation.

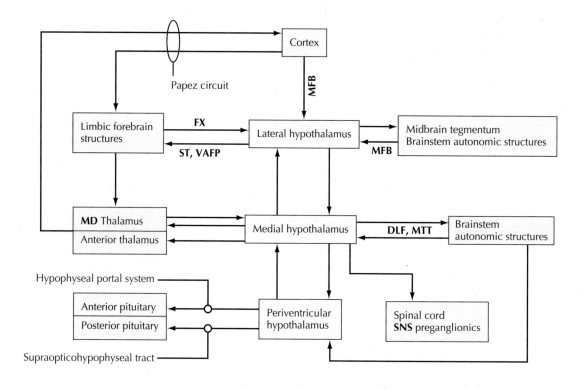

DLF = Dorsal longitudinal fasciculus
FX = Fornix
MD = Medial dorsal nucleus of thalamus
MFB = Median forebrain bundle

MTT = Mammillothalamic tract
SNS = Sympathetic nervous system
ST = Stria terminalis
VAFP = Ventral amygdalofugal pathway

16.11 SUMMARY OF GENERAL HYPOTHALAMIC CONNECTIONS

The lateral, medial, and periventricular zones of the hypothalamus have specific connections with the cerebral cortex, limbic forebrain structures, thalamus, and widespread areas of the brainstem. Extensive efferent projections of the hypothalamus are directed toward regulation of preganglionic sympathetic and parasympathetic neurons and toward release and regulation of hormones of the anterior and posterior pituitary. The anterior pituitary hormones regulate hormonal secretion and functional activities of many target structures throughout the body.

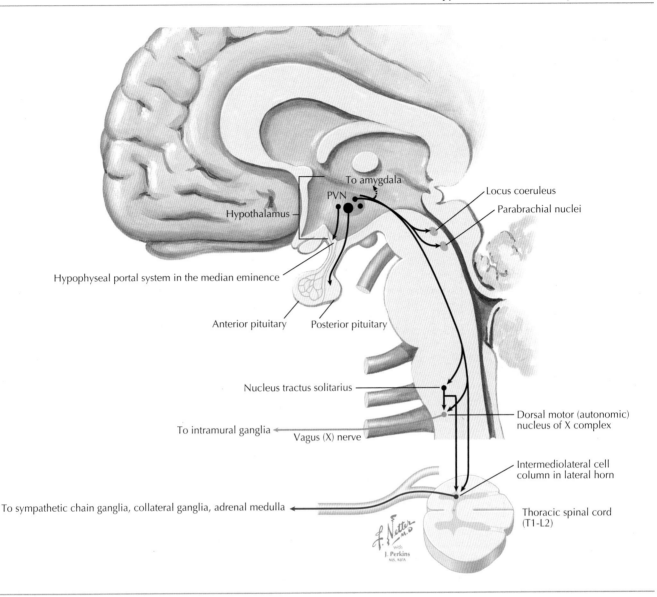

To amygdala

PVN

Hypothalamus

Locus coeruleus

Parabrachial nuclei

Hypophyseal portal system in the median eminence

Anterior pituitary

Posterior pituitary

Nucleus tractus solitarius

To intramural ganglia

Vagus (X) nerve

Dorsal motor (autonomic) nucleus of X complex

Intermediolateral cell column in lateral horn

To sympathetic chain ganglia, collateral ganglia, adrenal medulla

Thoracic spinal cord (T1-L2)

16.12 PARAVENTRICULAR NUCLEUS OF THE HYPOTHALAMUS: REGULATION OF PITUITARY NEUROHORMONAL OUTFLOW, AUTONOMIC PREGANGLIONIC OUTFLOW, AND LIMBIC ACTIVITY

The PVN has many projections that help to coordinate pituitary neurohormonal outflow, autonomic preganglionic outflow, and limbic activity. **Magnocellular neurons** send axons to the posterior pituitary, releasing oxytocin and vasopressin into the general circulation. Corticotropin-releasing factor (CRF) neurons and some vasopressin neurons send axons to the median eminence; these axons release their hormones into the hypophyseal portal system, influencing the release of ACTH. PVN **parvocellular neurons** send direct descending projections to preganglionic neurons for the parasympathetics (dorsal motor nucleus of CN X) and sympathetics (intermediolateral cell column in the T1–L2 lateral horn of the spinal cord) and to the nucleus tractus solitarius. PVN parvocellular neurons also send axons to several important limbic-related structures, such as the amygdaloid nuclei, parabrachial nuclei, and locus coeruleus.

CLINICAL POINT

The PVN of the hypothalamus is a small region along the upper borders of the third ventricle in the dorsal hypothalamus. It contains a remarkable array of chemically specific neural populations. The magnocellular neurons produce oxytocin and vasopressin along with neurophysins and project to the median eminence. Some parvocellular neurons synthesize corticotropin-releasing hormone and send axons to the contact zone of the median eminence, where corticotropin- releasing hormone is released into the hypophyseal portal vessels. Parvocellular neurons also send descending projections to the brainstem (particularly the nucleus solitarius) and the intermediolateral cell column of the thoracolumbar spinal cord, where activation of the SNS can occur. The PVN therefore can coordinate the activation of both the neuroendocrine components (hypothalamic-pituitary-adrenal axis and cortisol secretion) and the autonomic components (sympathetic activation, diminished parasympathetic activity) of a stress response or activational response. The PVN receives inputs from many limbic regions and from brainstem sites (parabrachial nuclei, brainstem noradrenergic nuclei, nucleus tractus solitarius) that provide visceral information to the PVN. In addition, the PVN receives a variety of inputs that help it to monitor inflammatory mediators (IL-1β, IL-6, tumor necrosis factor [TNF]-α, prostaglandin E2 [PGE$_2$]), and other small molecules (nitric oxide) that reflect the outside chemical milieu. This information is received through the hypothalamus and circumventricular organs, and some of it through the vagus nerve afferents and nucleus tractus solitarius. Thus, PVN is a key regulatory site for behavioral responses that require autonomic reactivity.

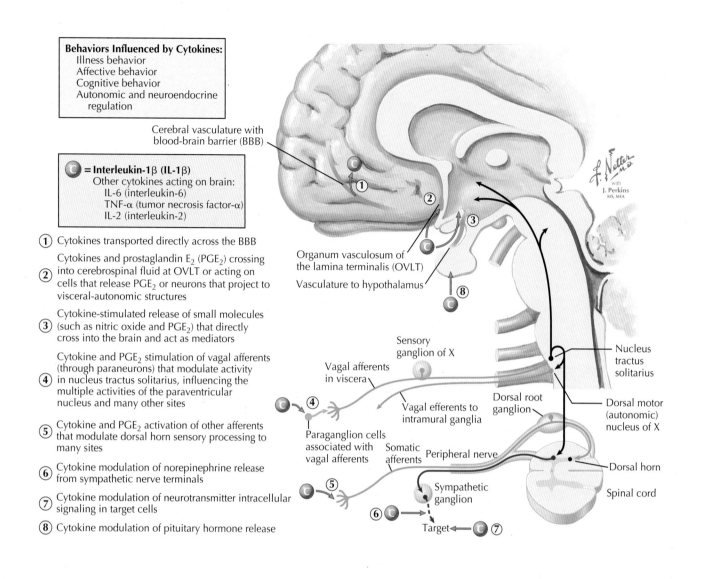

Behaviors Influenced by Cytokines:
Illness behavior
Affective behavior
Cognitive behavior
Autonomic and neuroendocrine
regulation

C = **Interleukin-1β (IL-1β)**
Other cytokines acting on brain:
IL-6 (interleukin-6)
TNF-α (tumor necrosis factor-α)
IL-2 (interleukin-2)

(1) Cytokines transported directly across the BBB

(2) Cytokines and prostaglandin E_2 (PGE$_2$) crossing into cerebrospinal fluid at OVLT or acting on cells that release PGE$_2$ or neurons that project to visceral-autonomic structures

(3) Cytokine-stimulated release of small molecules (such as nitric oxide and PGE$_2$) that directly cross into the brain and act as mediators

(4) Cytokine and PGE$_2$ stimulation of vagal afferents (through paraneurons) that modulate activity in nucleus tractus solitarius, influencing the multiple activities of the paraventricular nucleus and many other sites

(5) Cytokine and PGE$_2$ activation of other afferents that modulate dorsal horn sensory processing to many sites

(6) Cytokine modulation of norepinephrine release from sympathetic nerve terminals

(7) Cytokine modulation of neurotransmitter intracellular signaling in target cells

(8) Cytokine modulation of pituitary hormone release

Cerebral vasculature with blood-brain barrier (BBB)

Organum vasculosum of the lamina terminalis (OVLT)
Vasculature to hypothalamus

Sensory ganglion of X
Vagal afferents in viscera
Vagal efferents to intramural ganglia
Paraganglion cells associated with vagal afferents
Somatic afferents   Peripheral nerve
Sympathetic ganglion
Target

Nucleus tractus solitarius
Dorsal root ganglion
Dorsal motor (autonomic) nucleus of X
Dorsal horn
Spinal cord

16.13 MECHANISMS OF CYTOKINE INFLUENCES ON THE HYPOTHALAMUS AND OTHER BRAIN REGIONS AND ON BEHAVIOR

Cytokines, including IL-1β, IL-6, TNF-α, and IL-2, can influence central neuronal activity and behavior. This figure illustrates IL-1β access to the brain: (1) directly crossing the blood-brain barrier into the brain (especially in cortical regions); (2) acting on circumventricular organs (the OVLT) to release small mediators such as PGE$_2$; (3) acting on vascular endothelial cells to release nitric oxide, which acts in the CNS; (4) activating vagal afferents that project into the nucleus tractus solitarius via paraganglion cells; and (5) activating other afferent nerve fibers. IL-1β can evoke illness behavior (fever, induction of slow-wave sleep, decreased appetite, lethargy, classical illness symptoms), can influence autonomic and neuroendocrine regulation, and can influence both affective and cognitive functions and behavior.

CLINICAL POINT
There is a **widespread influence of cytokines**, especially inflammatory cytokines (IL-1β, IL-6, TNF-α), as well as prostaglandin E$_2$ (PGE$_2$), on the nervous system. A key target of these influences is the PVN of the hypothalamus. Inflammatory cytokines can provoke a robust activation of cortisol secretion (through the hypothalamo-pituitary-adrenal axis) and SNS activation (via descending projections of the PVN). The consequences of prolonged stress activation include increased risk for many chronic diseases, such as cardiovascular disease and stroke, metabolic syndrome, type II diabetes, and many cancers. The cytokines can influence the PVN and other central neurons through several mechanisms, including some direct transport into the forebrain, actions on neurons of the OVLT that release PGE$_2$ and signal the PVN, release of nitric oxide and PGE$_2$ from vascular endothelial cells, and activation of vagal afferents and other afferents that send neural signals to the PVN. Inflammatory cytokines also can stimulate the release of some hormones from pituitary cells, can alter neurotransmitter release in both the CNS and the autonomic nervous system (especially sympathetic norepinephrine), and can interact with neurotransmitter effects on target cells of autonomic innervation. Other cytokines such as IL-2 also appear to have central effects; the infusion of IL-2 in immunotherapy for some cancers was curtailed because of adverse effects of IL-2 on the brain, including depression and suicidal behavior.

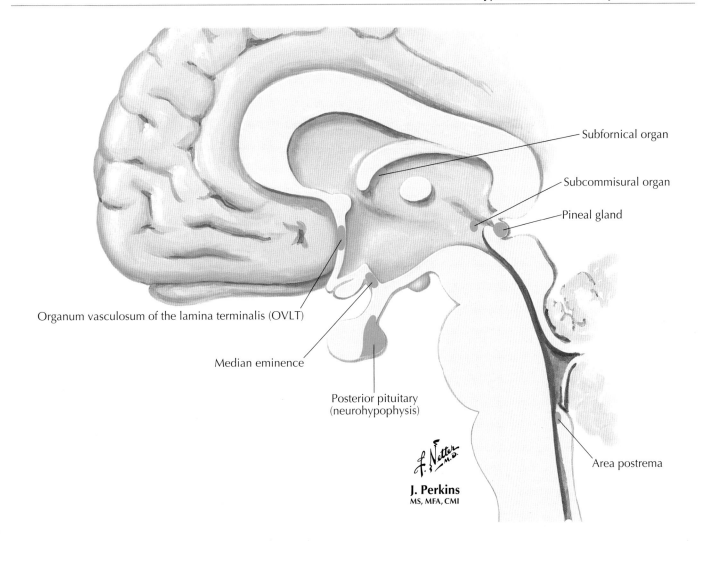

Subfornical organ

Subcommisural organ

Pineal gland

Organum vasculosum of the lamina terminalis (OVLT)

Median eminence

Posterior pituitary
(neurohypophysis)

Area postrema

J. Perkins
MS, MFA, CMI

16.14 CIRCUMVENTRICULAR ORGANS

Circumventricular organs are "windows on the brain" that are devoid of the usual tight junction endothelial appositions and instead have fenestrated vasculature. Thus, the circumventricular organs have no blood-brain barrier. Some of these organs (the OVLT, the subfornical organ, and the area postrema) have associated neurons that project to the hypothalamic and other visceral structures. They also have cells that can release small molecules such as PGE_2 into the cerebrospinal fluid, thus affecting target structures at a distance. The neurohypophysis is a site of axonal release (from PVN and SON magnocellular neurons) of oxytocin and arginine vasopressin into the general circulation. The median eminence is a zone of neuroendocrine transduction for the secretion of releasing factors and inhibitory factors into the hypophyseal portal vasculature; these factors influence the release of anterior pituitary hormones. The pineal gland synthesizes and releases the hormone melatonin.

CLINICAL POINT

The CNS is protected from damage caused by many potentially harmful substances in the periphery by the blood-brain barrier. The CNS capillary endothelial cells contain tight junctions as well as specific transport mechanisms for the uptake of certain important substances (such as amino acids needed for neurotransmitter synthesis, glucose). Brain capillaries also can actively pump some substances out of the brain. Some regions of the brain contain fenestrated capillaries, and this permits the sampling of circulating substances. These are the circumventricular organs. The area postrema contains neurons that project to the nucleus tractus solitarius and activate the vomiting reflex. The subfornical organ contains neurons that respond to salt content in the blood and elicit protective neuroendocrine responses. The OVLT contains neurons that help to regulate blood pressure through an angiotensin II mechanism; these neurons also regulate PGE_2 availability to the PVN and other central areas to influence activation of the hypothalamo-pituitary-adrenal axis and the SNS. The OVLT and subfornical organ also respond to pyrogens and help to regulate hypothalamic responses for control of body temperature. At the median eminence, circulating hormones and other substances can interact with the projecting axonal terminals that secrete releasing hormones and inhibitory hormones at the contact zone for regulation of anterior pituitary hormonal secretion. The posterior pituitary and the pineal gland also have fenestrated capillaries, enabling their secretion of hormones directly into the systemic circulation.

Circumventricular Organs: Functional Considerations	
Structure	**Location and Functional Roles**
Organum vasculosum of the lamina terminalis (OVLT)	• Location: anteroventral region of the third ventricle • Contains osmoreceptors, responds to osmotic factors; helps to regulate vasopressin secretion from magnocellular paraventricular nucleus (PVN) and supraoptic nucleus (SON) neurons. Projects to median preoptic nucleus to help control thirst • Angiotensin II stimulates OVLT (and subfornical organ), elevating blood pressure (BP) • Produces IL-1β during fever; helps provoke illness behavior • Responds to Na$^+$ and increases lumbar sympathetic and adrenal catecholamine reactivity, elevating BP
Subfornical organ	• Location: just below the fornix at rostral end of the third ventricle • Senses Na$^+$ concentration and dehydration; controls water intake • Excited by angiotensin II and cholecystokinin; influences water intake and BP, triggers drinking behavior • Angiotensin II may help to drive chronic hypertension • Responds to glucose during hyperglycemia • Responds to ghrelin to increase food intake, responds to satiety signal molecules amylin and leptin, providing a dual feeding response
Subcommissural organ (SCO)	• Location: dorsal caudal region of third ventricle, near the aqueduct • Ependymal cells produce transthyretin, which helps to move cerebrospinal fluid (CSF), transport thyroid hormone in the blood • Secretes transthyretin and other glycoproteins, and basic fibroblast growth factor into adult and fetal CSF; may regulate neuronal stem cell production, neuronal differentiation, and axonal growth and extension • Secretes basic fibroblast growth factor: a mitogenic factor and brain repair molecule • Secretes SCO-spondin: helps commissural axonal connectivity • May be involved in water balance • Receives extensive inputs from dopamine, norepinephrine, neuropeptides, CSF factors
Area postrema	• Location: at the inferior and posterior limit of fourth ventricle, near obex • Detects toxins in the blood, triggers nausea and vomiting; integrates humoral and neural signaling; a lesion prevents detection of poisons and vomiting response, impairs taste aversion • Integrates visceral information from vagal and sympathetic afferent inputs; area postrema connects with nucleus solitarius, triggers nausea and vomiting • Integrates cardiovascular, feeding, and metabolic responses, osmoregulation and electrolyte balance, and BP control • Responds to opiates to trigger nausea and vomiting • Transports many substances into and out of the CSF (as do tanycytes)
Pineal	• Location: in epithalamus, near the center of the brain • Pinealocytes synthesize melatonin (stimulated in dark, inhibited in light) • Melatonin synthesized from serotonin, through a rate-limiting enzyme (serotonin N-acetyl transferase), regulated by sympathetic norepinephrine input from superior cervical ganglion; pathway for control is retina to suprachiasmatic nucleus to PVN of the hypothalamus to preganglionic neurons in T1–T2 lateral horn or directly to pineal • Modulates sleep patterns in circadian rhythms and seasonal rhythms • Modulates follicle-stimulating hormone and luteinizing hormone as an "antigonadotropin" response • Exogenous melatonin may help to entrain new sleep patterns in jet lag • Brainstem parasympathetics and PVN and other hypothalamic nuclei may directly innervate the pineal, in addition to sympathetics
Median eminence	• Location: upper part of the infundibular stem (stalk); lacks neurons • Provides a contact zone of capillary loops onto which nerve terminals of the tuberoinfundibular tract secrete hypophysiotropic hormones (releasing and inhibitory factors for anterior pituitary hormones) into the hypophyseal-portal closed vascular system • Hypophysiotropic hormones: CRF, gonadotropin-releasing hormone, thyrotropin-releasing hormone, growth hormone–releasing hormone, dopamine (prolactin inhibitory factor), vasopressin, and many other neuromodulators
Neurohypophysis (posterior pituitary)	• Location: posterior region of the pituitary gland, beneath hypothalamus • A site where oxytocin and vasopressin are secreted by axon terminals from neurons of PVN and SON into the systemic circulation

16.15 CIRCUMVENTRICULAR ORGANS: FUNCTIONAL CONSIDERATIONS

Blood Supply of Hypothalamus and Pituitary Gland

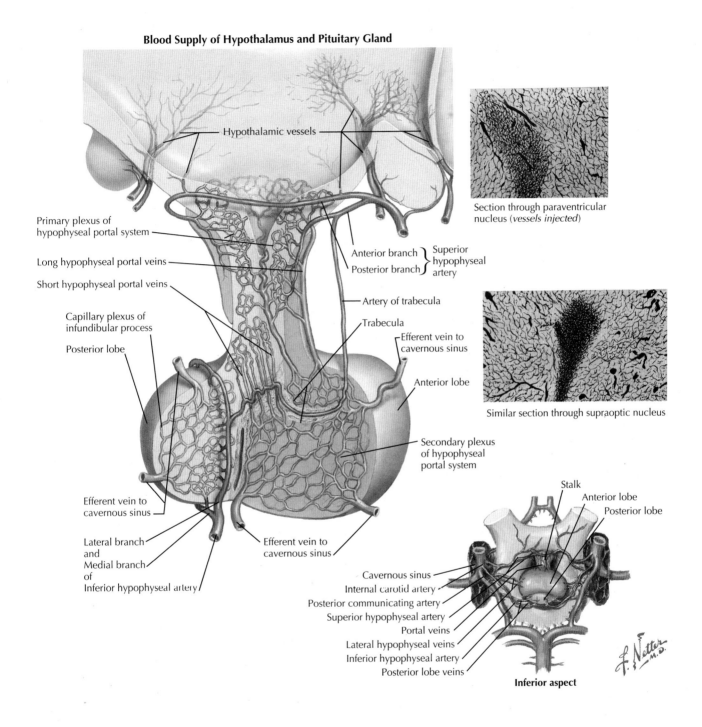

Hypothalamic vessels

Section through paraventricular nucleus (*vessels injected*)

Primary plexus of hypophyseal portal system

Long hypophyseal portal veins

Short hypophyseal portal veins

Capillary plexus of infundibular process

Posterior lobe

Anterior branch ⎫ Superior
Posterior branch ⎬ hypophyseal
　　　　　　　　⎭ artery

Artery of trabecula

Trabecula

Efferent vein to cavernous sinus

Anterior lobe

Similar section through supraoptic nucleus

Secondary plexus of hypophyseal portal system

Efferent vein to cavernous sinus

Lateral branch and Medial branch of Inferior hypophyseal artery

Efferent vein to cavernous sinus

Stalk
Anterior lobe
Posterior lobe

Cavernous sinus
Internal carotid artery
Posterior communicating artery
Superior hypophyseal artery
Portal veins
Lateral hypophyseal veins
Inferior hypophyseal artery
Posterior lobe veins

Inferior aspect

16.16 THE HYPOPHYSEAL PORTAL VASCULATURE

The hypophyseal portal vascular system derives from arterioles coming into the median eminence at the base of the hypothalamus. The primary capillary plexus is a site where releasing and inhibitory factors that influence the secretion of anterior pituitary hormones are released from axons (neurocrine secretion) whose neurons reside in the hypothalamus and other CNS sites. These releasing and inhibitory factors then travel through venules into the secondary capillary plexus in very high concentrations and act directly on anterior pituitary cells that synthesize and secrete the hormones of the anterior pituitary.

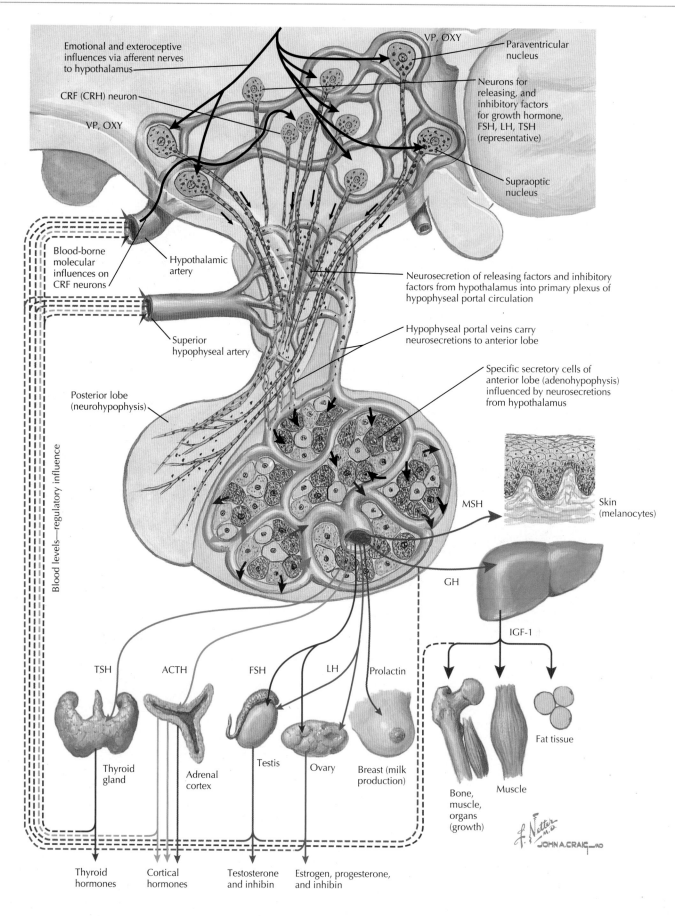

Emotional and exteroceptive
influences via afferent nerves
to hypothalamus

VP, OXY — Paraventricular nucleus

CRF (CRH) neuron

VP, OXY

Neurons for releasing, and inhibitory factors for growth hormone, FSH, LH, TSH (representative)

Supraoptic nucleus

Blood-borne molecular influences on CRF neurons

Hypothalamic artery

Neurosecretion of releasing factors and inhibitory factors from hypothalamus into primary plexus of hypophyseal portal circulation

Superior hypophyseal artery

Hypophyseal portal veins carry neurosecretions to anterior lobe

Specific secretory cells of anterior lobe (adenohypophysis) influenced by neurosecretions from hypothalamus

Posterior lobe (neurohypophysis)

Blood levels—regulatory influence

MSH — Skin (melanocytes)

GH

IGF-1

TSH   ACTH   FSH   LH   Prolactin

Testis   Ovary   Breast (milk production)

Fat tissue

Thyroid gland

Adrenal cortex

Bone, muscle, organs (growth)

Muscle

Thyroid hormones   Cortical hormones   Testosterone and inhibin   Estrogen, progesterone, and inhibin

16.17 REGULATION OF ANTERIOR PITUITARY HORMONE SECRETION

See next page.

16.17 REGULATION OF ANTERIOR PITUITARY HORMONE SECRETION

Neurons that synthesize releasing and inhibitory factors for control of anterior pituitary hormones send axons that terminate on the primary plexus of the hypophyseal portal system (the zone of neuroendocrine transduction) and release these factors into the hypophyseal portal blood. These factors then flow into the secondary hypophyseal portal plexus and regulate the release of anterior pituitary hormones. The major anterior pituitary hormones are thyroid-stimulating hormone (TSH), adrenal corticotropic hormone (ACTH), follicle-stimulating hormone (FSH), luteinizing hormone (LH), prolactin (LTH), growth hormone (GH), and melanocyte-stimulating hormone (MSH). These anterior pituitary hormones act on peripheral target organs to effect release of target organ hormones or to influence metabolic and functional activities. For example, CRF neurons release CRF (CRH, corticotropin-releasing hormone) into the hypophyseal portal blood, regulating the release of ACTH, which in turn regulates the release of cortisol from the adrenal cortex. Magnocellular neurons of the PVN and SON send axons directly to the posterior pituitary and release oxytocin and arginine vasopressin directly into the systemic circulation.

CLINICAL POINT

The term **hypopituitarism** refers to the deficiency or absence of one or more anterior **pituitary hormones**. The process of pituitary dysfunction can be very slow in onset because of the great reserve; more than 75% of the anterior pituitary must be destroyed before symptoms become evident. Pituitary damage may result from tumors, ischemia and infarction, infiltrative lesions (e.g., sarcoidosis), head injury, immunological damage during pregnancy, or other causes. With some tumors such as pituitary adenomas initial symptoms may occur because of disruption of releasing hormones, such as gonadotropin-releasing hormone (GnRH), leading to elevated secretion of prolactin, FSH, LH, and ACTH and cortisol, producing gonadal dysfunction. With progressive pituitary insufficiency, the first hormones to markedly fall generally are growth hormone (GH), which is highly conspicuous in children whose growth is impaired, and gonadotropins, causing amenorrhea in women and impotence or sexual dysfunction in men. At a later stage, impairment of TSH, ACTH, prolactin, and other hormones occurs; hormonal replacement therapy is necessary. Diabetes insipidus caused by posterior pituitary damage also may accompany pituitary insufficiency.

Many pituitary tumors secrete anterior pituitary hormones, leading to symptoms of **pituitary hypersecretion**. Prolactinomas (adenomas) result in excess prolactin secretion, gonadal dysfunction, and galactorrhea. GH-secreting adenomas result in gigantism if they are present before the epiphyseal plates of the long bones are closed and in acromegaly in adults, with soft tissue enlargement, enlarged hands and feet, and coarse facial features. ACTH-secreting adenomas lead to Cushing's disease. Pituitary tumors commonly impinge on the optic chiasm and produce bitemporal visual field defects (bitemporal hemianopia), usually starting in the upper outer fields.

CLINICAL POINT

The hypothalamus and anterior pituitary gland are subject to **extensive hormonal feedback**. In the **hypothalamo-pituitary-adrenal (HPA) axis**, cortisol acts via a negative long feedback loop to inhibit the secretion of both ACTH and CRH (CRF). ACTH acts via a short feedback loop to inhibit the secretion of CRH. Exogenous administration of corticosteroids also results in feedback inhibition of ACTH and CRH. High cortisol levels can result in hypertension, muscle weakness, mood alterations, polydipsia and polyuria, weight gain, moon-like facies, and other symptoms.

The **regulation of thyroid hormone secretion** involves hypothalamic thyrotropin-releasing hormone (TRH) stimulating the release of TSH from the anterior pituitary, which acts on the thyroid gland to stimulate the release of the thyroid hormones triiodothyronine (T3) and thyroxine (T4). T3 and T4 feed back on the anterior pituitary and hypothalamus to inhibit the secretion of TRH and TSH. Administration of exogenous thyroid hormone produces the same negative feedback loop. Thyroid-binding globulin (TBG) is a human protein that helps to transport T3 and T4 into the blood. Thus, thyroid hormones in the blood can be free T3 and T4 as well as bound T3 and T4.

Sex steroids are regulated through the hypothalamus and the anterior pituitary. Hypothalamic GnRH stimulates the release of LH and FSH from the anterior pituitary, which act on the testes in males to produce testosterone and on the ovaries in females to produce estradiol and progesterone, which regulate menstruation and the reproductive cycle. Long-term exogenous testosterone in males may exert initial desirable effects on muscle mass, libido, and other characteristics but also may act in a negative manner to diminish spermatogenesis, shrink the testes, increase the risk of clotting, and increase the risk of strokes and heart attacks.

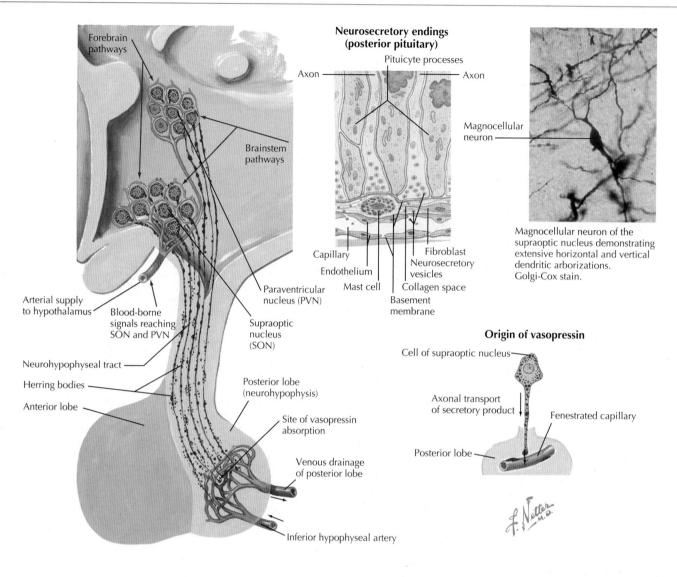

Neurosecretory endings (posterior pituitary)

Pituicyte processes

Axon — — Axon

Magnocellular neuron

Capillary
Endothelium
Mast cell
Fibroblast
Neurosecretory vesicles
Collagen space
Basement membrane

Paraventricular nucleus (PVN)

Supraoptic nucleus (SON)

Arterial supply to hypothalamus

Blood-borne signals reaching SON and PVN

Neurohypophyseal tract

Herring bodies

Anterior lobe

Posterior lobe (neurohypophysis)

Site of vasopressin absorption

Venous drainage of posterior lobe

Inferior hypophyseal artery

Magnocellular neuron of the supraoptic nucleus demonstrating extensive horizontal and vertical dendritic arborizations. Golgi-Cox stain.

Origin of vasopressin

Cell of supraoptic nucleus

Axonal transport of secretory product

Fenestrated capillary

Posterior lobe

16.18 POSTERIOR PITUITARY (NEUROHYPOPHYSEAL) HORMONES: OXYTOCIN AND VASOPRESSIN

Magnocellular neurons in the paraventricular nucleus (PVN) and supraoptic nucleus (SON) send axons directly through the infundibular region and the pituitary stalk to terminate on the vasculature in the posterior pituitary. Neurons from both nuclei synthesize and release oxytocin and arginine vasopressin into the systemic vasculature. Brainstem and forebrain pathways terminate on the magnocellular neurons and regulate their secretion of oxytocin and vasopressin. These magnocellular neurons possess extensive protein synthesis capacity and transport the vesicles in which their hormones are packaged to the axon terminals with very fast axoplasmic transport. The hormones are released from the terminals and diffuse through the fenestrated capillaries directly into the systemic vasculature (see inset of neurosecretory efferent endings from magnocellular neurons in PVN and SON).

CLINICAL POINT

The SON and magnocellular neurons of the PVN of the hypothalamus synthesize and secrete both oxytocin and arginine vasopressin (antidiuretic hormone, or ADH), along with their neurophysin

carrier proteins. A majority of vasopressin comes from the SON, and a majority of oxytocin comes from magnocellular PVN. These neuronal groups send axons (the supraopticohypophyseal tract) into the posterior pituitary, where they terminate on fenestrated capillaries and secrete their hormones directly into the systemic circulation. These neurons are called neuroendocrine transducer cells. Oxytocin cells respond to estrogen and to afferent signals caused by suckling, and they stimulate milk let-down (milk ejection reflex) and uterine contraction in pregnancy. Vasopressin neurons respond to changes in blood osmolarity, secreting vasopressin in the presence of high osmolarity. This causes the collecting tubules in the kidney to increase water resorption and prevent diuresis. If the supraopticohypophyseal tract or associated neurons (seen in congenital disorders) are damaged, as happens with pituitary stalk sectioning, diabetes insipidus results. **Diabetes insipidus** involves the loss of vasopressin secretion and the production of huge amounts (10+ liters per day) of dilute urine, provoking marked polydipsia. Vasopressin replacement therapy is necessary. Alcohol consumption, some antiseizure drugs (phenytoin), and anticholinergic agents may also inhibit vasopressin secretion. Excessive vasopressin secretion (called **inappropriate secretion of ADH, or SIADH**) may occur because of partial damage to the hypothalamus, a vasopressin-secreting tumor in the periphery (e.g., lung carcinoma), or as the result of treatment by chemotherapeutic and other pharmacological agents. SIADH results in hypo-osmolar serum, hyponatremia, and high urine osmolarity.

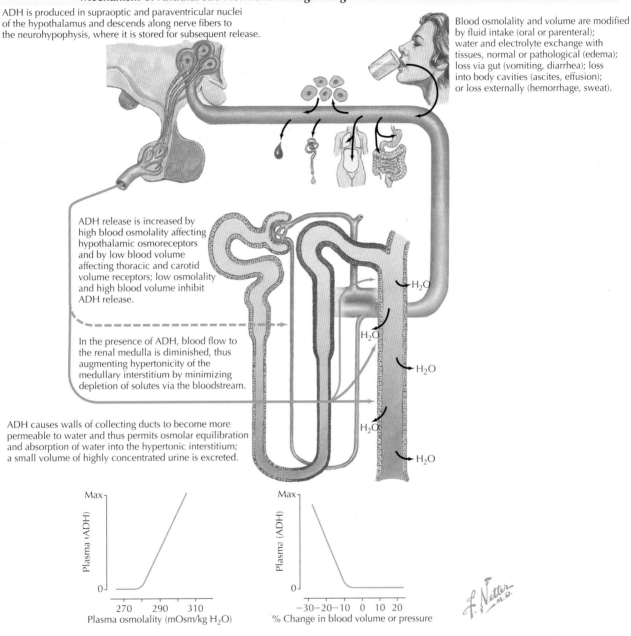

Mechanism of Antidiuretic Hormone in Regulating Urine Volume and Concentration

ADH is produced in supraoptic and paraventricular nuclei of the hypothalamus and descends along nerve fibers to the neurohypophysis, where it is stored for subsequent release.

Blood osmolality and volume are modified by fluid intake (oral or parenteral); water and electrolyte exchange with tissues, normal or pathological (edema); loss via gut (vomiting, diarrhea); loss into body cavities (ascites, effusion); or loss externally (hemorrhage, sweat).

ADH release is increased by high blood osmolality affecting hypothalamic osmoreceptors and by low blood volume affecting thoracic and carotid volume receptors; low osmolality and high blood volume inhibit ADH release.

In the presence of ADH, blood flow to the renal medulla is diminished, thus augmenting hypertonicity of the medullary interstitium by minimizing depletion of solutes via the bloodstream.

ADH causes walls of collecting ducts to become more permeable to water and thus permits osmolar equilibration and absorption of water into the hypertonic interstitium; a small volume of highly concentrated urine is excreted.

H_2O

Plasma (ADH) — Max — 0
270 290 310
Plasma osmolality (mOsm/kg H_2O)

Plasma (ADH) — Max — 0
−30 −20 −10 0 10 20
% Change in blood volume or pressure

16.19 VASOPRESSIN (ANTIDIURETIC HORMONE) REGULATION OF WATER BALANCE AND FLUID OSMOLALITY

Vasopressin regulates the volume of water secreted by the kidneys. Its secretion is regulated by the osmolality of body fluids and by blood volume and pressure. Changes in body fluid osmolality of a small percentage are sufficient to significantly alter vasopressin secretion.

Decreases in blood volume and pressure of 10% to 15% or more are needed to affect vasopressin secretion. The blood volume and pressure sensors are found in the large pulmonary vessels, the carotid sinus, and the aortic arch. These baroreceptors respond to the stretching of the vessel wall, which is dependent on blood volume and pressure. The figure shows the mechanisms of action of vasopressin on the kidney, with resultant effects on urine volume and concentration.

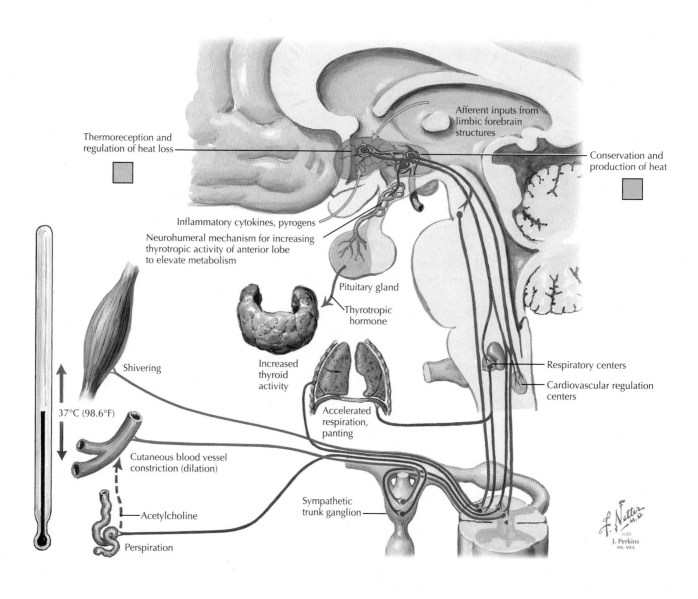

Thermoreception and regulation of heat loss

Afferent inputs from limbic forebrain structures

Conservation and production of heat

Inflammatory cytokines, pyrogens

Neurohumeral mechanism for increasing thyrotropic activity of anterior lobe to elevate metabolism

Pituitary gland

Thyrotropic hormone

Increased thyroid activity

Respiratory centers

Cardiovascular regulation centers

Shivering

37°C (98.6°F)

Accelerated respiration, panting

Cutaneous blood vessel constriction (dilation)

Acetylcholine

Sympathetic trunk ganglion

Perspiration

16.20 THE HYPOTHALAMUS AND THERMOREGULATION

The preoptic area of the hypothalamus contains heat-sensitive neurons, and the posterior hypothalamic area contains cold-sensitive neurons. The preoptic area and the anterior hypothalamic area initiate neuronal responses for heat dissipation (parasympathetic); the posterior hypothalamic area initiates neuronal responses for heat generation (sympathetic). Neuronal pathways arising from the brainstem and limbic forebrain areas can modulate the activity of these thermoregulatory systems. The preoptic area is responsive to pyrogens and the inflammatory cytokine IL-1β; this area can generate an increased set point for temperature regulation, thus initiating a disease-associated fever. Extensive hypothalamic connections with the brainstem and spinal cord are used to initiate appropriate heat-dissipation or heat-generation responses. Appropriate behavioral responses also are initiated to optimize thermoregulation (e.g., going to a warmer or cooler location).

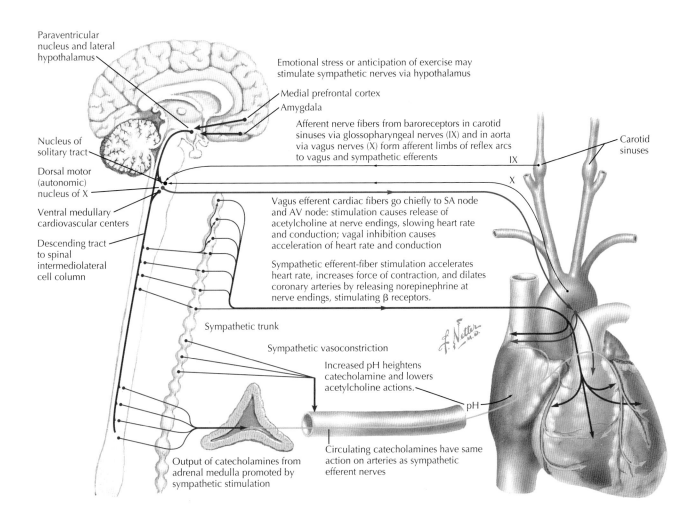

Paraventricular nucleus and lateral hypothalamus

Emotional stress or anticipation of exercise may stimulate sympathetic nerves via hypothalamus

Medial prefrontal cortex

Amygdala

Afferent nerve fibers from baroreceptors in carotid sinuses via glossopharyngeal nerves (IX) and in aorta via vagus nerves (X) form afferent limbs of reflex arcs to vagus and sympathetic efferents

Carotid sinuses

Nucleus of solitary tract

Dorsal motor (autonomic) nucleus of X

Ventral medullary cardiovascular centers

Descending tract to spinal intermediolateral cell column

IX

X

Vagus efferent cardiac fibers go chiefly to SA node and AV node: stimulation causes release of acetylcholine at nerve endings, slowing heart rate and conduction; vagal inhibition causes acceleration of heart rate and conduction

Sympathetic efferent-fiber stimulation accelerates heart rate, increases force of contraction, and dilates coronary arteries by releasing norepinephrine at nerve endings, stimulating β receptors.

Sympathetic trunk

Sympathetic vasoconstriction

Increased pH heightens catecholamine and lowers acetylcholine actions.

pH

Output of catecholamines from adrenal medulla promoted by sympathetic stimulation

Circulating catecholamines have same action on arteries as sympathetic efferent nerves

16.21 HYPOTHALAMIC REGULATION OF CARDIAC FUNCTION

Regulation of cardiovascular (CV) function by the brain involves several domains of neuronal control. In the forebrain, medial prefrontal cortex, limbic cortical areas, and amygdaloid nuclei mediate emotional and behavioral responses and influence cardiovascular function. These forebrain areas act through projections to the hypothalamus (lateral hypothalamic area, paraventricular nucleus, preoptic and anterior hypothalamic areas for parasympathetic control, and the posterior hypothalamic area for sympathetic control).

These hypothalamic regulatory regions send projections to many brainstem sites, including the parabrachial nuclei, ventral medullary cardiovascular centers, nucleus solitarius, the dorsal

motor (autonomic) nucleus or X, and the intermediolateral cell column of the thoracic spinal cord lateral horn.

The parabrachial nuclei also respond to visceral afferent input and nociceptive input to regulate CV responses to pain, respiratory challenges, and gastrointestinal activity. The ventromedial CV medullary area generates CV responses needed for thermogenesis, and the ventrolateral CV medullary area helps to maintain blood pressure and CV responses during an upright posture and is responsive to baroreceptor reflexes.

The nucleus solitarius is a major integrative center for descending (limbic and hypothalamic), local brainstem, and ascending regulation of autonomic preganglionic responses (dorsal motor [autonomic] nucleus of X for parasympathetic, intermediolateral cell column for sympathetic).

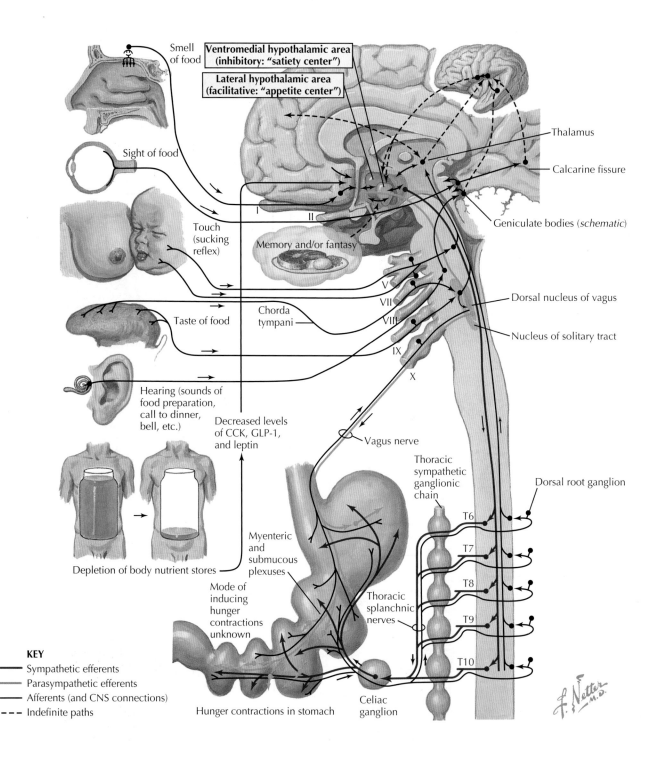

Smell of food

Ventromedial hypothalamic area (inhibitory: "satiety center")

Lateral hypothalamic area (facilitative: "appetite center")

Thalamus

Calcarine fissure

Sight of food

Geniculate bodies (*schematic*)

Touch (sucking reflex)

Memory and/or fantasy

Dorsal nucleus of vagus

Chorda tympani

Nucleus of solitary tract

Taste of food

Hearing (sounds of food preparation, call to dinner, bell, etc.)

Decreased levels of CCK, GLP-1, and leptin

Vagus nerve

Thoracic sympathetic ganglionic chain

Dorsal root ganglion

T6

T7

T8

T9

T10

Depletion of body nutrient stores

Myenteric and submucous plexuses

Mode of inducing hunger contractions unknown

Thoracic splanchnic nerves

KEY
— Sympathetic efferents
— Parasympathetic efferents
— Afferents (and CNS connections)
---- Indefinite paths

Hunger contractions in stomach

Celiac ganglion

16.24 NEURAL CONTROL OF APPETITE AND HUNGER

The sensations of hunger and satiety are complex and include multiple neural pathways and circulating hormones. This figure depicts pathways involved in the sensation of hunger. Although our understanding is incomplete, the hypothalamus is known to play a critical role in controlling appetite and food intake. When food is ingested, cholecystokinin (CCK) and glucagon-like peptide (GLP-1) are released from neuroendocrine cells in the intestine. These hormones suppress appetite and give the sensation of satiety. In the absence of food, the levels of these hormones are low. Long-term regulation of food intake involves the hormone leptin, which is produced by fat cells. When fat stores are high, leptin is released and appears to act on the hypothalamus to suppress appetite. When body nutrient stores are depleted, leptin levels are low. Other hormones such as ghrelins also are involved with control of hunger and satiety. Both the cerebral cortex and limbic forebrain structures have regulatory connections with this hypothalamic circuitry, permitting cognitive and emotional factors to influence appetite and eating behavior.

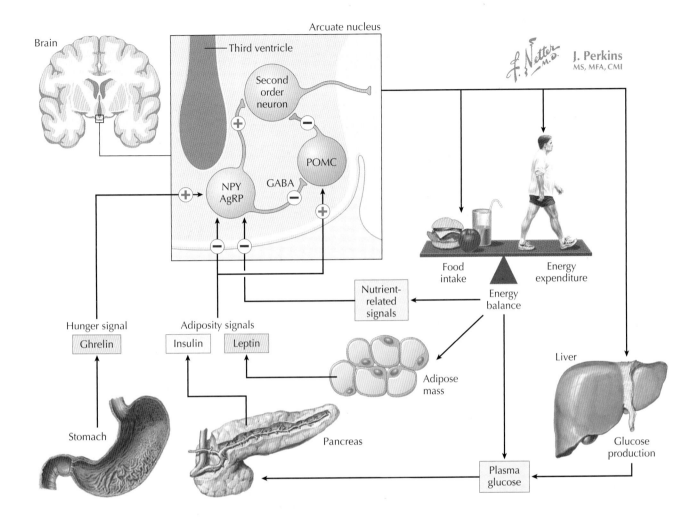

16.25 SIGNALING SYSTEMS INVOLVED IN REGULATION OF FOOD INTAKE, BODY WEIGHT, AND METABOLISM

The hypothalamus regulates food intake, body weight, and metabolism. The hormone ghrelin is produced by the gastric mucosa of the stomach when it is empty and stimulates cells in the arcuate nucleus of the hypothalamus to bring about increased food intake. The hormone leptin is made by white adipose tissue during robust metabolic activity and also acts on cells in the arcuate nucleus. High levels of ghrelin and low levels of leptin stimulate food intake, but high levels of leptin do not suppress eating activity.

Ghrelin and leptin have access to the arcuate nucleus neurons through the hypophyseal portal vessels, which are devoid of a blood-brain barrier. These hormones act on cells of the arcuate nucleus that use neuropeptide Y (NPY) and agouti-related protein (AgRP) as neurotransmitters. These arcuate neurons act through connections in the hypothalamus with the paraventricular nucleus, ventromedial nucleus, dorsomedial nucleus, and lateral hypothalamic area, and with descending connections with the parabrachial nuclei, and can activate feeding behavior.

Other neurons in the arcuate nucleus, using proopiomelanocortin (POMC) derivatives such as alphamelanocyte-stimulating hormone and beta-endorphin, have connections with these same hypothalamic and brainstem targets and can suppress feeding behavior. Circadian-related circuits from the suprachiasmatic nucleus project to these same hypothalamic nuclei, superimposing circadian influences on feeding behavior.

Superimposed on this circuitry are limbic and cortical connections, including olfactory projections, which can provide emotional, behavioral, or volitional components to the control of food intake and appetite.

Ascending arousal pathways

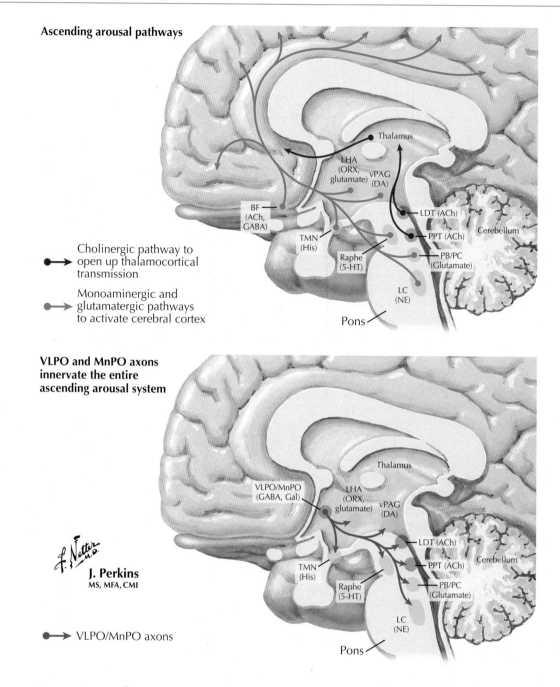

→ Cholinergic pathway to
open up thalamocortical
transmission

→ Monoaminergic and
glutamatergic pathways
to activate cerebral cortex

**VLPO and MnPO axons
innervate the entire
ascending arousal system**

J. Netter M.D.

J. Perkins
MS, MFA, CMI

→ VLPO/MnPO axons

16.26 HYPOTHALAMIC REGULATION OF SLEEP AND WAKING STATES

The state of alertness or wakefulness is dependent on neuronal systems that originate from the rostral pons and caudal midbrain and include cholinergic neurons (pedunculopontine tegmental nucleus [PPT] and the laterodorsal tegmental nucleus [LDT]), noradrenergic neurons (locus coeruleus), serotonergic neurons (dorsal raphe nucleus, central superior nucleus), dopamine neurons (ventral periaqueductal gray), histaminergic neurons (tuberomammillary nucleus), and glutaminergic neurons (parabrachial nucleus, pre-coeruleus nucleus). Projections from this collection of chemically specific neurons funnel into the lateral hypothalamic area and are joined by axons originating from this area (orexin neurons and glutaminergic neurons). This array of axons then is joined in the basal forebrain by cholinergic and

γ-aminobutyric acid (GABA)-ergic neurons to collectively activate cortical neurons for processing information. The more caudal cholinergic projections inhibit the sheet-like reticular nucleus of the thalamus, which helps to activate the thalamic relay nuclei projecting to the cortex.

During sleep, the activity of these multiple pathways diminishes. During REM sleep, some cholinergic and glutaminergic neurons demonstrate rapid firing, while the monoaminergic neurons cease firing.

Sleep is regulated by hypothalamic neurons in the median preoptic (MnPO) nucleus and ventrolateral preoptic (VLPO) nucleus, whose neurons begin firing at the onset of sleep. VLPO communicates with the ascending systems above, using GABA and galanin to diminish arousal.

Neural, Neuroendocrine and Systemic Components of Rage Reaction

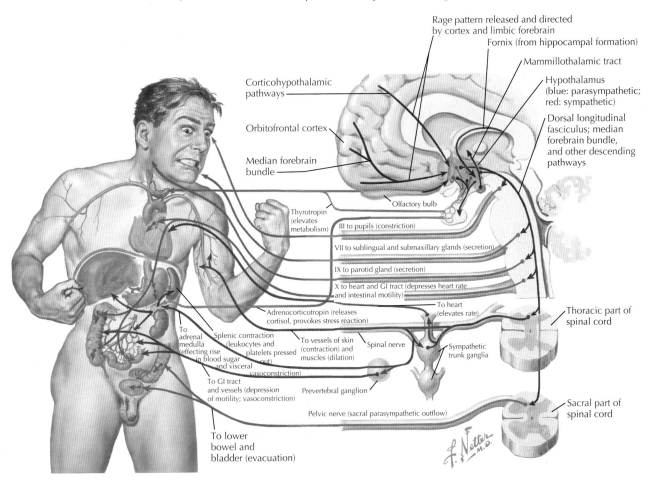

Rage pattern released and directed by cortex and limbic forebrain

Fornix (from hippocampal formation)

Mammillothalamic tract

Hypothalamus (blue: parasympathetic; red: sympathetic)

Dorsal longitudinal fasciculus; median forebrain bundle, and other descending pathways

Corticohypothalamic pathways

Orbitofrontal cortex

Median forebrain bundle

Olfactory bulb

Thyrotropin (elevates metabolism)

III to pupils (constriction)

VII to sublingual and submaxillary glands (secretion)

IX to parotid gland (secretion)

X to heart and GI tract (depresses heart rate and intestinal motility)

To heart (elevates rate)

Thoracic part of spinal cord

Adrenocorticotropin (releases cortisol, provokes stress reaction)

To adrenal medulla (effecting rise in blood sugar and visceral vasoconstriction)

Splenic contraction (leukocytes and platelets pressed out)

To vessels of skin (contraction) and muscles (dilation)

Spinal nerve

Sympathetic trunk ganglia

To GI tract and vessels (depression of motility; vasoconstriction)

Prevertebral ganglion

Pelvic nerve (sacral parasympathetic outflow)

Sacral part of spinal cord

To lower bowel and bladder (evacuation)

16.27 NEURAL AND NEUROENDOCRINE ROLES IN THE FIGHT-OR-FLIGHT RESPONSE

The classic sympathetic fight-or-flight response, shown here as a rage response, involves the secretion of neuroendocrine "stress hormones," including cortisol from the hypothalamo-pituitary-adrenal (HPA) axis and norepinephrine and epinephrine from sympathetic nerve terminals and the adrenal medulla. Sympathetic connections with the viscera initiate physiological changes to support the integrated fight-or-flight response. These changes include diversion of blood from the viscera and skin to the muscles, increased heart rate and cardiac output and contractility, bronchodilation, pupillary dilation, decreased gastrointestinal activation, decreased renal activity, glycogenolysis from the liver with increased blood glucose for fuel, and many other actions. Inputs from limbic forebrain regions, the cerebral cortex, and the brainstem regulate the complex hypothalamic control of neuroendocrine and autonomic outflow and are key in initiating the classic fight-or-flight response. In this response, the brainstem parasympathetic neurons are inhibited.

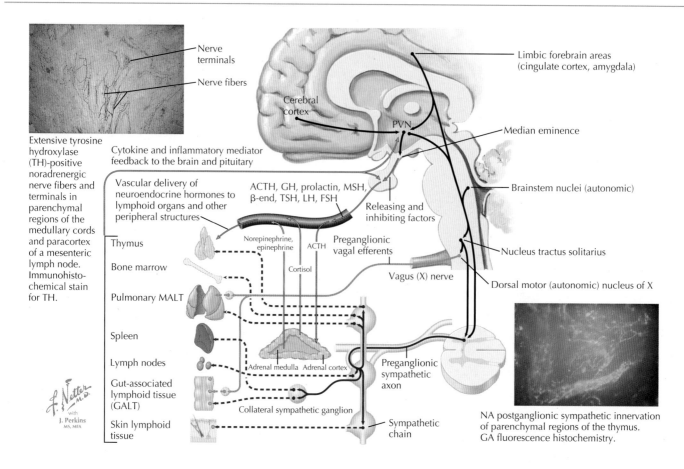

Extensive tyrosine hydroxylase (TH)-positive noradrenergic nerve fibers and terminals in parenchymal regions of the medullary cords and paracortex of a mesenteric lymph node. Immunohistochemical stain for TH.

Nerve terminals

Nerve fibers

Cytokine and inflammatory mediator feedback to the brain and pituitary

Vascular delivery of neuroendocrine hormones to lymphoid organs and other peripheral structures

ACTH, GH, prolactin, MSH, β-end, TSH, LH, FSH

Releasing and inhibiting factors

Cerebral cortex

PVN

Limbic forebrain areas (cingulate cortex, amygdala)

Median eminence

Brainstem nuclei (autonomic)

Nucleus tractus solitarius

Dorsal motor (autonomic) nucleus of X

Thymus

Bone marrow

Pulmonary MALT

Spleen

Lymph nodes

Gut-associated lymphoid tissue (GALT)

Skin lymphoid tissue

Norepinephrine, epinephrine

ACTH

Cortisol

Adrenal medulla   Adrenal cortex

Collateral sympathetic ganglion

Preganglionic vagal efferents

Vagus (X) nerve

Preganglionic sympathetic axon

Sympathetic chain

NA postganglionic sympathetic innervation of parenchymal regions of the thymus. GA fluorescence histochemistry.

16.28 NEUROIMMUNOMODULATION

Connections from the cerebral cortex, limbic forebrain, hypothalamus, and brainstem can exert extensive modulation of autonomic preganglionic outflow and neuroendocrine outflow. Hormones and neurotransmitters from this outflow target lymphoid organs and cells of the immune system. This circuitry provides the substrate for behavior, emotional responsiveness, chronic stressors, and positive complementary and behavioral interventions to influence immune responses. Sympathetic postganglionic noradrenergic fibers directly innervate virtually all organs of the immune system, including (1) primary lymphoid organs (bone marrow, thymus), (2) secondary lymphoid organs (spleen, lymph nodes), (3) mucosa-associated lymphoid organs (gut and lung), and (4) skin-associated lymphoid cells. Vagal postganglionic nerve fibers innervate pulmonary- and gut-associated lymphoid tissue. Pituitary hormones in the circulation (e.g., CRF, ACTH, prolactin, GH, endorphins) and their target organ hormones (cortisol, thyroid hormone) modulate immune reactivity in all lymphoid organs. Cortisol, norepinephrine, and epinephrine are particularly important in mediating chronic stress responses related to immune reactivity. Circulating and local cytokines and inflammatory mediators act on the brain and pituitary to provide feedback information from lymphoid organs (immune-neural signaling) and can modulate CNS neurotransmitter turnover, inflammatory responses, and illness behavior. The gene expression of hormones from secretory cells, cytokines from cells of the immune system, and neurotransmitters from neurons innervating lymphoid organs can be regulated by the presence of multiple signal molecules in the local environment. Some mediators are produced by neurons, paracrine cells, and cells of the immune system and modulate all of these systems. GALT, gut-associated lymphoid tissue; MALT, mucosa-associated lymphoid tissue.

CLINICAL POINT

The **PVN of the hypothalamus** is a key regulatory site for neural modulation of immune responses; it acts through both hormonal secretion and autonomic regulation. The principal neural outflow systems that act on peripheral immunocytes are the HPA axis and the SNS connections to organs of the immune system and secretion into the general circulation. Activation of the HPA and the SNS can block some immune defenses, leading to greater susceptibility to viral infections (10-fold in experimental models of murine influenza). Other anterior pituitary hormones also exert immunomodulatory effects. Chronic stressors can influence neural-immune outflow via cortical and limbic connections to the hypothalamus (especially the PVN); chronic stressors exert both HPA and SNS effects that produce diminished cell-mediated immunity and natural killer cell activity. Both immune-inhibiting and immune-enhancing responses can be classically conditioned, a process that requires forebrain involvement and subsequent neural and hormonal outflow (but not cortisol; conditioned immunosuppression occurs in adrenalectomized animals). Both circulating cytokines and endogenous brain cytokines, including IL-1β, IL-6, and TNF-α, can act on the PVN and other CNS sites involved in neuroendocrine and SNS outflow to immune targets, markedly activating cortisol production and catecholamine secretion. In adults, the regulation of secretion of dangerous inflammatory mediators as well as behavioral and lifestyle influences on the HPA axis and SNS may be important components of maintaining robust antiviral and antitumor immunity (anti-metastatic spread) and may aid in protection from many chronic diseases. These mediators are key components targeted in integrative medical treatment, directed toward enhancing PSNS activity and diminishing SNS activity.

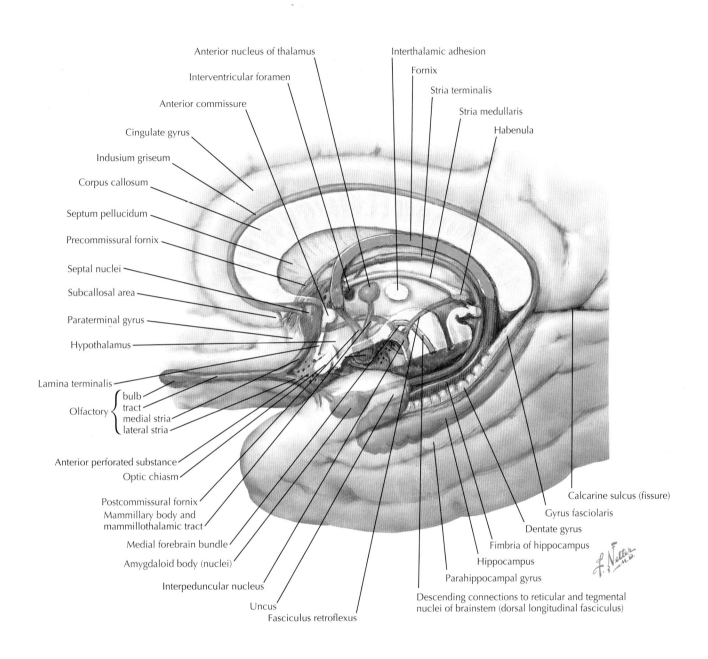

Anterior nucleus of thalamus

Interventricular foramen

Anterior commissure

Cingulate gyrus

Indusium griseum

Corpus callosum

Septum pellucidum

Precommissural fornix

Septal nuclei

Subcallosal area

Paraterminal gyrus

Hypothalamus

Lamina terminalis

Olfactory { bulb / tract / medial stria / lateral stria

Anterior perforated substance

Optic chiasm

Postcommissural fornix

Mammillary body and mammillothalamic tract

Medial forebrain bundle

Amygdaloid body (nuclei)

Interpeduncular nucleus

Uncus

Fasciculus retroflexus

Interthalamic adhesion

Fornix

Stria terminalis

Stria medullaris

Habenula

Calcarine sulcus (fissure)

Gyrus fasciolaris

Dentate gyrus

Fimbria of hippocampus

Hippocampus

Parahippocampal gyrus

Descending connections to reticular and tegmental nuclei of brainstem (dorsal longitudinal fasciculus)

LIMBIC SYSTEM

16.29 ANATOMY OF THE LIMBIC FOREBRAIN

Structures of the limbic forebrain are found in a ring (limbus) that encircles the diencephalon. Two major temporal lobe structures, the hippocampal formation with its fornix and the amygdala with its stria terminalis, send C-shaped axonal projections through the forebrain, around the diencephalon, and into the hypothalamus and septal region. The amygdala also has a more direct pathway (the ventral amygdalofugal pathway) into the hypothalamus. The septal nuclei sit just rostral to the hypothalamus and send axons to the habenular nuclei via the stria medullaris thalami. The cingulate, prefrontal, orbito-frontal, entorhinal, and periamygdaloid areas of the cortex interconnect with subcortical and hippocampal components of the limbic forebrain and are often considered part of the limbic system. The limbic system is thought to be a major substrate for regulation of emotional responsiveness and behavior, for individualized reactivity to sensory stimuli and internal stimuli, and for integrated memory tasks.

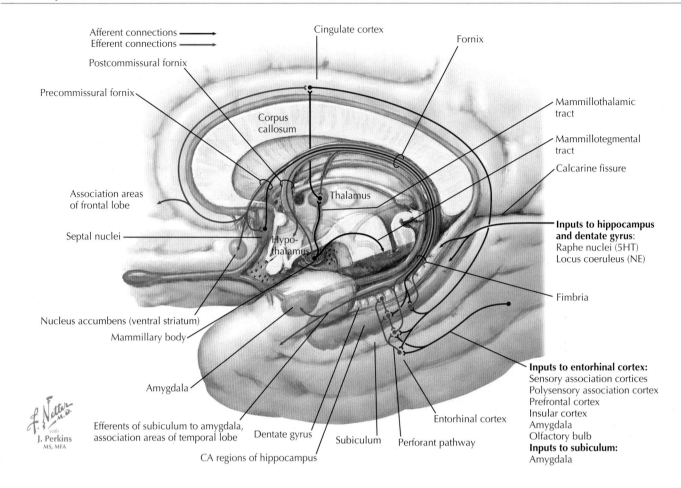

Afferent connections ⟶
Efferent connections ⟶

Postcommissural fornix

Precommissural fornix

Cingulate cortex

Fornix

Corpus callosum

Mammillothalamic tract

Mammillotegmental tract

Calcarine fissure

Association areas of frontal lobe

Thalamus

Septal nuclei

Inputs to hippocampus and dentate gyrus:
Raphe nuclei (5HT)
Locus coeruleus (NE)

Hypo-thalamus

Fimbria

Nucleus accumbens (ventral striatum)

Mammillary body

Amygdala

Inputs to entorhinal cortex:
Sensory association cortices
Polysensory association cortex
Prefrontal cortex
Insular cortex
Amygdala
Olfactory bulb
Inputs to subiculum:
Amygdala

Efferents of subiculum to amygdala, association areas of temporal lobe

Dentate gyrus

Subiculum

Entorhinal cortex

Perforant pathway

CA regions of hippocampus

16.32 MAJOR AFFERENT AND EFFERENT CONNECTIONS OF THE HIPPOCAMPAL FORMATION

Pyramidal neurons in the subiculum and hippocampal regions CA1 and CA3 give rise to the efferent fornix. The subiculum projects axons to hypothalamic nuclei (especially mammillary nuclei) and thalamic nuclei via the postcommissural fornix. CA1 and CA3 of the hippocampus send axons to the septal nuclei, the nucleus accumbens, the preoptic and anterior hypothalamic regions, the cingulate cortex, and association areas of the frontal lobe. Afferent cholinergic axons from septal nuclei traverse the fornix to supply the dentate gyrus and hippocampal CA regions. Massive inputs arrive in the hippocampal formation from sensory association cortices, polysensory association cortices, the prefrontal cortex, the insular cortex, the amygdaloid nuclei, and the olfactory bulb via projections to the entorhinal cortex. The entorhinal cortex is fully integrated into the internal circuitry of the hippocampal formation. The subiculum is connected reciprocally with the amygdala and also sends axons to cortical association areas of the temporal lobe. 5HT, 5-hydroxytryptamine [serotonin]; NE, norepinephrine.

CLINICAL POINT

Explicit memory is acquisition of information about objects, stimuli, and information that is consciously noted and recallable, and it includes information about personal events, factual knowledge, and information about which cognitive assessment takes place. **Explicit memory** involves structures in the medial temporal lobe, including the hippocampal formation. Implicit memory is the process of learning how to perform tasks or acquire skills that are not recallable by conscious processes; this form of memory depends upon other brain circuitry and is not lost in classic cases of hippocampal lesions. Explicit memory recall depends upon reassembly of information stored in the brain and involves reconstruction that depends upon sensory perceptions. It is not a video record of the precise external events and can be markedly different from reality, which raises serious questions about the accuracy of "recovered memory" of past events. Explicit memory requires the formation of new synaptic connections and gene expression for new sets of neuronal proteins. The consolidation of immediate and short-term explicit memory into long-term traces involves a process of **long-term potentiation**, which involves a burst of activity in a specific temporal pattern from an incoming axon that enhances the likelihood that the target neuron will be activated by this same input and other incoming inputs, providing an increased response to the same magnitude of excitation. Thus, a brief, sustained pattern of input makes it more likely that future synaptic activity will occur. Long-term potentiation occurs in dentate granule cells, CA1 neurons, and CA3 neurons. In the former two neurons, it requires N-methyl-D-aspartate receptor activation, depolarization, Ca^{++} influx, and communication between pre- and postsynaptic elements. In CA3 neurons, long-term potentiation depends on presynaptic Ca^{++} influx and subsequent cyclic adenosine monophosphate–dependent protein kinase production.

Afferent and efferent cortical connections of entorhinal cortex

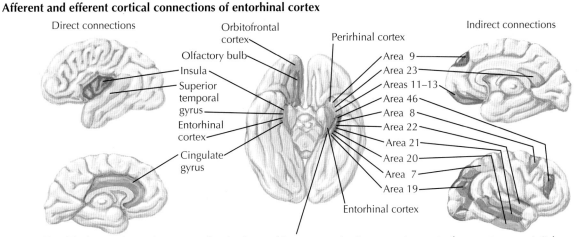

Direct connections

Orbitofrontal cortex

Olfactory bulb

Insula

Superior temporal gyrus

Entorhinal cortex

Cingulate gyrus

Perirhinal cortex

Indirect connections

Area 9
Area 23
Areas 11–13
Area 46
Area 8
Area 22
Area 21
Area 20
Area 7
Area 19

Entorhinal cortex

Entorhinal cortex is a major source of projections to hippocampus (major processing center for recent memory). Polysensory association cortices project directly to entorhinal cortex or indirectly via perirhinal cortex or parahippocampal gyrus. Association cortices receive reciprocal projections from entorhinal cortex. Area numbers refer to Brodmann classifications.

Possible processing circuit for recent memory

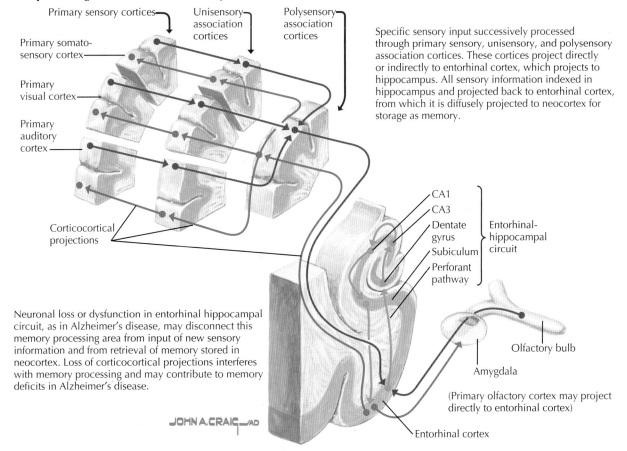

Primary sensory cortices

Unisensory association cortices

Polysensory association cortices

Primary somato-sensory cortex

Primary visual cortex

Primary auditory cortex

Corticocortical projections

CA1
CA3
Dentate gyrus
Subiculum
Perforant pathway

Entorhinal-hippocampal circuit

Olfactory bulb

Amygdala

(Primary olfactory cortex may project directly to entorhinal cortex)

Entorhinal cortex

Specific sensory input successively processed through primary sensory, unisensory, and polysensory association cortices. These cortices project directly or indirectly to entorhinal cortex, which projects to hippocampus. All sensory information indexed in hippocampus and projected back to entorhinal cortex, from which it is diffusely projected to neocortex for storage as memory.

Neuronal loss or dysfunction in entorhinal hippocampal circuit, as in Alzheimer's disease, may disconnect this memory processing area from input of new sensory information and from retrieval of memory stored in neocortex. Loss of corticocortical projections interferes with memory processing and may contribute to memory deficits in Alzheimer's disease.

JOHN A. CRAIG—AD

16.33 AFFERENT AND EFFERENT CONNECTIONS OF THE ENTORHINAL CORTEX

The entorhinal cortex is located in the medial temporal lobe and is integrated into the hippocampal formation circuitry related to memory formation and consolidation and declarative and spatial memory.

Afferents project to the entorhinal cortex from both cortical and subcortical sources. Cortical inputs include the association cortex (from all sensory modalities), perirhinal cortex, parahippocampal cortex, orbitofrontal and prefrontal cortex, cingulate cortex, and the hippocampus (to layers V and VI). Subcortical inputs derive from the septal region (especially the cholinergic medial septal nucleus via the fornix), basal forebrain (substantia innominate, nucleus of the diagonal band, the olfactory bulb), amygdala (basolateral nuclei), claustrum, thalamus (mainly midline nuclei), and brainstem monoaminergic nuclei (dopaminergic ventral tegmental area, noradrenergic locus coeruleus, and serotonergic rostral raphe nuclei).

Efferent projections are directed to components of hippocampal circuitry, polysensory association cortex, and subcortical regions. For hippocampal circuitry, neurons in layer II project to the dentate gyrus and the CA3 region, and neurons in layer III project to the CA1 region and the subiculum. Efferents to subcortical regions project to the claustrum, nucleus accumbens, and thalamus (medial dorsal nucleus, lateral dorsal nucleus, medial pulvinar).

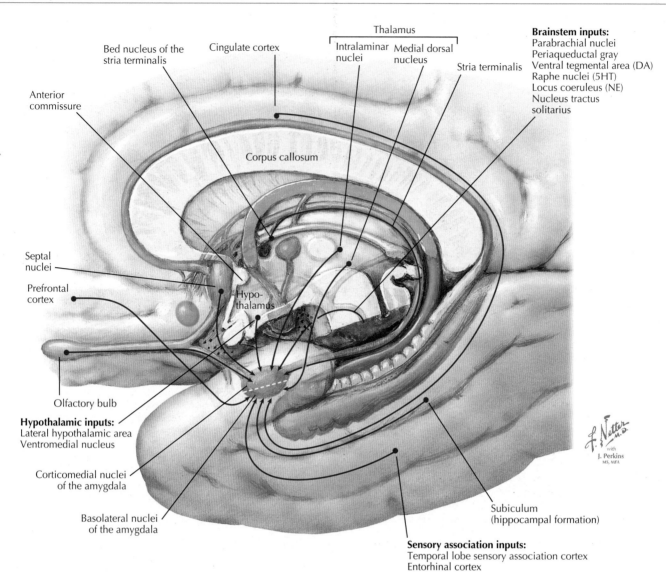

Brainstem inputs:
Parabrachial nuclei
Periaqueductal gray
Ventral tegmental area (DA)
Raphe nuclei (5HT)
Locus coeruleus (NE)
Nucleus tractus solitarius

Thalamus
Intralaminar nuclei   Medial dorsal nucleus
Stria terminalis

Cingulate cortex

Bed nucleus of the stria terminalis

Anterior commissure

Corpus callosum

Septal nuclei

Prefrontal cortex

Hypo-thalamus

Olfactory bulb

Hypothalamic inputs:
Lateral hypothalamic area
Ventromedial nucleus

Corticomedial nuclei of the amygdala

Basolateral nuclei of the amygdala

Subiculum (hippocampal formation)

Sensory association inputs:
Temporal lobe sensory association cortex
Entorhinal cortex
Insular cortex
Medial frontal lobe

16.34 MAJOR AFFERENT CONNECTIONS OF THE AMYGDALA

The amygdala is an almond-shaped collection of nuclei in the medial portion of the anterior temporal lobe. It is involved in the emotional interpretation of external sensory information and internal states. It provides individual-specific behavioral and emotional responses, particularly those involving fear and aversive responses. The amygdala is subdivided into corticomedial nuclei and basolateral nuclei (which receive afferents and project axons to target structures) and the central nucleus, which provides mainly efferent projections to the brainstem. Afferents to the corticomedial nuclei arrive primarily from subcortical limbic sources, including the olfactory bulb, septal nuclei, and hypothalamic nuclei (VM, LHA); the thalamus (intralaminar nuclei); the bed nucleus of the stria terminalis; and extensive numbers of autonomic nuclei and monoamine nuclei of the brainstem. Afferents to the basolateral nuclei arrive mainly from cortical areas, including extensive sensory association cortices, the prefrontal cortex, the cingulate cortex, and the subiculum. 5HT, 5-hydroxytryptamine [serotonin]; NE, norepinephrine.

CLINICAL POINT

The amygdala is a subcortical collection of nuclei in the medial anterior temporal lobe. It is involved in the emotional interpretation and "flavoring" of external sensory information and internal states. Afferents to corticomedial nuclei come from subcortical limbic structures, and afferents to basolateral nuclei derive mainly from cortical structures. Most cases in humans of bilateral destruction of the amygdala occur with trauma or temporal lobe surgery for seizures, and they involve destruction of more than just amygdaloid nuclei. On the basis of primate studies and observations in humans, it appears that **amygdaloid** lesions result in placid behavior, lack of fear even when confronted with normally fear-provoking stimuli, and withdrawal from social contacts. The normal integration of emotional reactive and cognitive processing is disrupted. Studies have found that patients with bilateral amygdaloid damage cannot recognize facial expressions in others that indicate fear and do not learn or remember events with strong emotional context better than those without such emotional context, as is normally the case. In patients with bilateral temporal lobe damage involving extensive cortical and subcortical neuronal destruction, **Klüver-Bucy syndrome** can occur. This syndrome is characterized by placid behavior, loss of fear of potentially dangerous objects, compulsive exploration of the environment (particularly orally), visual agnosias, inappropriately directed hyperphagia (of nonedible items), and hypersexuality. In some cases, loss of consolidation of memory (hippocampal involvement) and cognitive deficits are also seen.

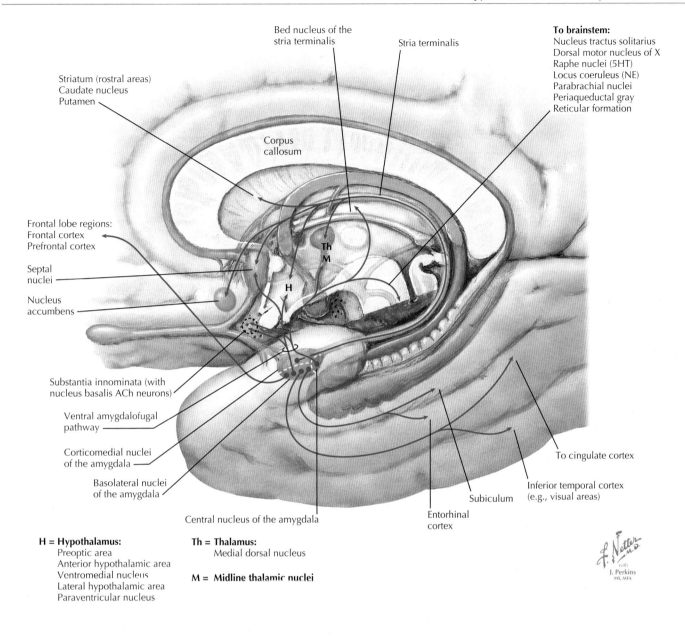

Bed nucleus of the stria terminalis

Stria terminalis

To brainstem:
Nucleus tractus solitarius
Dorsal motor nucleus of X
Raphe nuclei (5HT)
Locus coeruleus (NE)
Parabrachial nuclei
Periaqueductal gray
Reticular formation

Striatum (rostral areas)
Caudate nucleus
Putamen

Corpus callosum

Th
M

Frontal lobe regions:
Frontal cortex
Prefrontal cortex

Septal nuclei

H

Nucleus accumbens

Substantia innominata (with nucleus basalis ACh neurons)

Ventral amygdalofugal pathway

Corticomedial nuclei of the amygdala

Basolateral nuclei of the amygdala

To cingulate cortex

Inferior temporal cortex (e.g., visual areas)

Subiculum

Central nucleus of the amygdala

Entorhinal cortex

H = Hypothalamus:
Preoptic area
Anterior hypothalamic area
Ventromedial nucleus
Lateral hypothalamic area
Paraventricular nucleus

Th = Thalamus:
Medial dorsal nucleus

M = Midline thalamic nuclei

16.35 MAJOR EFFERENT CONNECTIONS OF THE AMYGDALA

Efferents from the corticomedial nuclei project through the stria terminalis and are directed mainly toward subcortical nuclei, such as septal nuclei, the mediodorsal (medial dorsal) nucleus of the thalamus, the hypothalamic nuclei, the bed nucleus of the stria terminalis, the nucleus accumbens, and the rostral striatum. Efferents from the basolateral nuclei project through the ventral amygdalofugal pathway to cortical regions, including the frontal cortex, the cingulate cortex, the inferior temporal cortex, the subiculum, and the entorhinal cortex, and to subcortical limbic regions, including hypothalamic nuclei, septal nuclei, and the cholinergic nucleus basalis in substantia innominata. The central amygdaloid receives input mainly from internal amygdaloid connections and sends extensive efferents through the ventral amygdalofugal pathway to autonomic nuclei and monoaminergic nuclei of the brainstem, the midline thalamic nuclei, the bed nucleus of the stria terminalis, and the cholinergic nucleus basalis.

CLINICAL POINT

Efferents from the corticomedial nuclei are directed mainly to subcortical limbic nuclei. Efferents from the basolateral nuclei are directed through the ventral amygdalofugal pathway to extensive cortical regions and subcortical structures. The central amygdaloid nucleus sends extensive efferents to brainstem nuclei associated with the machinery of emotional responsiveness provoked by amygdaloid activation. This central nucleus receives its input mainly from other amygdaloid nuclei. Amygdaloid stimulation has been performed in humans (for epilepsy surgery) and in experimental animals. Corticomedial stimulation produces a **freezing response** (cessation of voluntary movement), automated gestures (lip smacking), and parasympathetic activation that leads to voiding and defecation. Basolateral stimulation produces the **vigilance responses** of becoming alert and scanning the environment. These responses most likely reflect the outflow of the amygdala to brainstem circuitry that coordinates behavior appropriate to the emotional context of the stimuli. Conditioned fear responses and reactions to stressors require coordinated interaction of neuroendocrine outflow, autonomic reactivity, and behavioral activity. In humans, amygdaloid stimulation results in feelings associated with fear and anxiety. 5HT, 5-hydroxytryptamine [serotonin]; NE, norepinephrine.

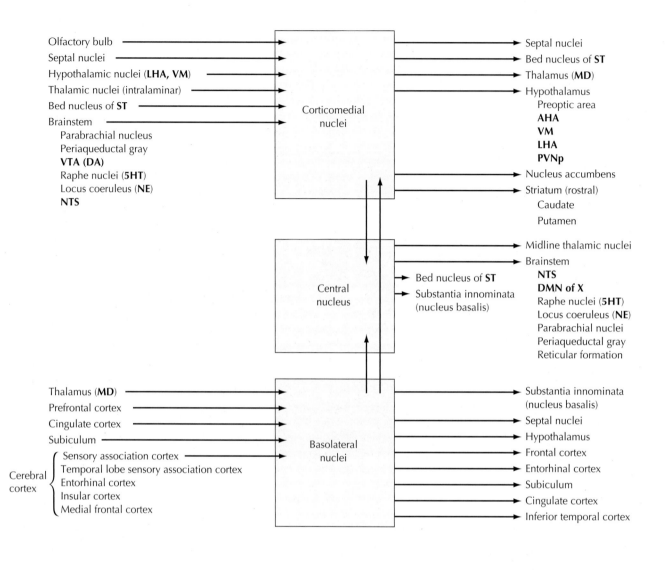

AHA = Anterior hypothalamic area
DA = Dopamine
DMN of X = Dorsal motor (autonomic) nucleus of X
5HT = 5-Hydroxytryptamine (serotonin)
LHA = Lateral hypothalamic area
MD = Medial dorsal nucleus of thalamus

NE = Norepinephrine
NTS = Nucleus tractus solitarius
PVNp = Paraventricular nucleus, parvocellular
ST = Stria terminalis
VM = Ventromedial
VTA = Ventral tegmental area

16.36 SUMMARY OF MAJOR AFFERENTS, EFFERENTS, AND INTERCONNECTIONS OF THE AMYGDALA

The corticomedial amygdala is connected reciprocally mainly with subcortical limbic forebrain structures and receives extensive additional inputs from brainstem autonomic and monoaminergic nuclei. The basolateral amygdala is connected reciprocally with extensive regions of limbic and association cortex and has additional efferents to subcortical limbic forebrain regions. Both the corticomedial and basolateral nuclei send axons to the central nucleus of the amygdala. The central nucleus has massive descending efferents to extensive autonomic and monoaminergic nuclei of the brainstem as well as to some subcortical limbic forebrain regions. These interconnections with extensive regions of the cortex, the limbic forebrain regions, and the autonomic/limbic brainstem nuclei provide the integrated circuitry that permits analysis of both external and internal information and provides an emotional and interpretive context for the initiation and control of appropriate behavioral and emotional responses. See Fig. 15.26 for a brief discussion of the extended amygdala, including the bed nucleus of the stria terminalis and nucleus accumbens.

AFFERENTS

Major afferents from:
Hippocampal CA pyramidal cells
Amygdaloid nuclei
    Corticomedial nuclei via stria terminalis
    Basolateral nuclei via ventral
        amygdalofugal pathway
Ventral tegmental area
Hypothalamus
    Preoptic area
    Anterior hypothalamic area
    Paraventricular nucleus
    Lateral hypothalamic area
Locus coeruleus (NE; not shown)

EFFERENTS

Major efferents to:
Hippocampal CA regions ⎤
Dentate gyrus (ACh path) ⎦ Via fornix
Habenular nuclei ⎤ Via stria
Medial dorsal nucleus ⎥ medullaris
    of the thalamus ⎦ thalami
Ventral tegmental area — Via median
Hypothalamus   forebrain bundle
    Preoptic area
    Anterior hypothalamic area
    Ventromedial nucleus
    Lateral hypothalamic area

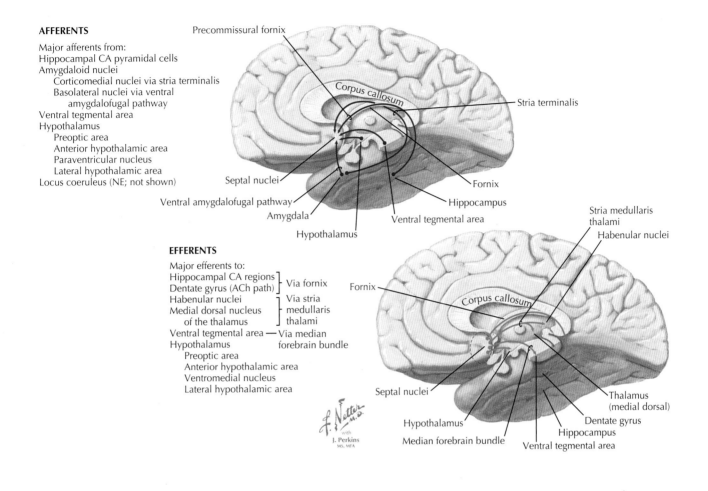

16.37 MAJOR AFFERENT AND EFFERENT CONNECTIONS OF THE SEPTAL NUCLEI

The septal nuclei are subcortical nuclei initially implicated by early ablation and stimulation studies in the regulation of emotional responsiveness such as rage behavior. In experimental studies, the septal nuclei appear to play a role in emotional behaviors, sexual behavior, aggressive behavior, modulation of autonomic functions, and attention and memory functions (from the cholinergic neurons). Afferents to the septal nuclei arrive mainly from the hippocampus, the corticomedial and basolateral amygdala, the ventral tegmental nucleus in the midbrain, and several hypothalamic nuclei. Efferents from the septal nuclei distribute mainly to the hippocampus and dentate gyrus (via the fornix), the habenular nuclei (via the stria medullaris thalami), the medial dorsal nucleus of the thalamus (via the stria medullaris thalami), the ventral tegmental area (via the median forebrain bundle), and several hypothalamic nuclei.

CLINICAL POINT

In some humans with ischemic damage involving the septal area, rage behavior has been observed. This is consistent with early experimental studies in rodents in which septal lesions resulted in exaggerated reactivity to both appropriate and innocuous stimuli (sham rage). In contrast, implanted electrodes in the septal nuclei for electrical self-stimulation studies resulted in prolonged and repeated stimulation, indicative of pleasurable responses.

Efferent connections to the habenula and, via its efferent pathways to the brainstem such as the fasciculus retroflexus (habenulopeduncular tract), and connections to the hypothalamus and brainstem through the descending median forebrain bundle represent the descending regulatory circuitry from the septal nuclei through which some of the associated behaviors are accomplished. The recent findings that a cholinergic cell group in the septum, along with the bed nucleus of the stria terminalis, sends axons via the fornix to the hippocampal formation, and that these are commonly found to have degenerated in the brains of patients with AD, raise the possibility that these cholinergic neurons are contributors to the process of consolidation of immediate and short-term memory into long-term traces. Damage to the entire collection of cholinergic neurons (including nucleus basalis of Meynert) produces such memory deficits, but experimental studies of selective lesions of cholinergic neurons in the septal nucleus and bed nucleus of the stria terminalis did not result in profound loss of such memory function. It is likely that the cholinergic projections to the hippocampal formation and the cerebral cortex function as a distributive system and affect memory function through an influence on the entire circuitry involved in cognitive and memory functions.

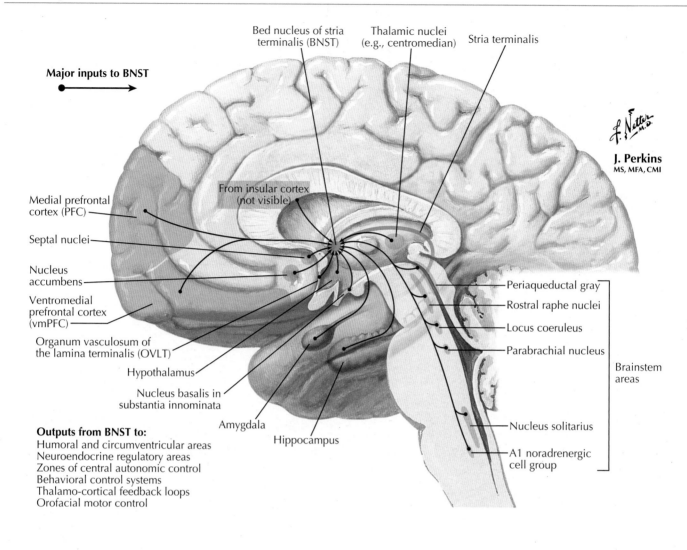

Major inputs to BNST ●————▶

Bed nucleus of stria terminalis (BNST)

Thalamic nuclei (e.g., centromedian)

Stria terminalis

Medial prefrontal cortex (PFC)

From insular cortex (not visible)

Septal nuclei

Nucleus accumbens

Ventromedial prefrontal cortex (vmPFC)

Organum vasculosum of the lamina terminalis (OVLT)

Hypothalamus

Nucleus basalis in substantia innominata

Amygdala

Hippocampus

Periaqueductal gray

Rostral raphe nuclei

Locus coeruleus

Parabrachial nucleus

Brainstem areas

Nucleus solitarius

A1 noradrenergic cell group

Outputs from BNST to:
Humoral and circumventricular areas
Neuroendocrine regulatory areas
Zones of central autonomic control
Behavioral control systems
Thalamo-cortical feedback loops
Orofacial motor control

J. Perkins
MS, MFA, CMI

16.38 BED NUCLEUS OF THE STRIA TERMINALIS

The bed nucleus of the stria terminalis (BNST), a limbic forebrain structure, consists of multiple clusters of neurons surrounding the caudal portion of the anterior commissure. Its caudal region, at the end of the stria terminalis, is adjacent to the amygdala, and its rostral region is ventral to the septal area and the dorsal preoptic area. Its interconnections coordinate physiological functions and behaviors related to autonomic, neuroendocrine, and motor systems. The BNST is an integrative site where descending cortical information and ascending exteroceptive and interoceptive information come together.

Major inputs to the BNST derive from cortical areas (medial prefrontal, infralimbic, and insular), forebrain areas (nucleus accumbens, substantia innominata, lateral septal area), hippocampus, amygdala (basomedial and central nuclei, which connect reciprocally), circumventricular organs (subfornical organ, organum vasculosum of the lamina terminalis), thalamic regions (centromedian, other nonspecific regions), numerous hypothalamic areas, and brainstem areas (periaqueductal gray, rostral raphe nuclei, parabrachial nuclei, locus coeruleus, nucleus solitarius, A1 noradrenergic cell group). The BNST monitors inputs related to stressors, blood pressure, blood volume, and other ongoing physiological parameters.

Projections from the BNST include humoral and circumventricular areas, neuroendocrine regulatory areas, zones of central autonomic control, behavioral control systems, thalamo-cortical feedback loops, and orofacial motor control sites.

Behavioral involvement of the BNST includes monitoring uncertain, nonimminent fear states (amygdala involved in defined fear states), and modulating aggressive behaviors, social attachment, mating and parental activities, goal-directed and addictive behaviors (through the dopamine connections from the midbrain ventral tegmental area), pain reactivity, and visceral regulatory functions. The BNST has been identified as a component of psychiatric-related disorders such as anxiety, social dysfunction, posttraumatic stress, mood disorders, and others.

BNST neurons utilize many neurotransmitter systems, including norepinephrine, serotonin, acetylcholine, nitric oxide, opioid peptides, endocannabinoids, and others.

See the reference for an excellent review:

Dong HW, Swanson LW: Projections from bed nuclei of the stria terminalis, anteromedial area: cerebral hemisphere integration of neuroendocrine, autonomic, and behavioral aspects of energy balance. *J Comp Neurol* 494:75–107, 2006.

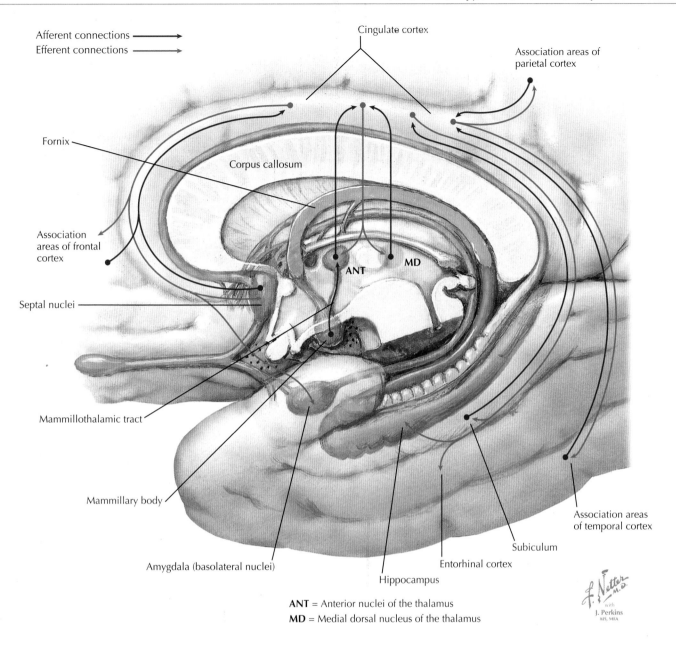

Afferent connections ⟶
Efferent connections ⟶

Cingulate cortex

Association areas of
parietal cortex

Fornix

Corpus callosum

Association
areas of frontal
cortex

Septal nuclei

ANT   **MD**

Mammillothalamic tract

Mammillary body

Association areas
of temporal cortex

Subiculum

Amygdala (basolateral nuclei)

Entorhinal cortex

Hippocampus

ANT = Anterior nuclei of the thalamus
MD = Medial dorsal nucleus of the thalamus

16.39 MAJOR CONNECTIONS OF THE CINGULATE CORTEX

The cingulate cortex is located above the corpus callosum. This cortical region is involved in the regulation of autonomic functions (respiratory, digestive, cardiovascular, pupillary), some somatic functions (motor tone, ongoing movements), and emotional responsiveness and behavior. Lesions in the cingulate cortex, like lesions in the orbitofrontal cortex, result in indifference to pain and other sensations that have emotional connotations, and in social indifference. Afferents to the cingulate cortex arrive from association areas of the frontal, parietal, and temporal lobes; the subiculum; the septal nuclei; and the thalamic nuclei (mediodorsal, anterior). Efferents from the cingulate cortex project to association areas of frontal, parietal, and temporal lobes and to limbic forebrain regions, such as the hippocampus, the subiculum, the entorhinal cortex, the amygdala, and septal nuclei. These limbic forebrain regions send extensive projections to the hypothalamus for regulation of autonomic and somatic regions of the brainstem and spinal cord.

CLINICAL POINT

The anterior cingulate cortex may participate in selecting **appropriate responses to conflicting stimuli.** Inputs to the cingulate cortex derive from many regions of frontal, parietal, and temporal cortex, the subiculum; the septal nuclei; and the medial dorsal thalamus (prefrontal connections). Efferent connections project back to many of these same regions as well as to the amygdala, subiculum, and entorhinal cortex. Through these efferent connections, circuitry to the brainstem can coordinate appropriate autonomic and somatic functions. Lesions in the cingulate cortex result in indifference to pain and other sensations that have strong emotional connotations; they produce social indifference and apathy, eliminate emotional intonation in speech, and cause personality changes. Bilateral anterior cingulate lesions, or cingulotomies, have been done as "psychosurgery" to alleviate intractable pain and to incapacitate anxiety, obsessive-compulsive behavior, and intractable depression. Lesions in the posterior cingulate cortex result in diminished ability to perform spatial navigation.

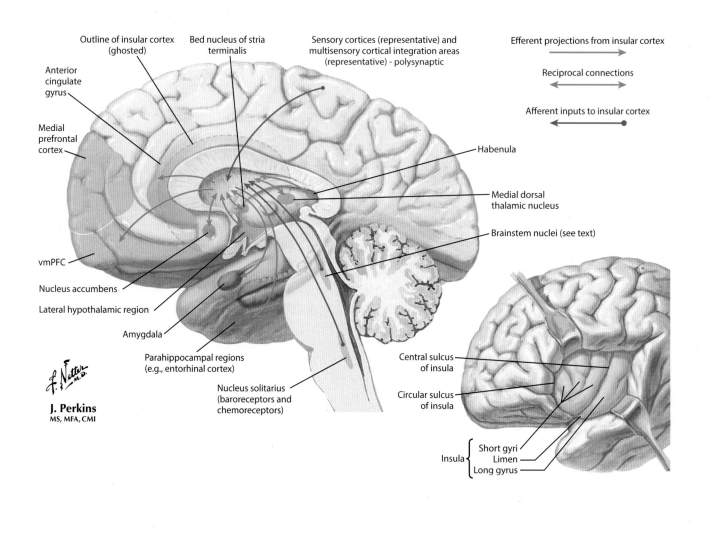

Outline of insular cortex (ghosted)

Bed nucleus of stria terminalis

Sensory cortices (representative) and multisensory cortical integration areas (representative) - polysynaptic

Efferent projections from insular cortex

Reciprocal connections

Afferent inputs to insular cortex

Anterior cingulate gyrus

Medial prefrontal cortex

Habenula

Medial dorsal thalamic nucleus

Brainstem nuclei (see text)

vmPFC

Nucleus accumbens

Lateral hypothalamic region

Amygdala

Parahippocampal regions (e.g., entorhinal cortex)

Nucleus solitarius (baroreceptors and chemoreceptors)

Central sulcus of insula

Circular sulcus of insula

Insula { Short gyri / Limen / Long gyrus

J. Perkins
MS, MFA, CMI

16.40 INSULAR CORTEX

The insular cortex, sometimes called the "fifth lobe of the brain," is a viscerosensory cortex located deep in the lateral fissure, continuous anteriorly with the ventromedial prefrontal cortex (vmPFC), also called the orbitofrontal cortex. Afferent projections to the insular cortex include (1) viscerosensory inputs and inputs from chemoreceptors and baroreceptors; (2) multisensory inputs, through the thalamus and cortex, for somatosensory, trigeminal, taste, olfaction, vision, and some interoceptors; (3) nucleus basalis (cholinergic) in substantia innominata; (4) cortical areas involved in multisensory integration; and (5) numerous brainstem nuclei and sites (periaqueductal gray, parabrachial nuclei, dopaminergic ventral tegmental area, noradrenergic locus coeruleus, and serotonergic raphe nuclei).

Efferent projections from the insular cortex are mainly reciprocal interconnections with (1) limbic structures (basolateral amygdala, lateral BNST), (2) parahippocampal regions such as the lateral entorhinal cortex, (3) cortical regions (medial prefrontal, anterior cingulate), (4) nucleus accumbens, (4) medial dorsal (MD) thalamic nucleus, (5) lateral hypothalamic region, and (6) habenula.

The insular cortex links sensory processing and emotional recognition and feelings and can assist with subsequent motor and autonomic reactivity. The insular cortex also aids in risk prediction and decision making related to addictive behaviors and uncertain situations. It participates, with several other limbic and cortical structures, with fear responses and anxiety responses, social interactions, and complex emotional responses such as empathy.

In situations where the insular cortex is damaged or disrupted, the patient can perceive sensory information, such as pain, but is unable to react emotionally to it, showing altered or absent emotions.

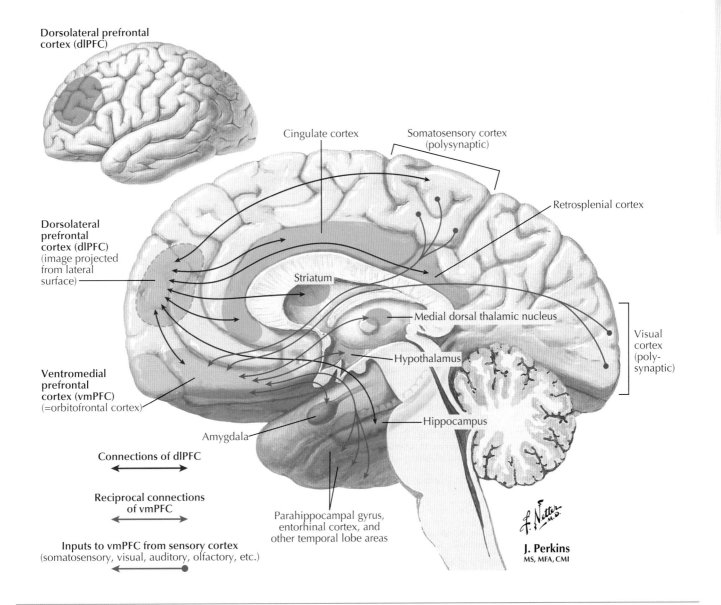

Dorsolateral prefrontal cortex (dlPFC)

Cingulate cortex

Somatosensory cortex (polysynaptic)

Retrosplenial cortex

Dorsolateral prefrontal cortex (dlPFC) (image projected from lateral surface)

Striatum

Medial dorsal thalamic nucleus

Visual cortex (poly-synaptic)

Ventromedial prefrontal cortex (vmPFC) (=orbitofrontal cortex)

Hypothalamus

Hippocampus

Amygdala

Connections of dlPFC

Reciprocal connections of vmPFC

Inputs to vmPFC from sensory cortex
(somatosensory, visual, auditory, olfactory, etc.)

Parahippocampal gyrus, entorhinal cortex, and other temporal lobe areas

J. Perkins
MS, MFA, CMI

16.41 PREFRONTAL CORTEX

The prefrontal cortex (PFC) consists of two major anatomical and functional regions, the ventromedial (vmPFC), also called the orbitofrontal cortex, and the dorsolateral (dlPFC).

VENTROMEDIAL (ORBITOFRONTAL) PREFRONTAL CORTEX

The vmPFC is reciprocally connected with medial dorsal (MD) thalamic nucleus, cortical areas (entorhinal, perirhinal, parahippocampal, some temporal lobe area), amygdala (central and basolateral), and some hypothalamic areas. Inputs to the vmPFC also include sensory integration cortex (pyriform cortex) and many sensory cortical areas (olfactory [uncus], taste, somatosensory SI and SII, visual, and auditory).

The vmPFC participates in reward and emotional reactivity in decision making, expectations, and adaptive learning and can regulate autonomic reactivity via the dopamine mesocortical system. It also is a component of perception of pleasure, aggressive behavior, and complex sensory integration. Damage to the vmPFC, which occurs in traumatic brain injury (TBI), can result in behavioral disinhibition and aggression and abuse, poor decision making, poor social interactions, compulsive behaviors (addictive behaviors), and lack of empathy.

The vmPFC is involved in psychiatric disorders such as schizophrenia, mood disorders, obsessive-compulsive disorder, addictive behaviors, and borderline personality disorder.

DORSOLATERAL PREFRONTAL CORTEX

The dlPFC is connected with cortical areas (vmPFC, primary and secondary sensory association cortical areas, cingulate cortex [anterior and posterior, retrosplenial cortex, premotor cortex), hippocampus, striatum thalamic areas, and the lateral cerebellum.

The dlPFC is the "Mr. Spock" of Star Trek, the rational decision maker, carrying out logical cognitive assessment in an unemotional manner. The dlPFC directs executive functions, abstract reasoning, and complex planning and is able to inhibit impulsive amygdaloid-driven activities and behaviors. It is a major site for working memory and deductive reasoning, as well as behavioral strategies such as lying and deception. The dlPFC directs many activities that people define as "intelligence."

Damage to the dlPFC results in a loss of drive, ambition, and motivation, leading to disinterest and loss of attention. Spontaneous activities and conversation are often lost. There is an increase in addictive behaviors, depression, and indications of major life stress.

Pathways for communication from the more rostral regions of PFC include the cingulum, the extreme capsule, and the uncinate fasciculus. Pathways for communication from the more caudal regions of PFC include the superior longitudinal fasciculus, the occipitofrontal fasciculus, and the arcuate fasciculus. The activation of the dlPFC and vmPFC is inversely correlated.

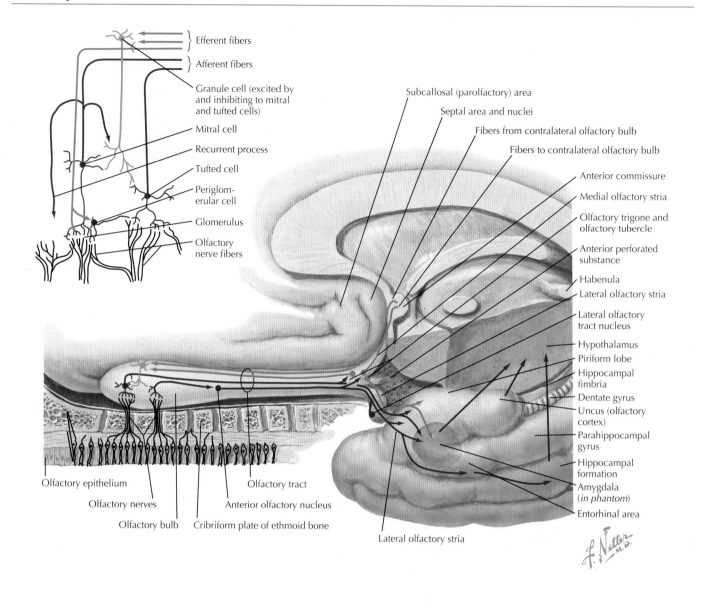

Efferent fibers

Afferent fibers

Granule cell (excited by
and inhibiting to mitral
and tufted cells)

Mitral cell

Recurrent process

Tufted cell

Periglom-
erular cell

Glomerulus

Olfactory
nerve fibers

Subcallosal (parolfactory) area

Septal area and nuclei

Fibers from contralateral olfactory bulb

Fibers to contralateral olfactory bulb

Anterior commissure

Medial olfactory stria

Olfactory trigone and
olfactory tubercle

Anterior perforated
substance

Habenula

Lateral olfactory stria

Lateral olfactory
tract nucleus

Hypothalamus

Piriform lobe

Hippocampal
fimbria

Dentate gyrus

Uncus (olfactory
cortex)

Parahippocampal
gyrus

Hippocampal
formation

Amygdala
(*in phantom*)

Entorhinal area

Olfactory epithelium

Olfactory nerves

Olfactory bulb

Olfactory tract

Anterior olfactory nucleus

Cribriform plate of ethmoid bone

Lateral olfactory stria

16.44 OLFACTORY PATHWAYS

Primary sensory axons from bipolar neurons pass through the cribriform plate and synapse in the olfactory glomeruli in the glomerular layer of the olfactory bulb. The glomeruli are the functional units for processing specific odor information. The olfactory nerve fibers synapse on the dendrites of the tufted and mitral cells, the secondary sensory neurons that give rise to the olfactory tract projections. Periglomerular cells are interneurons that interconnect the glomeruli. Granule cells modulate the excitability of tufted and mitral cells. Centrifugal connections (from serotonergic raphe nuclei and the noradrenergic locus coeruleus) modulate activity in the glomeruli and periglomerular cells. The olfactory tract bypasses the thalamus and projects to the anterior olfactory nucleus, the nucleus accumbens, the primary olfactory cortex (in the uncus), the amygdala, the periamygdaloid cortex, and the lateral entorhinal cortex. The olfactory cortex has interconnections with the orbitofrontal cortex, the insular cortex, the hippocampus, and the lateral hypothalamus.

CLINICAL POINT

The olfactory bulb and tract can be damaged by meningiomas of the olfactory groove or, less commonly, of the sphenoid ridge. These tumors produce **Foster-Kennedy syndrome**, which consists of ipsilateral anosmia, ipsilateral optic atrophy resulting from direct pressure, and papilledema caused by increased intracranial pressure. If the ipsilateral optic nerve is completely atrophic, papilledema will not be observed on that side. The olfactory bulb and tract also can be damaged by tumors of the frontal bone, pituitary tumors with frontal extension, frontal tumors such as gliomas that act as mass lesions, aneurysms at the circle of Willis, and meningitis. These conditions are distinguished from the olfactory groove meningiomas by the additional symptoms they cause.

Section IV GLOBAL BRAIN FUNCTIONS

17. Global Brain Functions

17

GLOBAL BRAIN FUNCTIONS

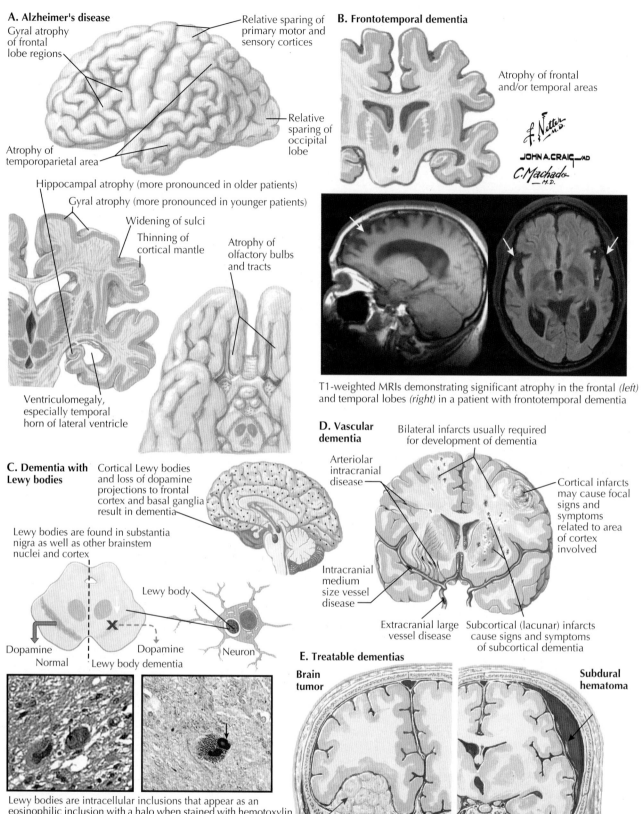

A. Alzheimer's disease

Gyral atrophy of frontal lobe regions

Relative sparing of primary motor and sensory cortices

Atrophy of temporoparietal area

Relative sparing of occipital lobe

Hippocampal atrophy (more pronounced in older patients)

Gyral atrophy (more pronounced in younger patients)

Widening of sulci

Thinning of cortical mantle

Atrophy of olfactory bulbs and tracts

Ventriculomegaly, especially temporal horn of lateral ventricle

B. Frontotemporal dementia

Atrophy of frontal and/or temporal areas

T1-weighted MRIs demonstrating significant atrophy in the frontal *(left)* and temporal lobes *(right)* in a patient with frontotemporal dementia

C. Dementia with Lewy bodies

Cortical Lewy bodies and loss of dopamine projections to frontal cortex and basal ganglia result in dementia

Lewy bodies are found in substantia nigra as well as other brainstem nuclei and cortex

Lewy body

Dopamine Normal

Dopamine Lewy body dementia

Neuron

Lewy bodies are intracellular inclusions that appear as an eosinophilic inclusion with a halo when stained with hemotoxylin and eosion *(left)*. Newer immunostaining techniques using antibodies to alpha-synuclein densely label Lewy bodies *(right)*.

D. Vascular dementia

Bilateral infarcts usually required for development of dementia

Arteriolar intracranial disease

Intracranial medium size vessel disease

Extracranial large vessel disease

Cortical infarcts may cause focal signs and symptoms related to area of cortex involved

Subcortical (lacunar) infarcts cause signs and symptoms of subcortical dementia

E. Treatable dementias

Brain tumor

Subdural hematoma

17.1 DEMENTIA

17.1 DEMENTIA (CONTINUED)

Dementia is a group of symptoms affecting memory, thought processes, and social interactions to a sufficient extent to interfere with daily life. It is accompanied by cognitive changes such as memory loss, confusion, getting lost, inattention, diminished problem-solving ability, impaired reasoning, loss of organizational skills, and loss of coordination. Psychological changes also are seen, such as depression, anxiety, agitation, anger, inappropriate behaviors, and personality changes. The onset of dementia is usually subacute or chronic. Altered consciousness does not occur until late in the disease. Psychotic behavior is uncommon in dementia.

Alzheimer's disease (AD) is the most common form of dementia. The cortex commonly demonstrates atrophy, with sparing of sensory, motor, and occipital cortices. The cortex and other areas such as the hippocampus demonstrate aberrant amyloid-beta deposits, extracellular neuritic plaques, and intracellular neurofibrillary tangles. See Plates 17.2 and 17.3 for details of AD and its pathology.

Frontotemporal dementia is characterized by frontal and temporal lobe atrophy, with loss of neurons and neuronal connections. Patients demonstrate altered cognition, altered decision making and judgment, disinhibition and impulsivity, altered language capabilities, and personality and behavioral changes.

Dementia with Lewy bodies, constituting 10% to 15% of dementias, is accompanied by abnormal changes in the synaptic protein alpha-synuclein (Lewy bodies) in the brainstem (especially substantia nigra, pars compacta) and many areas of cerebral cortex. Lewy bodies are sometimes found with plaques and neurofibrillary tangles in AD. Patients often experience visual hallucinations and striking images of animate objects and may exhibit cognitive impairment. Symptoms of Parkinson's disease (rigidity, resting tremor, bradykinesia, postural instability) may occur, along with depression, anxiety, and autonomic dysfunction (orthostatic hypotension, dizziness, syncope).

Vascular dementia is the second most common form of dementia and may accompany small and/or large vessel disease. A single stroke may precipitate dementia. Gradual occurrence of small vessel disease may precipitate damage to subcortical white matter from multiple lacunar infarcts and bring about progressive cognitive impairment, including loss of attention and ability to focus, slowed thinking, impaired organizational ability, and diminished problem-solving ability. Vascular dementia is sometimes referred to as *multi-infarct dementia* (caused by multiple strokes) or *Binswanger's disease* (subcortical arteriosclerotic encephalopathy [SAE]), small vessel disease caused by damage to white matter, such as seen in longstanding hypertension.

Treatable dementias, appearing with cognitive decline and intellectual impairment, may occur from other causes such as traumatic brain injury (TBI), brain tumors, subdural hematomas, normal-pressure hydrocephalus, metabolic encephalopathy, or depression. Such dementias may be accompanied by headache, seizures, gait disturbances, past history of TBI, changes in consciousness or presence of sleepiness, and incontinence.

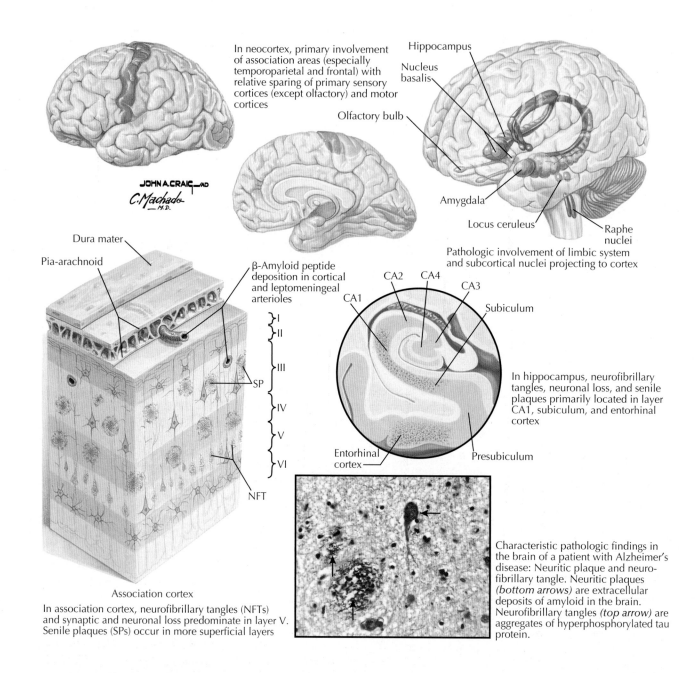

In neocortex, primary involvement of association areas (especially temporoparietal and frontal) with relative sparing of primary sensory cortices (except olfactory) and motor cortices

JOHN A. CRAIG—AD
C. Machado—M.D.

Hippocampus
Nucleus basalis
Olfactory bulb
Amygdala
Locus ceruleus
Raphe nuclei
Pathologic involvement of limbic system and subcortical nuclei projecting to cortex

Dura mater
Pia-arachnoid
β-Amyloid peptide deposition in cortical and leptomeningeal arterioles
I
II
III
IV
V
VI
SP
NFT

CA2   CA4
CA1   CA3
Subiculum

In hippocampus, neurofibrillary tangles, neuronal loss, and senile plaques primarily located in layer CA1, subiculum, and entorhinal cortex

Entorhinal cortex
Presubiculum

Association cortex

In association cortex, neurofibrillary tangles (NFTs) and synaptic and neuronal loss predominate in layer V. Senile plaques (SPs) occur in more superficial layers

Characteristic pathologic findings in the brain of a patient with Alzheimer's disease: Neuritic plaque and neurofibrillary tangle. Neuritic plaques (bottom arrows) are extracellular deposits of amyloid in the brain. Neurofibrillary tangles (top arrow) are aggregates of hyperphosphorylated tau protein.

17.2 ALZHEIMER'S DISEASE: DISTRIBUTION OF PATHOLOGY IN THE BRAIN

The characteristic pathology in the brain in AD is neuritic (amyloid) plaques (extracellular deposits) and neurofibrillary tangles (intracellular aggregates of hyperphosphorylated tau protein in neurons). Although these are described as the characteristic pathologic features of AD, some severely cognitively impaired individuals have normal amounts of plaques and tangles, and some individuals with extensive autopsy-confirmed plaques and tangles were cognitively intact before death.

Neuritic plaques are usually abundant in AD, particularly in frontal and parietal cortical regions, found particularly in upper layers of the cortex. Neurofibrillary tangles are abundant in neurons in AD, starting in the medial temporal lobe (amygdaloid region, entorhinal cortex), expanding into the hippocampal formation and cingulate cortex, and in late stages affecting widespread areas. Neurons with intracellular tangles are abundant in layer V of affected regions of cortex.

Clinical findings accompanying these pathologies include cognitive impairment, memory deficits, poor judgment and decision making, disorientation, and language impairment.

In early stages of AD, the CA1 sector of the hippocampus, the subiculum, and the entorhinal cortex are susceptible to neuronal damage from both plaques and tangles; hence the early presence of memory deficits, especially short-term memory deficits.

Some cortical areas remain relatively spared from pathology from plaques and tangles in AD, including sensory cortices (somatosensory, auditory, visual) and motor cortex. See Plate 16.31 Clinical Point.

Selective loss of corticocortical and subcorticocortical projections

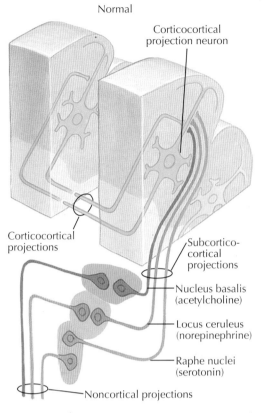

Corticocortical projection neurons project to neurons in distant areas of cortex. They receive subcorticocortical projections from neurons in subcortical nuclei.

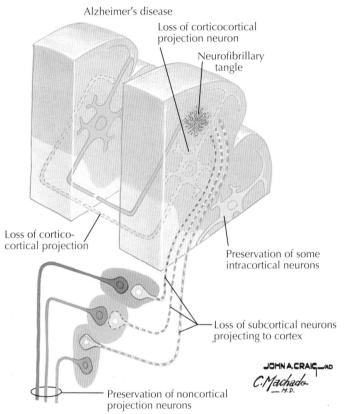

Alzheimer-related loss of subcorticocortical projection neurons results in loss of those circuits and cognitive dysfunction.

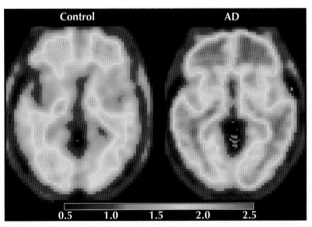

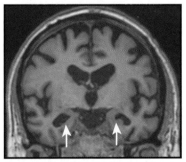

PET imaging with florbetapir reveals the presence of amyloid plaque deposits in the brain of an individual with a clinical diagnosis of Alzheimer disease (shades of red) compared to a cognitively normal older adult with little to no evidence of amyloid (lighter red and yellow).

Coronal T1-weighted MRI scan showing atrophy of the hippocampus bilaterally *(arrows)*, with enlargement of the temporal horns of the lateral ventricles. Global atrophy is evident with widening of the sulci and enlargement of sub-arachnoid spaces.

17.3 ALZHEIMER'S DISEASE: PATHOLOGY

Pathological changes seen in AD include enlarged ventricles and the lateral fissure, with significant cortical atrophy and hippocampal atrophy, loss of cortico-cortical connections, and widened cortical sulci. Cellular pathology includes amyloid-beta deposits, extracellular neuritic plaques, and intracellular neurofibrillary tangles. Also present is a significant subcortical loss of serotonergic (raphe nuclei), noradrenergic (locus coeruleus), and cholinergic (nucleus basalis) nuclei and their projections to the cortex.

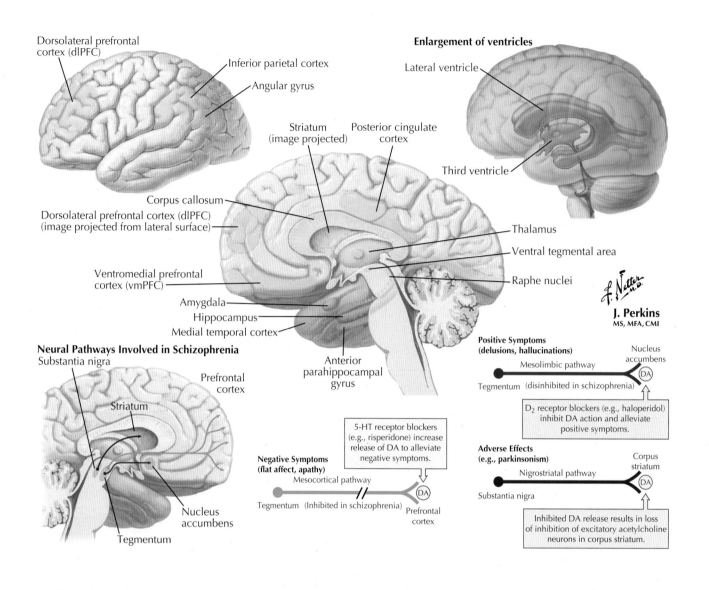

Dorsolateral prefrontal cortex (dlPFC)

Inferior parietal cortex

Angular gyrus

Striatum (image projected)

Posterior cingulate cortex

Enlargement of ventricles

Lateral ventricle

Third ventricle

Corpus callosum

Dorsolateral prefrontal cortex (dlPFC) (image projected from lateral surface)

Thalamus

Ventral tegmental area

Ventromedial prefrontal cortex (vmPFC)

Raphe nuclei

Amygdala

Hippocampus

Medial temporal cortex

Anterior parahippocampal gyrus

J. Perkins
MS, MFA, CMI

Neural Pathways Involved in Schizophrenia

Substantia nigra

Prefrontal cortex

Striatum

Nucleus accumbens

Tegmentum

Positive Symptoms (delusions, hallucinations)

Mesolimbic pathway

Nucleus accumbens

Tegmentum   (disinhibited in schizophrenia)

D$_2$ receptor blockers (e.g., haloperidol) inhibit DA action and alleviate positive symptoms.

5-HT receptor blockers (e.g., risperidone) increase release of DA to alleviate negative symptoms.

Negative Symptoms (flat affect, apathy)

Mesocortical pathway

Tegmentum   (Inhibited in schizophrenia)

Prefrontal cortex

Adverse Effects (e.g., parkinsonism)

Nigrostriatal pathway

Corpus striatum

Substantia nigra

Inhibited DA release results in loss of inhibition of excitatory acetylcholine neurons in corpus striatum.

17.4 NEUROPSYCHIATRIC DISORDERS: SCHIZOPHRENIA

Schizophrenia is a major psychiatric disorder, with a genetic component, characterized by delusions, hallucinations, disorganized speech and thoughts, psychomotor disturbances, and often cognitive impairment. Positive symptoms (delusions and hallucinations) and negative symptoms (catatonic behavior, social withdrawal, blunted affect, alogia, and avolition) are seen. Patients sometimes have difficulty distinguishing fantasy from reality and show reduced insight and awareness of their illness. Cognitive impairment may include deficits in episodic memory, attention, executive functions, and intellectual ability. These many symptoms may be variable in their appearance and severity but usually have a drastic effect on personal relationships and business and professional relationships. Schizophrenia has a lifetime prevalence of approximately 1%, typically appears at 20 to 35 years of age, and is more frequent in men than in women. Approximately 15% of patients with schizophrenia commit suicide.

Areas of the brain involved in schizophrenia include:

1. Prefrontal cortex (both ventromedial prefrontal cortex [vmPFC] and dorsolateral prefrontal cortex [dlPFC]) and its connections with temporal cortex, parietal cortex, and striatum
2. Medial temporal cortex
3. Other cortical areas—posterior cingulate cortex, inferior parietal cortex, angular gyrus, anterior parahippocampal gyrus, and cortico-cortical excitatory pathways
4. Corpus callosum—slower interhemisphere processing
5. Hippocampus—disorganized pyramidal neurons in CA1, CA2, subiculum, entorhinal cortex
6. Amygdala—diminished emotionality
7. Thalamus—especially dorsal and medial dorsal (MD) regions
8. Striatum—striatal enlargement may result from antipsychotic meds
9. Enlarged lateral and third ventricles—may be the consequence of neuronal loss
10. Ventral tegmental area (VTA) and its mesolimbic and mesocortical pathways
11. Raphe nuclei—dorsal raphe nucleus, central superior nucleus

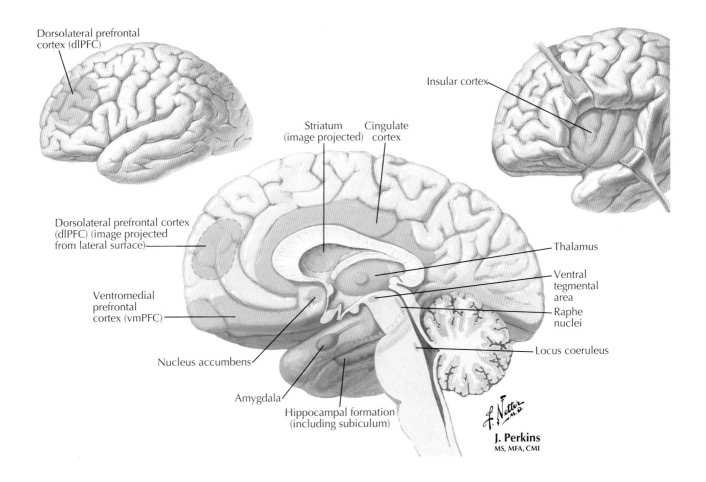

Dorsolateral prefrontal cortex (dlPFC)

Insular cortex

Striatum (image projected) Cingulate cortex

Dorsolateral prefrontal cortex (dlPFC) (image projected from lateral surface)

Thalamus

Ventral tegmental area

Raphe nuclei

Ventromedial prefrontal cortex (vmPFC)

Locus coeruleus

Nucleus accumbens

Amygdala

Hippocampal formation (including subiculum)

J. Perkins
MS, MFA, CMI

17.5 NEUROPSYCHIATRIC DISORDERS: MAJOR DEPRESSIVE DISORDER AND BIPOLAR DISORDER

Major depressive disorder (MDD) is a common neuropsychiatric disorder, with onset often in early adulthood, that occurs in approximately 5% of the population. MDD is more prevalent in women and is associated with a genetic component. Many medical conditions may provoke MDD. The clinical onset includes at least 2 weeks with sadness and a loss of pleasure (anhedonia), accompanied by at least five of the following symptoms: (1) diminished concentration, (2) lethargy and fatigue, (3) altered appetite and weight changes, (4) sleep dysfunction, (5) restlessness, (6) feelings of worthlessness or guilt, (7) difficulty making decisions or thinking, and (8) suicidal thoughts or an actual attempt. MDD is a chronic illness with a tendency to recur, sometimes becoming worse at it progresses. A major treatment approach is pharmacologic, such as the use of selective serotonin reuptake inhibitors (SSRIs).

Brain areas involved in MDD include:
1. Prefrontal cortex—both vmPFC and dlPFC
2. Insular cortex
3. Cingulate cortex and its connections regulating autonomic and neuroendocrine systems
4. Corticolimbic connections
5. Hippocampal formation, including the subiculum

6. Amygdala
7. MD thalamus and its connections to PFC, amygdala, and striatum
8. Striatum
9. Nucleus accumbens and its midbrain dopaminergic (DA) mesolimbic connections for reward and motivation
10. Raphe nuclei—dorsal raphe nucleus and central superior nucleus (serotonergic)
11. Locus coeruleus and its noradrenergic connections
12. VTA and its dopaminergic mesolimbic and mesocortical connections

Bipolar disorder often appears as recurrent manic episodes seen before a major depressive disorder. Bipolar I disorder is the occurrence of one or more full-blown manic episodes, accompanied by expansive or irritable mood, grandiosity, racing thoughts, excess energy and a decreased need for sleep, distractibility, poor judgment, and risk-taking. Bipolar II disorder involves prior hypomanic behavior and depressive episodes but no major manic episode. In some situations, both manic/hypomanic and depressive components may occur together.

Areas of the brain involved in bipolar disorder include many of the areas noted above for MDD, including PFC, cingulate cortex, reduced cortical thickness (frontal, temporal, and parietal), hippocampal CA regions, amygdala, and ventral striatum.

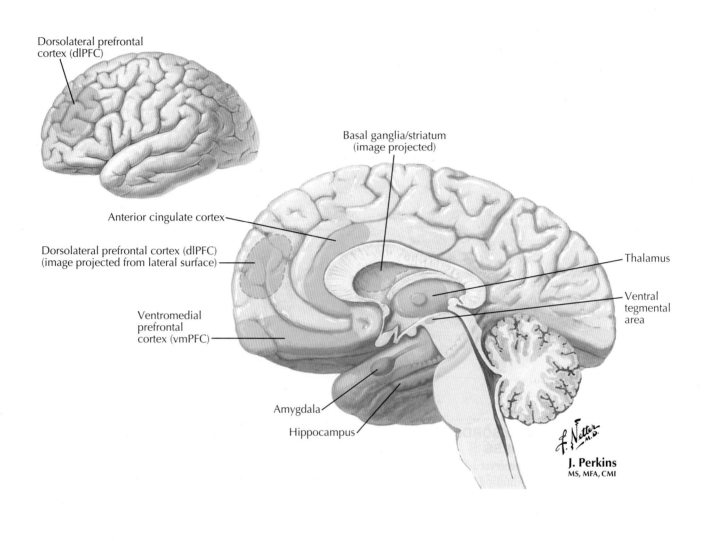

Dorsolateral prefrontal cortex (dlPFC)

Basal ganglia/striatum (image projected)

Anterior cingulate cortex

Dorsolateral prefrontal cortex (dlPFC) (image projected from lateral surface)

Ventromedial prefrontal cortex (vmPFC)

Thalamus

Ventral tegmental area

Amygdala

Hippocampus

J. Perkins
MS, MFA, CMI

17.8 NEUROPSYCHIATRIC DISORDERS: OBSESSIVE-COMPULSIVE DISORDER

Obsessive-compulsive disorder (OCD) is characterized by intrusive and unwanted thoughts and obsessions, which provoke activities and rituals that are meaningless and inappropriate. The obsessive thoughts and compulsive behaviors are disturbing to the patient and greatly interfere with normal life. Obsessions often relate to cleanliness and fear of the presence of "germs," resulting in endless handwashing and cleaning rituals. Some obsessions center on detailed organization and orderliness of objects in the environment, with repeated checking to ensure that everything is exactly as desired. OCD also may lead to hoarding and accumulation of clutter. OCD sometimes is accompanied by anxiety and mood disorders, such as bipolar disorder. OCD is often chronic and disrupts behavioral life and daily activities. The lifetime prevalence is approximately 2%. Early onset of OCD may be foreshadowed by Tourette's syndrome and tic disorders. There may be a genetic component to OCD.

Several neural structures and brain circuits are associated with OCD:

1. Prefrontal cortex (PFC)–basal ganglia–thalamus–cerebral cortex loops. The dlPFC, head of the caudate nucleus, corticostriate circuitry, and thalamic circuitry demonstrate heightened metabolic activity. Diminished executive functions from the dlPFC may occur, leading to compulsive and impulsive activity.
2. vmPFC—increased activity may underlie intrusive thoughts
3. Anterior cingulate cortex—activation may lead to anxiety
4. Hippocampus—may be associated with short-term memory dysfunction
5. Amygdala
6. Midbrain VTA and its DA mesolimbic and mesocortical pathways
7. Increased glutamate neural activity—increased in the caudate nucleus and diminished in the anterior cingulate cortex

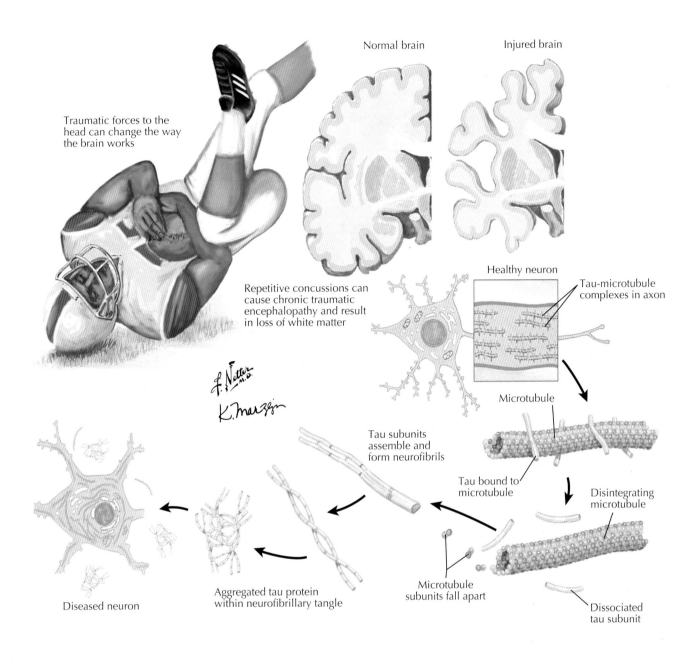

Traumatic forces to the head can change the way the brain works

Normal brain

Injured brain

Repetitive concussions can cause chronic traumatic encephalopathy and result in loss of white matter

Healthy neuron

Tau-microtubule complexes in axon

Microtubule

Tau subunits assemble and form neurofibrils

Tau bound to microtubule

Disintegrating microtubule

Aggregated tau protein within neurofibrillary tangle

Microtubule subunits fall apart

Dissociated tau subunit

Diseased neuron

17.9 TRAUMATIC BRAIN INJURY

A concussion is a TBI caused by forces impinging on the head that alter brain function but usually do not cause loss of consciousness. More than 1.5 million concussions occur per year during sports activities. Repeated concussions can result in **chronic traumatic encephalopathy** (CTE), with serious physical, emotional, and cognitive consequences.

Symptoms of concussion include memory impairment, altered thinking, emotional changes, and physical problems such as nausea, headaches, and visual impairment. A second concussion or trauma occurring before the resolution of the initial concussion can escalate the problems, contributing to cerebral edema, severe neurological impairment, coma, or death. A problematic consideration is the lack of an accurate indicator for the full recovery from an initial concussion or vulnerability to a subsequent trauma.

CTE may occur in former athletes or individuals who have experienced repeated concussions or head trauma. CTE involves progressive brain deterioration and degenerative brain changes, including chronic accumulation of tau protein within neurofibrillary tangles, similar to what is observed in the brains of patients with AD. In addition to alterations in gray matter, CTE may be accompanied by white matter loss, even in young athletes.

Significant numbers of TBI cases are seen in military combat theaters from high-velocity rifle injuries, from shrapnel and blast injuries, and as consequences of improvised explosive devices. These patients experience severe acute edema and increased intracranial pressure, and they sometimes require mechanical ventilation. Advances in field treatment of these military personnel have led to lives being saved, but at the expense of severe sequelae from the resultant injuries.

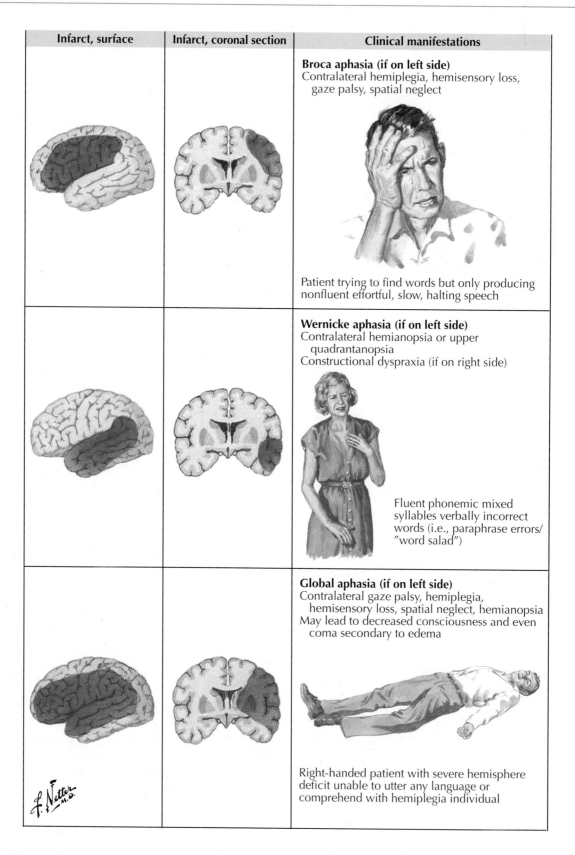

Infarct, surface	Infarct, coronal section	Clinical manifestations
		Broca aphasia (if on left side) Contralateral hemiplegia, hemisensory loss, gaze palsy, spatial neglect Patient trying to find words but only producing nonfluent effortful, slow, halting speech
		Wernicke aphasia (if on left side) Contralateral hemianopsia or upper quadrantanopsia Constructional dyspraxia (if on right side) Fluent phonemic mixed syllables verbally incorrect words (i.e., paraphrase errors/"word salad")
		Global aphasia (if on left side) Contralateral gaze palsy, hemiplegia, hemisensory loss, spatial neglect, hemianopsia May lead to decreased consciousness and even coma secondary to edema Right-handed patient with severe hemisphere deficit unable to utter any language or comprehend with hemiplegia individual

17.10 APHASIAS AND CORTICAL AREAS OF DAMAGE

Cerebral infarcts and other damage to cortical gray matter and cortical white matter (long association pathways) can result in language disorders called aphasias. This chart presents the location and clinical manifestations of major types of aphasia, including Broca (expressive) aphasia, Wernicke's (receptive) aphasia, and global aphasia. The location and clinical characteristics of conduction aphasia are discussed in Plate 13.26 Clinical Point.

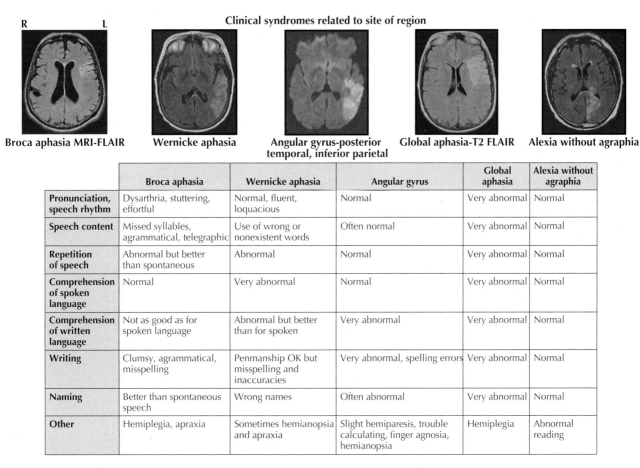

Clinical syndromes related to site of region

Broca aphasia MRI-FLAIR   Wernicke aphasia   Angular gyrus-posterior temporal, inferior parietal   Global aphasia-T2 FLAIR   Alexia without agraphia

	Broca aphasia	Wernicke aphasia	Angular gyrus	Global aphasia	Alexia without agraphia
Pronunciation, speech rhythm	Dysarthria, stuttering, effortful	Normal, fluent, loquacious	Normal	Very abnormal	Normal
Speech content	Missed syllables, agrammatical, telegraphic	Use of wrong or nonexistent words	Often normal	Very abnormal	Normal
Repetition of speech	Abnormal but better than spontaneous	Abnormal	Normal	Very abnormal	Normal
Comprehension of spoken language	Normal	Very abnormal	Normal	Very abnormal	Normal
Comprehension of written language	Not as good as for spoken language	Abnormal but better than for spoken	Very abnormal	Very abnormal	Normal
Writing	Clumsy, agrammatical, misspelling	Penmanship OK but misspelling and inaccuracies	Very abnormal, spelling errors	Very abnormal	Normal
Naming	Better than spontaneous speech	Wrong names	Often abnormal	Very abnormal	Normal
Other	Hemiplegia, apraxia	Sometimes hemianopsia and apraxia	Slight hemiparesis, trouble calculating, finger agnosia, hemianopsia	Hemiplegia	Abnormal reading

Images reprinted with permission from Jones RH, et al. The Netter Collection of Medical Illustrations, Part I, Brain, 2nd Edition. Philadelphia: Elsevier, 2014.

17.11 APHASIAS: MAGNETIC RESONANCE IMAGES AND CHARACTERISTIC LANGUAGE DYSFUNCTION

Aphasia is a language disorder affecting language use and language comprehension. It does not include dysarthrias, characterized by impaired articulation and the loss of ability to speak, or dysphonia, characterized by the inability to speak due to dysfunction of structures in the oral cavity or the vocal cords. The presence of aphasia is associated with dysfunction of the dominant hemisphere for language, usually the left side. The evaluation of language function includes the capabilities on the left side of the chart. The major types of aphasia considered in this chart include Broca aphasia (expressive aphasia), Wernicke aphasia (receptive aphasia), angular gyrus aphasia, global aphasia, and alexia without agraphia. MRIs, with typical lesions for these aphasias, are included at the top of the chart. Alexia without agraphia is a disconnect syndrome in which patients can write but not read; it usually occurs with strokes in the left occipital cortex that also disrupt the transfer of visual information from the right visual cortex to the left, language-dominant hemisphere. Another type of aphasia (not represented in the table) is conduction aphasia, in which communication between Broca's area and Wernicke's area is disrupted, resulting in the patient's loss of ability to repeat words, phrases, or sentences that are spoken to them. Conduction aphasia occurs with the disruption of the arcuate fasciculus (interconnecting the frontal and temporal lobes) or the supramarginal gyrus.

CLINICAL POINT

Nondominant cortical hemispheric dysfunction. Damage to the nondominant hemisphere, usually the right hemisphere, often leads to left-sided hemiplegia and many additional problems:

1. Left-sided neglect for objects, people, written material, and sound, involving the right frontal and parietal lobes and associated thalamic connections.
2. Anosognosia—failure to recognize one's own left-sided hemiplegia and weakness. These individuals are susceptible to increased falls.
3. Flat affect and blunted emotional responses—unconcerned about physical deficits and future problems.
4. Altered prosody of speech, including tone, loudness, rhythm, intonation, timbre, and word emphasis. This problem also affects music production and appreciation.
5. Prosopagnosia—difficulty recognizing familiar faces.
6. Social communication problems, including the inability to perceive emotional content of facial expression, missing nonverbal cues, and diminished abstract understanding.
7. Attention issues and difficulty focusing on tasks.
8. Cognitive difficulty with reasoning and problem solving.
9. Memory problems with recall and learning new information.
10. Disorientation to place, date, time, and topographic locations.
11. Constructional apraxia for drawing simple configurations such as a clock face. The drawing is incomplete and tails off to the left. Other apraxias (motor, ideomotor, ideational) involve damage to the dominant hemisphere.

Right-sided strokes and damage demonstrate poorer recovery than damage elsewhere, with functionally disabling problems persisting.

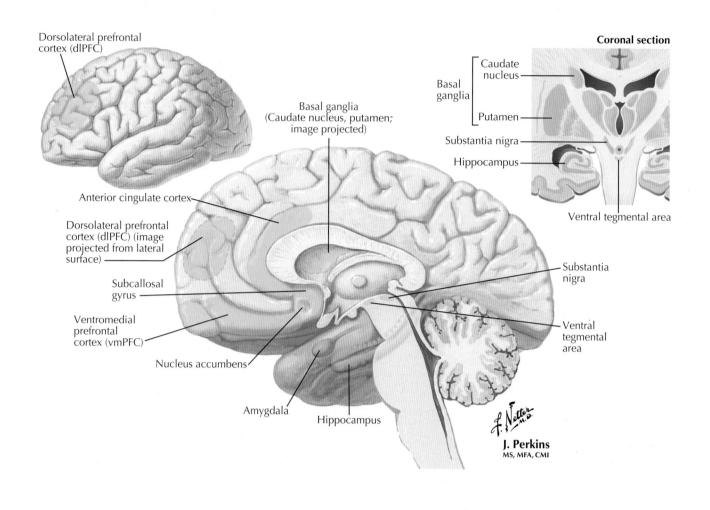

Dorsolateral prefrontal cortex (dlPFC)

Anterior cingulate cortex

Dorsolateral prefrontal cortex (dlPFC) (image projected from lateral surface)

Subcallosal gyrus

Ventromedial prefrontal cortex (vmPFC)

Nucleus accumbens

Amygdala

Hippocampus

Basal ganglia (Caudate nucleus, putamen; image projected)

Substantia nigra

Ventral tegmental area

Coronal section

Caudate nucleus

Basal ganglia

Putamen

Substantia nigra

Hippocampus

Ventral tegmental area

J. Netter M.D.

J. Perkins
MS, MFA, CMI

17.12 BRAIN SUBSTRATES OF ADDICTIVE BEHAVIORS

Addiction is a compulsion for the need or use of a habit-forming substances (cocaine, fentanyl, other opiates, alcohol, nicotine) or activities (smoking, gambling). Addiction is driven by physiological and neurological processes interacting with environmental influences, with a genetic component. Addiction involves the repeated activation of brain reward circuitry in the presence of the addicting substance or activity. There is a three-phase reaction with addicting substances: (1) the rush and binge (high, intoxication, euphoria), (2) withdrawal and adverse effects, and (3) anticipation and then preoccupation with the next high. These three phases utilize the same brain circuitry, but with significantly different activation or inactivation; these changes may persist even after cessation of use of the addicting substance. Addictive substances provoke greater reward, motivation, and drive than other positive stimuli.

Addiction is associated with several brain circuits:

1. Reward circuitry—nucleus accumbens, ventral pallidum
2. Motivation and drive circuitry—vmPFC, subcallosal gyrus
3. Cortical circuitry—dlPFC, anterior cingulate cortex
4. Learning and memory circuitry—amygdala (basolateral) and hippocampus

5. Habit-learning circuitry—caudate nucleus, putamen, and DA input from the substantia nigra, pars compacta, and its nigrostriatal pathway
6. DA circuitry from the VTA and its mesolimbic (major DA projections to nucleus accumbens, amygdala, and hippocampus) and mesocortical (PFC) components

With the rush and euphoria of drug use, high amounts of DA release activate nucleus accumbens (mood), the vmPFC (motivation), and amygdala and hippocampus (emotion, learning, memory). The cognitive control circuitry of the dlPFC and anterior cingulate cortex cannot block or counter this DA surge, which reinforces the compulsive substance use. The anticipation of subsequent drug use can be even more powerful for DA release than use of the drug itself.

During prolonged drug use, and especially during withdrawal, DA release plummets, removing the pleasurable and euphoric effects and initiating the negative effects. Subsequent anticipation of the next use can then reverse the DA crash and enhance DA release. Superimposed on this cycle is the influence of environment, which can modulate the DA activity. Susceptibility to addiction and the large DA activation may be partially driven by individual variation in DA D2 receptor numbers and expression.

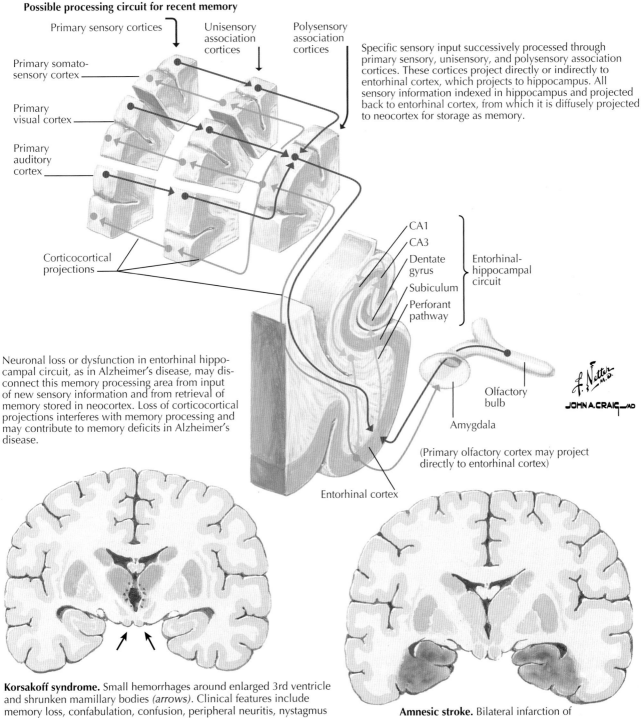

Possible processing circuit for recent memory

Primary sensory cortices

Unisensory association cortices

Polysensory association cortices

Primary somato-sensory cortex

Primary visual cortex

Primary auditory cortex

Specific sensory input successively processed through primary sensory, unisensory, and polysensory association cortices. These cortices project directly or indirectly to entorhinal cortex, which projects to hippocampus. All sensory information indexed in hippocampus and projected back to entorhinal cortex, from which it is diffusely projected to neocortex for storage as memory.

Corticocortical projections

CA1
CA3
Dentate gyrus
Subiculum
Perforant pathway

Entorhinal-hippocampal circuit

Neuronal loss or dysfunction in entorhinal hippo-campal circuit, as in Alzheimer's disease, may dis-connect this memory processing area from input of new sensory information and from retrieval of memory stored in neocortex. Loss of corticocortical projections interferes with memory processing and may contribute to memory deficits in Alzheimer's disease.

Olfactory bulb

Amygdala

(Primary olfactory cortex may project directly to entorhinal cortex)

Entorhinal cortex

Korsakoff syndrome. Small hemorrhages around enlarged 3rd ventricle and shrunken mamillary bodies *(arrows)*. Clinical features include memory loss, confabulation, confusion, peripheral neuritis, nystagmus and opthalmoplegia.

Amnesic stroke. Bilateral infarction of hippocampus and medial temporal lobes

17.13 MEMORY CIRCUITS

Memory circuits involve multiple regions of the temporal lobe, hippocampal formation (including the entorhinal cortex), and sensory/polysensory cortical areas. Conditions such as Korsakoff syndrome and amnestic strokes can result in damage to this circuitry.

Full Outline of UnResponsiveness Score (FOUR)

Eye response

4 = eyelids open or opened, tracking, or blinking to command
3 = eyelids open but not tracking
2 = eyelids closed but open to loud voice
1 = eyelids closed but open to pain
0 = eyelids remain closed with pain

Motor response

4 = thumbs-up, fist, or peace sign
3 = localizing to pain
2 = flexion response to pain
1 = extension response to pain
0 = no response to pain or generalized myoclonus status

Brainstem reflexes

4 = pupil and corneal reflexes present
3 = one pupil wide and fixed
2 = pupil or corneal reflexes absent
1 = pupil and corneal reflexes absent
0 = absent pupil, corneal, and cough reflex

Respiration

4 = not intubated, regular breathing pattern
3 = not intubated, Cheyne-Stokes breathing pattern
2 = not intubated, irregular breathing
1 = breathes above ventilator rate
0 = breathes at ventilator rate or apnea

Interpretation: Minimum score = 0, Maximum score = 16. The lower the score the greater the coma.

Reprinted with permission from Wijdicks EFM, Bamlet WR, Maramattom BV. Validation of a new coma scale: the FOUR score. Ann Neurol 58:585-593, 2005.

17.14 CONSCIOUSNESS AND COMA ASSESSMENT

A new coma scale assesses eye response, motor responses, brainstem reflexes, and respiratory responses. The original classic coma scale is the Glasgow Coma Scale, using eye, motor, and verbal responses.

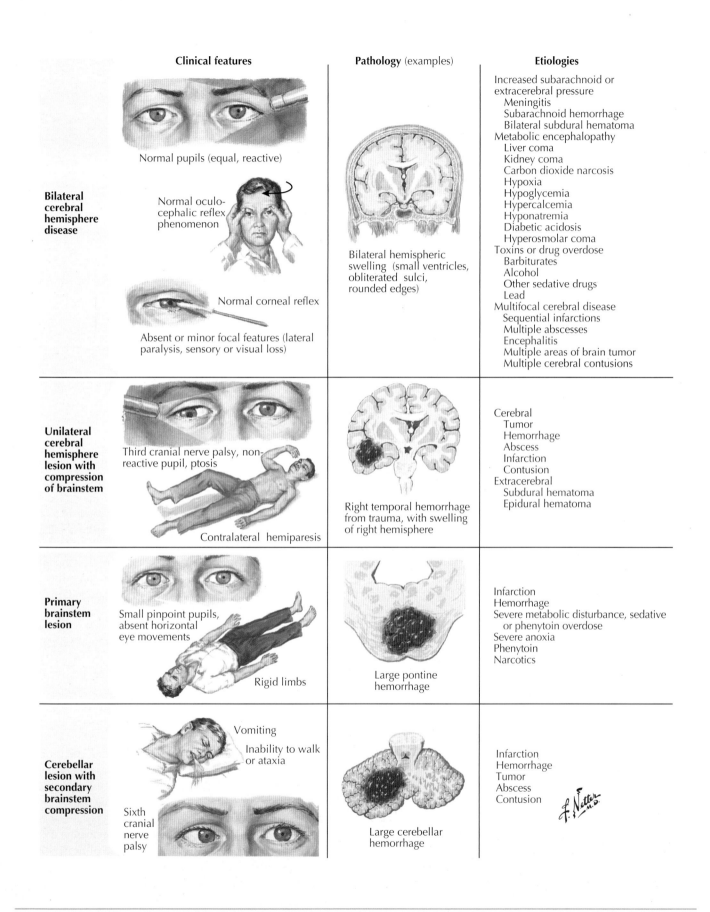

Clinical features	Pathology (examples)	Etiologies

Bilateral cerebral hemisphere disease — Normal pupils (equal, reactive); Normal oculo-cephalic reflex phenomenon; Normal corneal reflex; Absent or minor focal features (lateral paralysis, sensory or visual loss)	Bilateral hemispheric swelling (small ventricles, obliterated sulci, rounded edges)	Increased subarachnoid or extracerebral pressure
		  Meningitis
		  Subarachnoid hemorrhage
		  Bilateral subdural hematoma
		Metabolic encephalopathy
		  Liver coma
		  Kidney coma
		  Carbon dioxide narcosis
		  Hypoxia
		  Hypoglycemia
		  Hypercalcemia
		  Hyponatremia
		  Diabetic acidosis
		  Hyperosmolar coma
		Toxins or drug overdose
		  Barbiturates
		  Alcohol
		  Other sedative drugs
		  Lead
		Multifocal cerebral disease
		  Sequential infarctions
		  Multiple abscesses
		  Encephalitis
		  Multiple areas of brain tumor
		  Multiple cerebral contusions

Unilateral cerebral hemisphere lesion with compression of brainstem — Third cranial nerve palsy, non-reactive pupil, ptosis; Contralateral hemiparesis	Right temporal hemorrhage from trauma, with swelling of right hemisphere	Cerebral
		  Tumor
		  Hemorrhage
		  Abscess
		  Infarction
		  Contusion
		Extracerebral
		  Subdural hematoma
		  Epidural hematoma

Primary brainstem lesion — Small pinpoint pupils, absent horizontal eye movements; Rigid limbs	Large pontine hemorrhage	Infarction Hemorrhage Severe metabolic disturbance, sedative or phenytoin overdose Severe anoxia Phenytoin Narcotics
Cerebellar lesion with secondary brainstem compression — Vomiting; Inability to walk or ataxia; Sixth cranial nerve palsy	Large cerebellar hemorrhage	Infarction Hemorrhage Tumor Abscess Contusion

17.15 DIFFERENTIAL DIAGNOSIS OF COMA

This chart depicts the differential diagnosis of coma.

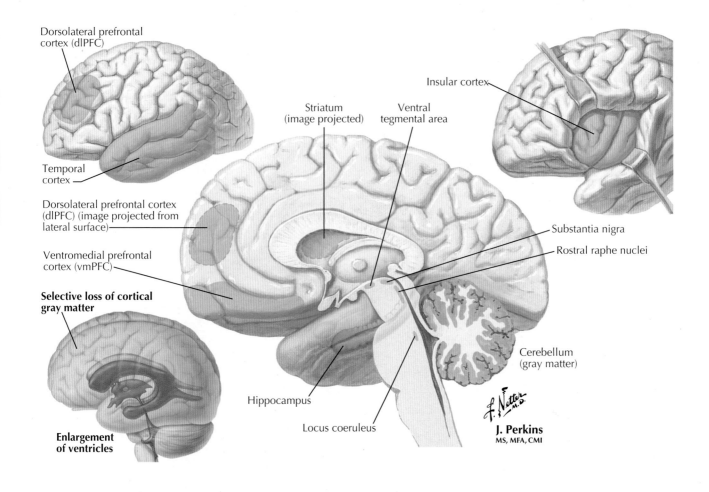

Dorsolateral prefrontal cortex (dlPFC)

Temporal cortex

Dorsolateral prefrontal cortex (dlPFC) (image projected from lateral surface)

Ventromedial prefrontal cortex (vmPFC)

Selective loss of cortical gray matter

Enlargement of ventricles

Striatum (image projected)

Ventral tegmental area

Insular cortex

Substantia nigra

Rostral raphe nuclei

Cerebellum (gray matter)

Hippocampus

Locus coeruleus

J. Perkins
MS, MFA, CMI

17.16 AGING AND THE NERVOUS SYSTEM

The aging human shows great variation in the consequences of changes, usually due to genetic background, medical history and conditions, and environmental factors. The MacArthur Commission on Successful Aging noted the three most significant factors contributing to successful aging: (1) stay socially engaged, (2) stay physically active, and (3) avoid disease (refrain from smoking, substance abuse, obesity, damaging stress, and other factors that can bring about diabetes, cardiovascular disease, and other adverse health conditions).

Numerous alterations in brain and brain function have been reported in normal aging (differing from Alzheimer's disease, other dementias, and neurodegenerative diseases):

1. Diminished brain volume and gray matter loss, accompanied by enlargement of the ventricles. This loss is not uniform and most significantly affects the prefrontal cortex, striatum, temporal cortex (especially on the left side), insular cortex, cerebellum, and hippocampus. The occipital cortex and cingulate cortex appear to be least affected.

2. Increased susceptibility to neurodegenerative disease (Alzheimer's disease, Parkinson's disease, amyotrophic lateral sclerosis), cerebrovascular disease, mild cognitive impairment, and dementia. It should be noted than many aging individuals have no evidence of any of these problems.

3. Increased damage to noradrenergic (NA), dopaminergic (DA), and serotonergic (5HT) systems due to oxidative stress and the production of damaging free radicals. Highly toxic derivatives of these monoamines can be produced by the release and subsequent reuptake into the monoamine nerve terminals, leading to gradual destruction. DA and 5HT receptors also decline with

age. NA terminals in the postganglionic sympathetic peripheral systems also can be damaged by monoamine-derived free radical production and subsequent uptake. This can lead to loss of optimal sympathetic interactions with the cardiovascular system and with secondary lymphoid organs and natural immune cells such as natural killer cells and some T lymphocytes. Accelerated DA release, as occurs in Parkinson's disease, or NA release, as occurs in chronic sympathetic activation during chronic stress, can accelerate this damaging process.

4. Diminished presence of other neurotransmitters such as glutamate (in parietal cortex, basal ganglia, and frontal cortex), and diminished N-acetyl aspartate.

5. Physiological changes, including diminished brain glucose metabolism, cerebrovascular changes from ischemia, white matter lesions with some loss of myelin, and some diminished dendritic arborizations of neurons in important structures such as prefrontal cortex and hippocampus.

6. Diminished performance on tasks requiring attention and executive functions (prefrontal cortex–basal ganglia–thalamic circuitry). Deficits also occur in processing speed and problem-solving ability, and in spatial orientation.

7. Diminished memory function, including episodic memory (e.g., recalling places and occurrences) and semantic memory (memory for meanings), both components of declarative or explicit memory. Working memory (briefly retaining a password or phone number) also may be diminished. Procedural memory (implicit memory), which aids in accomplishing some activities without conscious awareness (e.g., tying shoes or riding a bike), remain intact.

Index

Page numbers followed by *b* indicate box (Clinical Point) and *f* indicate figure.